Contents

OXFORD MEDICAL PUBLICATIONS

Oxford Handbook of Clinical Specialties

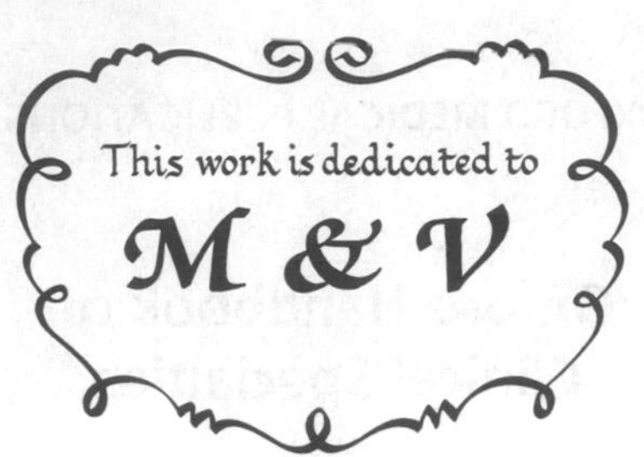
This work is dedicated to
M & V

Oxford Handbook of Clinical Specialties

FIFTH EDITION

J. A. B. COLLIER

J. M. LONGMORE

and

T. J. DUNCAN BROWN

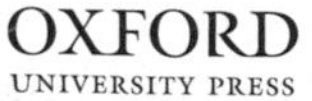

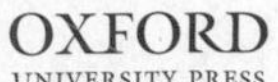

Great Clarendon Street, Oxford OX2 6DP

Oxford University Press is a department of the University of Oxford and furthers the University's aim of excellence in research, scholarship, and education by publishing worldwide in

Oxford New York

Athens Auckland Bangkok Bogota Buenos Aires Calcutta Cape Town Chennai Dar es Salamm Delhi Florence Hong Kong Istanbul Karachi Kuala Lumpur Madrid Melbourne Mexico City Mumbai Nairobi Paris São Paulo Singapore Taipei Tokyo Toronto Warsaw

and associated companies in Berlin Ibadan

Published in the United States by Oxford University Press Inc., New York

First published 1987
Second edition 1989
Third edition 1991
Fourth edition 1995
Fifth edition 1999

A catalogue record for this book is available from the British Library.

Library of Congress Cataloging in Publication Data

ISBN 0 19 2629433

Typeset by J M L; film by AMA DataSet Limited, Preston; printed in China

Translations and adaptations

—Spanish translation 1991—

—German translation 1991, 1994—

—Hungarian translation 1992—

—Polish translation 1993—

—Indian impression (hardback) 1994—

—Romanian translation 1997—

Multimedia electronic versions updatable via the Internet

(Containing
Still & Moving Images from the Archives of
Oxford Medical Illustration & OUP
and the
EMIS Intelligent Index of Differential Diagnoses
and text from the
Oxford Handbook of Clinical Medicine
and the
Oxford Handbook of Clinical Specialties
and the
Oxford Handbook of Clinical Rarities
with electronic links to the
World Wide Web
and the
Oxford Textbook of Medicine—eOTM
and the
British National Formulary—eBNF):

—Oxford Clinical Mentor 1.1 (16 bit), OUP 1997 & 1999—

—Oxford Clinical Mentor PLUS^{html} *(32 bit), OUP 1999—*

Preface to the fifth edition

The text of this edition has been entirely reset, in what is a larger, and, we hope, more readable font, while, at the same time, we have extended the level of detail for the most important topics, as well as providing a series of plates in *Ophthalmology*. This edition also sees innumerable additions: so many grains and nuggets from libraries and bedsides we now lay before our readers who must judge in their own clinics and surgeries how rich our harvest has been. As a foretaste we mention the following additions and major changes in just one field—namely obstetrics and gynaecology—to illustrate our commitment to provide timely and concise answers to those difficult questions which have a habit of cropping up *anywhere*, and often when we least expect them:

–Options in emergency contraception (p 63).
–The dangers of ovarian hyperstimulation (p 75).
–The failure rate of sterilization (p 69).
–Exams—those starting prenatally (p 166–8).
–Risks of breast cancer in HRT (p 19).
–Bleeding mothers refusing transfusion (p 139).
–Recurrent spontaneous abortion (p 23).
–Emergency management of pre-eclampsia (p 97).
–Thrombo-embolism prevention after Caesarean section (p 133).
–Thrombocytopenia in pregnancy (p 142).
–Using psychotropics safely in pregnancy (p 152).
–Nuchal translucency elucidated (p 167).
–Hyperemesis gravidarum causing Wernicke's encephalopathy (p 91).
–Discussing antenatal tests without causing nightmares (p 167).

Such a list could be continued for the rest of this volume. However, to do so would be to risk putting in the shade another element, newly-developed for this edition—namely a change, where appropriate, to a more discursive and speculative approach to the complexities and unlimited possibilities of the doctor–patient relationship. The psychotherapy section of *Chapter 4* particularly exemplifies this approach.

How has this been possible to achieve all this extra material, while keeping the book's dimensions the same? The answer, to borrow a phrase introduced by T. S. Eliot to describe the still point of our turning world, is '*concentration without elimination*'–a kind of paradox, it might be assumed, that has no real meaning until it is remembered that it is only the mind which can concentrate in this way. In the preparation of this text we hope we have been able to achieve this degree of concentration in our own minds.

Ferring
1999

J.A.B.C.
J.M.L.

Drugs (and how to keep abreast of chang

While every effort has been made to check this text, it is still possible that drug or other errors have been missed. Also, dosage schedules are continually being revised and new side-effects recognized. Oxford University Press makes no representation, express or implied, that drug dosages in this book are correct. For these reasons, the reader is strongly urged to check with the most up to date published product information and *Data sheets* provided by the manufacturers, and the most recent codes of conduct and safety regulations. The authors and the publishers do not accept responsibility or legal liability for any errors in the text, or for the misuse or misapplication of material in this work.

Except where otherwise stated, drug doses and recommendations are for the **non-pregnant adult** who is **not breast feeding**.

Corrections and peer-reviewed updatings are posted on the Internet at http://www.mentor-update.com. Not all software can access this site: if you are experiencing problems, try unpeer-reviewed material at http://www.zyworld.com/ohcm/new.htm.

See also http://www.oup.co.uk/OHCS & http://www.oup.co.uk/scimed. More detailed electronic updatings are an integral part of our *Oxford Clinical Mentor* (see p 446).

Readers are also reminded of the need to keep up to date, and that this need can only ever be *partly* addressed by printed texts such as this.

Drug nomenclature

This volume uses British[uk] approved names, followed, where there is a difference, by the recommended international non-proprietary name (rINN; usually there is no difference). A European Directive requires use of rINNs throughout the European Union; there is a 5-year change-over period (from 1988, our next edition will employ only rINNs). Exceptions to our rule of giving both names occur where the change is minute, eg amoxycillin[uk]/amoxicillin, where the rINN is used, to avoid tedious near-duplications. Among the new rINNs used are:

Alimemazine	(trimeprazine[uk])	Epinephrine	(adrenaline[uk])
Amoxicillin	(amoxycillin[uk])	Furosemide	(frusemide[uk])
Bendroflumethiazide	(bendrofluazide[uk])	Lidocaine	(lignocaine[uk])
Ciclosporin	(cyclosporin[uk])	Chlormethine	(mustine[uk])
Clomifene	(clomiphene[uk])	Norepinephrine	(noradrenaline[uk])
Diethylstilbestrol	(stilboestrol[uk])	Sulfonamides (all)	(sulphonamides[uk])
Dosulepin	(dothiepin[uk])	Trihexyphenidyl	(benzhexol[uk])

In addition, rINNs for cefalosporins (formerly cephalosporins) now all start with *cef*... (not *ceph*). For consistency, and to avoid distracting variations in adjacent usages, we have spelt sulphur (and its derivatives) *sulfur* as all *sulphonamides* have a rINN starting *sulf*... Problems remain with oestrogens such as ethinyl(o)estradiol and (o)estradiol: here we use the shorter spelling, as far as drugs are concerned, so that we abide by the directive, while retaining the UK spelling of oestrogens in non-pharmacological contexts.

ce to the first edition

someone says that he is 'doing obstetrics'—or whatever, this d not hide the fact that much more is being done besides, not just ttle of each of medicine, psychiatry, gynaecology and paediatrics, but so a good deal of work to elicit and act upon the patient's unspoken hopes and fears. At the operating table he must concentrate minutely on the problem in hand; but later he must operate on other planes too, in social and psychological dimensions so as to understand how the patient came to need to be on the operating table, and how this might have been prevented. All the best specialists practise a holistic art, and our aim is to show how specialism and holism may be successfully interwoven, if not into a fully watertight garment, then at least into one which keeps out much of the criticism rained upon us by the proponents of alternative medicine.

We hope that by compiling this little volume we may make the arduous task of learning medicine a little less exhausting, so allowing more energy to be spent at the bedside, and on the wards. For a medical student coming fresh to a specialty the great tomes which mark the road to knowledge can numb the mind after a while, and what started out fresh is in danger of becoming exhausted by its own too much. It is not that we are against the great tomes themselves—we are simply against reading them too much and too soon. One starts off strong on 'care' and weak on knowledge, and the danger is that this state of affairs becomes reversed. It is easier to learn from books than from patients, yet what our patients teach us may be of more abiding significance: the value of sympathy, the uses of compassion and the limits of our human world. It is at the bedside that we learn how to be of practical help to people who are numbed by the mysterious disasters of womb or tomb, for which they are totally unprepared. If this small book enables those starting to explore the major specialties to learn all they can from their patients, it will have served its purpose—and can then be discarded.

Because of the page-a-subject format, the balance of topics in the following pages may at first strike the reader as being odd in places. However, it has been our intention to provide a maximally useful text rather than one which is perfectly balanced in apportioning space according to how common a particular topic is—just as the great *Terrestrial Globes* made by George Phillips in the 1960s may seem at first to provide an odd balance of place names, with Alice Springs appearing more prominently than Amsterdam. To chart a whole continent, and omit to name a single central location out of respect for 'balance' is to miss a good opportunity to be useful. George Phillips did not miss this opportunity, and neither we hope, have we. It is inevitable that some readers will be disappointed that we have left out their favoured subjects (the Phillips' Globe does not even mention Oxford!). To these readers we offer over 300 blank pages by way of apology.

Ferring
1987

J.A.B.C.
J.M.L.

Symbols and abbreviations

►	This is important
►►	Don't dawdle! Prompt action saves lives
◇	Reference to evidence-based medicine (p 433). Examples appear on p 19, 102, 186, 624
💾	More details available in the electronic version of this text (see p 446)
💣	Conflict (controversial topic)
☎	Internet address
♂/♀	Male to female ratio
#	Fracture
∵	On account of
~	Approximately
–ve	Negative
+ve	Positive
↓	Decreased (eg plasma level)
↑	Increased (eg plasma level)
↔	Normal (eg plasma level)
ac	Ante cibum (before food)
ACE(i)	Angiotensin-converting enzyme (inhibitor)
ACLS	Advanced Cardiac Life Support
ACTH	Adrenocorticotrophic hormone
ADH	Antidiuretic hormone
AFP	α-fetoprotein
AIDS	Acquired immunodeficiency syndrome
Alk	Alkaline (Phos = phosphatase)
ANF	Antinuclear factor
AP	Anteroposterior
APH	Antepartum haemorrhage
A(P)LS	Advanced (Paediatric) Life Support *Manuals* (269)
ASO	Antistreptolysin O (titre)
ATLS	Advanced Trauma Life Support *Manual* reference
AV	Atrioventricular
BMJ	*British Medical Journal*
BP	Blood pressure
ca	Carcinoma
CCF	Combined (right & left sided) cardiac failure
ChVS	Chorionic villus sampling
CI	Contraindications
CMV	Cytomegalovirus
CNS	Central nervous system
CoC	Combined oral contraceptive
CPR	Cardiopulmonary resuscitation
CRP	C-reactive protein
CSF	Cerebrospinal fluid
CVP	Central venous pressure
CVS	Cardiovascular system
CXR	Chest x-ray
D	Dimension
D&C	Dilatation (cervix) & curettage
dB	Decibel
DIC	Disseminated intravascular coagulation
DIP	Distal interphalangeal
dL	Decilitre
DM	Diabetes mellitus
DoH	Department of Health
D&V	Diarrhoea and vomiting
DVT	Deep venous thrombosis
E-BM	*Evidence-based Medicine*
ECG	Electrocardiogram
ECT	Electroconvulsive therapy
EEG	Electroencephalogram
ENT	Ear, nose and throat
ESR	Erythrocyte sedimentation rate
ET	Endotracheal
FB	Foreign body
FBC	Full blood count
FH	Family history
FSH	Follicle-stimulating hormone
G	Gauge
g	Gram
G6PD	Glucose-6-phosphate dehydrogenase
GA	General anaesthesia
GI	Gastrointestinal
GP	General practitioner
GGT	Gamma glutamyl transpeptidase
GU	Genitourinary
h	Hour
Hb	Haemoglobin
HBsAg	Hepatitis B surface antigen
HDL	High-density lipoprotein
HIV	Human immunodeficiency virus
HRT	Hormone replacement therapy
HVS	High vaginal swab
Ib/ibid	Ibidem (in the same place)
ICP	Intracranial pressure
IE	Infective endocarditis
Ig	Immunoglobulin
IHD	Ischaemic heart disease
IM	Intramuscular
INR	International normalized ratio of prothromin time

IP	Interphalangeal
IPPV	Intermittent +ve pressure ventilation
iu	International unit
IUCD	Intrauterine contraceptive device
IV	Intravenous
IVI	Intravenous infusion
IVU	Intravenous urography
JRCGP	*Journal of the Royal College of General Practitioners*
JVP	Jugular venous pressure
K^+	Potassium
kg	Kilogram
kPa	Kilopascal
l	Litre
LA	Local anaesthesia
LDH	Lactate dehydrogenase
LFT	Liver function test
LH	Luteinizing hormone
LMP	First day of the last menstrual period
LP	Lumbar puncture
LVH	Left ventricular hypertrophy
µg	Micrograms
MAOI	Monoamine oxidase inhibitor
MCP	Metacarpophalangeal
MCV	Mean cell volume
mg	Milligrams
mL	Millilitre
mmHg	Millimetres of mercury
MRI	Magnetic resonance imaging
MSU	Midstream urine (culture of)
MTP	Metatarsophalangeal
NaCl	Sodium chloride
NBM	Nil by mouth
NEJM	*New England Journal of Medicine*
NGT	Nasogastric tube
NHS	National Health Service
NMR	Nuclear magnetic resonance scan
N_2O	Nitrous oxide
NSAIDs	Non-steroidal anti-inflammatory drugs
OHCM	*Oxford Handbook of Clinical Medicine* 4th ed, OUP
ORh-ve	Blood group O, Rh negative
PA	Posteroanterior
PAN	Polyarteritis nodosa
P_aCO_2	Partial pressure of CO_2 in arterial blood
P_aO_2	Partial pressure of oxygen in arterial blood
pc	Post cibum (after food)
PCV	Packed cell volume
PET	Pre-eclamptic toxaemia
PID	Pelvic inflammatory disease
PIP	Proximal interphalangeal
PO	Per os (by mouth)
PoP	Progesterone-only pill
PPH	Postpartum haemorrhage
PR	Per rectum
PTR	Prothrombin ratio
PE	Pulmonary embolism
PUO	Pyrexia of unknown origin
PV	Per vaginam
RBC	Red blood cell
RCGP	Royal College of General Practitioners
RA	Rheumatoid arthritis
RTA	Road traffic accident(s)
RUQ	Right upper quadrant
RVH	Right ventricular hypertrophy
R_x	Treatment (prescribing drugs)
SBE	Subacute bacterial endocarditis
SC	Subcutaneous
SCBU	Special care baby unit
SE	Side-effects
sec	Seconds
SpO_2	Oximetry estimation of capillary blood oxygen saturation (also SaO_2)
STD	Sexually transmitted disease
SVC	Superior vena cava
$t_{1/2}$	Half life
T°	Temperature
T_3	Triiodothyronine
T_4	Thyroxine
TB	Tuberculosis
TIA	Transient ischaemic attack
TFT	Thyroid function tests
TPR	Temperature, pulse, and respirations
TSH	Thyroid-stimulating hormone
u (or U)	Units
U&E	Urea and electrolytes
UTI	Urinary tract infection
UV	Ultraviolet
VSD	Ventricular septal defect
WCC	White blood cell count
wt	Weight
yrs	Years

Note: other abbreviations are given in full on the pages where they occur.

Acknowledgements

We thank the British Lending Library, Ms Susan Merriott, and Mrs Thelma Royce for their diligence in supplying us with hard-to-find references—without their tireless and much appreciated help this publication would not have been possible. We also thank Dr T Toma (USA/Romanian fax correspondant) for his timely updates. For typographic expertise, we thank Mr Simon Mather, and Mr Andrew Mather.

For their invaluable help we thank Mr G Bates, Mr J Braithwaite, Mr A Carr, Dr G Caldwell, Dr T Chalmers-Watson, Dr J Colston, Dr R Downes, Dr S Eccles, Dr S Holmes, Mr G Knepil, Professor Mackie, Dr C Moulton, Dr P Muthusamy, Ms A Peattie, Dr B Phillips, Dr A Pittaway, Professor C Redman, Mr T Lavy, and Dr M Too-Chung.

Dr Sunil Jain has most generously put his considerable knowledge at our disposal. The fruits of his updatings have enriched every chapter.

For peer reviewing and underpinning of our electronic version, we are grateful to Dr Paul Scott, Dr John Cox, Dr David Ward, Dr Stephanie Hart, Dr Tim Kenny, Dr Sean King, Dr Laurence Knott, Dr J Orrell, Dr Simon Huins, Mr Carl Westerman, and Dr Huw Thomas. Dr Tudor Toma's fax updates have also been very useful.

Readers' participation We have been very fortunate to receive communications via our reader's comments card (enclosed with this volume); these comments have contributed greatly to this edition. We acknowledge and thank them here: N Abcod; S Abedin; K Abou-Elhmd; A Adiele; R Adley; A Agbobee; M Al-Amin; A Alaraji; H Albrecht; Zulfiqar Ali; A Alwael; anonymous readers from Hinckley and District Hospital; V Atamyan; M Azam; N Balasuriyar; D Bansevicius; S Beasley; D Boddie; B Bourke; P Piotr Brykalski; C Budd; K Burn; I Cardozo; P Cliffe; P Collins; S Corcoran; H Constantinides; J Crane; D Dharmi; J Dart; T Davies; H Dormand; S Dunarchie; J Eduardien; S Eley; J Fagan; O Fenton; P Fanagan; M Fry; D Foss; E France; D Groneberg; J Guznan; P Hausserman; J Hazlewood; S Helmy; T Hennigan; J Hill; S Holliday; R William Howe; G Hutchison; M Ip; A Juanroyee; H Kabil; B Kloft; A Kuber; C Law; N Lees; J Lehane; A McBride; J McFazdean; R McLaughlin; S Mcpartlin; K Mandana; A Martin; C Maytum; E Miller; D Moskopp; M Naraen; K Narayanan; K O'Driscoll; E Odumenya; F Olson; J Olson; A Omorojor; A Madkhana; B & S Manidas; R Payne; R Price; S Ranka; A Rees; J Rees P Rees; R Reynolds; J Revilla; C Robertson; A Rodgers; E Russell; R Pyper; D Shukla; H Soren; M Stryan; S Swiig; L Tait; N Tseraidi; M Tsolaks; M Turur; F Udoh; A Uqaili; C Vandenbussche; D Warren; S Western; E Wright; P Zack.

We particularly thank all staff at Oxford University Press for their help.

We thank the following authors, publishers and editors for permission to reproduce images: D Kinshuck; A Land; K O'Driscoll; A Swain; the *British Journal of Hospital Medicine*; the *British Medical Journal*; *General Practitioner*; the *Journal of Pediatrics*; the Association for Consumer Research; Baillière Tindall; John Wright; Edward Arnold; Lange; Churchill Livingstone.

Pronouns For brevity, the pronoun *he* or *she* has been used in places where *he or she* would have been appropriate. Such circumlocutions do not aid the reader in forming a vivid visual impression, which is one of the leading aims of good authorship. Therefore, for balance and fairness, and where sense allows, we have tried alternating *he* with *she*.

Most of the time we chug along treating patients quite well, without ever really understanding them. The idea that we should strive to understand and empathize with *all* our patients is ultimately unsustainable. Out-patient clinics and surgeries would grind to a halt, and urgent visits would never get done. It is also possible that to do so would be counter-productive from the patient's point of view. For two human beings to understand each other's inner life is a rare event, and if we offered this understanding to all our patients they might become addicted to us, and be unable to get on with the rest of their lives. Nevertheless, it is good practice to have a go, on occasion, at trying to understand *some* patients. Doing so may entail swallowing an alien world and digesting it rather slowly. Paradoxically, to achieve this, we very often need to keep our mouths *shut*, particularly with those in whom we have reached a therapeutic impasse—for example if the illness is untreatable, or the patient has rejected our treatment, or if the patient seems to be asking or appealing for something more. Eye contact is important here. One of the authors (JML) recalls forever his very first patient—found on a surgical ward recovering from the repair of a perforated duodenal ulcer: a nice simple surgical patient, ideal for beginners. I asked all the questions in the book, and knew all his answers and his physical features: even the colour of his eyes. Luckily, the house officer who was really looking after him did not ask so many questions, and knew how to interpret the appeal for help behind those eyes, and in his busy day found space to receive the vital clue beyond my grasp—that my patient was a drug addict and under great stress as he could no longer finance his activity.

So, the first step in trying to understand a patient is to sit back and listen. Next, if possible, it is very helpful to see your patient often, to establish rapport, and mutual respect. If the relationship is all one way, with the doctor finding out all about the patient, but revealing nothing of him- or herself, this mutual respect can take a very long time to grow. But beware of sharing too much of your own inner life with your patients: you may overburden them, or put them off. Different patients respond to different approaches. Understanding patients inevitably takes time, and it may be hard in a series of short appointments. A visit to the patient's home may be very revealing, but for many doctors trapped in hospital wards or clinics, this is impossible. But it is usually possible to have a longish, private interview, and take whatever opportunity turns up. We once worked with a consultant who infuriated his junior staff on busy ward rounds by repeatedly selecting what seemed to us the most boring and commonplace medical 'cases' (such as someone with a stroke) and proceeding to draw the curtain around the patient's bed to exclude us, and engage in what seemed like a long chat with the patient, all in very hushed voices, so that we never knew what he said—until Sister told us that he never said anything much, and simply received anything that was on the patient's mind. For the most part, he was swallowing their world in silence. We came to realize that there was nothing these patients, robbed as they were of health and wholeness, appreciated more in their entire hospital stay.

Contents

Note: The content of individual chapters is detailed on each chapter's first page.

Tolstoy describes the uselessness of medical books (and Natásha illustrates the pitfalls of pure specialisms)

Doctors came to see her singly and in consultation, talked much in French, German, and Latin, blamed one another, and prescribed a great variety of medicines for all the diseases known to them, but the simple idea never occurred to any of them that they could not know the disease Natásha was suffering from, as no disease suffered by a live man can be known, for every living person has his own peculiarities and always has his own peculiar, personal, novel, complicated disease unknown to medicine—not a disease of the lungs, liver, skin, heart, nerves, and so on mentioned in medical books, but a disease consisting of one of the innumerable combinations of the maladies of those organs. This simple thought could not occur to the doctors (as it cannot occur to a wizard that he is unable to work charms), because the business of their lives was to cure, and they received money for it and had spent the best years of their lives on that business. But above all that thought was kept out of their minds by the fact that they saw they were really useful. . . They satisfied that eternal human need for hope of relief, for sympathy. . . the need seen in its most elementary form in a child when it wants to have a place rubbed that has been hurt.

Leo Tolstoy, *War & Peace* Book ix ch xvi, tr L & A Maude, OUP

1. Gynaecology

Relevant pages in other chapters

Puberty p 200; virilism and hirsutism *OHCM* p 556

Relevant web sites

http://www.obgyn.net/

History and examination

History Let her tell the story, but remember that she may be reluctant to admit some problems, particularly if you are a man, so make sure to cover them in your questions.

1 *Menstrual history:* ►Note date of last menstrual period (LMP), ie first day of bleeding, or menopause. Was the last period normal? Cycles: number of days bleeding/number of days from day 1 of one period to day 1 of next (eg 5/26). Are periods regular? If heavy, are there clots or flooding? How many pads/tampons are needed (this may not be a reliable guide)? Are periods painful? Is there bleeding between periods, postcoitally, or since the menopause? Age at menarche?

2 *Obstetric history:* How many children? Antenatal problems, delivery, gestation, outcome (and weights of babies) and puerperium of each pregnancy? Terminations and miscarriages—at *what* stage, *why* and (terminations) *how*?

3 *Symptoms:* If she has *pain* what is it like? Uterine pain tends to be colicky and felt in the sacrum and groins. Ovarian pain tends to be felt in the iliac fossa and radiates down front of the thigh to the knee. Ask about *dyspareunia* (painful intercourse). Is it superficial (round the outside) or deep inside? If she has *vaginal discharge* what is it like (amount, colour, smell, itch); when does she get it? Ask about *prolapse* and *incontinence*. When? How bad?

4 *Sex and contraception:* Is she sexually active? Are there physical or emotional problems with sex? What contraception is she using and is she happy with it? What has she tried previously? Has she had problems conceiving? If so, has she had treatment for infertility? What about sexually transmitted diseases? Date and result of last smear?

5 *Other:* General health, smoking. Previous gynaecological treatment.

Examination ►Many women find pelvic examination painful and undignified, and particularly embarrassing if you are male. Explain what you are going to do. Be gentle. Use a chaperone.

General: Is she well or ill? Is she shocked? If so, treat it.

Abdomen: Look for tenderness and peritonism. If there is a mass, could it be a pregnancy? Listen for a fetal heart (p 84).

Vaginal examination: (p 6). Use your eyes to inspect the vulva, a *speculum* to examine the vagina and cervix and your *fingers* to assess the uterus and adnexae bimanually. Examination is usually done with the patient on her back or in the left lateral position (preferable for detecting prolapse). *Sims' speculum* has 2 right-angle bends, and is used for inspecting the vaginal walls, eg for prolapse and incontinence.

Cusco's (bivalve) speculum is used for inspecting the cervix with the aid of a light. Insert the speculum closed (warmed under a tap) with the blades parallel to the labia; lubricating jelly makes it easier. When it is in, rotate it and open it. The speculum should achieve its full length before opening and usually the cervix will pop into view. If it doesn't, do a bimanual to check the position of the cervix and try again. Do swabs (p 48) and a cervical smear (p 32) if indicated. Close the speculum gradually as you withdraw it, to avoid trapping the cervix.

Sexual health

Sexual health is the enjoyment of sexual activity of one's choice, without causing or suffering physical or mental harm.[1] Of course there is more to sex than enjoyment. 'Perhaps the sexual life is the great test. If we can survive it with charity to those we love, and affection to those we have betrayed, we needn't worry so much about the good and the bad in us. But jealousy, distrust, cruelty, revenge, recrimination. . . then we fail. The wrong is in that failure even if we are the victims and not the executioners. Virtue is no excuse. . .'[2]

Enemies of sexual health include:

- Disharmony in personal relationships, or simply *too many* relationships.
- Pain, or any medical, or gynaecological condition.
- Anxiety (whether or not related to fear of failure); depression; fatigue.
- Drugs (eg tamoxifen; the Pill; cyproterone; antidepressants; narcotics).
- A multiplicity of irreconcilable rôles (if your patient is trying to achieve ascendency in her work, as well as being chief shopper, cook, housewife, mother and friend, then the rôle of lover may be eclipsed—all the more so if she also finds herself in the rôle of being chief person to blame if things go wrong—if the fridge is empty, if the money runs out, if the children don't get to school on time, or if her partner loses his job).
- Myths about sexual performance (eg that all physical contact must lead to sex, that sex equals intercourse, and that sexual relations should come naturally and easily).[3]

1 P Greenhouse 1995 BMJ i 1468 2 G Greene 1965 *The Comedians*, Penguin, p139, ISBN 0-14-018494-5
3 J Butcher 1999 BMJ i 41

Gynaecological anatomy

The vulva comprises the entrances to the vagina and urethra, the structures which surround them (clitoris, labia minora and fourchette), and the encircling labia majora and perineum. The hymen, when broken (by tampons, or intercourse) leaves tags at the mouth of the vagina.
Look for: Rashes; atrophy; ulcers; lumps (p 28–30); deficient perineum (you can see the back wall of the vagina).

The vagina is a potential space with distensible folded muscular walls. The contents of the rectum, which runs behind the posterior wall, may be palpated through the vagina. The cervix projects into the vault at the top which forms a moat around it, deepest posteriorly, conventionally divided into anterior, posterior and two lateral fornices. From puberty until the menopause lactobacilli in the vagina keep it acid, discouraging infection.
Look for: Inflammation; discharge (p 48); prolapse (p 54).

The cervix is mostly connective tissue. It feels firm, and has a dent in the centre (the opening, or os, of the cervical canal). Mucin-secreting glands on its surface lubricate the vagina. The os is circular in nulliparous women, but is a slit in the parous.
Look for: Pain on moving the cervix (excitation—p 24 & p 50); ectopy; cervicitis and discharge; polyps, carcinoma (p 32).

The uterus has a thick muscular-walled *body* lined internally with columnar epithelium (the endometrium) connected to the cervix or neck. It is supported by the uterosacral ligaments. The peritoneum is draped over the uterus. The valley so formed between it and the rectum is the rectovaginal pouch (of Douglas), and the fold of peritoneum in which the Fallopian tubes lie is known as the broad ligament. The *size* of the uterus is by convention described by comparison with its size at different stages of pregnancy. Since that is variable, estimates are approximate, but the following is a guide: nonpregnant—plum-sized; 6 weeks—egg; 8 weeks—small orange; 10 weeks—large orange; 14 weeks—fills pelvis.

In most women the uterus is *anteverted*, ie its long axis is directed forward and the cervix points backwards. The body then flops forwards on the cervix—*anteflexed*. An anteverted uterus can be palpated between the two hands on bimanual examination (unless the woman is obese or tense).

In 20% it is *retroverted and retroflexed* (p 6).
Look for: Position (important to know for practical procedures); mobility (especially if retroverted); size; tenderness (p 24 & p 50).

Adnexae These are the *Fallopian tubes, ovaries* and associated connective tissue (parametria). They are palpated bimanually in the lateral fornices, and if normal cannot be felt. The ovaries are the size of a large grape and may lie in the rectovaginal pouch.
Look for Masses (p 42) and tenderness (p 50).

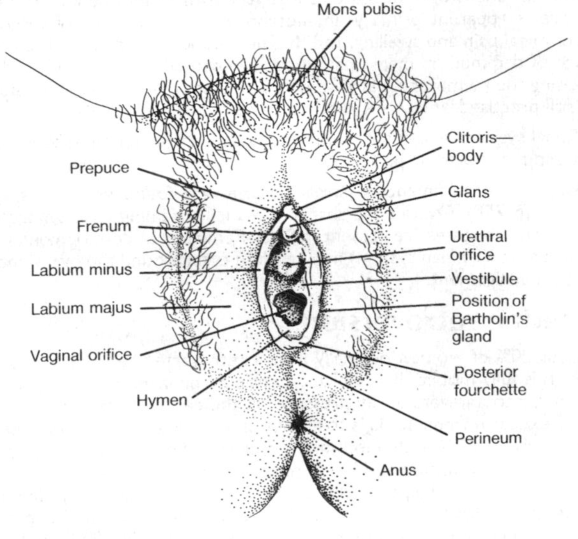
Mons pubis
Prepuce
Clitoris—body
Glans
Frenum
Urethral orifice
Labium minus
Vestibule
Labium majus
Position of Bartholin's gland
Vaginal orifice
Posterior fourchette
Hymen
Perineum
Anus

Genital abnormalities

Vagina and uterus These are derived from the Müllerian duct system and formed by fusion of the right and left parts. Different degrees of fail-
6 ure to fuse lead to duplication of any or all parts of the system.

Vaginal septae are quite common (and often missed on examination).

Duplication of the cervix and/or uterus may also be missed, eg until the woman becomes pregnant in the uterus without the IUCD!

A partially divided (*bicornuate*) uterus or a uterus where one side has failed to develop (*unicornuate*) may present as recurrent miscarriage, particularly in the second trimester, or as difficulties in labour. Such abnormalities are diagnosed by *hysterosalpingogram*.

An absent uterus or a rudimentary uterus with absent endometrium are rare. They present with primary amenorrhoea.

An absent or short vagina is uncommon but can be corrected by plastic surgery. The membrane at the mouth of the vagina where the Müllerian and urogenital systems fuse (the hymen) may be imperforate. There is apparent primary amenorrhoea, with a history of monthly abdominal pain and swelling, and the membrane bulging under the pressure of dammed up menstrual blood (haematocolpos). It is relieved by incising the membrane. NB: in some communities, female 'circumcision'* is still practised, and this is another cause of haematocolpos.

►Renal system abnormalities often coexist with genital ones, so IVU and ultrasound should be performed.

Ovary Thin, rudimentary 'streak' ovaries are found in Turner's syndrome (p 758). Ovaries are absent in testicular feminization syndrome, but primitive testes are present (p 222). Remnants of developmental tissue (eg the Wolffian system) may result in cysts around the ovary and in the broad ligament.

Uterine retroversion

About 20% of women normally have a retroverted retroflexed uterus which is fully mobile. It is difficult to palpate bimanually unless you can push it into anteversion by pressure on the cervix. It causes no problems except (rarely) if it fails to lift out of the pelvis at 12 weeks of pregnancy, presenting with discomfort and retention of urine, eg at 14 weeks; catheterization and lying prone may relieve it.

Inflammation in the pelvis (due to infection or endometriosis) can cause adhesions which tether the uterus in a retroverted position. The patient may present with dysmenorrhoea, dyspareunia, or infertility—problems which can only be relieved by treatment of the underlying disease.

*Circumcision is a misnomer, as it implies a parallel with male circumcision, which is incorrect: the female 'operation' is carried out later (at 5–7yrs) and may be much more damaging and extensive, eg as practised in Somalia. Procedures include clitoridectomy ± infundibulation (removal of the clitoris, labia minora and labia majora, with oversewing or aposition by thorns). Even the milder Sunna entails removal of part of the clitoris, and more may be removed than intended. At betrothal, an attendant cuts the scar tissue to allow intercourse. Longterm problems include very slow urination, haematocolpos, dyspareunia or non-consummation, obstructed labour, as well as emotional trauma. *See* H Gordon 1998 *Diplomate* 5 86.

1. Gynaecology

Normal menstruation

Puberty is the development of adult sexual characteristics. The sequence: breast buds develop, then growth of pubic hair, then axillary hair. Then menses begin (**menarche**) from 10½ years onwards (mean ~13yrs; age was falling in the UK, but no longer); it is earlier if short and overweight; investigate if no periods by 16yrs (p 10). A growth spurt (p 200) is the first change in puberty and is usually completed 2yrs after menarche when the epiphyses fuse.

The menstrual cycle The cycle is controlled by the 'hypothalamic-pituitary-ovarian (HPO) axis'. Pulsatile production of gonadotrophin-releasing hormones by the hypothalamus stimulates the pituitary to produce the gonadotrophins: follicle stimulating hormone (FSH) and luteinizing hormone (LH). These stimulate the ovary to produce oestrogen and progesterone. The ovarian hormones modulate the production of gonadotrophins by feeding back on the hypothalamus and pituitary.

Day 1 of the cycle is the first day of menstruation. Cycle lengths vary greatly; only 12% are 28 days. Cycles soon after menarche and before the menopause are most likely to be irregular and anovulatory. In the first 4 days of the cycle, FSH levels are high, stimulating the development of a primary follicle in the ovary. The follicle produces oestrogen, which stimulates the development of a glandular 'proliferative' endometrium and of cervical mucus which is receptive to sperm. The mucus becomes clear and stringy (like raw egg white) and if allowed to dry on a slide produces 'ferning patterns' due to its high salt content. Oestrogen also controls FSH and LH output by positive and negative feedback.

14 days before the onset of menstruation (on the 16th day of the cycle of a 30-day cycle) the oestrogen level becomes high enough to stimulate a surge of LH. This stimulates ovulation. Having released the ovum, the primary follicle then forms a corpus luteum and starts to produce progesterone. Under this influence, the endometrial lining is prepared for implantation: glands become convoluted ('secretory phase'). The cervical mucus becomes viscid and hostile to sperm and no longer ferns. If the ovum is not fertilized the corpus luteum breaks down, so hormone levels fall. This causes the spiral arteries in the uterine endothelial lining to constrict and the lining sloughs—hence menstruation.

Menstruation This is the loss of blood and uterine epithelial slough. It lasts 2–7 days and is usually heaviest at the beginning. Normal loss is 20–80mL, median 28mL.

Climacteric The ovaries fail to develop follicles. Without hormonal feedback from the ovary, gonadotrophin levels rise. Periods cease (menopause), usually at ~50 years of age (p 18).

Postponing menstruation (eg on holiday) Try norethisterone 5mg/12h PO from 4 days before the period is due until bleeding is acceptable, or take 2 packets of combined contraceptive Pills without a break.

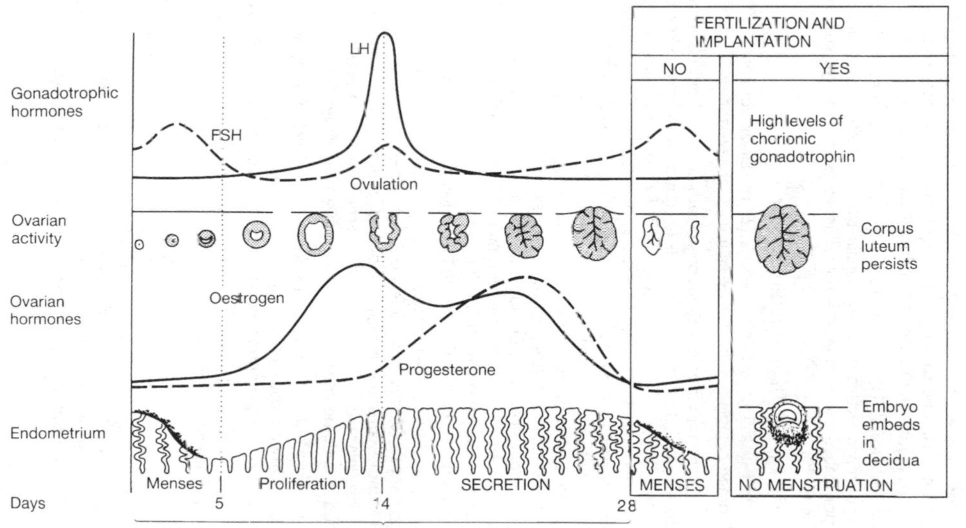
Gonadotrophic hormones
LH
FSH
Ovulation
Ovarian activity
Ovarian hormones
Oestrogen
Progesterone
Endometrium
Menses
Proliferation
SECRETION
Days
5
14
28
One menstrual cycle
FERTILIZATION AND IMPLANTATION
NO
YES
High levels of chorionic gonadotrophin
Corpus luteum persists
Embryo embeds in decidua
MENSES
NO MENSTRUATION

Abnormal menstruation

Primary amenorrhoea (see p 12) This is failure to start menstruating. It needs investigation in a 16-year-old, or in a 14-year-old who has no breast development. For normal menstruation to occur she must be structurally normal with a functioning control mechanism (hypothalamic-pituitary-ovarian axis).

Secondary amenorrhoea (see p 12) This is when periods stop for >6 months, other than due to pregnancy. Hypothalamic-pituitary-ovarian axis disorders are common, ovarian and endometrial causes rare.

Oligomenorrhoea This is infrequent periods. It is common at the extremes of reproductive life when regular ovulation often does not occur. A common cause throughout the reproductive years is polycystic ovary syndrome (p 44).

Menorrhagia (p 14) This is excessive blood loss.

Dysmenorrhoea This is painful periods (± nausea or vomiting). 50% of British women complain of moderate pain, 12% of severe disabling pain.

Primary dysmenorrhoea is pain without organ pathology—often starting with anovulatory cycles after the menarche. It is crampy with ache in the back or groin, worse during the first day or two. Excess prostaglandins cause painful uterine contractions, producing ischaemic pain. *Treatment:* Prostaglandin inhibitors, eg mefenamic acid 500mg/8h PO during menstruation reduce contractions and hence pain. Paracetamol is a good alternative to NSAIDs. In pain with ovulatory cycles, ovulation suppression with the combined Pill can help (thus dysmenorrhoea may be used as a covert request for contraception). Smooth muscle antispasmodics (eg alverine 60–120mg/8h PO) or hyoscine butylbromide (20mg/6h PO) give unreliable results. Cervical dilatation in childbirth may relieve it but, surgical dilatation may render the cervix incompetent and is no longer used as therapy.

Secondary dysmenorrhoea: Associated pathology: adenomyosis, endometriosis, chronic sepsis (eg chlamydial infection), fibroids—and so it appears later in life. It is more constant through the period, and may be associated with deep dyspareunia. Treatment of the cause is the best plan. Antiemetics may be needed in endometriosis. IUCDs increase dysmenorrhoea.

Intermenstrual bleeding This may follow a midcycle fall in oestrogen production. Other causes: cervical polyps; ectropion; carcinoma; cervicitis and vaginitis; hormonal contraception (spotting); IUCD; pregnancy-related.

Postcoital bleeding *Causes:* Cervical trauma, polyps, cervical carcinoma; cervicitis and vaginitis of any cause.

Postmenopausal bleeding This is bleeding occurring later than 1yr after the last period. It must be considered due to endometrial carcinoma until proved otherwise (p 40). Other causes: vaginitis (often atrophic); foreign bodies, eg pessaries; carcinoma of cervix or vulva; endometrial or cervical polyps; oestrogen withdrawal (hormone replacement therapy or ovarian tumour). She may confuse urethral, vaginal and rectal bleeding.

1. Gynaecology

11

Amenorrhoea

►*Always ask yourself 'Could she be pregnant?'*

Primary amenorrhoea (see also p 10). This may cause great anxiety. In most patients puberty is just late (often familial), and reassurance is all that is needed. A few causes will be structural or genetic, so check:

- Has she got normal external secondary sexual characteristics? If so, are the internal genitalia normal (p 6)?
- If she is not developing normally, examination and karyotyping may reveal Turner's syndrome (p 758) or testicular feminization (p 222). The aim of treatment is to help the patient to look normal, to function sexually, and, if possible, to enable her to reproduce if she wishes.

Causes of secondary amenorrhoea

- Hypothalamic-pituitary-ovarian causes are very common as control of the menstrual cycle is easily upset, eg by emotions, exams, weight loss, excess prolactin (30% have galactorrhoea), other hormonal imbalances, and severe systemic disease, eg renal failure. Pituitary tumours and necrosis (Sheehan's syndrome) are rare.
- Ovarian causes: polycystic ovary syndrome (p 44), tumours, ovarian failure (premature menopause), are uncommon.
- Uterine causes: pregnancy-related, Asherman's syndrome (uterine adhesions after a D&C). 'Post-Pill amenorrhoea' is generally oligomenorrhoea masked by regular withdrawal bleeds.

Tests Serum LH and testosterone (↑in polycystic ovary syndrome), FSH (very high in premature menopause), prolactin (↑by stress, prolactinomas and drugs, eg phenothiazines) and TFT are the most useful blood tests. 40% of those with hyperprolactinaemia have a tumour so do skull x-ray ± CT scan (p 58).

Treatment is related to cause. Premature ovarian failure cannot be reversed but hormone replacement (p 18) is necessary to control symptoms of oestrogen deficiency and protect against osteoporosis and heart disease. Pregnancy can be achieved with oocyte donation and *in vitro* fertilization techniques.

Hypothalamic-pituitary axis malfunction: If mild (eg stress, moderate weight loss): there is sufficient activity to stimulate enough ovarian oestrogen to produce an endometrium (which will be shed after a progesterone challenge, eg norethisterone 5mg/8h for 7 days), but the timing is disordered so cycles are not initiated. If the disorder is more severe the axis shuts down (eg in severe weight loss). FSH and LH and hence oestrogen levels are low. Reassurance and advice on diet or stress management, or psychiatric help if appropriate (p 348), and time may solve the problem. She should be advised to use contraception as ovulation may occur at any time. If she wants fertility restored now, or the reassurance of seeing a period, mild dysfunction will respond to clomifene (=clomiphene) but a shut-down axis will need stimulation by gonadotrophin-releasing hormone (see p 58 for both).

1. Gynaecology

Menorrhagia

This is excessive menstrual blood loss (defined as >80mL lost/cycle), but in reality loss is rarely measured so management deals with those women whose significant menstrual loss interferes with their normal life. Consider ►hypothyroidism (look for weight gain, constipation, dislike of cold, bradycardia, dry skin, goitre, oedema—see *OHCM* p 544; do FBC, T_4).

Causes The most likely cause changes with age. In girls, pregnancy and dysfunctional uterine bleeding are likely. With increasing age, think also of IUCD, fibroids, endometriosis and adenomyosis, pelvic infection, polyps. In *perimenopausal women*, consider endometrial carcinoma. Ask about general bleeding problems as she may have a blood dyscrasia, eg von Willebrand's. Do a pelvic examination—which may reveal polyps, fibroids, or endometriosis.

Tests None may be needed. FBC, TFT, ultrasound or laparoscopy if pelvic pathology suspected; D&C if perimenopausal to exclude endometrial cancer.

Dysfunctional uterine bleeding (DUB) This is heavy and/or irregular bleeding in the absence of recognizable pelvic pathology. It is associated with anovulatory cycles, so is common at the extremes of reproductive life or it may be ovulatory (eg with inadequate luteal phase). If PV is normal and organic pathology is ruled out, this is the diagnosis, by exclusion.

Treatment of menorrhagia Treat any underlying condition. Where the diagnosis is dysfunctional uterine bleeding, treatment depends on age. Reassurance helps. Teenage menorrhagia generally settles without interference as cycles become ovulatory. Those with unacceptable loss should be offered treatment.

Drugs *Antifibrinolytics* These are taken during bleeding and reduce loss—eg *tranexamic acid* 1g/6–8h PO. CI: thromboembolic disease—but this is no more common in those on tranexamic acid. *Antiprostaglandins*, eg *mefenamic acid* 500mg/8h PO pc (CI: peptic ulceration) are taken during days of bleeding and are particularly helpful if there is also dysmenorrhoea. *Hormones* such as cyclical progestogens, eg *norethisterone* 5mg/8h PO, are traditional, eg days 12–26; or days 5–26 (she then has a period). Studies have proved them minimally effective.[1] SE: weight↑, breast tenderness, bloating. The *combined Pill* is effective but may be contraindicated in older women—(eg smokers >35 years). *Danazol* 100mg/6–24h PO is effective, and expensive, but side-effects may be unacceptable: weight gain, acne, muscle pain, amenorrhoea. It inhibits ovulation (unreliably, so advise condoms as it masculinizes the ♀ fetus).

Progesterone-containing IUCDs, eg the Mirena® are suitable for those not wishing to get pregnant and do reduce bleeding<2> (by up to 86% at 3 months, 97% at 1 year). They are effective in dysfunctional uterine bleeding and should possibly be considered for first line management of menorrhagia (although not specifically licensed as treatment). They have also been shown to reduce fibroid volume after 6–18 months use.[3]

For those women who have completed their families consider endometrial resection or hysterectomy (p 72). Endometrial resection removes the first few millimetres thickness of endometrium; eg by laser or rollerball electrode (safest)[4] or by electrocautery loop (most side-effects).[4] Ablation is more likely to be effective if the endometrium is thin, and pretreatment with leuproprelin (p 52) may be better than using a progestogen or danazol. About 30% become amenorrhoeic and a further 50% have reduced flow after any method of ablation.

1 R Hart 1996 *Prescriber* **4** 17 <2> P Haukkamaa 1999 E-BM 4 18 (the need for hysterectomy is ↓) **3** F Sturridge 1997 *Br J Obs Gynae* **104** 285 **4** C Overton 1998 *Br J Obs Gynae* **105** 1351

1. Gynaecology

The premenstrual syndrome (PMS)

Most women notice that their mood or physical state may be worse premenstrually. The symptoms may be mild one month and severe the next, perhaps depending on external events. Symptoms tend to be worse in the 30s and 40s and improve on the combined Pill. About 3% of women regularly have cyclical symptoms so severe that they cause major disruption to their lives: premenstrual syndrome (PMS) or tension (PMT).

Causes See opposite.

Symptoms Commonest symptom patterns are tension and irritability; depression; bloating and breast tenderness; carbohydrate craving and headache; clumsiness; libido↓.[1] Almost any symptom may feature.

Diagnosis Suggest symptom diary. If she has PMS her symptoms are worst before periods, are relieved by menstruation and there is at least one symptom-free week afterwards. Diaries may also reveal psychiatric disorders (which may be worse premenstrually) or menstrual disorders.

Treatment Simply to acknowledge her problem, listen, and reassure may be all that is needed to enable her to cope. Are her partner and children understanding? Can she rearrange work schedules to reduce stress premenstrually? Some women find self-help groups supportive. Health measures, eg improved diet, reducing smoking and drinking, increased exercise and relaxation, often help. Herbal remedies are not scientifically tested but some find them helpful, eg sage and fennel for irritability. Any drug evokes a big placebo effect, improving 90% in some studies. Pyridoxine (vit B_6) 10mg/24h PO for the symptomatic period or continuously, may help low mood and headache (DoH says higher, more effective, doses cause neuropathy—but the evidence is flimsy[2]). For severe *cyclical mastalgia* consider:

1 Reduce saturated fats eaten: these increase the affinity of oestrogen-receptors for oestrogen.[3]
2 Gamolenic acid 120mg/12h PO. 1 capsule = 40mg in evening primrose oil.
3 Bromocriptine 2.5mg/12h PO days 10–26, even if prolactin normal.
4 Danazol 100–200mg/12h PO for 7 days before menstruation (see below).

Premenstrual progestogens, eg progesterone suppositories 200mg/12h PR or PV, or dydrogesterone 10mg/12h PR/PV, may provide general relief. Some benefit from suppression of ovulation with the combined Pill, oestrogen patches or implants, with cyclical progesterone, or danazol 200mg/24h (SE nausea, weight gain, masculinization of the ♀ fetus, so advise barrier contraception). Avoid diuretics unless fluid retention is severe (when spironolactone 25mg/6h PO days 18–26 of the cycle is the drug of choice).

For psychological symptoms, fluoxetine 20mg/day PO helps, with ~30% experiencing remission.[4] Alprazolam (0.25mg/day PO during the luteal phase) also helps, with apparently low risk of dependence. Other treatments for PMT include mefenamic acid (250–500mg/8h PO from day 16 until 3 days into period). This may help fatigue, headache, pains, and mood. Goserelin (*OHCM* p 392) may help severe PMT but symptoms return when ovarian activity recommences and after 6 months' use bone thinning can be detected. It is better used to predict the severely affected women who may benefit from hysterectomy with oophorectomy (these women can then have oestrogen replacement).[5]

Follow-up: it is not 'cheating' to ensure that her next appointment will *not* be in the premenstrual phase—more objectivity may be forthcoming.

1 J Butcher 1999 BMJ i 41 2 A Beckett 1998 *Lancet* **352** 62 3 *Drug Ther Bul* 1992 **30** 1
4 D Menkes 1992 BMJ **ii** 346 5 P O'Brien 1992 in *Gynaecology*, Churchill, 325-39

The Rapkin hypothesis and putative pathways in PMS[1]

Some physiological and pharmacological observations:

- There is no evidence that ovarian events cause premenstrual syndrome: models presupposing progesterone deficiency have not been confirmed (and progesterone suppositories are no panacea for the condition).
- Artificially altering circulating progesterone and oestradiol (estradiol) does not induce premenstrual symptoms in previously well women—only in those already prone to PMS.
- Studies with psychoactive compounds suggest that the key events are occuring in the brain, not the ovary—eg an abnormal CNS response to normal progesterone excursions occurring in the luteal phase.
- Allopregnanolone and pregnenolone (metabolites of progesterone) are psychoactive, interacting, eg with γ-aminobutyric acid A (GABA-A) receptors.
- Allopregnanolone is anxiolytic, so low levels may cause anxiety.

Putative conclusion: Neurones or glia in those with PMS preferentially metabolize progesterone to pregnenolone (which heightens anxiety) rather than allopregnanolone (which is anxiolytic and up-regulates serotonin receptors, so ameliorating depression). On this view, alprazolam, by augmenting GABA-A-receptor function, is a substitute for allopregnanolone.

1 A Rapkin 1997 *Obstet Gynaecol* **90** 709–14 & S Berga 1998 *Lancet* **351** 465

The menopause and HRT

The climacteric is the time of waning fertility leading up to the last period (which is the menopause). Problems are related to falling oestrogen levels:

- Menstrual irregularity as cycles become anovulatory, before stopping.
- Vasomotor disturbances cause hot flushes, sweating and palpitations. Flushes are brief but unpleasant and may occur every few minutes for more than 10 years, disrupting life and sleep.
- Atrophy of oestrogen-dependent tissues (genitalia, breasts) and skin. Vaginal dryness can lead to vaginal and urinary infection, dyspareunia, traumatic bleeding, stress incontinence and prolapse.
- Osteoporosis. The menopause accelerates bone loss which predisposes to fracture of femur neck, radius and vertebrae in later life (p 676).
- Arterial disease becomes more common after the menopause.
- Attitudes to the menopause vary widely, and partly depend on irritability, depression, 'empty nest syndrome'—all exacerbated by the menopause.

Management ≥20% of women seek medical help.

- Is it the menopause? Thyroid and psychiatric problems may present similarly. Measure FSH in younger women (very high in menopause).
- Counselling helps psychosocial *and* physical symptoms. Enlist family's support.
- Menorrhagia may respond to treatment (p 14). A D&C is required if irregular bleeding is abnormal (it may be difficult to decide).
- Continue contraception for 1yr after the last period, eg POP, IUCD, condoms.
- Hot flushes may respond to clonidine 50–75μg/12h PO, HRT, or tibolone.
- Vaginal dryness responds to oestrogen.

Hormone replacement therapy (HRT) Oestrogen is not a panacea for all problems, but it is effective for flushes and atrophic vaginitis. It postpones menopausal bone loss and *may* protects from cardiovascular disease (controversial[1,2]), ovarian cancer, and Alzheimer's disease; it can ↑breast cancer risk (below). Benefits of HRT are many; most women should at least consider it.

Women with a uterus should also receive progestogens, eg norgestrel 150μg/24h, PO for 12 days out of 28 to reduce risk of endometrial carcinoma; this produces withdrawal bleeds—if unacceptable, consider tibolone 2.5mg/day PO, a preparation which aims not to cause bleeds—or continuous combined oestrogen/progestogen combinations, eg Kliofem®, estradiol (=oestradiol) 2mg and norethisterone 1mg.[3] For both these, either wait for 1yr after the last period, or, if changing from cyclical HRT, wait until after 54yrs of age; bleeding is common, in the 1st 4 months of use–reassure; if after 8 months, do an endometrial biopsy. Kliofem® may be useful if cyclical HRT causes 'premenstrual' symptoms. There *may* be advantages in using natural 'lipid-friendly' progestogen, dydrogesterone (no androgenic, mineralocorticoid, or oestrogenic action), eg Femoston 2/10® or (2/20 tabs, ie 2mg 17β (o)estradiol tabs, each with added 20mg dydrogesterone after day 14), but see p 66 for possible SE (DVT). Raloxifene, a selective (o)estrogen receptor modulator (SERM) protects bones while *reducing* breast and endometrial cancer risk. It is ineffective for flushes.[4]

HRT contraindications: •Oestrogen-dependent cancer •Undiagnosed PV bleeding •LFTs↑ •Pregnancy •Breast feeding •Phlebitis •Past pulmonary embolus Avoid or monitor closely in Dubin–Johnson/Rotor syndromes (*OHCM* p 696). BP↑ is *not* a CI. If past spontaneous DVT/PE: *is there thrombophilia* (*OHCM* p 626)?

Side-effects: Weight↑; 'premenstrual' syndrome; cholestasis; vomiting.

Annual check-up: Breasts; weight; any abnormal bleeding?

Creams, pessaries, & rings are useful for vaginal symptoms, eg Ovestin®, ie (o)estriol 0.1%, 1 applicator-full PV daily for 3 weeks, then twice weekly They are absorbed but, if used intermittently, progestogens are probab unnecessary. If creams are unacceptable, consider an oestrogen-containing vaginal ring (eg Estring®) replaced every 3 months, for up to 2yrs. Vagifem® is an estradiol (=oestradiol) 25μg vaginal tablet daily for 2 weeks, and then twice weekly, with reassessment every 3 months.

Transdermal patches are less 'medical' but are expensive and women with wombs still need progestogen, eg as tablets or Estracombi® patches. Estradiol (=oestradiol) patches supply 25–100μg/24h for 3–4 days. SE: dermatitis.

(O)estradiol implants (Surgical) 25mg lasts ~36 weeks, 100mg lasts ~1yr.

(O)estradiol gel 2 measures are applied daily to arms shoulders or inner thighs. Women with a womb using gel or implants also require progestogens for 12 days per cycle.

When is HRT *particularly* desirable? ►Make a point of offering HRT to:
- Those who have had premenopausal bilateral oophorectomy.
- Hysterectomy (ovaries often fail, eg by 5yrs after a hysterectomy).
- Those with ↑risk of osteoporosis (eg smokers or if inactive); see p 676.
- Those with ischaemic heart disease or risk factors such as hypercholesterolaemia or diabetes mellitus.
- Those with rheumatoid arthritis.

HRT and breast cancer This is the most serious question mark over HRT. If HRT is used for ≥5yrs, relative risk increases by 1.023/yr of HRT use.[5] For this reason our policy on HRT is:
- To discuss the risk of breast cancer with each patient starting HRT.
- To document this discussion in the patient's notes.
- To air issues about breast-awareness during normal activities such as bathing and dressing, and to explain, if necessary, that formal breast examination by nurses may give false reassurance (advice of the UK's chief medical officer). The rôle of mammography in preventing HRT-induced breast cancer is unknown. It is difficult if aged 40–50yrs (breast density↑).
- To encourage women to bring up problems with therapy at an early stage.
- Not to prescribe HRT in a blanket fashion just because a woman wants it.
- To be wary about HRT in those with a family history of breast cancer.
- To consider stopping HRT before 6 completed years of therapy.

An alternative *for those wanting HRT only for their bones* may be raloxifene (new HRT which *decreases* risk of breast cancer: it is related to tamoxifen).[4]

HRT and venous thromboembolism The number of extra cases is only about 1 in 500 users per year. Risk may be concentrated in new users, rather than those who have been taking HRT for many years.[6] The UK commitee on safety of medicines (CSM) suggests reviewing need for HRT in those with predisposing factors, such as prolonged immobility, surgery, obesity, past or family history of DVT or embolism, or *severe* varicose veins.[7]

S Hulley 1999 *E-BM* **4** 16 2 M Duncan 1994 *BMJ* ii 191 3 M Rees 1994 *Lancet* **343** 250
Beardsworth 1999 *Prescriber* **10** 83 (*N*=7705) 5 V Beral 1997 *Lancet* **350** 1047 (*N*=52,705)
Colditz 1995 *NEJM* **332** 1589 6 M Vessey 1996 *Lancet* **348** 977 7 *BMJ* 1996 ii 1102

Termination of pregnancy (ToP)

►Under UK law, no one *has* to have an abortion, and no one *has* to do one. Worldwide, 30% of pregnancies are terminated. Good contraceptive services reduce but do not abolish demand. *Incidence:* ~170,000 ToPs/yr in UK.

Legal (UK) constraints The 1967 and 1990 Human Fertilization/ Embryology Acts allow termination *before 24 weeks* if this reduces the risk:
1 To the woman's life, or: 2 To her physical or mental health—or:
3 Of adverse physical or mental health to her existing children, or:
4 Of the baby's being seriously handicapped, mentally or physically.
90% of ToPs are carried out via *Clause 2* ('social'). 2 doctors must sign form HSA 1. Parental consent (and the patient's) is needed for those under 16.
There is no upper time limit if there is: •Risk to the mother's life.
- Risk of grave, permanent injury to the mother's physical/mental health (allowing for reasonably foreseeable circumstances).
- Substantial risk that if the child were born he or she would suffer such physical or mental abnormalities as to be seriously handicapped.

<1% of ToPs are done after 20 weeks, usually after amniocentesis, or when very young or menopausal mothers have concealed, or not recognized, pregnancy. ToPs after 24 weeks may only be carried out in NHS hospitals.

Before ToP ►She has to live with the decision for the rest of her life.
- Counselling to help her reach the decision she will least regret.
- Is she definitely pregnant? Do a VE or scan to confirm dates.
- Is ToP what she really wants? Why? Has she considered alternatives—discuss their implications. What about her partner? Ideally give her time to consider and bring her decision to a further consultation. If she chooses ToP:
- Screen for chlamydia. Untreated, 25% get post-op salpingitis, p 50.
- Routine tetracycline prophylaxis ↓post-op infections (from 10 to 6%).
- Discuss contraception (eg start Pill next day if she wishes).
- Arrange follow-up. If RhD–ve she needs anti-D (p 109). The time that she would have delivered may particularly raise emotions.

Methods The commonest method for first trimester abortions is dilatation of the cervix followed by curettage or vacuum aspiration of uterine contents. Mortality is low (1:100,000), as is infection risk.

For second trimester abortions, labour is induced using intravaginal prostaglandin gel, or pessaries, eg gemeprost 1mg/3h to a maximum of 5 in 24h. Oxytocin to stimulate contractions and surgical removal of retained placenta may be required. The procedure may be prolonged, painful and distressing. Alternatively the uterus may be evacuated surgically using forceps. It is unpleasant to do and the considerable dilatation of the cervix required may damage it, even after prostaglandin priming. After 14 weeks mortality and morbidity rise steeply with gestation.

4-stage medical ToP with an antigestagen + prostaglandin (Only if gestation <9 weeks, in fully licensed clinics): •Counselling and ultrasound •Supervised mifepristone 600mg PO (RU486, an antiprogesterone) disimplants the conceptus (CI: smokers >35yrs old; avoid aspirin and NSAIDs for 12 days) •A gemeprost 1mg pessary PV 36–48h later completes abortion. Observe for 6h post-gemeprost (risk of BP↓↓). Only 3% abort before this stage. •Follow-up and scan at 12 days. Surgery is needed in 5%. Psychiatric morbidity appears to be the same as with surgical ToP.

Complications Infection, later miscarriages, breast cancer (*JAMA* 1996 **275** 283) and other imponderables such as coarsening of attitudes to life and death when ToP is done lightly. We all dream* of a time when no one needs our services, but for those who do, today, we must show a willingness to help and console.

* *'You dream', he said, 'because of the child*
Asleep in the nest of your body, who dreams...' Stephen Spender, *The Drea*

Recommendations of the 1994–96 Confidential Enquiry into Maternal Mortality

- Ideally all women should undergo ultrasound prior to termination to establish gestational age, viability, and site of pregnancy.
- Failure to obtain tissue at suction termination of a sonagraphically intrauterine pregnancy suggests abnormal implantation, eg cornual.
- Laparoscopy and/or laparotomy is essential if perforation of the uterus occurs during suction termination to assess any bowel damage.
- Questions remain as to whether dilatation and evacuation is safe and appropriate for second-trimester terminations—when effective medical alternatives exist.

Abortion (miscarriage)

Abortion is the loss of a pregnancy before 24 weeks' gestation. 20–40% of pregnancies miscarry, mostly in the first trimester. Most present with bleeding PV. Diagnosis may not be straightforward (consider ectopics p 24): have a low threshold for doing an ultrasound scan. Pregnancy tests remain +ve for several days after fetal death.

Management of early pregnancy bleeding Consider the following:
- ►Is she shocked? There may be blood loss, or products of conception in the cervical canal (remove them with sponge forceps).
- Has pain and bleeding been worse than a period? Have products of conception been seen? (Clots may be mistaken for products.)
- Is the os open? The external os of a multigravida usually admits a fingertip.
- Is uterine size appropriate for dates?
- Is she bleeding from a cervical lesion and not from the uterus?
- What is her blood group? If RhD–ve she will need anti-D (p 109).

If symptoms are mild and the cervical os is closed it is a *threatened abortion*. Rest is advised but probably does not help. 75% will settle. Threatened abortion (especially second trimester) is associated with risk of subsequent preterm rupture of membranes[1] and preterm delivery—so book mother at a hospital with good neonatal facilities.

If symptoms are severe and the os is open it is an *inevitable abortion* or, if most of the products have already been passed, an *incomplete abortion*. If bleeding is profuse, consider ergometrine 0.5mg IM. If there is unacceptable pain or bleeding, or much retained tissue on ultrasound, arrange evacuation of retained products of conception (ERPC)—otherwise an expectant policy is justified for most (>75%) women if gestation is <13 weeks.<2>

Missed abortion: The fetus dies but is retained. There has usually been bleeding and the uterus is small for dates. Confirm with ultrasound. ERPC or prostaglandin (possibly with mifepristone) evacuation is required.

Mid-trimester abortion This is usually due to mechanical causes, eg cervical incompetence (rapid, painless delivery of a live fetus), uterine abnormalities; or chronic maternal disease (eg DM, SLE).

After a miscarriage ►Miscarriage may be a bereavement. Give the parents space to grieve, and to ask why it happened and if it will happen again.

Most early pregnancy losses are due to aneuploidy and abnormal fetal development; 10% to maternal illness, eg pyrexia. 2nd trimester loss may be due to infection, eg CMV (p 98–100). Bacterial vaginosis has been implicated. Most subsequent pregnancies are normal although at increased risk.

Recurrent miscarriage 3 abortions without a normal pregnancy merit referral for genetic, immunological and anatomical investigation. See p 23. If lupus anticoagulant, phospholipid antibodies, or cardiolipin antibodies are present, giving aspirin and heparin in the next pregnancy may help. The dose in one study was aspirin 75mg/24h PO from the day of the +ve pregnancy test plus heparin (unfractionated self-administered Calciparine®) 5000u/12h SC—as soon as the fetal heart is seen (eg vaginal scan at 5 weeks) until 34 weeks' gestation.[3] Get expert advice.

An incompetent cervix may be strengthened with a cervical encirclage suture at ~16 weeks of pregnancy. It is removed prior to labour.
The right time to try again is when the parents wish to do so.

Septic/'backstreet' abortion Presents as acute salpingitis (p 50) and is treated similarly. Start broad-spectrum antibiotics 1h prior to uterine curettage, eg co-amoxiclav (ampoules are 1.2g; 1g is amoxicillin and 200mg clavulanic acid; give 1.2g/6h IV) + metronidazole (eg a 1g suppository/8h).

1 J Konje 1992 *J Obs Gynae* **12** 150 <2>S Nielsen 1995 *Lancet* **345** 84 & E-BM **1** 13 3 R Rai 1997 BMJ **i** 253 (Live births with aspirin alone were 42%; with aspirin + heparin: 71%; this study is criticized because of the unexpectedly high rate of fetal loss overall; also no cytogenic analysis was done: NB: heparin has serious SEs: osteoporosis & platelets↓

Causes of recurrent spontaneous miscarriage (RSM)[1]

This is loss of 3 or more consecutive pregnancies. It affects 1% of women.

Possible causes

Endocrine: Polycystic ovaries (found in 58% on ultrasound; the effect is possibly mediated by high luteinizing hormone levels); poorly controlled diabetes; thyroid antibody presence.

Infection: The rôle of bacterial vaginosis (p 48) is being assessed.

Exposure to chemicals: Smoking, for example, increases abortion rates.[2]

Parental chromosome abnormality: ~4% of those with RSM. It is usually a balanced reciprocal or Robertsonian translocation. Refer to a geneticist.

Uterine abnormality: Rates are similar to those in women without RSM so it is probably not a cause.[1] Traditionally, it is said to be a cause.

Antiphospholipid antibodies: (lupus anticoagulant and anticardiolipin antibodies) These are present in 15% of women with RSM. Most women with antibodies miscarry in the first trimester. For treatment see opposite.

Alloimmune causes: The theory is that these women share human leukocyte alleles (HLA) with their partners and do not mount the satisfactory protective response to the fetus. Treatment by paternal or third party leukocyte maternal immunization (immunotherapy) is contentious.

1 R Rai 1996 *Br J Obs Gynae* **103** 106 2 B Roberta 1999 NEJM **340** 333

Ectopic pregnancy

The fertilized ovum implants outside the uterine cavity. The UK incidence is 9:1000 pregnancies and rising; worldwide rates are higher. ~7% of maternal deaths are due to ectopics (0.3 deaths/1000 ectopic pregnancies).

Predisposing factors Anything slowing the ovum's passage to the uterus increases risk: damage to the tubes (salpingitis; previous surgery); previous ectopic; endometriosis; the presence of an IUCD; the POP (p 66), GIFT (p 58).

Site of implantation 97% are tubal. Most implant in the ampulla, 25% in the narrow inextensible isthmus (so tend to present early and to rupture). 3% implant on the ovary, cervix or peritoneum.

Natural history The trophoblast invades the tubal wall, weakening it and producing haemorrhage which dislodges the embryo. If the tube does not rupture, the blood and embryo are shed or converted into a tubal mole and absorbed. Rupture can be sudden and catastrophic, or gradual, giving increasing pain and blood loss. Peritoneal pregnancies may survive into the third trimester, and may present with failure to induce labour.

Clinical presentation ►Always think of ectopics in a sexually active woman with abdominal pain or bleeding.

There is generally ~8 weeks' *amenorrhoea* but an ectopic may present before a period is missed. Tubal colic causes *abdominal pain* which may precede *vaginal bleeding*. Blood loss may be dark ('prune juice', as the decidua is lost from the uterus) or fresh. The ectopic may rupture the tube with sudden severe pain, peritonism, and shock. More often there is gradually increasing vaginal bleeding, and bleeding into the peritoneum producing shoulder-tip pain (diaphragmatic irritation) and pain on defecation and passing water (due to pelvic blood). The patient may be faint, with a tender abdomen (95%), enlarged uterus (30%), cervical excitation (50%), adnexal mass (63%). Examine gently, to reduce risk of rupture; preferably with an IVI *in situ*.

Management[1] Early diagnosis is vital. Quantitative βHCG (human chorionic gonadotrophin); do ultrasound. If βHCG >6000iu/L and an intrauterine gestational sac is not seen, ectopic pregnancy is very likely, as is the case if βHCG 1000–1500iu/L and no sac is seen on *transvaginal* ultrasound. The higher the index of suspicion, the quicker the progress to laparoscopy (the final diagnostic aid). The pregnancy is removed at laparotomy or laparoscopy, conserving the tube (eg by laparoscopic injection of methotrexate), if possible. Is anti-D needed? (p 109). When conservative surgery has been possible monitor βHCG weekly to exclude persistent ectopic (occurs in ~13%. This is trophoblastic tissue persisting which then grows and can cause later rupture). If βHCG remains raised have low threshold for further surgery.[2]

►►Shock from a ruptured ectopic can be fatal. *Immediate* laparotomy is necessary as only clamping the bleeding artery will relieve it. If you suspect an ectopic, put up an IVI; if already shocked put up 2 (14 or 16G). Give colloid as fast as possible (use pressure bag to ↑flow), followed by blood—O–ve if desperate, but usually better to wait for group compatible. Inform your consultant.[3] Take immediately to theatre.

Measures to reduce missing ectopic pregnancies[1]

- Always send uterine curettings at ERPC (p 72) for histology.
- If histology does not confirm uterine failed pregnancy, recall the patient. (Ensure rapid return of histology results.)
- When ultrasound reports suggest a missed abortion but the fetus has not been seen—think: could this be an ectopic?

1 S Norman 1991 *Br J Obs Gynac* **98** 1267 2 L Dwarakanath 1996 *Br J Obs Gynae* **103** 1021
3 DoH 1996 *Confidential Enquiry into Maternal Deaths in the United Kingdom 1991-93* HMSO p68

Avoiding maternal mortality from ectopics

(Advice from the *1994–96 Confidential Enquiries into Maternal Deaths*)

- Thinks of an ectopic *whenever* a possibly fertile woman has abdominal pain.
- Assume that *any* fertile woman who faints is exsanguinating from an ectopic.
- Have a low threshold for β-HCG testing, even if she's not missed a period.
- If shocked from an ectopic, *take to theatre* **NOW** (IVI resuscitation may fail).
- *Classical features may be absent.* Diarrhoea and painful defacation may be prominant features.
- An *ultrasonically empty uterus* suggests that PV bleeding is from an ectopic.
- Deaths from ectopics are often in socially disadvantaged people: give the your especial care. Get an interpreter as needed.

When may laparoscopy replace laparotomy for ectopics?

The main absolute indications for laparotomy in tubal pregnancy are excessive bleeding and haemodynamic instability. In other instances, if there is sufficient skill, laparoscopy may be appropriate, and can maintain tubal viability. With expert advice there are other options—briefly discussed here.

Some tubal pregnancies end themselves without any problem, so conservative management *may* be an option (if striving for maximum fertility), but *only* if the patient has no acute symptoms and βHCG levels are falling. It is also helpful if transvaginal colour Doppler shows poor vascularity in the trophoblast.[1] ***Get expert help.*** IM methotrexate, eg 50mg/m^2, (or, possibly, tubal injection at laparoscopy) are also options, eg if the pregnancy is <3.5cm in the greatest diameter.[2]

1 B Kemp 1997 *Lancet* 349 26 April 2 L Mascarenhas 1997 BMJ ii 141

Trophoblastic disease

This comprises hydatidiform mole and choriocarcinoma. A fertilized ovum forms abnormal trophoblast tissue, but no fetus. The growth may appear 'benign' (mole) or 'malignant' (choriocarcinoma)—but these terms are confusing because *normal* trophoblast shows some features of malignancy (invasion and metastasis: in most normal pregnancies trophoblastic tissue ends up, for example, in the mothers lungs—so it may be better to think of the tissue as a failed pregnancy rather than a true neoplasia[1]).

The trophoblast is usually genetically paternal but has a 46XX karyotype. Rarely, a triploid, partial mole is found with a fetus (usually abnormal). Partial moles do not seem to develop into choriocarcinoma.

Hydatidiform mole The tumour consists of proliferated chorionic villi which have swollen up and degenerated. Since it derives from chorion, it produces human chorionic gonadotrophin (HCG) in large quantities. This gives rise to exaggerated pregnancy symptoms and a strongly +ve pregnancy test. Incidence is 1.54:1000 births (UK). It is more common at extremes of maternal age, after a previous mole, and in non-Caucasians. A woman who has had a previous mole is at increased risk for future pregnancies; 0.8–2.9% after one mole, 15–28% after 2 moles.

Presentation is usually with a pregnancy which is 'not quite right': she may have severe morning sickness or first-trimester pre-eclampsia (20%); the uterus is large for dates in 50% and feels doughy instead of firm. There is no fetal heart. Ultrasound: 'snowstorm' in the uterus.

50% present with vaginal bleeding which is often heavy and prolonged. Molar tissue is likely to be aborted. It looks like a mass of frogspawn.

Abdominal pain may be due to huge theca-lutein cysts in both ovaries. These may rupture or tort. They take ~4 months to resolve after molar evacuation. HCG resembles TSH, and may cause hyperthyroidism. ►Tell the anaesthetist as thyrotoxic storm can occur at evacuation.

Treatment of moles is by removal of molar tissue. The uterus, which is soft and liable to perforation, is evacuated using gentle suction, followed by a repeat evacuation ~10 days later. She should then avoid pregnancy for a year while HCG levels are monitored. Levels should return to normal within 6 months. If levels dropped rapidly to normal, oral contraceptive pills may be used after 6 months. If they do not, either the mole was invasive (myometrium penetrated) or has given rise to choriocarcinoma (10%). Invasive mole may metastasize, eg to lung, vagina, brain, liver and skin. Both conditions respond to chemotherapy.

Choriocarcinoma This highly malignant tumour occurs in 1:40000 deliveries. 50% follow a benign mole, 20% follow abortions and 10% follow normal pregnancy. *Presentation:* May be many years after pregnancy, with general malaise (due to 'malignancy' and to raised HCG); or uterine bleeding; or with signs and symptoms from metastases, which may be very haemorrhagic, eg haematoperitoneum, or cannonball shadows on CXR. Pulmonary artery obstruction via tumour emboli may lead to pulmonary artery hypertension (haemoptysis and dyspnoea).[2]
Treatment: Choriocarcinoma in UK is treated at 3 specialist centres and is extremely responsive to combination chemotherapy based on methotrexate. Outlook is excellent and fertility is usually retained.

►Persistent vaginal bleeding after a pregnancy requires investigation to exclude choriocarcinoma.

1 H Fox 1997 *BMJ* i 1363 2 M Seckl 1991 *Lancet* ii 1313

1. Gynaecology

The vulva

Pruritus vulvae Vaginal itch is distressing and embarrassing. *Causes:* There may be a disorder causing general pruritus (p 578) or skin disease (eg psoriasis, lichen planus). The cause may be local: infection and vaginal discharge (eg candida); infestation (eg scabies, pubic lice, threadworms); or vulval dystrophy (lichen sclerosis, leukoplakia, carcinoma). Symptoms may be psychogenic in origin. Obesity and incontinence exacerbate symptoms. Postmenopausal atrophy does not cause itch.

The history may suggest the cause. Examine general health and look for widespread skin conditions. Examine the vulva and genital tract, under magnification if possible, and take a cervical smear. Take vaginal and vulval swabs and test for diabetes. Biopsy if in doubt about diagnosis. ►Scratching and self-medication may have changed the appearance.

Treatment: This is often unsatisfactory.[1] Treat the cause if possible. Reassurance can be very important. Advise her to avoid nylon underwear, chemicals and soap (use aqueous cream) and dry with a hair dryer. A short course of topical steroids, eg betamethasone valerate cream 0.1% may help. Avoid any topical preparation which may sensitize the skin, so give antipruritics orally if needed, eg promethazine 25–50mg/24h.

Lichen sclerosis This is due to elastic tissue turning to collagen after middle age—or, occasionally, before puberty, where the 'bruised' red, purpuric signs appear, to the ignorant, to suggest abuse—particularly if there are bullae, erosions, and ulcerations. The vulva gradually becomes white, flat and shiny. There may be an hourglass shape around the vulva and anus. It is intensely itchy. It may be pre-malignant and long-term surveillance is desirable.[2] *Treatment:* Betamethasone valerate cream 0.1% may help; vulval ablation may be needed to relieve itch. In children, 50% resolve by menarche.[2]

Leukoplakia There are white patches on and around the vulva due to skin thickening and hypertrophy. It is itchy. It should be biopsied as it may be a pre-malignant lesion. *Treatment:* Topical corticosteroids (problems: mucosal thinning, absorption); psoralens with ultraviolet phototherapy; methotrexate; ciclosporin.[2]

Carcinoma of the vulva 95% are squamous. They are rare and occur mostly in the elderly.

Vulval malignancy has a pre-invasive phase, vulval intra-epithelial neoplasia (VIN), which may be itchy. ~6% progress to invasive carcinoma. VIN is associated with human papilloma virus (HPV) infection. There may not be visible warts but 5% acetic acid stains affected areas white. If VIN is found on biopsy, examine the cervix and check the breasts (>10% have coexistent neoplasia elsewhere, most commonly cervical). *Treatment* is aimed at symptom control by wide local excision[3] or laser ablation. Avoid topical steroids[3]. Recurrence is common so follow up regularly.

An indurated ulcer with an everted edge suggests carcinoma. It may not be noticed unless it causes pain and bleeding, so it often presents late (50% already have inguinal lymph node involvement).

Treatment: Stage I and 2 disease (ie tumour <2cm without nodal involvement) may be treated by 'triple incision surgery'. Radical vulvectomy (wide excision of the vulva + removal of inguinal glands) is used if more extensive disease. Post-operative healing may require skin grafts. 5-yr survival is 75% for lesions <2cm without node involvement; otherwise <50%.

1 Because of the not uncommonly recalcitrant nature of chronic vulval itch and chronic vulval pain (often ignored, or inappropriately diagnosed as candida)—and because of its effects on mood and sexuality, a patients' group (with professional input) has been set up in the UK (Vulval Pain Society, PO Box 514, Slough, Berkshire, SL1 2BP) 2 H Bell 1998 *The Diplomate* 5 112
3 D McConnell 1998 *The Diplomate* 5 118

Vulval lumps and ulcers

Causes of vulval lumps Local varicose veins; boils; sebaceous cysts; keratoacanthomata (rare); viral warts (condylomata acuminata); condylomata lata (syphilis); primary chancre; molluscum contagiosum; Bartholin's cyst or abscess; uterine prolapse or polyp; inguinal hernia, varicocele; carcinoma.

Vulval warts Human papilloma virus (HPV)—is usually spread by sexual contact.) Incubation: weeks. Her partner may not have obvious penile warts. The vulva, perineum, anus, vagina or cervix may be affected. Warts may be very florid in the pregnant and immunosuppressed. HPV types 16, 18 and 33 can cause vulval and cervical intra-epithelial neoplasia, so she needs annual cervical smears and observation of the vulva. Warts may also cause anal carcinoma (*OHCM* p 154). Treat both partners. Exclude other genital infections. Warts may be destroyed by diathermy, cryocautery or laser. Vulval and anal warts (condylomata acuminata) may be treated weekly in surgeries and GU clinics with 15% podophyllin paint, washed off after 30min (CI: pregnancy). Only treat a few warts at once, to avoid toxicity. Self-application with 0.15% podophyllotoxin cream (Warticon® 5g tubes—enough for 4 treatment courses—is supplied with a mirror): use every 12h for 3 days, repeated up to 4 times at weekly intervals if the area covered is $<4\text{cm}^2$. Relapse is common. NB: HPV types 6 and 11 may cause laryngeal or respiratory papillomas in the offspring of affected mothers (risk 1:50–1:1500; 50% present at <5yrs old).

Exclude other genital infections. Treat both partners.

Urethral caruncle This is a small red swelling at the urethral orifice. It is caused by meatal prolapse. It may be tender and give pain on micturition. *Treatment:* Excision or diathermy.

Bartholin's cyst and abscess The Bartholin's glands and their ducts lie under the labia minora. They secrete thin lubricating mucus during sexual excitation. If the duct becomes blocked a painless cyst forms; if this becomes infected the resulting abscess is extremely painful (she can't sit down) and a hugely swollen, hot red labium is seen. *Treatment:* The abscess should be incised, and permanent drainage ensured by marsupialization, ie the inner cyst wall is folded back and stitched to the skin. *Tests:* Exclude gonococcal infection.

Vulvitis Vulval inflammation may be due to infections, eg candida (p 48), herpes simplex; chemicals (bubble-baths, detergents). It is often associated with, or may be due to, vaginal discharge.

Causes of vulval ulcers: Always consider syphilis. *Herpes simplex* is common in the young. Others: carcinoma; chancroid; lymphogranuloma venereum; granuloma inguinale; TB; Behçet's syndrome; aphthous ulcers; Crohn's.

Herpes simplex Herpes type II, sexually acquired, classically causes genital infection, but type I transferred from cold sores can be the cause.
The vulva is ulcerated and exquisitely painful. Urinary retention may occur. *Treatment:* Strong analgesia, lidocaine (=lignocaine) gel 2%, salt baths (and micturating in the bath) help. Exclude coexistent infections. Aciclovir topically and 200mg 5 times daily PO for 5 days shortens symptoms and infectivity. Reassure that subsequent attacks are shorter and less painful. Prescribe acilovir cream for use when symptoms start. For herpes in pregnancy, see p 100.

1. Gynaecology

The cervix

This is is the part of the uterus below the internal os. The endocervical canal is lined with mucous columnar epithelium, the vaginal cervix with squamous epithelium. The transition zone between them—the squamo-columnar juction—is the area which is predisposed to malignant change.

Cervical ectropion This is often called erosion, an alarming term for a normal phenomenon. There is a red ring around the os because the endo-cervical epithelium has extended its territory over the paler epithelium of the ectocervix. Ectropions extend temporarily under hormonal influence during puberty, with the combined Pill, and during pregnancy. As columnar epithelium is soft and glandular, ectropion is prone to bleeding, to excess mucus production and to infection. *Treatment:* Cautery will treat these if they are a nuisance; otherwise no treatment is required.

Nabothian cysts These mucus retention cysts found on the cervix are harmless. *Treatment:* Cautery if they are discharging.

Cervical polyps These pedunculated benign tumours usually arise from the endocervical epithelium and so may cause increased mucus discharge or postcoital bleeding. *Treatment:* In young women they may be simply avulsed, but in older women treatment usually includes D&C to exclude intrauterine pathology.

Cervicitis This may be follicular or mucopurulent, presenting with discharge. *Causes:* Chlamydia (up to 50%),[1] gonococci, or herpes (look for vesicles). Chronic cervicitis is usually a mixed infection and may respond to antibacterial cream. Cervicitis may mask neoplasia on a smear.

Cervical screening Cervical cancer has a pre-invasive phase: cervical intra-epithelial neoplasia (CIN—not to be pronounced 'sin'). Papanicolaou smears collect cervical cells for microscopy for dyskaryosis (abnormalities which reflect CIN). A smear therefore identifies women who need cervical biopsy. The degree of dyskaryosis approximates to the severity of CIN (Table, p 34). ~50% of CIN I lesions return to normal but most CIN III lesions progress to invasive carcinoma. This may take ~10yrs, but may happen much faster in young women.

A programme of 2 smears in the first year of sexual activity, then 3-yearly smears should reduce the incidence of invasive carcinoma by 90%. The trouble is, those most at risk are the hardest to trace and persuade to have screening, eg older women, smokers, and those in inner cities. One of the great achievements of UK primary care and its software houses is that these women are now being reached: 83% of the eligible UK population is now screened, a figure which no other country exceeds, and mortality here is starting to fall; this depends critically on being able to retain skilled lab staff.

Taking a smear Explain to the woman the nature and purpose of the test, and how results will be conveyed to her. It may be sensible to warn that results are not categoric or unequivocal.

The cervix is visualized with a speculum (p 2). Are there any suspicious areas? If so, carry on with the smear and indicate this on the referral form, but do not wait for its results before arranging further care.

Cells are scraped from the squamo-columnar transformation zone with a special spatula or brush, then transferred to a slide and fixed at once. Good technique is needed (make sure that all 4 quadrants of the cervix are sampled); it is best to learn by instruction from an expert at the bedside.

1 D Taylor-Robinson 1994 *BMJ* i 150

Cervical carcinoma

►*Aim to detect pre-invasive disease.* ~1600 women die yearly of cervical carcinoma in the UK. Many have had no smear, but this is changing: see p 32.

Risk factors Smoking, HIV, many sexual partners (in both sexes) spreading human papilloma virus (HPV 16, 18 and 33). HPV oncogenes (E6) bind to the tumour-suppressor gene *p53* (the genome guardian, see p 752) so promoting tumorigenesis. Those with atypical versions of *p53* (*p53Arg*, 'double arginine') are at 7-fold ↑risk of cervical cancer. Thus cervical carcinoma is a sexually transmitted disease. (Neither partner may have visible warts.)

Management of abnormal smears (Guidelines below) Either a repeat smear or colposcopy and biopsy are needed, depending on likelihood of the smear reflecting CIN III or microinvasive disease (<3mm).

►Abnormal smears cause anxiety and guilt. Explain. Give support.

Treatment of pre-invasive carcinoma The cervix is examined using a colposcope (×10 binocular microscope). Abnormal epithelium has characteristic blood vessel patterns and stains white with acetic acid. Punch biopsies are taken for histology. CIN is destroyed by cryotherapy, laser, cold coagulation or electrodiathermy (the latter requires general anaesthesia). These give ~90% cure rates with one treatment. She needs annual smears for at least 10 years. If the squamo-columnar junction cannot be seen, or if microinvasive carcinoma is found on histology, the abnormal tissue is removed by cone biopsy, which may be curative. Colposcopy does not detect adenocarcinoma.

Invasive disease Once a disease of the over-50s, this is now seen in under-40s. Most are squamous cancers. ~5% are adenocarcinomas (from endocervical epithelium, with unknown risk factors). Spread is local and lymphatic. *Stage I* tumours are confined to the cervix. *Stage II* have extended locally. *Stage III* have spread to pelvic wall & lower ⅓ of vagina. *Stage IV* have spread to bladder or rectum. Most present in stages I or II.

Diagnosis ►Overt carcinoma is rarely detected on a smear. Non-menstrual bleeding is the classic symptom. The early tumour is firm. It grows as a friable mass which bleeds on contact.

Treating invasive cancers Wertheims's hysterectomy or radiotherapy treat the tumour and lymph nodes, and achieve good cure rates at stages I (80% 5-yr survival) and II (60%). Radiotherapy causes vaginal stenosis: so encourage intercourse within 2 months of treatment (+ lubricant). Follow-up: annual smears. Stage III needs extensive radiotherapy and chemotherapy, eg 5-FU + cisplatin; exenteration is probably *not* indicated (p 73). Stage IV: ?palliation only. Terminal problems are pain, fistulae, and GI/GU obstruction.

Histology of cervical pre-malignant disease (CIN = cervical intra-epithelial neoplasia)

	Papanicolaou class	*Action*	*Histology*
I	Normal	Repeat in 3 years (Unless clinical suspicion)	0.1% CIN II–III
II	Inflammatory	Repeat in 6 months (Colposcopy after 3 abnormal)	6% CIN II–III
	Mild atypia	Repeat in 4 months (Colposcopy after 2 abnormal)	20–37% CIN II–III
III	Mild dyskaryosis	Colposcopy	50% CIN II–III
	Moderate dyskaryosis	Colposcopy	50–75% CIN II–III
IV	Severe dyskaryosis 'Positive' 'Malignant cells'	Colposcopy	80–90% CIN II–III 5% Invasion
V	Invasion suspected	Urgent colposcopy	50% Invasion
	Abnormal glandular cells	Urgent colposcopy	?Adenocarcinoma or endometrium

CIN I = mild dysplasia; CIN II = moderate dysplasia; CIN III = Severe dysplasia/carcinoma-*in-situ*

The table above shows comparative terms and the recommended action. The third column, headed histology, shows the percentage of smears in each Papanicolaou (cytological) class which have more serious lesions (CIN II or III) on histology. 6% of inflammatory smears have serious pathology, hence the recommendation for colposcopy if inflammation persists.

In 1986, the term *borderline nuclear abnormality* was introduced to use when in doubt as to the neoplastic nature of any change. New guidelines are issued[1] for labs to request recall, eg at 3–6 months, or to advise colposcopy referral, eg after 2 smears with borderline nuclear abnormality, in which the number of affected cells has not reduced over time; colposcopy in these cases should be seen as part of the screening process, and should not necessarily prompt treatment. This goes part of the way to avoid false negatives, as well as to avoid the problems of overtreatment.

In the UK, 5–6 million smears are done each year—and the death rate from cervical carcinoma has fallen to <1900/yr (a fall of ~15% in the last decade). 2.4% of smears are reported as mild dyskaryosis, and 2.2% as borderline nuclear abnormalities. Because most of these will eventually need colposcopy because of further smear results and 48% can be expected to have CIN II or III, and as a significant proportion may be lost to follow-up, it is suggested that *immediate* colposcopy with directed biopsy is indicated.[2] However, this would be very expensive, and anxiety-provoking. The cost in the USA of adopting this policy is ~$1 billion, and the benefits are uncertain as no randomized trials have been done.[3]

Terminology used in reporting smears changed in the '80s, and different countries use different nomenclature—eg the Bethesda system.[4]

Neural networks for cervical smears? Until recently, computers in the lab and surgery have acted as no more than glorified filing clerks and secretaries; but as reading smears is labour-intensive, and boring, mistakes are inevitably made, particularly false negatives, and exaggeration of abnormalities (perhaps to avoid blame if time reveals malignancy to have been present). Neural network systems such as PAPNET realize the advantages of a machine (speed—1 slide/min with objectivity, thoroughness, freedom from boredom, and 24h/day operation) without allowing machines to take over. The program bar-codes slides, focuses them, digitizes images, selects the most interesting/difficult parts of the slide, records their *x–y* coordinates, and, if needed, signals that this is the area the cytologist should look at, whether they be individual cells, or clusters. Neural networks such as our own brain have ~10^{15} connections, whereas man-made systems have only up to one-billionth of this number, but this is still sufficient for reasonable accuracy, tolerance of conflicting information in a single specimen, and the ability to learn from experience. It is this ability which sets these networks apart from statistical or rule-based systems (if X is present find out if Y is also present). The disadvantage of rule-based systems is the rules have to be explicit—and in cervical cytology this is too tough a prerequisite to be realized.[5,6] For severe dysplasia, ca-*in-situ*, and suspected invasive carcinoma, PAPNET gives accuracy rates (compared with histology) of 38%, 35% and 72% respectively, compared with 40%, 20% and 62% for conventional analysis. PAPNET will also go though your negative slides, and tell you which ones may be false –ves and need reviewing by a cytologist.

The disadvantage of these networks are that they are difficult (and expensive) to train, and are only as good as the experience they have.

1 BMJ 1998 **i** 1628 2 Work. Part. Rep. 1994 *J Clin Path* **34** 481–92 & W Souter 1994 BMJ **ii** 591 3 M Shafi 1994 BMJ **ii** 590 4 JAMA 1989 **262** 931 5 R Dybowski 1995 *Lancet* **346** 1203 6 J Wyatt 1995 *Lancet* **346** 1175

The uterus

Endometritis Uterine infection is uncommon unless the barrier to ascending infection (acid vaginal pH and cervical mucus) is broken, eg after abortion and childbirth, IUCD insertion or surgery. Infection may involve Fallopian tubes and ovaries.

Presentation: Lower abdominal pain and fever; uterine tenderness on bimanual palpation. Low-grade infection is often due to chlamydia. *Tests:* Do cervical swabs and blood cultures. *Treatment:* Give antibiotics (eg doxycyline 100mg/24h PO with metronidazole 400mg/8h PO).

Endometrial proliferation Oestrogen stimulates proliferation of the endometrium during the first half of the menstrual cycle; it then comes under the influence of progesterone and is shed at menstruation. A particularly exuberant proliferation is associated with heavy menstrual bleeding and polyps.

If high oestrogen levels continue (eg anovulatory cycles) the endometrium becomes hyperplastic ('cystic glandular hyperplasia'—a histological diagnosis after D&C). Eventually it will break down, causing irregular bleeding (dysfunctional uterine bleeding). *Treatment:* Cyclical progestogens (p 14).

In older women proliferation may contain foci of atypical cells which may lead to endometrial carcinoma (p 40).

Pyometra This is a uterus distended with pus. Salpingitis may produce pyosalpinx and pyometra, or outflow blockage may lead to inflammation and secondary infection in the uterus. *Treatment:* It is relieved by drainage and treatment of the cause.

Haematometra This is a uterus filled with blood due to outflow obstruction. It is rare. The blockage may be an imperforate hymen in the young (p 6); carcinoma; or iatrogenic cervical stenosis, eg after cone biopsy.

Endometrial tuberculosis Genital tract tuberculosis is rare in Britain, except among high-risk groups (Asian immigrants). It is blood-borne and usually affects first the Fallopian tubes, then the endometrium.

It may present with acute salpingitis if disease is very active, or with infertility, pelvic pain and menstrual disorders (eg amenorrhoea, oligomenorrhoea). There may be pyosalpinx.

Exclude pulmonary disease with CXR. *Treatment* is medical with antituberculous therapy as for disease elsewhere (*OHCM* p 198–200). Repeat endometrial histology after one year.

Vaginal carcinoma

These tumours are usually squamous. They are commonest in the upper third of the vagina. Presentation is usually with bleeding. Clear cell adenocarcinoma was thought to be associated with intrauterine exposure to diethylstilboestrol but risk is low (0.1–1:1000). Spread is local and by lymphatics. Treatment is usually radiotherapy.

Fibroids

Fibroids are benign tumours of the smooth muscle of the uterus (leiomyomas). They are often multiple, and may vary in size from seedling size to large tumours occupying a substantial part of the abdomen. They start as lumps in the wall of the uterus but may grow to bulge out of the wall so that they lie under the peritoneum (subserosal, 20%) or under the endometrium (submucosal, 5%), or become pedunculated. Fibroids are common (20% of women have fibroids), increasing in frequency with age, and in non-Caucasians.

Natural history Fibroids are oestrogen-dependent. Consequently they enlarge in pregnancy and on the combined Pill and atrophy after the menopause. They may degenerate gradually or suddenly (red degeneration). Occasionally they calcify ('womb stones'). Rarely, they undergo sarcomatous change—usually causing pain, malaise, bleeding, and increase in size in a postmenopausal woman.

Presentation Many are asymptomatic.

- *Menorrhagia:* Fibroids often produce heavy and prolonged periods. They do not generally cause intermenstrual or postmenopausal bleeding.
- *Fertility problems:* Submucosal fibroids may interfere with implantation ('natural IUCD'). Large or multiple tumours which distort the uterine cavity may cause abortion should pregnancy occur.
- *Pain:* This may be due to torsion of a pedunculated fibroid, producing symptoms similar to that of a torted ovarian cyst. 'Red degeneration' following thrombosis of a fibroid's blood supply usually only happens in pregnancy and produces severe pain, fever and local tenderness until degeneration is complete.
- *Mass:* Large fibroids may be felt abdominally. They may press on the bladder, causing frequency, or on the veins, causing oedematous legs and varicose veins. Pelvic fibroids may obstruct labour or cause retention of urine.

Treatment In many women treatment is not needed.

Menorrhagia due to fibroids tends to respond poorly to antiprostaglandins, progestogens or danazol. Women who have completed their families may opt for hysterectomy. In younger women a reversible menopausal state may be induced with analogues of LHRH (leutinizing hormone releasing hormone), eg buserelin nasal spray 100μg/4h (expensive)[1] or goserelin 3.6mg by monthly subcutaneous injection (preferred method—intermittent buserelin use can increase their size rather than shrink them). Bone demineralization can occur with their use, so their place is in shrinking fibroids prior to surgery (to reduce blood loss at surgery and make surgery easier); those unfit for surgery; or those desiring later pregnancy. They reduce bulk by 40% over 12 weeks, but no further reduction occurs after 24 weeks use.[1] Side-effects are menopausal symptoms; fertility (and fibroids) return when the drug is stopped. Alternatively the fibroids may be surgically shelled out (myomectomy); torrential bleeding necessitating hysterectomy is a complication and postoperative adhesions notorious.[1] Laparoscopic surgery with or without use of lasers is possible but requires considerable patience.[1]

Red degeneration requires only analgesia until symptoms settle.

Torsion may resemble an acute abdomen, requiring urgent surgery.

1 C Sutton 1996 *Br J Obs Gynae* **103** 494

Endomentrial carcinoma

►Postmenopausal vaginal bleeding must be investigated as the cause may be endometrial carcinoma.

Carcinoma of the uterine body is less common than carcinoma of the cervix. It usually presents after the menopause. Most tumours are adenocarcinomas and are related to excessive exposure to oestrogen unopposed by progesterone. There is marked geographical variation: North American:Chinese ratio = 7:1.

Risk factors •Obesity •Nulliparity •Diabetes •Unopposed oestrogen therapy •Late menopause •Pelvic irradiation •Functioning ovarian tumour •Tamoxifen[1]* •FH of breast, ovary, colon cancer

Presentation This is usually as postmenopausal bleeding (PMB). Any woman with a history of PMB has a 10–20% risk of genital cancer. It is initially scanty and occasional, perhaps with a watery discharge. Over time, bleeding becomes heavier and more frequent. Pre-menopausal women may have intermenstrual bleeding, but 30% have only menorrhagia.

Diagnosis Postmenopausal bleeding is an early sign, and generally leads a woman to see her doctor, but examination is usually normal. Endometrial carcinoma can sometimes be seen on a smear. The diagnosis is made by uterine sampling (p 41) or curettage. All parts of the uterine cavity must be sampled; send *all* material for histology. Hysteroscopy enables visualization of abnormal endometrium to improve accuracy of sampling. Sceptics claim it may cause spread through the Fallopian tubes to the peritoneum.

Pathology Most tumours start in the fundus of the uterine cavity. The tumour spreads slowly to the uterine muscle. With time, it may reach the cervix or peritoneum and may metastasize to the vagina (5%), ovary (5%), and any of the pelvic lymph nodes (7%).

Staging

I: Tumour is confined to the body of the uterus.
II: As for I but with cervical involvement.
III: Tumour has extended beyond the uterus but not beyond the pelvis.
IV: Extension outside the pelvis. Bowel and bladder may be affected.

Treatment Stages I and II may be cured by total hysterectomy with bilateral salpingo-oophorectomy and/or radiotherapy if unfit for surgery (5-yr survival: stage I = 72%, stage II = 56%). Post-operative vault irradiation reduces vault recurrence. In advanced disease consider radiotherapy and/or high-dose progestogens, eg medroxyprogesterone acetate 250mg/24h PO, which shrinks the tumour (SE: fluid retention). Radiotherapy may either be given pre-operatively (caesium or radium rods inserted into the uterus and upper vagina) or post-operatively (external radiation).

Recurrent disease usually presents in the first 2–3yrs. Common sites are pelvic (in nonirradiated patients), lung, bone, inguinal and supraclavicular nodes, vagina, liver, peritoneal cavity. Surgical exenteration, radiotherapy, and medroxyprogesterone may all be of use. Cytotoxics may be used for those who fail to respond to the above.

*Note: tamoxifen 20mg daily reduces annual risk of breast cancer recurrence by 27%.[2] Risk of endometrial carcinoma from taking tamoxifen is 1.2 per 1000 person-years.[2] Counsel to report abnormal vaginal bleeding.

1 FE van Leeuwen 1994 *Lancet* **343** 448 2 1994 *Current Problems in Pharmacovigilance* (CSM) **20** 13

Endometrial sampling in outpatients

This relatively new bedside technique is replacing D&C (p 72) in the investigation of postmenopausal bleeding, perimenopausal irregular bleeding, and unexpected bleeding patterns in women on hormone replacement therapy because it is cheap, reliable, and gives quick results without the need for anaesthesia.[1] It is less useful in menorrhagia in women with regular cycles, as pathology is less common. It is not indicated if <35 years old.

A sample is obtained using a side-opening plastic cannula in which a vacuum is created by withdrawal of a stopped central plunger mechanism. As the cannula is then withdrawn and rotated within each quadrant of the uterine cavity, endometrial tissue is sucked into its interior, through the hole in the side of the cannula. Successful insertion is possible in 90–99% of women (D&C is possible in 99%). Adequate samples will be obtained in 91% of these, and in 84% of those for whom postmenopausal bleeding (PMB) was the indication (at D&C an adequate sample is only achieved in 68%, and only in 45% if the indication was PMB). 95% of endometrial cancers will be detected by either procedure. Abandon the procedure if it is impossible to enter the uterus successfully, or if it causes too much pain.

Technique

1 Bimanual examination to assess size and position of uterus (p 2).
2 Bend cervical cannula to follow the curve of the uterus.
3 Insert device, watching the centimetre scale on the side; observe resistance on entering the internal os (at 3–4 cm) and then as the tip reaches the fundus (eg at 6cm if postmenopausal or 8cm in an oestrogenized uterus).
4 When the tip is in the fundus, create a vacuum by withdrawing plunger until the stopper prevents further withdrawal. Then move sampler up and down in uterus, rotate and repeat to sample whole cavity.
5 Remove cannula, and expel tissue into formalin. Send for histology.

Management Reassure those in whom the results show normal or atrophic endometrium and those in whom tissue was insufficient for diagnosis. If those with PMB re-bleed refer for hysteroscopy (polyps or a fibroid will be present in 20%). Those with simple hyperplasia on histology can be treated with cyclical progesterones (but refer if >55yrs to search for exogenous oestrogen source). Refer those with polyps or necrotic tissue on histology for hysteroscopy and curettage; and those with atypical hyperplasia or carcinoma for hysterectomy and bilateral salpingo-oophorectomy. Those in whom endometrial sampling was impossible or abandoned should have transvaginal uterine ultrasound to establish endometrial thickness (<5mm normal in the postmenopausal; refer if >5mm).

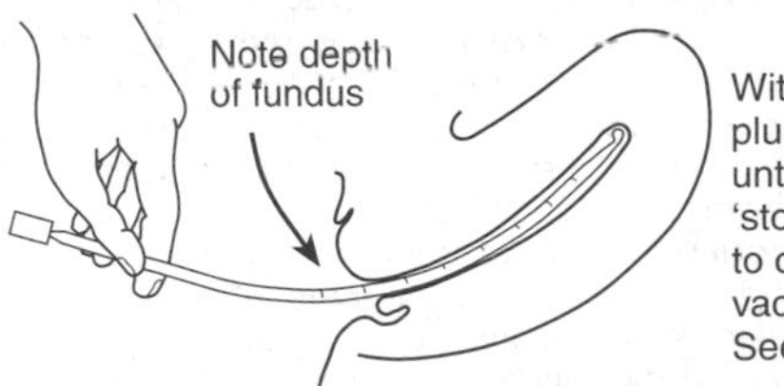

We thank Genesis Medical Ltd for permission to reproduce the diagram

1 A Coulter 1993 BMJ i 236

Ovarian tumours

Any of the ovary's many tissue types may become neoplastic.

Benign tumours (94%). They are usually cystic. 24% of all ovarian tumours are functional cysts. Others: endometriotic cysts (5%—p 52); theca-lutein cysts (p 26); epithelial cell tumours (serous and mucinous cystadenomas—40%); mature teratomas (from germ cells—20%); fibromas (solid—5%).

Malignant tumours (6%). 5% are cystadenomas which have become malignant. 0.5% are a group of rare germ cell or sex cord malignancies (p 44). 0.5% are secondaries, eg from the uterus, or the stomach (Krukenberg tumours—in which spread is transcoelomic, ie, in the case of the abdomen, via the peritoneum).

Risk markers of ovarian malignancy: Nulliparity (risk$\uparrow \times 1.5$); infertility; early menarche; +ve family history (p 46); no past use of the Pill/HRT with progesterone; ovulation-inducing treatments of infertility (eg carcinomas, teratomas, and stromal tumours).[1]

Presentations are varied, depending on size, form and histological type:
Asymptomatic—chance finding (eg on doing a bimanual for a smear test).
Swollen abdomen—with palpable mass arising out of the pelvis which is dull to percussion (and does not disappear if the bladder is catheterized).
Pressure effects (eg on bladder, causing urinary frequency).
Infarction/haemorrhage—this mimics torsion (see below).
Rupture ± local peritonism. Rupture of a large cyst may cause peritonitis and shock. Rupture of a malignant cyst may disseminate malignant cells throughout the abdomen. Rupture of mucinous cystadenomas may disseminate cells which continue to secrete mucin and cause death by binding up the viscera (pseudomyxoma peritonei). See p 44. Pseudomyxoma peritonei is treated by surgical debulking. 10-year survival is 30–50%.[2]
Ascites—shifting dullness suggests malignancy or Meigs' syndrome (p 44). If tense, ascites may be hard to distinguish from a mass.
Torsion—to twist, a tumour must be small, and free on a pedicle. Twisting occludes the venous return but the arterial supply continues to engorge the tumour, and cause great pain (with a high WBC). Tumours may twist and untwist, giving a history of intermittent pain. If the pain is not too severe, a firm tender adnexal swelling may be felt.
Endocrine or metastatic effects—Hormone-secreting tumours may cause virilization, menstrual irregularities or postmenopausal bleeding.

Management *Ultrasound* may confirm the presence of a mass (though, as with bimanual examination, it can be difficult to tell an ovarian mass from a uterine one). It may show whether it is cystic or solid.
Laparoscopy may distinguish a cyst from an ectopic pregnancy or appendicitis. Note: laparoscopy is not advised if malignancy is possible, due to seeding along the surgical tract. *Fine needle aspiration* may be used to confirm the impression that a cyst is benign. Urgent *laparotomy* is required when a cyst problem presents as an acute abdomen.

Any cyst not positively identified as non-neoplastic should be removed, as seemingly benign tumours may be malignant. In younger women *cystectomy* may be preferable to oöphorectomy. In postmenopausal women, if one ovary is pathological both are removed. For management in pregnancy see p 150.

1 K Tewari 1998 *Lancet* **351** 957 2 H Fox 1996 *Br J Obs Gynae* **103** 197

1. Gynaecology

Ovarian tumours: pathology

Functional cysts These are enlarged or persistent follicular or corpus luteum cysts. They are so common that they may be considered normal if they are small (<5cm). They may cause pain by rupture, failing to rupture at ovulation, or bleeding.

Polycystic ovary syndrome (PCOS) The cause of this common (5–10% of premenopausal women affected), poorly understood syndrome is unknown—but may be related to insulin resistance (*OHCM* p 529). The result appears to be a vicious circle of ovarian, hypothalamic-pituitary, and adrenal dysfunction. Insulin resistance and hyperinsulinaemia are features. Hormonal cycling is disrupted and the ovaries become enlarged by follicles which have failed to rupture.

The patient may be obese, virilized, with acne and irregular or absent menses (Stein–Leventhal syndrome). She may present with infertility. Investigation may show LH↑, testosterone↑. Any feature may be normal. Laparoscopy or ultrasound show characteristic ovaries.

Treatment is symptomatic: clomifene (=clomiphene) will induce ovulation (p 58), the combined Pill will control bleeding and reduce risk of unopposed oestrogen on the endometrium. Hirsutes may be treated cosmetically, or with an anti-androgen, eg cyproterone 2mg/day, as in Dianette® (avoid pregnancy). Weight loss helps. Metformin improves insulin sensitivity, menstrual disturbance and ovulatory function.[1]

Serous cystadenomas These develop papillary growths which may be so prolific that the cyst appears solid. They are commonest in women aged 30 to 40 years. About 30% are bilateral and about 30% are malignant.

Mucinous cystadenomas These are the commonest large ovarian tumours and may become enormous. They are filled with mucinous material and rupture may rarely cause pseudomyxoma peritonei (p 42). They may be multilocular. They are commonest in the 30–50 age group. About 5% will be malignant. Remove the appendix at operation in those with suspected mucinous cystadenoma and send for histology.[1] (Interestingly men can get pseudomyxoma from intestinal or appendicular neoplasms; most women with pseudomyxoma peritonei do not have overt rupture of ovarian tumours and 90% have concurrent intestinal or appendicular tumours and it is now thought that the ovarian tumours may be secondary to GI ones).[2]

Fibromas These are small, solid benign fibrous tissue tumours. They are associated with Meigs' syndrome (*OHCM* p 704) and ascites.

Teratomas These arise from primitive germ cells. A benign mature teratoma (dermoid cyst) may contain well differentiated tissue, eg hair, teeth. 20% are bilateral. They are most common in young women. Poorly differentiated, malignant teratomas are rare.

Other germ cell tumours (all malignant and all rare): nongestational choriocarcinomas (secrete HCG); ectodermal sinus tumours (yolk sac tumours—secrete α-fetoprotein); dysgerminomas which are histologically similar to seminomas of testis.

Sex-cord tumours (rare and usually of low-grade malignancy): These arise from cortical mesenchyme. Granulosa-cell and theca-cell tumours produce oestrogen and may present with precocious puberty, menstrual problems or postmenopausal bleeding. Arrhenoblastomas secrete androgens.

1 N Sattar 1998 *Lancet* **351** 305 2 H Fox 1996 *Br J Obs Gynae* **103** 197

Ovarian carcinoma

This is rare, but more women die from it (it is the fourth commonest cause of cancer-related death in Western women) than from carcinoma of the cervix and uterine body combined because in 75% it causes few symptoms until it has metastasized, often to the pelvis with omental and peritoneal seedlings (± lymphatic spread via the para-aortic glands).

Incidence 1 in 2500 women >55yrs; 1 in 3800 if >25yrs. 1% have familial disease. If your daughter has ovarian cancer, your relative risk (RR) is 1.1; if your mother, RR=6; if just your sister, RR=3.8.[1] Women with 2 *close relatives* affected have a 40% risk of ovarian cancer (liaise with a gynaecologist; see below). It is commoner in those with many ovulations (*early menarche, nullipara*) and after infertility treatment (p 58).

Presentation Symptoms are often vague and insidious and include abdominal pain, discomfort and distension.

Diagnosis This is made at laparotomy, although malignancy is likely if ultrasound scan shows an irregular or solid tumour, bilateral disease, or the presence of ascites.

Staging at laparotomy

Stage I: Disease limited to 1 or both ovaries.
Stage II: Growth extends beyond the ovaries but confined to the pelvis.
Stage III: Growth involving ovary and peritoneal implants outside pelvis (eg superficial liver), or +ve retroperitoneal or inguinal nodes.
Stage IV: Those with distant metastases (including liver parenchyma).

80% present with stage III or IV disease. 5-yr survival: Stage I, 67%; Stage II, 42%; Stage III and IV, 14.4%.

Treatment This depends on the type of tumour. Cystadenocarcinomas (80%) are treated with surgery and chemotherapy which aims for cure. Surgery removes as much tumour as possible: the less left, the more effective is chemotherapy and the better the prognosis. In a young woman with early disease, the uterus and other ovary may be left, for fertility; if the tumour involves both ovaries, uterus and omentum are removed.

Chemotherapy for ~6 months post-op is usual. Cisplatin (eg ≥50mg/m^2) or carboplatin IV are used (± doxorubicin & cyclophosphamide; but one good trial found that these increased side-effects, not survival—eg alopecia, WCC↓, nausea).[2] Carboplatin causes less nausea, vomiting and neuropathy and is not renally toxic, and may not require hospital admission. Relapse is common, and we note that substituting the cyclophosphamide for paclitaxel (from Pacific yew trees) may be better.[3] Radiotherapy may be tried.

Further treatment may involve a 'second look' laparotomy, further chemotherapy, or radiotherapy. Colloidal gold may control ascites.

Palliative care involves relief of symptoms which are generally due to extensive peritoneal disease.

Screening and prevention There is no really good screening test. Transvaginal, but not abdominal, ultrasound combined with measurement of tumour blood flow, can differentiate between benign and malignant neoplasms at an early stage, but is time-consuming. Carcino-embryonic antigen 125 is insufficiently sensitive or specific. A blood test based on a 2-allele polymorphism in intron 3 of gene *p*53 (explained on p 752) has given a specificity of 98% and a sensitivity of 16%.[4]

Some advocate prophylactic oophorectomy when an older woman is having abdominal surgery. The combined oral contraceptive Pill reduces the risk of ovarian malignancy by up to 40%.

1 J Stratton 1998 *Br J Obs Gyn* **105** 493 2 ICON group 1998 *Lancet* **352** 1571 & M Gore 1994 *Lancet* **343** 339 3 W McGuire 1996 E-BM **1** 152 4 I Runnebaum 1995 *Lancet* **345** 994

Vaginal discharge

A inoffensive discharge may be physiological. Most discharges are smelly and itchy and due to infection. A very foul discharge may be due to a foreign body (eg forgotten tampons, or beads in children).

Note the details of the discharge. Is she at risk of, or afraid of, a sexually transmitted disease (STD)? See *OHCM* p 216–220. If she has an STD, contact-tracing is needed—consult a genito-urinary clinic.

Do a speculum examination and take swabs: endocervical (and special medium) for chlamydia; cervical swabs for gonorrhoea (*OHCM* p 220). ►Discharges rarely resemble their classical descriptions.

Physiological discharge Its increase with puberty, sexual activity, pregnancy and the combined Pill. It may cause much anxiety.

Thrush (*Candida albicans*) Thrush is the commonest cause of discharge, which is classically white curds. The vulva and vagina may be red, fissured and sore, especially if there is an allergic component. Her partner may be asymptomatic. Pregnancy, contraceptive and other steroids, immunodeficiencies, antibiotics and diabetes are risk factors—check for glycosuria. *Diagnosis:* Microscopy reveals strings of mycelium or typical oval spores. Culture on Sabouraud's medium.

Treatment: A single imidazole pessary, eg clotrimazole 500mg, plus cream for the vulva (and partner) is convenient. She may need reassurance that thrush is not necessarily sexually transmitted.

Thrush is often recurrent; consider nystatin vaginal pessaries for 14 nights (messy) or fluconazole 150mg PO as a single dose (avoid if pregnant). Candida elsewhere (eg mouth, natal cleft) of both partners may cause re-infection. Live yoghurt (on a tampon) or acetic acid jelly pH 4, eg Aci-Jel® may prevent or relieve mild attacks. Avoidance of chemicals around the vulva (no bathsalts); wiping the vulva from front to back; cotton underwear, double rinsed; and vinegar baths, may help.

Trichomonas vaginalis (TV) This produces vaginitis and a thin, bubbly, fishy smelling discharge. It is sexually transmitted. Exclude gonorrhoea, which often coexists. The motile flagellate may be seen on a wet film (×40 magnification), or cultured. *Treatment:* Metronidazole 200mg/8h PO for 7 days or 2g PO stat; treat the partner; if pregnant, use the 7-day regimen.

Bacterial vaginosis There is offensive discharge with fishy odour, from cadaverine and putrescine. Vaginal pH is >5.5. The vagina is not inflamed and pruritus is uncommon. Mixed with 10% potassium hydroxide on a slide under the nose, a whiff of ammonia may be emitted. Stippled vaginal epithelial 'clue cells' may be seen on wet microscopy. There is altered bacterial flora—overgrowth, eg of *Gardnerella vaginalis*, *Mycoplasma hominis*, peptostreptococci, *Mobiluncus* and anaerobes, eg *Bacteroides* species—with too few lactobacillae. There is increased risk of preterm labour and intra-amniotic infection in pregnancy; a 2-fold risk of cervical dysplasia[1] and a 2–4-fold increase in post-abortion sepsis. *Diagnosis:* By culture. *Treatment:* Metronidazole 2g PO once or clindamycin 2% vaginal cream, 1 applicatorful/night PV for 7 doses. If recurrent, treating the partner may be helpful. If pregnant, use metronidazole alone at 200mg/8h PO for 7 days.

Discharge in children may reflect infection from *faecal flora*, associated with alkalinity from lack of vaginal oestrogen (prepubertal atrophic vaginitis). *Staphs* and *streps* may cause pus. *Threadworms* cause pruritus. Always consider *sexual abuse*. Gentle rectal examination may exclude a *foreign body*. *Tests:* Do a vulval ± vaginal swab. MSU: *is there glycosuria?* For prolonged or bloody discharge, examination under anaesthesia may be needed (a paediatric laryngoscope can be used as a speculum) ± ultrasound or x-rays. *Management:* •Discuss hygiene •If an antibiotic is needed, erythromycin is a good choice. •An oestrogen cream may be tried (≤1cm strip).[2]

1 R Lamont 1995 *Br J Obs Gynae* **102** 424   2 R Jones 1996 *Family Practice* **13** 369–72

Pelvic infection

Pelvic infection affects the Fallopian tubes (salpingitis) and may involve ovaries and parametra. 90% are sexually acquired, mostly chlamydia: 60% of these are asymptomatic (♀/♂ = 1 : 1)[1] but infertility or ectopic pregnancy may be the result, *which is why screening has been proposed*—eg by a urine ligase chain reaction DNA: see opposite. Other causes, eg the gonococcus are rarer. Organisms cultured from infected tubes are commonly different from those cultured from ectocervix, and are usually multiple. 10% follow childbirth or instrumentation (insertion of IUCD, ToP) and may be streptococcal. Infection can spread from the intestinal tract during appendicitis (Gram –ve and anaerobic organisms) or be blood-borne (tuberculosis).

Salpingitis Patients with *acute salpingitis* may be most unwell, with pain, fever, spasm of lower abdominal muscles (she may be most comfortable lying on her back with legs flexed) and cervicitis with profuse, purulent or bloody vaginal discharge. Heavy menstrual loss suggests endometritis. Nausea and vomiting suggest peritonitis. Look for suprapubic tenderness or peritonism, cervical excitation, and tenderness in the fornices. It is usually bilateral, but may be worse on one side. *Subacute infection* can be easily missed, and laparoscopy may be needed to make either diagnosis.

Management ▶ Prompt treatment and contact-tracing minimizes complications. Take endocervical and urethral swabs if practicable. Remember to check for chlamydia. Admit for blood cultures and IV antibiotics if very unwell. She needs bed rest, adequate fluid intake and antibiotics, eg a week of doxycycline 100mg/24h PO (substitute erythromycin 500mg/6h PO if pregnant) and metronidazole 400mg/8h PO. This covers gonococcus, but if that is cultured, it is advisable to add procaine penicillin 4.8g IM stat with probenecid 1g PO. Trace contacts and ensure they seek treatment (seek help of genito-urinary clinic).

NB: azithromycin is gaining ascendancy over doxycycline both in terms of patient compliance and cost-effectiveness (even though it is 4 times as expensive): one stat dose of 1g cures 90% of chlamydial infections.[2]

Complications If response to antibiotics is slow, consider laparoscopy. She may have an abscess (draining via the posterior fornix prevents perforation, peritonitis and septicaemia—but laparotomy may be needed). Inadequate or delayed treatment leads to chronic infection and to long-term tubal blockage (so 12% infertile after 1 episode, 23% after 2, 54% after 3). Advise that barrier contraception protects against infection. Ectopic pregnancy rate is increased 10-fold in those who do conceive.

Chronic salpingitis Unresolved, unrecognized or inadequately treated infection may become chronic. Inflammation leads to fibrosis, so adhesions develop between pelvic organs. The tubes may be distended with pus (pyosalpinx) or fluid (hydrosalpinx).

Pelvic pain, menorrhagia, secondary dysmenorrhoea, discharge and deep dyspareunia are some of the symptoms. She may be depressed. Look for tubal masses, tenderness and fixed retroverted uterus. Laparoscopy differentiates infection from endometriosis.

Treatment is unsatisfactory. Consider long-term broad-spectrum antibiotics (eg tetracycline 250mg/6h PO 1 hour before food for 3 months), short-wave diathermy and analgesia for pain, and counselling.[3] The only cures are menopause or surgical removal of infected tissue.

1 H Bower 1998 BMJ **i** 1479 2 Stamm *et al* 1995 JAMA **274** 545 3 C Douglas 1989 *Update* **38** 480

Urine screening tests to prevent chlamydial pelvic infection[1]

Current proposals are for opportunistic screening in family planning and TOP contexts, and routine GP appointments for all sexually active women aged up to 25yrs. This might miss up to 20% of infections (increasing the age limit to 30 might miss just 7%).[1] It is not clear how this screening is to be woven into routine appointments (which are already overfull), and whether patients will find screening acceptable.

1 F Boag 1998 BMJ i 1474

Endometriosis

Essence Foci of endometrial glandular tissue, looking like the head of a burnt match, are found beyond the uterine cavity, eg on an ovary ('chocolate cyst'), in the rectovaginal pouch, uterosacral ligaments, on the surface of pelvic peritoneum, and rarely in the umbilicus, lower abdominal scars and distant organs, eg lungs. If foci are found in the muscle of the uterine wall, the term *adenomyosis* is used. It occurs in ~12% of women; not all have symptoms, and in the asymptomatic, it may be physiological.

Cause Possibly retrograde menstruation (Sampson's theory) explaining its association with age—typically 40–44yrs, ie those with most menstrual exposure, its negative association with pregnancy and the Pill,[1] and its distribution in the pelvis—but not its appearance elsewhere. Women with endometriosis have raised autoantibody levels. Endometriotic foci are under hormonal influence so are suppressed during pregnancy, regress with the menopause, and bleed during menstruation. Blood may be confined in cysts (which look brown, hence 'chocolate cysts'). If the blood is free it is intensely irritating, provoking fibrosis and adhesions.

Presentation Endometriosis may be asymptomatic, even though extensive. Pelvic pain is the commonest symptom (classically cyclical, at the time of periods). It may be constant, eg if due to adhesions. Secondary dysmenorrhoea and deep dyspareunia are common. Periods are often heavy and frequent, especially with adenomyosis. Patients may present with infertility. Extra-pelvic endometriosis presents with pain or bleeding at the time of menstruation at the site of the pathology, eg haemothorax.

Diagnosis On vaginal examination a fixed retroverted uterus or nodules in the uterosacral ligaments+general tenderness suggest endometriosis. An enlarged, boggy, tender uterus is typical of adenomyosis. Typical cysts or peritoneal deposits at laparoscopy differentiates it from chronic infection.

Treatment If asymptomatic, then do not treat. Otherwise, try surgery or hormones (if not pregnant or lactating). In the UK, consider suggesting joining the Endometriosis Society,[3] as treatment can be long and difficult.

Hormonal treatment aims to suppress ovulation for 6–12 months during which time lesions atrophy. **Danazol** up to 400–800mg/24h PO is effective but SE may be unacceptable at high doses (it is a testosterone derivative with anabolic and androgenic effects so expect weight gain, acne, greasy skin, hirsutism, bloating and fluid retention). Advise barrier contraception as it masculinizes the female fetus. **Gestrinone** 2.5–5mg PO twice weekly is an alternative. LHRH analogues, eg **buserelin** nasal spray 300μg/8h or **goserelin** 3.6mg by monthly sc injection produce a reversible artificial menopause but bone demineralization occurs. SE: menopausal symptoms, headaches, depression, libido↓, breast tenderness, drowsiness, acne, dry skin, ovarian cysts (if so, stop), urticaria, changes in body hair, osteoporosis—so only give for <6 months. An alternative gonadotrophic-releasing hormone agonist with similar side-effects is **leuprorelin acetate**—dose: 3.75mg every 4 weeks IM or sc starting during the first 5 days of a cycle, for <6 months. Endometriotic resolution is similar to danazol, but SE are less (flushes, headaches, vaginal dryness, emotional lability). Progestogens, eg **norethisterone** (Primolut N®) 5–10mg/12h PO continuously for 9 months may suppress symptoms temporarily by mimicking pregnancy.[2]

Surgical treatment ranges from local excision or diathermy of endometriotic tissue, to total hysterectomy with bilateral salpingo-oophorectomy, depending on the site of lesions and the woman's wish for future fertility.

Prognosis Endometriosis is chronic or relapsing, being progressive in 50%. There is no evidence that treatment helps fertility.

1 D Limb 1995 *Update* **50** 158 2 M Vessey 1993 BMJ **ii** 182 3 50 Artillery Rd, London SW1 (0171 222 2776)

Prolapse

A prolapse occurs when weakness of the supporting structures allows the pelvic organs to sag within the vagina. The weakness may be congenital, but it usually results from stretching during childbirth. Poor perineal repair reduces support (p 146). Weakness is exacerbated by menopausal atrophy and by coughing and straining. They may cause distressing incontinence and be a nuisance but are not a danger to health—except for third degree uterine prolapse with cystocele when ureteric obstruction can occur.

Types of prolapse are named by the structures sagging. Several types may coexist in the same patient.

Cystocele The upper front wall of the vagina, and the bladder which is attached to it, bulge. Residual urine within the cystocele may cause frequency and dysuria.

Urethrocele If the lower anterior vaginal wall bulges, this will displace the urethra and impair the sphincter mechanisms (p 70), so leading to stress incontinence. Does she leak when she laughs?

Rectocele The middle posterior wall, which is attached to rectum, may bulge through weak levator ani. It is often symptomless, but she may have to reduce herniation prior to defecation by putting a finger in the vagina.

Enterocele Bulges of the upper posterior vaginal wall may contain loops of intestine from the pouch of Douglas.

Uterine prolapse With *first degree prolapse* the cervix stays in the vagina. In *second degree prolapse* it protrudes from the introitus when standing or straining. With *3rd degree prolapse* (procidentia) the uterus lies outside the vagina. The vagina becomes keratinized and the cervix may ulcerate.

Symptoms: 'Dragging' or 'something coming down' is worse by day. Cystitis, frequency, stress incontinence and difficulty in defecation may occur depending on the type of prolapse. Examine vaginal walls in left lateral position with a Sims' speculum, and ask the patient to bear down to demonstrate the prolapse.

Prevention: Lower parity; better obstetric practices.

Treatment: Mild disease may improve with reduction in intra-abdominal pressure, so encourage her to lose weight, stop smoking and stop straining. Improve muscle tone with exercises or physiotherapy, and, if post-menopausal, topical oestrogens, eg (o)estriol cream 0.1% as often as required (try twice weekly).

Severe symptomatic prolapse is best treated surgically. Incontinence needs to have the cause treated (so arrange urodynamic studies to plan the best type of surgery). Repair operations (p 72) excise redundant tissue and strengthen supports, but reduce vaginal width. Is she sexually active? If so, surgery must compromise between reducing prolapse and maintaining width. Marked uterine prolapse is best treated by hysterectomy.

Ring pessaries may be tried as a temporary measure or for the very frail. Use the smallest diameter which keeps the prolapse reduced. Insert into the posterior fornix and tuck above the pubic bone (easier if the ring has been softened in hot water first). Problems: discomfort, infection, ulceration (change every 6 months).

Infertility: causes and tests[1]

►*Infertility can be devastating to both partners:* its investigation a tremendous strain. Sympathetic management is crucial. 90% of young couples having regular intercourse conceive within a year. Fertility decreases with age. High fertility in one partner can compensate for low fertility in the other, so in many of the remaining 10% both partners are subfertile. Consider:

- Is she producing healthy ova? (Anovulation causes 21%.)
- Is he producing enough, healthy sperm? (Male factors cause 24%.)
- Are the ova and sperm meeting? (Tubal cause 14%, hostile mucus 3%, sexual dysfunction 6%.)
- Is the embryo implanting?

Endometriosis is thought to be the cause in 6%. The cause is 'unexplained' in 27% of couples. With 'unexplained' infertility 60–70% of women will achieve conception within 3 years.

Initial management It takes two to be infertile. See both partners. *Ask her about:* Menstrual history, previous pregnancies and contraception, history of pelvic infections or abdominal surgery. *Ask him about:* Puberty, previous fatherhood, previous surgery (hernias, orchidopexy, bladder neck surgery), illnesses (venereal disease and adult mumps), drugs, alcohol intake, job (is he home when ovulation occurs?). *Ask both about:* Technique, frequency, and timing of intercourse (nonconsummation is a rare problem); feelings about infertility and parenthood; previous tests.

Examination Check the woman's general health and sexual development and examine the abdomen and pelvis. If the sperm count is abnormal, examine the man for endocrine abnormalities, penile abnormalities, varicoceles; confirm there are 2 normal testes (size: 3.5–5.5 × 2.1–3.2cm).

Tests for ovulation If cycles are regular ovulation is likely. The only proof of ovulation is pregnancy. It is possible for a follicle to luteinize without rupturing, so tests may be +ve in the absence of an ovum. Negative results imply failure to ovulate. *Test examples:* Visualizing follicle development or change to secretory endometrium on ultrasound; finding 'ovulatory' mucus at midcycle (like raw egg white); detecting LH surge (eg Clearplan® kit); detecting a luteal rise in progesterone to >30nmol/L 7 days before the onset of menstruation[1] (eg day 21); detecting a rise in basal body temperature at midcycle (temperature charting is difficult to do and may create anxieties).

Blood tests Check rubella status and immunize if nonimmune. If you suspect anovulation check: •Blood prolactin (if high may be due to prolactinoma; do skull x-ray) •FSH (>10u/L indicates a poor response to ovarian stimulation; it may indicate primary ovarian failure) and LH (for polycystic ovary syndrome) •TFT.

Semen analysis Unless there has been a satisfactory postcoital test, analyse semen after 3 days' abstinence for: •Volume (mean 2.75mL now, formerly 3.4mL in the 1940s[1]) •Sperm count/morphology. •Antibodies. •Infection. Normal count >20 million sperm/mL, >40% motile and >60% normal form; mean count = 66 million/mL (113 million/mL in the 1940s; this average is falling at a rate of about 100 sperms/mL every hour—which may be due to an environmental influence[2]—or more frequent ejaculations[3]—or a data or geographical[4,5] artefact). Examine 2 specimens as variation may be considerable. Reduced counts require specialist referral.

1 T Hargreave 1998 BMJ **i** 1438 2 E Carlsen 1992 BMJ **ii** 609 3 H Menger 1994 BMJ **i** 14409 4 P Bromwich 1994 BMJ **ii** 19 5 More of the later sperm counts were Third World ones, where counts are lower anyway: *Fertil Steril* 1996 **65** 1009

Subfertility options: abbreviations[1]

FEC	Fetal egg child (offspring from an egg taken from the ovary of an aborted fetus)
ICSI	Intracytoplasmic sperm injection (directly into an egg)
IUIS	Intrauterine insemination with superovulation: a USA favourite
IVF	*In vitro* fertilization
GIFT	Gamete intrafallopian transfer
MESA	Microepididymal sperm aspiration (from testis, eg post-vasectomy)
NT(P)	Nuclear transfer procedure: the baby has 2 mothers: one (too old to conceive normally) provides the nucleus; the other provides fresher cytoplasm (+ mitochondrial DNA) for the ovum
PESA	Percutaneous epididymal sperm aspiration (rather like MESA, but using a 22G butterfly needle inserted into the epididymis—so scrotal exploration is not required).
POST	Peritoneal oozyte sperm transfer
SUZI	Subzonal sperm injection (directly into an egg)
TET	Tubal embryo transfer
TUFT	Transuterine fallopian transfer
ZIFT	Zygote intrafallopian transfer

1 E te Velde 1999 *NEJM* **340** 224

Ethical issues

Various national embryology authorities exist and pronounce on the ethical dimensions of fertility treatments—and their edicts can appear to be set in stone (although being mutually contradictory with those from other countries); one problem with this approach is that fertility treatments are constantly changing, as is society's views on what is acceptable—and it is not clear whether these views should lead, or simply be taken into account (an opaque phrase) or be trumped by appeal to some higher authority (God, or the conscience of a quango).

1 Y Khalifa 1996 *BMJ* i 5

Infertility: tests and treatment

Tests of tubal patency

1 Laparoscopy with dye. Pelvic organs are visualized and methylene blue dye injected through the cervix: if tubes are blocked proximally they don't fill with dye; with distal block there is no 'spill' into the peritoneal cavity.
2 A hysterosalpingogram (contrast x-ray) demonstrates uterine anatomy and tubal 'fill and spill'. It is unpleasant and requires premedication. False positives may occur with tubal spasm. Give antibiotics, eg cefradine 500mh/8h PO with metronidazole 1g/12h PR for 24h before and 5 days after procedure to prevent pelvic infection.

The postcoital test Carried out in the immediate pre-ovulatory phase (when cervical mucus is profuse, acellular and exhibits ferning and Spinnbarkeit—the ability for it to be drawn out), performed 6–12h after intercourse, cervical mucus is removed from the cervix and examined under high-power (×400) microscopy. A satisfactory test (ovulatory mucus, >10 motile sperm/high-power field) shows that his sperm are adequate, coitus is effective and the cervical mucus does not contain antibodies.

Treatment of infertility Treatment is directed at the cause.
Azoospermia is unresponsive to treatment. A low sperm count may be improved by avoiding tobacco and alcohol. Avoiding tight pants was advised, but experiments show no change in testis T° or semen paremeters.[1] Will they consider donor insemination (AID=artificial insemination by donor)?
Problems of sperm deposition (eg impotence) can be circumvented by artificial insemination using the partner's sperm (AIH).
Hyperprolactinaemia (*OHCM* p 562) is treated by removing the cause if one is found (pituitary macro-adenoma, drugs); if not, give bromocriptine 1mg/24h PO, increasing the dose until blood prolactin is normal.
Anovulation is managed by stimulating follicle development using clomifene (=clomiphene) 50–200mg/24h PO on days 2–6 inclusive. SE: visual disturbance, abdominal pain (ovarian hyperstimulation, p 75); warn about risk of multiple pregnancy ± excess risk of ovarian cancer (p 42). Aim to monitor the response to clomifene with luteal phase progesterone. Human chorionic gonadotrophin (HCG) resembles LH and may be needed to rupture a ripe follicle. If clomifene does not help, gonadotrophin injections or LHRH analogues may be tried.
Tubal problems may be remedied by surgery but results are poor.

Assisted fertilization[2] The couple require psychological stability (and finance). The 'take-home baby rate' averages 10% and fetal loss, ectopic pregnancy, obstetric problems, multiple births and fetal abnormality are all commoner than normal.

In vitro fertilization (IVF) is used for tubal (and other) problems. The ovaries are stimulated (see *hyperstimulation* p 75), and ova are collected (by transvaginal aspiration under transvaginal ultrasound guidance), fertilized, and embryos are returned to the uterus as an outpatient procedure.

Gamete intrafallopian transfer (GIFT) may be tried where tubes are patent, eg 'unexplained infertility'. Gametes are placed in the tubes by laparoscopic cannulation. Pregnancy rate ~28% per cycle treatment. ZIFT (zygote or early cleaved embryo transfer) can give higher pregnancy rates of up to 48% in women with unexplained fertility.

If there is severe oligospermia *intracytoplasmic sperm injection* may be possible (a spermatozoa is injected directly into the oocyte's cytoplasm). The source of sperm is the epididymis or testis in men with obstructive azoospermia; even if the problem is non-obstructive, sperm can be retrieved in ~50%.[3]

The possibility of adoption should not be forgotten. Those who remain childless may value counselling or a self-help group.[4]

1 *J Urol* 1998 160 1329–33 2 T Hargreave 1998 BMJ i 1438 3 *Hum Reprod* 1996 **11** s59 4 In UK, *National Association for the Childless*, 318 Summer Lane, Birmingham B19 3RL

Male infertility[1]

Normal spermatogenesis takes place in the seminiferous tubules of the testes. Undifferentiated diploid germ cells (spermatogonia) multiply and are then transformed into haploid spermatozoa. The total duration of a cohort of spermatogonia to develop into spermatozoa is 74 days. FSH and LH are both important for initiation of spermatogenesis at puberty. LH stimulates Leydig cells to produce testosterone. Testosterone and FSH stimulate Sertoli cells to produce essential substances for metabolic support of germ cells and spermatogenesis.

Spermatozoa A spermatozoon has a dense oval head (containing the haploid chromosome complement), capped by an acrosome granule (contains enzymes essential for fertilization) and is propelled by the motile tail. Seminal fluid forms 90% of ejaculate volume and is alkaline to buffer vaginal acidity. Only about 200 sperm from any ejaculate reach the middle third of the Fallopian tube, the site of fertilization.

Male infertility Male factors are the cause for infertility in ~24% of infertile couples. In reality, most are subfertile. Only a small number of men have an identifiable cause. Causes include (% cited in one study):

- Idiopathic oligo/azoospermia (16%): Testes are usually small and FSH ↑.
- Asthenozoospermia/teratozoospermia (17%): In asthenozoospermia sperm motility is reduced due to structural problems with the tails. Teratozoospermia indicates an excess of abnormal forms.
- Varicocele (17%): this is controversial for varicocele is found in 15% of males, most of whom have normal fertility.
- Genital tract infection (4%): gonococci, chlamydia and Gram –ve enterococci can cause adnexal infection (eg with painful ejaculation, urethral discharge, haematospermia, dysuria, tender epididymes, tender boggy prostate). Confirm by semen culture, urethral swab or finding >1 million peroxidase +ve polymorphs/mL semen. Treat both partners for 4 weeks with erythromycin, doxycycline, or norfloxacin (eg 400mg/12h PO).
- Sperm autoimmunity (1.6%): Risk factors for antibodies: vasectomy, testis injury, genital tract obstruction, family history of autoimmune disease. Most are on sperm membranes or in seminal fluid, but may occur in the woman. Prednisolone 20mg/12h PO on day 1–10 and 5mg on day 11 and 12 of his partner's cycle for 6 months reduces antibody levels.
- Congenital (cryptorchidism, chromosome disorders—2%): Klinefelter's account for 50% chromosome disorders. For optimal fertility undescended testes should be fixed in the scrotum before 2yrs of age.
- Genital tract obstruction (1.8%): Azoospermia, normal sized testes with normal or high FSH suggests this. It may follow infection, vasectomy, or be congenital (as in cystic fibrosis). It may be amenable to surgery, eg epididymovasostomy to bypass epididymal obstruction.
- Systemic/iatrogenic (1.3%). •Coital disorders (1%).
- Gonadotrophin deficiency (0.6%): This is the only cause of testicular failure consistently treatable by hormone replacement.

Examination Look at body form and secondary sexual characteristics. Any gynaecomastia? Normal testicular volume is 15–35mL (compare with Prader orchidometer). Rectal examination may reveal prostatitis.

Tests *Semen analysis* (p 56). *Postcoital tests* with midcycle cervical mucus may indicate antibody presence. *Plasma FSH* distinguishes primary from secondary testicular failure. *Testosterone and LH* levels are indicated if you suspect androgen deficiency. *Agglutination tests* to detect antibodies are available.

Treatment The treatment of treatable causes is given above.

1 F C Wu 1992 *Gynaecology*, Churchill Livingstone, 355-74

Contraception

►*Any method, even coitus interruptus, is better than none.* 90% of young women having regular unprotected intercourse become pregnant within a year. Properly used, contraception reduces this to <1% (combined Pill, injectables, sterilization); around 2% (POP, IUCD, cap, sheath); 12% (mucothermic)—success rates may be much higher; 15% (withdrawal). Failure rates may be much higher for user-dependent methods.

Barrier methods ►The main reason for failure is not using them. Sheaths reduce transmission of most STDs but not those affecting the perineum. Caps give some protection against gonorrhoea and chlamydia but not syphilis or herpes. Some spermicides inactivate HIV *in vitro*.

- **Sheaths** are effective when properly used and with spermicides. Unroll onto the erect penis with the teat or end (if teatless) pinched to expel air. This prevents bursting at ejaculation.
- **Caps** come in several forms. Diaphragms stretch from pubic bone to posterior fornix. She must check after insertion that the cervix is covered. Cervical caps fit over the cervix (so need a prominent cervix). Insert <2h before intercourse (keep in place >6h after sex). Use with a spermicide. Some find them unaesthetic. Problems: UTIs, rubber sensitivity.
- **Cervical sponges** These are simple but often fail.
- **The female condom** (eg Femidom®) Prescription and fitting are not needed. The manufacturer claims excellent barrier properties to HIV, bacteria and sperm. It might be suitable for contraception when a Pill has been missed, or if there is dyspareunia, or the perineum needs protection, eg post-childbirth—or if she is latex-allergic to condoms. One reason for failure is that the penis goes alongside it, rather than in it; another, that it gets pushed up in the vagina or may fall out. They can be noisy.
- **Spermicides**—Unreliable unless used with a barrier.

Natural (mucothermal) methods involve monitoring physiological phenomena to find fertile times (6 days prior to ovulation; the life of a sperm) to 2 days afterwards (the life of the ovum). Cervical mucus becomes clear and sticky at the beginning of the fertile time and dry at ovulation (but is altered by semen and vaginal infections). Basal body temperature ↑~0.3°C after ovulation (affected by fevers, drugs, recent food or drink). Additional observations (mittelschmerz, p 74 ± cervix changes) improve accuracy. Success is common if: •Regular cycles •Dedication •Self-control coexist. UK teachers are available (tel. 01222 754628).

High-technology natural methods Devices such as Persona® use solid-state urine chemistry on sticks for dual measurements of the oestrogen (o)estrone-3-glucuronide (E3G—peaks 24h pre-ovulation) and luteinizing hormone (LH—ovulation occurs within 36h of LH surge and sperm penetration through cervical mucus drops after the surge). Microtechnology builds up a database of the woman's natural variability over time, and this is used to to give her either a green light (almost infertile), a red light (fertile—typically days 6–10) or an orange light (do an early-morning urine test for E3G and LH). Usually, only 8 urine tests are needed per cycle. She needs to purchase sticks and one monitor (this houses a button to press the morning her period starts: she needs to check the lights on the monitor before passing urine each morning, in case a test is needed). *Reliability:* 93–95% (manufacturer's data, in motivated patients: it may be much less in practice; results must be regarded as only preliminary: explain uncertainty to your patient). *CI:* Cycle <23 or >35 days or variation >10 days; breast feeding; if already on hormones or tetracycline (minocycline is OK); menopausal; liver or kidney disease; polycystic ovary disease, or if pregnancy is definitely unwanted.

Further information: UK Family Planning Assoc^n, 2 Pentonville Rd, London N1 (0171 837 4044)

The ideal contraceptive—and the realities

An ideal contraceptive is: 100% *effective*, with only *desirable side-effects* (eg protection from sexually transmitted disease)—and it must be *readily reversible*, and be usable *unsupervised by professionals*. Try to find the best compromise for each person depending on age, health, and beliefs. Methods available:

- 'Natural methods' (no intercourse near time of ovulation)—acceptable to Catholic Church; also, the simplest are free, requiring no 'pollution of the body' with drugs—see opposite.
- Barrier methods (low health risk but need high user motivation—with some protection to HIV). See opposite.
- Hormonal (complex health risks but highly effective, p 64–8).
- IUCD (convenient and effective—if not contraindicated—p 62).
- Sterilization (very effective but effectively irreversible, p 69).

The intrauterine contraceptive device (IUCD)

IUCDs (loops, coils) are plastic shapes ~3cm long around which copper wire is wound, and carrying a plastic thread from the tail, eg Novagard®. They inhibit implantation and may impair sperm migration. Most need changing every 3–5 years. They have replaced the larger, noncopper-bearing 'inert' types (eg Lippes loop®), which caused more complications but did not need changing (and so are sometimes still found *in situ*).

Most of those who choose the IUCD (6%) are older, parous women in stable relationships, in whom the problem rate is low.

Problems with IUCDs 1 They tend to be expelled by a uterus which is nulliparous or distorted (eg by fibroids). 2 Ectopic pregnancy is more likely. 3 They are associated with pelvic infection and infertility, following sexually transmitted disease—or sometimes introduced during insertion. 4 They tend to produce heavy, painful periods. *Contraindications:* Aim to exclude women at high risk of these problems, also those who are immunosuppressed (eg HIV+ve), have Wilson's disease (*OHCM* p 712), or those with cardiac lesions (unless the coil is inserted under antibiotic cover).

Insertion Skilled insertion minimizes complications. Each device has its own technique, so read the instructions carefully and practise beforehand.

An IUCD can be inserted any time (and as postcoital contraception), as long as the woman is not pregnant, but it is more likely to be expelled during a period or shortly after childbirth. Determine the position of the uterus. Then insert a uterine sound to assess the length of the cavity. Then insert the IUCD, placing it in the fundus. This may cause crampy pains. Once the coil is in place, the threads are cut to leave 3cm visible in the vagina. Teach her to feel the threads after each period.

►Insertion of IUCDs may provoke 'cervical shock' (from increased vagal tone). Have IV atropine available.

Follow-up The first 3 months are the peak time for expulsion and the coil should be checked after the next period, then 6-monthly. Threads are often easier to feel than to see.

Lost threads The IUCD may have been expelled, so advise extra contraception and exclude pregnancy. Then sound the uterus. If you find the coil you may be able to bring down the threads with a special instrument. If you cannot find the threads, they may have dropped off. If you cannot find the coil, seek it on ultrasound. A coil may perforate the uterus, usually after insertion and often with little pain (remove, eg laparoscopically).

Infection This can be treated with the device in place, but if removed do not replace it for 6 months. Rarely, *Actinomyces* is found on smear test. Change the coil, cut threads off old one and send coil for culture. If positive, remove new coil and give penicillin V 250mg/6h PO for 90 days.

Pregnancy >90% are intrauterine. Remove coil, if you can as soon as pregnancy is diagnosed to reduce risk of miscarriage (20% if removed early, 50% if left), and to prevent risk of late septic abortion.

Removal Alternative contraception should be started (if desired) prior to removal, as there may be a fertilized ovum in the tubes. At the menopause, remove after at least 6 months' amenorrhoea.

IUCDs carrying hormones—eg Mirena® (carries levonorgestrel). Local effects make implantation less likely, and periods lighter; perhaps 20% may experience reversible amenorrhoea (reliability matchs that of sterilization, see p 69). It lasts ~3 years. There may be less risk of ectopic pregnancy. Risk of sexually transmitted infection is reduced. Warn about spotting ± heavy bleeding (NB: bleeding may become *scanty* or *absent* after a few cycles).

Emergency contraception[1]

This is for use after isolated episodes of unprotected intercourse, eg 'the split sheath' and should not be used regularly.

Management History of LMP; normal cycle; number of hours since unprotected intercourse; history of personal thromboembolism or focal migraine. Check BP. Explain that teratogenicity has not been demonstrated. Discuss future contraception. Give supply of oral contraceptives if day 1 start at next period is planned. Arrange follow-up at 3–4 weeks.

The Yuzpe method This must be initiated within 72 hours of unprotected intercourse. Absolute contraindications are migraine at presentation and previous thromboembolism. Past history of ectopic pregnancy is a relative contraindication. Dose: 2 tablets of 50μg ethinylestradiol and 250mg levonorgestrel, eg as Schering PC4® or Ovran® stat and 2 tablets 12 hours later (ideally timed so that the second dose can be within normal waking hours). If on liver enzyme inducers, eg rifampicin, rifabutin, griseofulvin, phenytoin, tropicamide, barbiturates including primidone, ritonavir, take 3 tablets each time. Risk of pregnancy with treatment ~3% (of which 10% may be ectopic).[2] Should pregnancy ensue there is no evidence of teratogenicity. 50% of women will experience nausea, 20% will vomit (if < 2 hours from taking the pills take two more after an antiemetic). Domperidone 10mg with or before each dose reduces nausea and vomiting, is unlikely to cause extrapyramidal side-effects, and has no reported adverse effects on pregnancy. Use precautions until next period (but continue oral contraceptive pills if taken for 'missed Pill' cover). Timing of the next period will be altered in 10%.[2]

The Ho and Kwan method This is with progesterone-only pills initiated within 72 hours of unprotected intercourse. It is suitable for those with focal migraine and past thromboembolism. Nausea occurs in 16%, vomiting in 2%. Two doses of 0.75mg levonorgestrel (ie 25 Microval® or Norgeston® tablets or 20 tablets Neogest®) taken 12 hours apart. The failure rate is as good as with the Yuzpe regimen; if not better (overall pregnancy rate 3.2% for Yuzpe regimen and 1.1% for levornorgestrel in one large study and levornorgestrel pregnancy rates were less than Yuzpe even up to 72 hours after unprotected intercourse).[3] With both regimens the earlier taken after unprotected intercourse, the fewer the pregnancies which occur.[3]

The emergency IUCD A copper IUCD can be inserted within 120 hours of unprotected intercourse. If exposure was more than 5 days previously it can be inserted up to 5 days after likely ovulation, so is useful in women who present later. Failure rates are extremely low. Infection is a risk (especially if the unprotected intercourse was sexual assault) and should be screened for, if suspected. It is possible to insert under antibiotic cover if suspected. It inhibits implantation.

1 A Kubba 1998 *Br J Family Planning* **23** 135 2 P Van Look 1993 *Br Med Bul* **49** 158
3 Task force on postovulatory methods of fertility regulation 1998 *Lancet* **352** 428

Hormonal contraception (the Pill)

~3 million women in the UK take the combined oral contraceptive (CoC)—the method of choice for 50% of younger users. CoCs contain oestrogen (usually ethinylestradiol) with a progestogen, either in fixed ratio or varying through the month (phased). Low-dose formulations (≤30µg oestrogen) are the norm. The combined Pill is taken daily for 3 weeks followed by a week's break. This inhibits ovulation and produces a withdrawal bleed in the Pill-free week. When prescribing CoCs, pay attention to these areas:

History Why does she want the Pill? Does she know about risks? These must be explained. Has she considered the alternatives? Are there any contraindications in her or her family, eg thrombotic disorders? Ask about smoking and drugs, and about contact lenses (Pill use may cause dry eyes). Does she have any anxieties, eg weight-gain?

The Pill, smoking, and thromboembolism Death due to the Pill in 35-year-olds is 8 times more common if they smoke (but still as safe as childbirth). Can she be helped to stop smoking? If not, stop the Pill at 30.

Contraindications Any disorder predisposing to venous or arterial problems, ie abnormal lipids; prothrombotic disorders such as quite common APC resistance (activated protein C);[1] many cardiovascular problems, except mild non-Pill related hypertension and varicose veins); liver disease; migraine with aura[1,2] (see opposite), migraine attacks for >72h (status migrainosus[3]) or requiring ergotamine; diseases exacerbated by sex steroids; recent trophoblast disease; undiagnosed uterine bleeding; gross obesity; immobility (stop Pill 4 weeks before until 2 weeks after very major surgery—provided alternative contraception is realistic, eg barrier methods or depot progesterone, p 67).

Special cautions Prescribe with caution if a family history of DVT, myocardial infarction, ↑BP or breast cancer; with severe migraine or migraine requiring sumatriptan;[3] epilepsy; sickle-cell disease; diabetes; oligomenorrhoea; illnesses causing diarrhoea (eg Crohn's); in heavy smokers and possibly those with abnormal cervical smears. NB: if a woman gets a first attack of migraine while on the combined Pill, stop it, and observe closely: restart cautiously only if there are no sequelae and if migraine attack was without aura[2] and there are no other arterial risk factors (see opposite).

Drugs interfering with the Pill *Liver enzyme inducers*, eg anticonvulsants, griseofulvin, and rifampicin reduce efficacy by ↓circulating oestrogen. If short-term use, take extra precautions (p 66) whilst used and for 7 days after (4 weeks for rifampicin). With long-term use consider using 50µg oestrogen Pills with higher doses of progesterone, eg Norinyl-1®. Use another type of contraceptive if on long-term rifampicin. *Antibiotics:* p 66.

Benefits of the Pill Very effective contraception; lighter, less painful 'periods'; reduced premenstrual syndrome. In long-term users, reduced risk of ovarian tumours (carcinoma ↓ 40%) and endometrial carcinoma (↓ 50%); less pelvic infection and endometriosis.

Serious disadvantages The risks of arterial and venous disease are increased, eg DVT, myocardial infarction. Risk of death due to the Pill increases sharply over 40yrs: 1:2500 for nonsmokers; 1:500 for smokers. The relationship with breast cancer is complex but rates in those <35yrs are increased (from ~0.2% to ~0.3%).

For contraception in those who are **HIV+ve**, see p 155.

1 C Chang 1999 BMJ i 13 & E MacGregor 1995 *Brit J Fam Plan* **21** 16 2 E Macgregor 1998 *Br J Fam Plan* **24** 55 3 J Guillebaud 1995 *Brit J Fam Plan* **21** 16 & 1994 **20** 24

Migraine, ischaemic stroke, and the Pill[1]

The problem is ischaemic stroke. The background annual incidence is 2 per 100,000 women aged 20, and 20 per 100,000 for those aged 40. Migraine itself is a risk factor. For those with migraine and CoC use incidence of ischaemic stroke becomes 8:100,000 if aged 20; and 80:100,000 in those aged 40. Low-dose CoCs only should be used. Those with migraine with aura are known to be at special risk precluding use of combined Pills in these women (however there is no problem with them using progesterone only or nonhormonal contraception). Other risk factors for ischaemic stroke include smoking, age >35 years, raised BP, obesity (body mass index >30), diabetes mellitus, hyperlipidaemia and family history of arterial disease <45 years. Women known to have migraine should be warned to stop pills immediately if they develop aura or worsening of migraine.

Diagnosing migraine with aura (Formerly called *classical* or *focal migraine*)
- Slow evolution of symptoms (see below) over several minutes
- Duration usually 10–30 minutes, resolving within 1 hour, and typically before onset of headache
- Visual symptoms (99% of auras), eg:
  - Bilateral homonymous hemianopia
  - Teichopsia and fortification spectra, eg a gradually enlarging C with scintillating edges)
  - Positive (bright) scotomata
- Sensory disturbance (31% of auras)
  - Usually associated with visual symptoms
  - Usually in one arm spreading from fingers to face (leg rarely affected)
- Speech disturbance (18% of auras):
  - Dysphasia; dysarthria; paraphasia
- Motor disturbances (6% of auras)

Both motor and speech disturbances are usually accompanied by visual and/or sensory disturbances.

Migraine without aura: (Formerly called *simple* or *common* migraine) includes symptoms of blurred vision, photophobia, phonophobia, generalized flashing lights affecting the whole visual field in both eyes, associated with headache.

Absolute contraindications to CoC use
- Migraine with aura
- Migraine without aura in women with >1 risk factor for stroke
- Severe migraine or status migrainosus
- Migraine treated with ergot derivatives

1 E McGregor 1998 *Br J Fam Plan* **24** 55

Hormonal contraception: further details

Do BP 6-monthly. Check weight and breasts—eg if >35yrs. Do a cervical smear if due (p 32). Adverse effects are dose-related: aim is to give the lowest dose Pill that gives good cycle control (ie no breakthrough bleeding).

Progesterone problems[1] Norethisterone and levonorgestrel-containing combined Pills may cause breakthrough bleeding, acne, headaches, weight↑), so prompting a search for newer progesterones such as gestodene (Femodene®, Marvelon®, Minulet®, Mercilon®, Triadene®, Triminulet®). These have their own problems with thrombosis from resistance to the blood's natural anticoagulation system—APC resistance, by about as much (relative risk 6–9-fold) as that induced by the V Leiden mutation (*OHCM* p 622), which is much less of a problem for older progesterones (relative risk 3–4). It is not clear if these Pills have a rôle in those with no risk factors for DVT (body mass index >30), immobility, marked varicose veins, past DVT, family history of unexplained thrombosis).[2] Overall, risk of death with the newer Pills from PE *is* higher than expected (≥1/100,000/yr in New Zealand).[3]

Switching from PoP: *If to a CoC*, start on day 1 of period. Use condoms for 7 days. *If to a progesterone-only Pill (PoP)*, start as the old pack finishes.

Switching from CoC: *If to a CoC*, start immediately with no Pill-free interval. *If to a PoP*, start immediately the CoC packet is finished.

Starting CoCs and PoPs Day 1 of cycle, or on the day of ToP, or 3 weeks postpartum or 2 weeks after full mobilization after major surgery.[1] With day 1–3 CoC starting regimen, contraceptive cover is immediate; use other precautions for 7 days with PoP and if CoC started day 4 or 5 of period.

Stopping the Pill Tell to stop at once if she develops: •Sudden severe chest pain •Sudden breathlessness (or cough with bloody sputum) •Severe calf pain •Severe stomach pain •Unusual severe prolonged headache. Smokers should stop at 30; low-risk nonsmokers may continue into their 40s. On stopping, 66% menstruate by 6 weeks, 98% by 6 months; women who are amenorrhoeic after the Pill were usually so before.

Special cases If >12h late (or diarrhoea), continue Pills but use condoms too for 7 days (+ days of diarrhoea); if this includes Pill-free days, start next pack *with no break*. Use condoms during and for 7 days after antibiotics. If a tablet from the 1st 7 days in pack is forgotten, consider postcoital contraception. *Vomiting <3h post Pill:* Take another. *Postcoital options:* p 63.

Progesterone only Pill (PoP, 'mini-pill') Low-dose progestogen renders cervical mucus hostile to sperm. In some women it also inhibits ovulation, improving efficacy but causing erratic bleeding, its worst side-effect. The risk of ectopics is increased. It is less effective than the combined Pill except in older, less fertile women. It can be used by most women with medical problems contraindicating the combined Pill, and by breast feeding mothers. Take at same time daily ± 3h, otherwise extra precautions are needed for 7 days. A regular lifestyle or using an alarm watch helps.

Postnatal Start 21 days after birth: eg CoC if not breast feeding; PoP, Depo-Provera® (or ?Norplant®) if breast feeding. IUCD: fit ~4 weeks postpartum.

At the menopause Stop PoP if >50yrs old with >1 year's amenorrhoea (2yrs if <50yrs old)—as a rough guide. In this last year, a spermicide and sponge is probably adequate due to declining fertility. As CoC masks the menopause, aim to stop all women at 50yrs, and replace with a nonhormonal method. An FSH >30IU/L indicates that the ovaries have retired.

Buying the Pill over the counter This might be safe for non-smokers with no hypertension who are having regular cervical smears. But it is hard to see how counter sales could be limited to this very low-risk group.[4]

1 J Guillebaud 1995 *BMJ* ii 1111 2 *Lancet* 1997 **349** 1113 3 *Lancet* 1999 **353** 389 4 D Skegg 1999 *BMJ* i 70

Depot and implant hormonal contraception

Depot progestogen ('the injection') is simple, safe and very effective but has suffered from adverse publicity. Two preparations are available: *medroxyprogesterone acetate* (Depo-Provera®) 150mg given deep IM 12-weekly; start during the first 5 days of a cycle (or at 5 days post-partum if bottle feeding; 6 weeks if breast feeding) or *norethisterone enanthate* (Noristerat®) 200mg into gluteus maximus 8-weekly (it is licensed for short-term use only, but can be given immediately postpartum when use of Depo-Provera® can cause very heavy bleeding). Exclude pregnancy biochemically and use condoms for 14 days after late injections (eg if she turns up one week late).

Contraindications: Pregnancy; abnormal undiagnosed vaginal bleeding; acute liver disease; severe cardiac disease.

Advantages of injectable progesterone injections:

- No oestrogen content
- Fewer ovarian cysts
- Reduces PMS (p 16)
- No compliance problems
- Reduced endometriosis
- Secret
- Good when GI disease
- Abolishes menorrhagia eventually
- Suppresses ovulation (so protects against ectopics)
- Can be used when breast feeding.
- 5-fold protective effect against endometrial carcinoma.

Problems: There may be irregular vaginal bleeding. This usually settles with more prolonged use and amenorrhoea often then supervenes, so encourage perseverance. With Depo-provera® 33% of women have amenorrhoea after 6-months use; 50% after 12 months, and 60% after 18 months (figures are 14%, 27%, and 33% respectively for Noristerat®). If very heavy bleeding occurs, exclude pregnancy; give injection early (but >4 weeks from previous dose) and give oestrogen if not contraindicated (eg Premarin® 1.25mg/24h PO for 21 days or a combined oral contraceptive pill). Fears that long-term use, especially in amenorrhoeic women with low serum oestrogen levels, may cause osteoporosis appear to be unfounded.[1] Other problems include weight gain and acne.

Special uses: Depot injections may be particularly useful:

- To cover major surgery. If given when stopping combined Pill 4 weeks before surgery it gives contraceptive cover for the next 8 or 12 weeks.
- Sickle-cell disease (reduces incidence of sickle-cell crises).
- Epileptics (inducement of liver enzymes from medication immaterial). If on rifampicin for TB give Depo-provera® injection every 10 weeks.
- After vasectomy while awaiting partner's sperm-free ejaculates.
- Where bowel disease may affect oral absorption.

There may be some delay in return of ovulation on stopping injections (median delay 10 months) but long-term fertility is not reduced.

Implants Progesterone implants are now available with the advantage that they give 5 years' contraception with one implantation. Norplant® consists of 6 capsules each containing levornogestrel 36mg which are implanted under local anaesthetic into the upper arm. If removed (may be difficult to do), plasma levornogestrel becomes undetectable within 2 days.[2] The main side-effect is irregular menstrual bleeding (during the first year this affects most women). Its action is by changing cervical mucus (ie similar to POP). Only 10% of users become amenorrhoeic. These therefore provide reversible long-term contraceptive cover with minimal medical intervention—except for those in whom suppression of ovulation leads to symptomatic ovarian cysts (these do not usually require surgery).

1 B Gbolade 1998 *Br J Obs Gyn* **105** 790 2 J Thompson 1993 *Brit J Fam Plan* **19** 195

Sterilization

Sterilization is popular, perhaps because it is reliable, without one having to think about it. ~100,000 women and ~90,000 men are sterilized annually in the UK. ~25% of women rely on sterilization for contraception.

Ideally see both partners and consider the following:

- Alternative methods. Do they know about the cap, the POP, depot progesterone injections, coils and implants?
- Consent. Is it the wish of both partners? Legally only the consent of the partner to be sterilized is required but the agreement of both is desirable.
- Who should be sterilized? Does she fear loss of her femininity? Does he see it as being neutered? If the woman is requesting sterilization, is she really wanting a hysterectomy or would she benefit from one?
- Irreversibility. Reversal is only 50% successful in either sex and tubal surgery increases the risk of subsequent ectopics, so the couple should see sterilization as an irreversible step. The sterilizations most regretted are those carried out on the young and at times of stress, or immediately after pregnancy (termination or delivery). Are their children healthy?
- If she wishes to be sterilized at Caesarean section, explain that it will only be done if the baby is normal and healthy.
- Failure rates—10-year follow-up of 10,863 USA women shows pregnancy rates of 18.5/1000 procedures[1], no better than new IUCDs (Copper T 380S®, Mirena®, GyneFIX®) and 10 fold *worse* than vasectomy.[2] ►Remember: IUCDs are reversible, conveniently mirroring many marriages: but sterilization is for ever. Warn that if pregnancy occurs it is likely to be ectopic (32.9%).[1]
- Side-effects. A women who has been on the Pill for many years may find her periods unacceptably heavy after sterilization.

►Record in the notes: *Knows it's irreversible; lifetime failure rate discussed*, eg 1:2000 for vasectomy, and 1:200 for Filshie clip ♀ sterilization: see above.

Female sterilization The more the tubes are damaged, the lower the failure rate and the more difficult reversal becomes. In the UK, most sterilizations are carried out laparoscopically with general anaesthesia. The commonest UK method used is Filshie clips.[2] The tubes may be clipped, ringed or diathermied. Alternatively the tubes may be divided and ligated through a mini-laparotomy incision, or clipped via the posterior fornix ('colpotomy'). Women should continue using effective contraception until the operation. An IUCD should be left in place until the next period in case an already fertilized ovum is present.

Vasectomy This is a simpler procedure than female sterilization and can be performed on an outpatient basis. The vas deferens is identified at the top of the scrotum, about 1cm is removed, and the cut ends doubled back before being ligated. Bruising and haematoma are complications.

The major disadvantage of vasectomy is that it takes up to 3 months before sperm stores are used up. Two ejaculates 'negative' for sperm should be obtained before other methods of contraception are stopped. Reversal is most successful if within 10 years of initial operation. **SE:** There is equivocal evidence of ↑risk of prostate cancer post-vasectomy. 6 papers report an association, and 4 do not.[3] None of the positive trials was on European men. The best trials looking at an association between testicular neoplasia and vasectomy have all proved negative.[3]

1 H Peterson 1996 *Am J Obs Gyn* **174** 1161 2 http://www.jr2.ox.ac.uk/bandolier/band52/b52-6.html (J Guillebaud) 2 V Brace 1998 *Diplomate* **5** 146 3 S McDonald 1997 *Brit J Gen Pract* **47** 381

Urinary malfunction

Control of bladder function Continence in women is maintained in the urethra by the external sphincter and pelvic floor muscles maintaining urethral pressure higher than bladder pressure. Micturition occurs when these muscles relax and the bladder detrusor muscle contracts.

Urge incontinence 'If I've got to go I've got to go', and she goes frequently. The bladder is 'unstable' with high detrusor muscle activity. It occurs in nulliparous and parous women. Usually no organic problem is found. Rarely, the cause is neurogenic.

Stress incontinence Small quantities of urine escape as intra-abdominal pressure rises, eg sneezing. It is much commoner in parous women as childbirth denervates the pelvic floor. Examination may reveal prolapse (p 54) or incontinence (ask her to cough).

Management
- Exclude a UTI and glycosuria.
- History and examination will not tell you whether the problem is stress or urge or both: arrange urodynamic studies.
- Urge improves with 'bladder training' (gradually increasing the time interval between voiding). She will need encouragement. Restricting fluids, and antimuscarinic drugs, eg oxybutynin 2.5mg/12h PO for 2 weeks; increasing stepwise to a maximum of 5mg/12h PO in the elderly (5mg/8h non-elderly) may help. (SE: dry mouth, constipation, blurred vision, arrhythmias; CI: glaucoma). Propantheline is an alternative.
- Mild stress incontinence responds well to pelvic floor exercises or physiotherapy, eg with weighted vaginal cones—insert the heaviest that can be retained (base up) for 15mins twice daily, graduating to heavier cones (max 100g) as tone improves, to improve muscle tone. A vaginal tampon supports the bladder neck, stopping leaks while playing sport.
- Surgery is required for severe stress symptoms to increase intraurethral pressure (by bringing the upper urethra into the zone of abdominal pressure when previously it was below the pelvic floor) and to reduce prolapse. Operations include: urethroplasty, transabdominal colposuspension.
- In some postmenopausal women urgency, increased frequency and nocturia may be helped by topical (o)estriol 0.1% cream PV used nightly for 3 weeks then twice weekly long term.
- When there is a mixed picture of stress/urge incontinence treat the detrusor instability first because this can be made worse by operations for stress incontinence.[1]

True incontinence Continuous leakage of urine may be due to congenital anatomical abnormalities, eg ectopic ureters, or to acquired problems, eg vesicovaginal fistula due to trauma (usually after abdominal hysterectomy in developed countries, after prolonged labour with vertex presentation in developing countries), malignancy or radiotherapy. If surgery is not possible, seek the help of the incontinence adviser.

Urethral syndrome Symptoms of cystitis occur with a –ve MSU, often associated with intercourse, and may be due to subinfective numbers of organisms being massaged into the urethra. Is she adequately lubricated? Try using Vaseline® over the urethra (but not if sheaths are used). Micturating before and after intercourse, different coital positions (her on top) and trimethoprim 100mg PO prior to intercourse may help.

1 L Cardozo 1994 *Prescribers' J* **34** 134

Voiding difficulties[1]

Symptoms

- Poor flow
- Straining to void
- Chronic retention
- Stress incontinence
- Intermittent stream
- Hesitancy
- Overflow incontinence
- Urge incontinence
- Incomplete emptying
- Acute retention
- UTI from residual urine

►*Remember faecal impaction as a cause of retention with overflow.* It is probably wise to classify stress incontinence and urge incontinence as symptoms, not diseases, as detrusor instability quite often (eg in 25% of patients[1]) manifests itself as stress incontinence, rather than as urge incontinence.

Causes

CNS: These may be suprapontine (eg stroke); due to cord lesions (cord injury, multiple sclerosis); peripheral nerve (prolapsed disc, diabetic or other neuropathy); or reflex, due to pain (eg with herpes infections).

Drugs: Especially epidural anaesthesia; also tricyclics, anticholinergics.

Obstructive: Early oedema after bladder neck repair is a common cause. A retroverted gravid uterus, fibroids, ovarian cysts, urethral foreign body, ectopic ureterocele, bladder polyp or carcinoma are other causes.

Bladder overdistension

Tests

- Do an MSU to exclude infection.
- Ultrasound for residual urine.
- Cystourethroscopy.
- Uroflowmetry (a rate of <15mL/sec for a volume of >150mL is abnormal). Do this test before any surgery is contemplated.

Treatment This depends upon the cause. Acute retention may require catheterization (using a suprapubic catheter if it is expected to be staying in place for several days). For persistent conditions (eg neurological conditions) self-catheterization techniques may need to be learned.[2,3] A silver catheter (not disposable!) may be ideal for this.

Drugs may be used to relax the urethral sphincter or stimulate the detrusor muscle (eg prazosin 0.5mg/12h PO, first dose given before bed, increasing to 2mg/12h PO after several days if needed; or indoramin 20mg/12h PO increasing every 2 weeks by 20mg to a maximum of 100mg/12h PO). Operative measures may overcome some of the obstructive causes, eg urethrotomy for distal urethral stenosis—although this is not often found in women.

For male voiding difficulty, see *Urinary retention and catheters*, OHCM p 134.

Agents for detrusor instability	*Symptoms which they may improve*
Oxybutynin 2.5mg/12h–5mg/12h SE: dry mouth, vision↓, drowsy, abdo. pain, flushes, arrhythmia	Frequency, urgency (tolterodine is an alternative) beware high doses if elderly or past cardiac disease/glaucoma
Imipramine 50mg PO at night	Nocturia, enuresis, coital incontinence
Propantheline 15mg/8h PO 1h ac	Frequency
Desmopressin nasal spray 20μg as a night-time dose	Nocturia/enuresis (↓urine production)
Oestrogens	Postmenopausal urgency, frequency and nocturia maybe by raising the bladder's sensory threshold
Surgery, eg clam ileocystoplasty	The bladder is bisected, opened like a clam and 25cm of ileum is sewn in
Hypnosis/psychotherapy	This requires good motivation

1 G Jarvis 1996 *BMJ* ii 112 2 G Hunt 1993 *The User's Guide to Intermittent Self Catheterisation*, BMA/Family Doctor Publications Ltd (Unit 14 Princeton Ct, SW15 (0181 780 5020) 3 *Drug Ther Bul* 1991 **29** 37

Gynaecological surgery

Hysterectomy *Abdominal hysterectomy* is usually total (uterine body + cervix removed), but may be *Wertheim's* (extended to include local lymph nodes and a cuff of vagina)—used for malignancy. If subtotal, the cervix is left behind—and may become malignant. At *vaginal hysterectomy* the uterus is brought down through the vagina. It is therefore performed for prolapse when the uterus is small. Healthy ovaries are usually conserved, especially in young women, unless the hysterectomy is for an oestrogen-dependent tumour. Complication: residual ovary syndrome (pain, deep dyspareunia, premature ovarian failure). *Laparoscopic hysterectomy* was developed for patients in whom problems with open surgery are anticipated (eg extensive adhesions with endometriosis), but it turns out that most of these patients can have a vaginal hysterectomy—which is much quicker (77min *vs* 131min[1]), with a similar complication rate.

Most hysterectomies are performed for dysmenorrhoea, and rates vary widely. Femininity and sexuality are bound up with the uterus. Reduced ability to produce orgasms after total abdominal hysterectomy is greater than after subtotal hysterectomy (leaving the cervix behind). Subtotal hysterectomy is also a faster and cleaner—but remember to go on smearing these cervixes. ► Women who are counselled, and make their own decision about surgery, are less likely to have regrets. Operative mortality: ~0.06%. A randomized trial (*N*=204) found hysterectomy does not cause ↑ psychological/sexual morbidity compared with ablation (below) at 1yr post-op.[2]

Manchester repair (Fothergill's operation) Pregnancy is still possible after this operation for uterine prolapse. The cervix is amputated and the uterus is supported by shortening the ligaments.

Dilatation and curettage (D&C) The cervix is dilated sufficiently to admit a curette to scrape out a sample of endometrium for histology. D&C is now largely a procedure for diagnosing abnormal bleeding (but outpatient endometrial sampling (p 44) may make D&C unnecessary). Evacuation of retained products of conception from the uterus after miscarriage (ERPC), or termination of early pregnancy, are carried out by **dilatation and suction**.

Hysteroscopy As an outpatient alternative to D&C, a hysteroscope can be inserted through the cervix into the uterus to visualize the endometrium. 'Blind' samples may then be taken using a sampler.

Hysteroscopic endometrial ablation by laser or diathermy (under GA or spinal ± paracervical block) reduces bleeding by achieving a deliberate Asherman's syndrome (p 12); as an alternative to hysterectomy, it has fewer complications.[3] Endometrium may be thinned pre-op by leuprorelin or danazol. By 4 months 10% have menorrhagia again. Complications: (major in 4% requiring further operation in 1%)[4] haemorrhage; infection (eg late necrotizing granulomatous endometritis); uterine perforation; haematometra, vesicovaginal fistula, fluid overload from irrigation fluid can cause ↑BP, ↓Na^+, pulmonary oedema, CNS symptoms, and haemolysis.[5] Some endometrium remains in the majority[6] (so give progesterone containing HRT later, if needed). See p 14.

Laparoscopy Gas (to separate the viscera) is inserted through a small umbilical incision and the laparoscope and instrumentation are inserted suprapubically. This procedure allows visualization of the pelvic organs and is used for diagnosis of pelvic pain and ectopic pregnancy. The patient is spared a full laparotomy unless needed for treatment. A 'lap and dye' demonstrates tubal patency. Sterilization and hysterectomy may be laparoscopically carried out, and ectopic pregnancies sometimes treated.

Colporrhaphy or **'repair'** The lack of support from the vaginal wall in cases of prolapse is rectified by excising a piece of the redundant mucosa and plicating levator ani. The operation may be combined with

Manchester repair or vaginal hysterectomy. The more mucosa is removed, the tighter the vagina. Enquire before surgery if she is sexually active. Catheterization circumvents post-operative retention of urine.

Cone biopsy A cone of tissue (point inwards) is cut out around the external cervical os, using knife or laser. This removes neoplastic tissue for histology, and may be curative. Complications: (immediate) bleeding, (long-term) cervical stenosis or incompetence.

Pelvic exenteration Consider this option when initial surgery fails to control neoplasia of the cervix, vulva, or vagina. It involves removal of the pelvic organs—ie ultra-radical surgery, which should only be contemplated if there is a chance of cure. Do your best to establish whether disease has spread to the pelvic sidewall or nodes, eg with MRI or CT scans and intra-operative biopsy with frozen section: if so, exenteration is probably not worthwhile. Only ~20% of possible candidates for surgery meet this criterion: in addition the patient should be quite fit, and ideally have a supportive partner. We know that palliative exenteration in those with unresectable disease is not worthwhile.[5] 5-yr survival: ~50%. Operative mortality: ~5%. Complications: GI obstruction/fistulae; urinary fistulae. Remember to give full pre-operative counselling about colostomies, and sexual function (refashioning of the vagina *may* be possible).

1 E Richardson 1995 *Lancet* **345** 36 2 DA Alexander 1996 BMJ **i** 280 3 S Pinion 1994 BMJ **ii** 979
3 N Dwyer 1993 *Br J Obs Gynae* **100** 237 4 A Thompson 1998 *The Diplomate* **5** 105
5 N Saunders 1995 *Lancet* **345** 5 6 L Turnbull 1997 *Br J Obs Gynae* **104** 934

Chronic pelvic pain

This can be a cause of much misery to women of reproductive age. The history is usually of longstanding pelvic pain with secondary dysmenorrhoea and deep dyspareunia. The pain may cause, or be exacerbated by, emotional problems. She may be depressed.

Laparoscopy may reveal a likely cause: chronic pelvic infection, endometriosis, adenomyosis, adhesions or congested pelvic veins. If it does not (or if all gynaecological causes have been surgically removed) the cause may be gastrointestinal: consider irritable bowel syndrome (OHCM p 518).

Pelvic congestion Lax pelvic veins become painfully congested with blood. The pain is worse when she is standing, walking (gravity fills the veins), and premenstrually. It is typically variable in site and intensity and there is unpleasant postcoital ache. She is maximally tender to deep palpation over the ovaries. The vagina and cervix may appear blue due to congestion and there may be associated posterior leg varicosities. The dilated veins may be demonstrated by venography or laparoscopically.

Relief may be difficult, though explanation helps ('pelvic migraine'). Medroxyprogesterone 50mg/24h PO for 3 months reduces pain (SE amenorrhoea, weight gain, bloating); migraine remedies (OHCM p 416) and relaxation may be tried.[1] When symptoms are very severe bilateral ovarian vein ligation may cure,[2] as may hysterectomy with bilateral salpingo-oophorectomy with hormone replacement therapy post-operatively.

Mittelschmerz this is mid-cycle menstrual pain which may occur in teenagers and older women around the time of ovulation—from the German 'mittel' (=middle) and 'Schmerz' (=pain).

Dyspareunia

This means pain during intercourse. There may be a vicious circle in which anticipation of pain leads to tense muscles and lack of lubrication, and so to further pain. ►*The patient may not volunteer the problem so ask about intercourse*. Her attitude to pelvic examination may tell you as much as the examination itself. Ask her to show you where the problem is. If the problem is actually vaginismus do not insist on examination and consider counselling and sex therapy (p 380). Was there 'female cicumsision' (p 6)?

Dyspareunia may be superficial (introital)—eg from infection so look for ulceration and discharge. Is she dry? If so is the problem oestrogen deficiency (p 18) or lack of sexual stimulation? Has she had a recent post-partum perineal repair? A suture or scar can cause well-localized pain which is cured by removing the suture and injection of local anaesthetic. If the introitus has been rendered too narrow, she may need surgery.

Deep dyspareunia is felt internally (deep inside). It is associated with endometriosis and pelvic sepsis; treat the cause if possible. If the ovaries lie in the rectovaginal pouch (or after hysterectomy), they may be subject to coital thrusts; try other positions or ventrosuspension if a 'cure' can be obtained with trial use of a Hodge pessary.

Dermatographism is a rare cause of dyspareunia: look for itchy wheals at the vulva some minutes after application of a calibrated dermatographometer. The thing to remember is that dermatographism can occur on any surface. It is the commonest physical cause of urticaria, and the clue to its presence is linear wheals with a surrounding bright red flare (but no angio-oedema) elsewhere on the skin, in response to a firm stroke. There are no known causes. Successful relief of dyspareunia in these cases has been achieved by 2% epinephrine (adrenaline) cream, and cetirizine 10mg/24h PO.[3]

1 C Farquar 1989 *Br J Obs Gyn* **96** 1153 2 J Hobbs 1990 *Br J H Med* **43** 200 3 A Lambiris 1997 *Lancet* **349** 28

Ovarian hyperstimulation[1]

Sudden multiplication of follicles in response to drugs, especially when gonadotrophin releasing hormone (GnRH) is used in assisted reproduction, gives diffuse lower abdominal pain and cystic ovarian enlargement on palpation. The incidence is 0.5–2% in women having ovarian stimulation. It is commoner in conception cycles. Associated complications are ascites, reduced intravascular volume, pulmonary effusions and (rare) pericardial effusions. Thromboembolic complications may ensue.

Management Admit to hospital. Give adequate analgesia (opiates if necessary). Check FBC, U&E, creatinine, LFTs and coagulation profile. Do CXR if chest pathology suspected; blood gases if tachypnoeic or dyspnoeic. Chart urine output (if oliguria suspected catheterize and measure fluid output hourly). Ovarian size is a guide to severity unless oocytes have been harvested.

Hyperstimulation is *severe* if haematocrit is >45%, WCC >15 x 10^9/L, there is massive ascites, oliguria, mild renal or liver dysfunction. Put up IVI, and consider CVP. Fluid replacement may be required, eg 500mL albumin over 2 hours. Paracentesis of ascites can improve renal function. To avoid thromboembolic complications use antiembolic stockings, encourage leg mobility and consider use of subcutaneous heparin.

The situation is *critical* if the haematocrit is >55% and WCC >25 x 10^9/L, there is tense ascites and renal failure. Thromboembolic phenomena and acute respiratory distress syndrome (*OHCM* p 350). Admit to ITU. Symptomatic pleural effusions may need drainage. Use antiembolic measures as above. Pay meticulous attention to fluid balance. Aim to maintain intake at 3L/24h using alternating normal and dextrose saline (but beware hyponatraemia).

The severity of effusions determines the time to recovery. In non-conception cycles with little ascites there will be resolution with menstruation. In conception cycles cysts may persist for weeks. Resolution usually occurs, but exceptionally termination of pregnancy may be needed.

1 J Jenkins 1995 *Br J Obs Gyn* **102** 2

2. Obstetrics

A world of made is not a world of born—pity poor flesh e. e. cummings

*The term *pregnancy-induced hypertension with proteinuria* is tending to replace the older term *pre-eclampsia*. We have not followed this trend here because to do so obscures the vital fact about pre-eclampsia: it may lead on to eclampsia. We favour *pre-eclampsia* because the term is short and sends the shadow of a shiver down our spines, being a constant reminder of how dangerous it can be.

The Cochrane Childbirth & Pregnancy Database Obstetrics is as much an art as a science, but when questioning standard practices, it is likely that someone somewhere has researched the issue, and one good starting point is to consult this database managed by the Cochrane Centre.[1,2]

1 *Via* Update Software, Oxford, OX44 7QB 2 RJ Lilford 1994 BMJ i 1448

The essence of reproductive health

Pregnancy is a risky affair, not only for babies, but also for mothers. The textbook causes of maternal mortality are pulmonary embolism, eclampsia, haemorrhage, and infection—with all the other causes being rare. But if an obstetrician could be granted one wish, it would not be to abolish these; rather it would be to make every pregnancy *planned* and *desired by the mother*. Worldwide, a woman dies every minute from the effects of pregnancy, and most of these women never wanted to be pregnant in the first place—but did not have to hand the means for contraception. So the real killers are poverty, ignorance, and the real solutions entail literacy and economic growth. Any obstetric or governmental initiatives in reproductive health which do not recognize these facts are doomed only to operate at the margins, and their good ideas are all too often vitiated by the reality operating in mothers' homes and workplaces.

School-based sex education This *can* be effective, especially when linked to easy access to contraceptive services. This is the conclusion of one good meta-analysis, taking into account cohort studies—but note that if meta-analyses confine themselves to the 15-or so randomized studies, no benefit could be demonstrated (*E-BM* 1997 **2** 150). It may be necessary to foster a knowledge-sharing, skill-promoting environment which is part of a continuing process, and not a 'one-off' affair—for educational programmes to work. *Adolescent pregnancy rates:* USA: 116/1000; UK: 57/1000; Canada: 50/1000. In the UK, 2,346,800 babies were born in 1991–3 (live and stillbirths), and 520,451 pregnancies were legally terminated.

Gravidity and parity—definitions

Gravidity refers to the number of pregnancies that a woman has had (to any stage). Parity refers to pregnancies that resulted in delivery beyond 28 weeks' gestation. An example of the shorthand way of expressing pregnancies before and after 28 weeks is: para 2+1. This means that she has had 2 pregnancies beyond 28 completed weeks' gestation, and 1 which terminated prior to 28 weeks. If she is not pregnant at the time of describing her she is gravida 3, but if she is pregnant now she is gravida 4. Twins present a problem as there is controversy as to whether they count as 1 for both parity and gravidity or should count as 2 for parity.

It is unclear whether the cut-off point in the above definitions should now be 24 weeks, to harmonize with the new definition of stillbirth (p 136). In general, aim to use proper English rather than the shorthand described above—which is open to varying interpretations. For example, when presenting a patient try something along these lines: 'Mrs Cottard is a 32-year-old lady who is 15 weeks into her fourth pregnancy; the third ended in a miscarriage at 17 weeks, and the others came to term with normal deliveries of children who are now 2 and 8.' The bald statement 'Para 2+1' is ambiguous, incomprehensible to the patient, and misses the point that the patient is now approaching the time when she lost her last baby.

Relevant pages in other chapters: Neonatology p 230–46; breast feeding p 176–8; rhesus haemolytic disease p 242; ectopic pregnancy p 24; abortion and termination of pregnancy p 20–2; trophoblastic disease p 26; examination of the neonate p 231; preterm and light-for-dates babies p 180; varicella (chickenpox) in pregnancy p 216; parvovirus B19 p 214; postnatal depression p 408.

The placenta

The placenta is the organ of respiration, nutrition and excretion for the fetus. It produces hormones for maternal wellbeing and immunologically protects the fetus by preventing rejection and allowing the passage of IgG antibodies from the mother.

Development Placental development is complete by 70 days after ovulation. At term the placenta weighs $\frac{1}{7}^{th}$ the weight of the baby. It has a blood flow of 600mL/min. The placenta changes throughout pregnancy as calcium is deposited in the villi and fibrin on them. Excess fibrin may be deposited in diabetes and rhesus disease, so decreasing fetal nutrients.

Placental types *Battledore* insertion is where the umbilical cord inserts into the side of the placenta. *Velamentous* insertion (1%) is where the umbilical vessels pass within the membranes before insertion. If these vessels break (as in vasa praevia) it is fetal blood which is lost. *Placenta succenturia:* (5%) There is a separate (succenturiate) lobe away from the main placenta which may fail to separate normally and cause a PPH or puerperal sepsis. *Placenta membranacea* (1/3000) is a thin placenta all around the baby. As some is in the lower segment it prediposes to APH. It may fail to separate in the third stage of labour. *Placenta accreta:* There is abnormal adherence of all or part of the placenta to the uterus, termed *placenta increta* where there is placental infiltration of the myometrium or *placenta percreta* if penetration reaches the serosa. These latter 3 types predispose to PPH and may necessitate hysterectomy.

Placenta praevia The placenta lies in the lower uterine segment. It is found in 0.5% of pregnancies. Risks are of significant haemorrhage by mother and fetus. *Associations:* Large placenta (eg twins); uterine abnormalities and fibroids; uterine damage (eg multiparity, former surgery including Caesarean section). Ultrasound at <24 weeks' gestation shows a low-lying placenta in 28% but lower segment development later in pregnancy results in only 3% being low-lying at term.

Terminology: Major (old III and IV degrees) with placenta covering the internal os requires Caesarean section for delivery. Minor (old I and II) where the placenta is in the lower segment but not across the internal os: aim for normal delivery. Presentation may be as APH (separation of the placenta as the lower segment stretches causes bleeding) or as failure for the head to engage with high presenting part. Problems are with bleeding and with mode of delivery as the placenta obstructs the os and may shear off during labour, or may be accreta (5%), especially after previous Caesarean section (>24%). Caesarean section should be consultant-performed or supervised.[1]

Placental function tests The placenta produces progesterone, human chorionic gonadotrophin, and human placental lactogen. Human chorionic gonadotrophin is used for detection of early pregnancy. Human placental lactogen assay (previously used to try to monitor placental function), and urinary oestrogens assay (to monitor the fetoplacental unit) have fallen out of favour due to lack of sensitivity, and are now being replaced by biophysical tests (p 118).

1 DoH 1994 *Report on Confidential Enquiries into Maternal Deaths in the United Kingdom 1988–90* HMSO

Physiological changes in pregnancy

Hormonal changes *Progesterone*, synthesized by the corpus luteum until 35 post-conception days and by the placenta mainly thereafter, decreases smooth muscle excitability (uterus, gut, ureters) and raises body temperature. *Oestrogens* (90% oestriol) increase breast and nipple growth, water retention and protein synthesis. *Human placental lactogen* promotes growth hormone release and insulin secretion, but decreases insulin's peripheral effects, liberating maternal fatty acids (so sparing maternal glucose use). It also stimulates mammary growth and maternal casein, lactalbumin and lactoglobulin production. The maternal thyroid often enlarges due to increased colloid production. Thyroxine levels, see p 158. Pituitary secretion of *prolactin* rises throughout pregnancy. Maternal *cortisol* output is increased but unbound levels remain constant.

Genital changes The 100g non-pregnant uterus weighs 1100g by term. Muscle hyperplasia occurs up to 20 weeks, with stretching after that. The cervix may develop ectropion ('erosions'). Late in pregnancy cervical collagen reduces. Vaginal discharge increases due to cervical ectopy, cell desquamation, and ↑ mucus production from a vasocongested vagina.

Haemodynamic changes *Blood:* From 10 weeks the plasma volume rises until 32 weeks when it is 3.8 litres (50% >non-pregnant). Red cell volume rises from 1.4 litres when non-pregnant to 1.64 litres at term if iron supplements not taken (↑18%), or 1.8 litres at term (↑30%) if supplements are taken—hence Hb falls due to dilution ('physiological anaemia'). WCC (mean 10.5×10^9/L), platelets, ESR (up 4-fold), cholesterol, β-globulin and fibrinogen are raised. Albumin and gamma-globulin fall.

Cardiovascular: Cardiac output rises from 5 litres/min to 6.5–7 litres/min in the first 10 weeks by increasing stroke volume (10%) and pulse rate (by ~15 beats/min). Peripheral resistance falls (due to hormonal changes). BP, particularly diastolic, falls during the first second trimesters by 10–20mmHg, then rises to non-pregnant levels by term. With increased venous distensibility, and raised venous pressure (as occurs with any pelvic mass), varicose veins may form. Vasodilatation and hypotension stimulates renin and angiotensin release—an important feature of BP regulation in pregnancy.

Other changes Ventilation increases 40% (tidal volume rises from 500 to 700mL), the increased depth of breath being a progesterone effect. O_2 consumption increases only 20%. Breathlessness is common as maternal P_aCO_2 is set lower to allow the fetus to offload CO_2. Gut motility is reduced resulting in constipation, delayed gastric emptying and with a lax cardiac sphincter, heartburn. Renal size increases by ~1cm in length during pregnancy.

Frequency of micturition emerges early (glomerular filtration rate↑ by 60%), later from bladder pressure by the fetal head. The bladder muscle is lax but residual urine after micturition is not normally present. Skin pigmentation (eg in linea nigra, nipples, or as chloasma—brown patches of pigmentation seen especially on the face), palmar erythema, spider naevi, and striae are common. Hair shedding from the head is reduced in pregnancy but the extra hairs are shed in the puerperium.

Pregnancy tests Positive from the first day of the first missed period, until ~20 weeks of pregnancy, they remain positive for ~5 days after abortion or fetal death. Otherwise, the false +ve rate is low. They detect the β-subunit of human chorionic gonadotrophin in early morning urine, so are positive in trophoblastic disease (p 26).

Plasma biochemistry in pregnancy[1,2,3]

Centile	*Non-pregnant* 2.5	97.5	*Trimester I* 2.5	97.5	*Trimester 2* 2.5	97.5	*Trimester 3* 2.5	97.5
Na^+ mmol/L	138	146	135	141	132	140	133	141
Ca^{2+} mmol/L	2	2.6	2.3	2.5	2.2	2.2	2.2	2.5
*corrected	2.3	2.6	2.25	2.57	2.3	2.5	2.3	2.59
Albumin g/L	44	50	39	49	36	44	33	41
$^{Free}T_4$ pmol/L	9	23	10	24	9	19	7	17

Other plasma reference intervals (not analysed by trimester)

	Non-pregnant	*Pregnant*
Alkaline phosphatase	3–300IU/L	up to 450IU/L **
Bicarbonate mmol/L	24–30	20–25
Creatinine µmol/L	70–150	24–68
Urea mmol/L	2.5–6.7	2–4.2
Urate µmol/L	150–390	100–270

*Calcium corrected for plasma albumin (see *OHCM* p 642).
**Occasionally very much higher in apparently normal pregnancies.[4]

C-reactive protein does not change much in pregnancy.
TSH may be low in the first half of a normal pregnancy (suppressed by HCG); for other thyroid changes see above and p 157.

1 B Berg 1984 *Acta Obstet Gynecol Scand* **63** 583–6 2 OTM 1987, OUP, 29.2 3 M de Swiet 1996 *Pulse* **56** 92
4 A Gowenlock 1988 Varley's *Practical Clinical Biochemistry* 1988, 535, Heinemann, London

Normal labour

From 30 weeks the uterus has Braxton-Hicks contractions. These are non-painful 'practice' contractions to ~15mmHg pressure (in labour pressure is ~60mmHg) and are commonest after 36 weeks.

Normal labour is that occurring after 37 weeks' gestation. It should result in the spontaneous vaginal delivery of the baby within 24h of the onset of regular spontaneous contractions. It is often heralded by a 'show', ie a plug of cervical mucus and a little blood as the membranes strip from the os. The membranes may then rupture.

The first stage of labour is the time from the onset of regular contractions until the cervix is fully dilated (no cervix felt around the head). The cervix initially *effaces* (becomes shorter and softer) before it dilates. A satisfactory rate of dilatation from 3cm dilated is 1cm/h. The first stage generally takes up to 12h in a primip, and 7.5h in a multip. During the first stage check maternal pulse, BP and T° half-hourly; assess the contractions every 15min, their strength (you should not be able to indent the uterus with the fingers during a contraction) and their frequency (ideally 3–4 per 10min, lasting up to 1min). Carry out vaginal examination every 4h to assess the degree of cervical dilatation, the position and the station of the head (measured in cm above the ischial spines) and note the degree of moulding (p 86). Note the state of the liquor (see p 128). Test maternal urine 4-hourly for ketones and protein. If the mother becomes ketotic set up an IVI and give her 10% dextrose. Measure the fetal heart rate (if not being continuously monitored) every 15min. Note the rate before, during and immediately after a contraction.

The second stage is the time from complete cervical dilatation until the baby is born (see Movement of head in labour, p 86).

The mother will have a desire to push and will use her abdominal muscles with the Valsalva manoeuvre to help move the baby. As the head descends, the perineum stretches and the anus gapes. Normal time for second stage is 45–120min in a primip, 15–45min in a multip. The aim is to prevent a precipitate delivery (and so intracranial bleeding) by pressure over the perineum.

The amount of delay before cutting the cord little affects term babies, but holding the baby 20cm below the introitus and delaying clamping for 30sec results in higher haematocrit levels, so reducing transfusion and oxygen supplement requirements in premature babies.[1]

The third stage is delivery of the placenta. As the uterus contracts to a 20-week size after the baby is born the placenta separates from the uterus through the spongy layer of the decidua basalis. It then buckles and a small amount of retroplacental haemorrhage aids its removal.

Signs of separation: Cord lengthens, rush of blood (retroplacental haemorrhage) from the vagina, uterus rises and contracts in the abdomen (felt with hand), and the uterus becomes more globular. Routine use of syntometrine (ergometrine maleate 500µg IM + oxytocin 5U IM) as the anterior shoulder of the baby is born has decreased third stage time (to ~5min), and has also decreased the incidence of PPH, but may cause problems for undiagnosed twins. Examine the placenta to check it is complete.

1 S Kimmond 1993 BMJ i 172

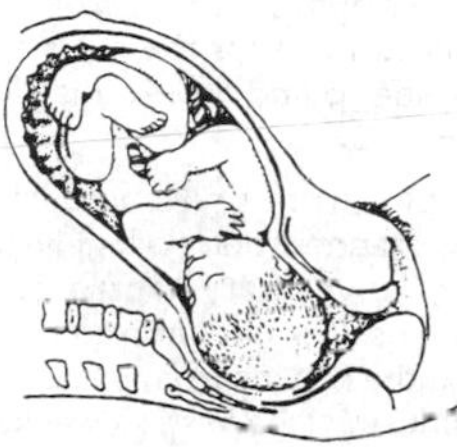

(1)
1st stage of labour. The cervix dilates. After full dilatation the head flexes further and descends further into the pelvis.

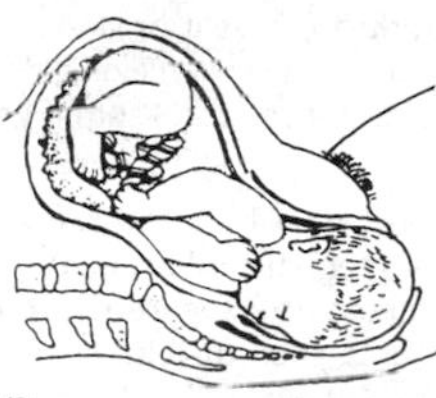

(2)
During the early second stage the head rotates at the level of the ischial spine so the occiput lies in the anterior part of pelvis.
In late second stage the head broaches the vulval ring (crowning) and the perineum stretches over the head.

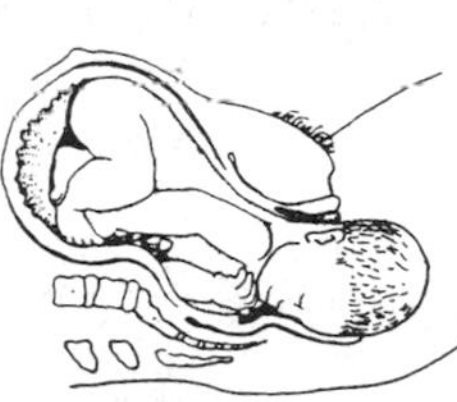

(3)
The head is born. The shoulders still lie transversely in the midpelvis.

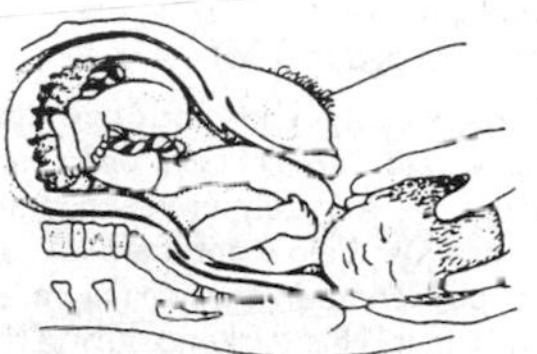

(4)
Birth of the anterior shoulder. The shoulders rotate to lie in the anteroposterior diameter of the pelvic outlet. The head rotates externally, 'restitutes', to its direction at onset of labour. Downward and backward traction of the head by the birth attendant aids delivery of the anterior shoulder.

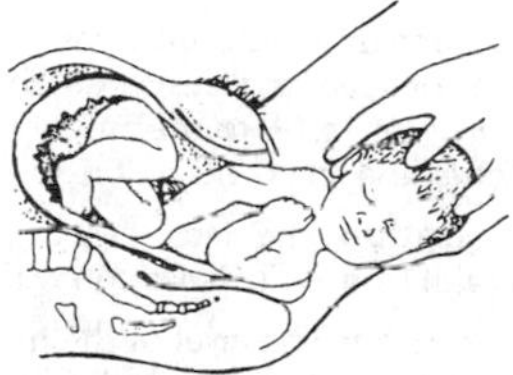

(5)
Birth of the posterior shoulder is aided by lifting the head upwards whilst maintaining traction.

Abdominal palpation

The uterus occupies the pelvis and cannot be felt *per abdomen* until 12 weeks' gestation. By 16 weeks it lies about half way between the symphysis pubis and the umbilicus. By 20–22 weeks it has reached the umbilicus. In a primigravida, the fundus lies under the ribs by 36 weeks. At term the uterus tends to lie a little lower than at 36 weeks due to the head descending into the pelvis. Some attendants prefer to measure the symphysis fundal height (SFH) in cm from the symphysis pubis. From 16 weeks the SFH increases ~1 cm/week. As a guide, the SFH is the gestation in weeks minus 3. It may be used as a rough guide to find babies small for gestational age (p 104).

On inspecting the abdomen note any scars from previous operations. Caesarean section scars are usually Pfannenstiel ('bikini-line'), although occasionally in very fat women they lie vertically. Laparoscopy scars are just below and parallel to the umbilicus. It is common to see a line of pigmentation, the linea nigra, extending in the midline from pubic hair to umbilicus. This darkens during the first trimester (the first 13 weeks).

Palpating the abdomen Measure the SFH and listen to the *fetal heart*. After 32 weeks palpate laterally to assess the lie, then bimanually palpate over the lower uterine pole for presentation and degree of engagement. Pawlik's grip (examining the lower pole of the uterus between the thumb and index fingers of the right hand) can also be used for assessing the degree of engagement. Watch the patient's face during palpation and stop if it causes pain. Obesity, polyhydramnios and tense muscles make it difficult to feel the fetus. Midwives are skilled at palpation, so ask them if you need help.

It is important to determine the *number of fetuses* (see p 122), the *lie* (longitudinal, oblique, or transverse), the *presentation* (cephalic or breech), and the *engagement*. Note the amount of liquor present, the apparent size of the fetus, and any contractions or fetal movements seen or felt.

Auscultation The fetal heart may be heard by Doppler ultrasound (Sonicaid) from ~12 weeks and with a Pinard stethoscope from ~24 weeks.

Engagement The level of the head is assessed in 2 ways—engagement, or fifths palpable abdominally. Engagement entails passage of the maximum presenting diameter through the pelvic inlet. Fifths palpable abdominally states what you can feel, and makes no degree of judgement on degree of engagement of the head. In primigravida the head is usually entering the pelvis by 37 weeks, otherwise causes must be excluded (eg placenta praevia or fetal abnormality). In multips the head may not enter the pelvis until the onset of labour.

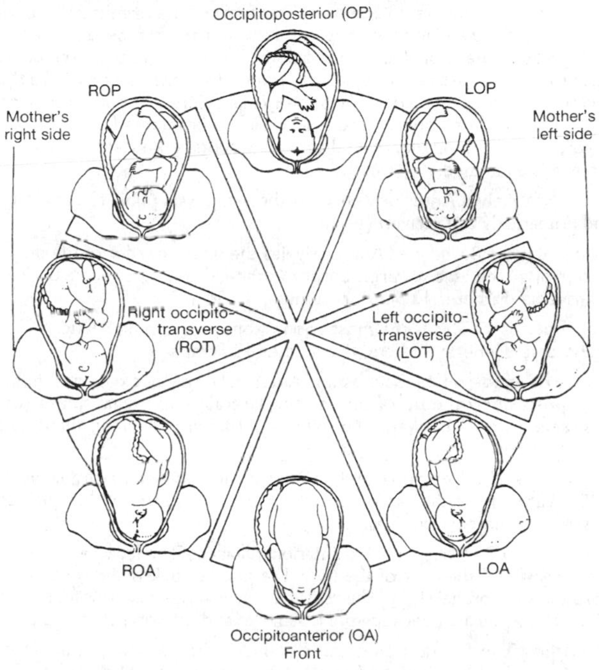

Position

Occipitoanterior	*Occipitolateral*	*Occipitoposterior*
Back easily felt	Back can be felt	Back not felt
Limbs not easily felt	Limbs lateral	Limbs anterior
Shoulder lies 2cm from midline on opposite side from back	Midline shoulder	Shoulder 6–8cm lateral, same side as back
Back from midline = 2–3cm	6–8cm	≥10cm

►The fetal heart is best heard over its back (left scapula).

Pelvis and head

The ideal pelvis This has an oval brim, a shallow cavity, non-prominent ischial spines, a curved sacrum with large sciatic notches and sacrospinous ligaments >3.5cm long. The angle of the brim is 55° to the horizontal, the AP diameter at least 12cm and transverse diameter at least 13.5cm. The subpubic arch should be rounded and the intertuberous distance at least 10cm. A *clinically favourable* pelvis is one where the sacral promontory cannot be felt, the ischial spines are not prominent, the suprapubic arch and base of supraspinous ligaments both accept 2 fingers and the intertuberous diameter accepts 4 knuckles when the woman is examined.

The true pelvis Anteriorly there is the symphysis pubis (3.5cm long) and posteriorly the sacrum (12cm long).

Zone of inlet *Boundaries:* Anteriorly lies the upper border of the pubis, posteriorly the sacral promontory, laterally the ileopectineal line. Transverse diameter 13.5cm; AP diameter 11.5cm.

Zone of cavity This is the most roomy zone. It is almost round. Transverse diameter 13.5cm; AP diameter 12.5cm.

Zone of mid-pelvis *Boundaries:* Anteriorly, the apex of the pubic arch; posteriorly the tip of the sacrum, laterally the ischial spines (the desirable distance between the spines is >10.5cm). Ovoid in shape, it is the narrowest part.

Zone of outlet The pubic arch is the anterior border (desirable angle >85°). Laterally lie the sacrotuberous ligaments and ischial tuberosities, posteriorly the coccyx.

Head terms The *bregma* is the anterior fontanelle. The *brow* lies between the bregma and the root of the nose. The *face* lies below the root of the nose and supraorbital ridges. The *occiput* lies behind the posterior fontanelle. The *vertex* is the area between the fontanelles and the parietal eminences.

Moulding The frontal bones can slip under the parietal bones which can slip under the occipital bone so reducing biparietal diameter. The degree of overlap may be assessed vaginally.

Presentation:	**Relevant diameter presenting:**	
Flexed vertex	suboccipitobregmatic	9.5cm
Partially deflexed vertex	suboccipitofrontal	10.5cm
Deflexed vertex	occipitofrontal	11.5cm
Brow	mentovertical	13cm
Face	submentobregmatic	9.5cm

Movement of the head in labour (normal vertex presentation)

1. Descent with increased flexion as the head enters the cavity. The sagittal suture lies in the transverse diameter of the brim.
2. Internal rotation occurs at the level of the ischial spines due to the grooved gutter of the levator muscles. Head flexion increases. (The head rotates 90° if occipitolateral position, 45° if occipitoanterior, 135° if occipitoposterior.)
3. Disengagement by extension as the head comes out of the vulva.
4. Restitution: as the shoulders are rotated by the levators until the bisacromial diameter is anteroposterior, the head externally rotates the same amount as before but in opposite direction.
5. Delivery of anterior shoulder by lateral flexion of trunk posteriorly.
6. Delivery of posterior shoulder by lateral flexion of trunk anteriorly.
7. Delivery of buttocks and legs.

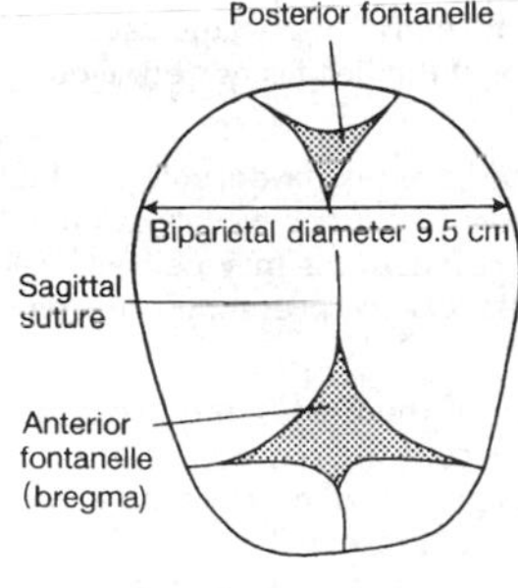

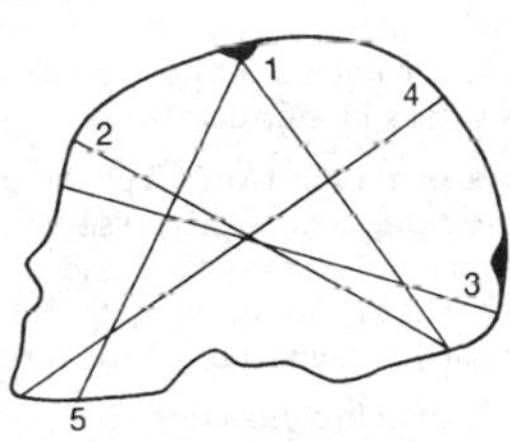

1 Suboccipitobregmatic 9.5 cm flexed vertex presentation
2 Suboccipitofrontal 10.5 cm partially deflexed vertex
3 Occipitofrontal 11.5 cm deflexed vertex
4 Mentovertical 13 cm brow
5 Submentobregmatic 9.5 cm face

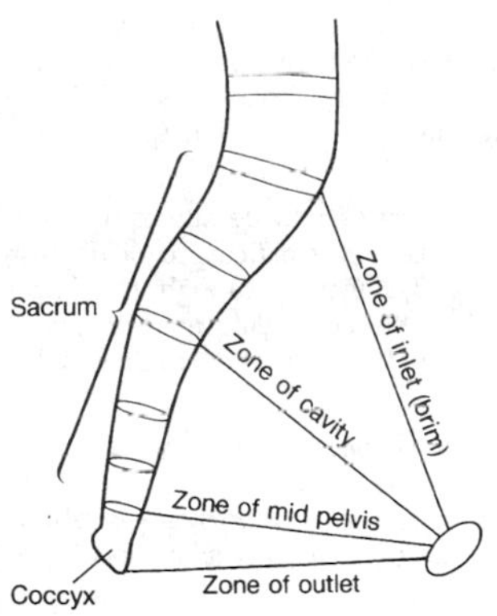

Dystocia

Dystocia is difficulty in labour. There may be problems with *the passenger* (large baby, see *shoulder dystocia*, p 128, abnormal presentation), *the passages* (for ideal pelvis see p 86) or of *propulsion* (the uterine powers). Cephalo-pelvic disproportion results if diameters are unfavourable (p 86).

The pelvis The ideal pelvis has a round brim (ie gynaecoid), but 15% of women have a long oval brim (anthropoid). A very flat brim is less favourable (platypoid); occurring in 5% of women over 152cm (5ft), it occurs in 30% of women < 152cm. Spinal scoliosis, kyphosis, sacralization of the L5 vertebra, spondylolisthesis and pelvic fractures may all affect pelvic anatomy. Rickets and polio were formerly important causes of pelvic problems. Suspect pelvic contraction if the head is not engaged by 37 weeks in a Caucasian primip.

The presentation Cephalic presentations are less favourable the less flexed the head. Transverse lie and brow presentations will always need Caesarean section: face and OP (p 126) presentations may deliver vaginally but are more likely to fail to progress. Breech presentation is particularly unfavourable if the fetus >3.5kg.

The uterine powers Contractions start in the fundus and propagate downwards. The intensity and duration of contractions are greatest at the fundus, but the contraction reaches its peak in all parts of the uterus simultaneously. Normal contractions occur at a rate of 3 per 10min, they should last up to 75sec, the contraction peak usually measures 30–60mmHg, and the resting uterine tone between them should be 10–15mmHg. Uterine muscle has the property of retraction. The shortening of the muscle fibres encourages cervical dilatation.

Uterine dysfunction Contractions may be hypotonic (low resting tone, low contraction peaks) or they may be normotonic but occur too infrequently. These dysfunctions can be corrected by augmentation with oxytocin (p 112). Whenever oxytocin is used discuss with a senior obstetrician. Pain and fear cause release of catecholamines which can inhibit uterine activity. Thus adequate analgesia is needed (p 114) and may speed the progress of labour.

Cervical dystocia Failure of cervical dilatation may be due to previous trauma, repair, cone biopsy and cauterization. It is difficult to distinguish from failure to dilate due to uterine dysfunction though the latter should respond to oxytocin (note the important difference between primips and multips, p 112). The treatment for cervical dystocia is delivery by Caesarean section.

Consequences of prolonged labour Neonatal mortality rises with prolonged labour as does maternal morbidity (especially infection). With modern management of labour, careful monitoring of progress in labour (p 112) takes place to diagnose delay early, and treat it as necessary, to prevent prolonged labour occurring.

►When there is dystocia, ask 'is safe vaginal delivery possible?'

Minor symptoms of pregnancy

►Before prescribing any drug, think—Is it necessary. Is it safe? Consult *Data-sheets* ± a national teratology information service (0191 232 1525)[uk].

Symptoms and signs in the first 10 weeks: Early symptoms are amenorrhoea, nausea, vomiting and bladder irritability. Breasts engorge, nipples enlarge (darken at 12 weeks), Montgomery's tubercles (sebaceous glands on nipples) become prominent. Vulval vascularity increases and the cervix softens and looks bluish (4 weeks). At 6–10 weeks the uterine body is more globular. Temperature rises (<37.8°C).

Headaches, palpitations, and fainting are all more common during pregnancy. Sweating and feeling hot are also common, and are due to a more dilated peripheral circulation. *Management:* Increase fluid intake and take plenty of showers.

Urinary frequency is due to pressure of the fetal head on the bladder in later pregnancy. Exclude UTI.

Abdominal pain: See p 135. *Breathlessness* is common. See p 80.

Constipation tends to occur as gut motility decreases. Adequate oral fluids and a high fibre diet help combat it. Avoid stimulant laxatives—they increase uterine activity in some women. Increased venous distensibility and pelvic congestion predispose to *haemorrhoids* (if they prolapse, rest the mother head down, apply ice packs and replace them), and *varicose veins*. Resting with feet up, and properly worn elastic stockings help.

Reflux oesophagitis and heartburn occur as pyloric sphincter relaxation allows irritant bile to reflux into the stomach. Cigarettes and spices should be avoided, small meals taken, and antacids used.

Third trimester backache: Due to pelvic ligament and muscle relaxation, pain tends to be worse at night. A firm mattress, flat shoes, standing with back straight and pelvic support from physiotherapy all help.

Carpal tunnel syndrome (p 662) in pregnancy is due to fluid retention. Advise wrist splints until delivery cures the problem.

Itch/itchy rashes are common (up to 25%) and may be due to the usual causes (*OHCM* p 50, check LFTs—see p 158) or to pruritic eruption of pregnancy (PEP = *prurigo of pregnancy*)—an intensely itchy papular/plaque rash on the abdomen and limbs. PEP is most common in first pregnancies beyond 35 weeks' gestation. Emollients and weak topical steroids ease it. Delivery cures it. If vesicles are present, think of *pemphigoid gestationis* (PG): a rare (1:50,000) condition which may cause fatal heat loss and cardiac failure; the baby may be briefly affected; refer early (prednisolone may be needed). PG recurs in later pregnancies, eg if there is a different father.

Ankle oedema: This is very common, almost normal manifestation of pregnancy. Measure BP and check urine for protein (pre-eclampsia, p 96). Check legs for DVT. It often responds to rest and leg elevation. Reassure that it is harmless (unless pre-eclampsia).

Leg cramps 33% get cramp, the latter half of pregnancy, severe in 5%, often worse at night. Raising the foot of the bed by 20cm will help.

Chloasma: This is a patch of darker pigmentation, eg on the face: p 578.

Nausea affects ~80%. *Vomiting* occurs in ~50%. It may start by 4 weeks and declines over the next weeks. At 20 weeks 20% may still vomit.[1] Most respond to frequent small meals, reassurance, and a stress-free environment. It is associated with good outcome (fewer fetal losses).

1 S Whitehead 1992 *J Obstet Gynae* **12** 364

Hyperemesis gravidarum

This is rare (1/1000). Risk is increased in youth, non-smokers, primips, working outside home, multiple or molar pregnancy (hence the idea that excessively high HCG levels may be the cause—whereas steeply rising oestrogens may cause the very common phenomenon of morning sickness).[1]

Presentation: Inability to keep food or fluids down; weight↓ (2–5kg) ± nutritional deficiency, dehydration, hypovolaemia, electrolyte disturbance with hyponatraemic shock, polyneuritis (B vitamins↓), behaviour disorders, liver and renal failure.

Tests: Do PCV and U&E to help guide IV fluid regimen. TFTs (there may be assocaited thyroid or adrenal dysfunction).[2] Chart losses. Exclude UTI. Ultrasound scan to exclude twins or hydatidiform mole.

Treatment: Admit to hospital. Spend time optimizing *psychological wellbeing*. Is she worried about how her other children are being cared for?

Most settle with due *care and attention*. If not, parenteral *anti-emetics* may be tried (eg metoclopramide 10mg/8h IV—but there are problems with extrapyramidal effects). Placing a Dobbhoff nasogastric tube for *enteral feeding* has proponents,[3] but note that iso-osmolar feeds are recommended, as is regular aspiration of the stomach (there is likely to be delayed gastric emptying); monitor plasma glucose (expect some insulin resistance).[1] If an IV infusion is used give IV thiamine to prevent Wernicke's encephalopathy (see *OHCM* p 712) developing.[4] Beware rapid reversal of hyponatraemia which can cause fatal central pontine myelinosis.[2] Those resistant to conventional treatments may respond to steroid treatment.[2]

Parenteral nutrition may be needed—*OHCM* p 106. ►Get a *dietition's help*.

1 CJM van de Ven 1997 *Lancet* **349** 445 2 C Nelson-Piercy 1994 *Br J Obs Gynae* **101** 1013 3 JJ Hsu 1996 *Obstet Gynecol* **88** 343–6 4 DoH 1996 *Report on Confidential Enquiry into Maternal Deaths in the United Kingdom 1991–93* HMSO

Booking criteria and home delivery

Most women in the UK have 'shared obstetric care'—ie most of their antenatal care is from the GP and community midwife, with limited (or no) visits (usually 2) to the hospital to see the consultant under whose care they are delivered, returning home (eg after 6–72h) for postnatal care. A minority receive their complete care from hospitals and the usual reasons for this would be that their GP did not provide obstetric services, or that the complications of pregnancy made full consultant care more desirable. Some women are cared for by community midwifery staff and their GP, but increasingly, low-risk women are receiving all their care from midwives, with medical staff involvement only if complications arise. Delivery may be at hospital, in GP units (which may or may not be geographically isolated from consultant units), or, rarely, at home. ►There is quite good evidence⟨1⟩ that consultant input into antenatal care of normal pregnancies achieves no added benefits (p 95)—but risk factors making specialist visits and booking desirable are generally agreed. They divide into those relating to the mother, to her previous deliveries, and to her pregnancy now, eg:

Features pertaining to the mother
- Nullips <20yrs old or >30yrs
- All women over 35yrs old
- From the 5th pregnancy onwards
- Height <154cm (158cm primips)
- Very obese; social deprivation
- +ve serology (HBsAg, HIV) p 98

Features pertaining to previous deliveries
- Preterm or small (<37 weeks, <2.5kg)
- Deformity, stillbirth, neonatal death
- Caesarean section or hysterotomy
- Retained placenta; abruption
- Births requiring pelvic floor repair
- Instrumental deliveries; PPH

Features of this pregnancy
- Cardiac or thyroid disease
- Multiple pregnancy
- Rh–ve with antibodies (p 242)
- Poor fetal growth or wellbeing
- Diabetes, ↑BP, anaemia
- Malpresentations after 34 weeks
- Raised serum α-fetoprotein

Is it safe for low-risk mothers to deliver in high-technology hospitals? Here interventions with their complications are more common. In the UK this question is usually academic as most GPs are reluctant to conduct births—and 6 months' Senior House Officer training in obstetrics gives scant skill. The rising birth rate and service pressures are putting these big hospitals under great strain. In places (eg New Zealand, Holland) where delivery outside of big hospitals is the norm, there is fairly clear (but not uncontested) evidence that on all measures, and in all but the highest risk groups, big hospitals come out less favourably.[2] The few trials seeming to favour high-technology are now recognized to be seriously flawed.[3]

Home delivery This is rare in the UK (~1% of births, of these only ⅔ are booked in advance for home delivery). We cannot draw statistical conclusions from the sparse data comparing morbidity and mortality in home *vs* hospital delivery, as home deliveries are so rare.[2] But an important observation is that rapid intervention is necessary to save life (maternal or fetal) in ~5% of low-risk pregnancies. This pinpoints the need for any domiciliary service to have good equipment available for home deliveries and good emergency back-up (provided in future by emergency obstetric ambulance units—specially trained ambulance personnel who, it is to be hoped, will liaise directly with senior medical obstetric staff in hospital).

Birthroom birth This offers a homely birth in congenial surroundings with labour ward facilities nearby, if needed. The mother is attended by her GP and community midwife. A randomized trial has shown that mothers' satisfaction is great, and nearly all requested this type of delivery for future births. This may offer a compromise to adherents of home delivery.

⟨1⟩ J Tucker 1996 *BMJ* i 312 & *E-BM* 1996 1 190 2 D Jewell 1989 *BMJ* i 690 3 R Campbell 1991 *BMJ* ii 1487

Issues surrounding home delivery

- In the UK, because of past hospital experience of many abnormal labours, GPs are are often *very* wary of home birth.
- Medico-legal aspects tend to dominate thoughts about worse-case scenarios—so that few GPs willingly take on intrapartum care.
- It's not clear who is to do the doctor's ordinary work when absent on a home delivery—if a mother particularly wants their GP present. Some small surgeries have had to close during delivery as no locum was available—an unacceptable consequence of offering mothers extra choice. NB: in the UK, midwives, but not GPs, have a statutory duty to help at home deliveries.
- It is not clear if there is a ready supply of doctors or midwives with the necessary experience in suturing and neonatal resuscitation. Where there is a good team, there is no doubt that home delivery can be a safe and rewarding experience.[1]
- It has to be remembered that decisions about the place of labour are dynamic, and need revising (eg in 29%) as events in pregnancy unfold. It is not always clear how these decisions are to be taken, and how they are to be communicated.
- Necessary equipment is not readily available, eg Entonox®, and mobile telephones—and we have not been able to get blood on site so as to be prepared for possible exsanguination.
- The key factor in increasing choice about home delivery is a good working relationship between the parents, the GP, and the midwife. Where this exists, ~70% of home delivery requests tend to come to fruition; where the GP is rated as being unsupportive, in a UK context, this figure drops to 54%.
- Everyone needs to know that transfer in labour is common in labours starting off as planned home deliveries (14%)—but that this need not mean that there is excess morbidity.[1]
- It is salutary to note that in 1994–5 only 18.5% of deliveries in England and Wales were considered 'normal' and without antenatal or postnatal complications.[2]

1 J Davies 1996 BMJ ii 1302 2 A Macfarlane 1998 BMJ 316 566

Pre-pregnancy counselling

The aim of pre-pregnancy care is to help parents embark upon pregnancy under conditions most likely to ensure optimal wellbeing for the fetus. At its simplest level this means ensuring that a woman is rubella (and chickenpox, p 216) immune prior to pregnancy, but areas covered include:

- Optimal control of chronic disease (eg diabetes) before conception.
- Discontinuation of teratogens prior to conception (p 159).
- Medication to protect the fetus from abnormality (eg folate supplements for neural tube defects, p 228 and below).
- Provision of expert information for those known to be at risk of abnormality so pregnancy or its avoidance is an informed choice and management of pregnancy with respect to any desirable tests (eg chorionic villus sampling, p 166) is planned. Regional genetic services give detailed pre-pregnancy counselling for a multitude of genetic conditions (p 210–2). In relevant ethnic populations take blood for thalassemia and sickle-cell tests (p 154).

For all women advice concerning the following may be relevant:

Diet To prevent neural tube defects and cleft lip all should have folate-rich foods and folic acid 0.4mg daily (eg Preconceive®) in the months before conception—until 13 weeks' gestation[1] (5mg/day PO if history of neural tube defect). These foods have >0.1mg of folic acid per serving: brussels sprouts, asparagus, spinach, kale, blackeye beans, fortified breakfast cereals. Avoid liver and vitamin A (vitamin A embryopathy risk).[2] Other vitamins at the time of conception may help prevent malformation.[3]

Cigarette smoking may decrease ovulations, result in abnormal sperm production, reduce sperm penetrating capacity, ↑rates of miscarriage (2-fold), and is associated with preterm labour and lighter-for-dates babies (mean is 3376g in non-smoker; smoker: 3200g). Reduced reading ability in smokers' children up to 11yrs shows that longer term effects may be important. About 17% of smoking mothers stop before or in pregnancy.

Alcohol consumption High levels of consumption are known to cause the fetal alcohol syndrome (p 226). Moderate drinking has not been shown to adversely affect the fetus but alcohol does cross the placenta and may affect the fetal brain. Miscarriage rates are higher among drinkers of alcohol. How to cut consumption: see p 454.

Spontaneous abortion (SA) At least 12% of first pregnancies spontaneously abort. Rates after 1 SA are increased to ~24%; after 2 SA to ~36%; after 3 to ~32% and after 4 to ~25%, so chances of a future pregnancy succeeding are ~2 in 3. Pregnancy order of SA/live pregnancies is also relevant: the more recent a live birth the more likely next time will be successful.

Recurrent spontaneous abortion Defined as ≥3 spontaneous recurrent abortions. See p 23. A potential cause may be found in ~50% and many of these are treatable.

Pre-pregnancy counselling is best done out by those who will look after the pregnant woman, but those with chronic medical conditions may require liaison between obstetrician and physician. In computerized practices it may be worth looking for likely beneficiaries of pre-pregnancy counselling by carefully perusing lists generated for these conditions:

- Diabetes mellitus
- Tropical travelers
- Frequent abortion
- Epilepsy
- Rubella-susceptible
- Pet-owners (toxoplasmosis)
- BP↑
- SLE
- PKU

Genetic history eg:
- Spina bifida etc
- Thalassaemia
- Duchenne's
- Cystic fibrosis

1 DoH 1992 Letter from Chief Medical Officer PL/CMO(92) 18 and G Shaw 1995 *Lancet* **346** 393
2 DoH 1990 Letter from Chief Medical Officer PL/CMO(90)10 3 A Czeizel 1993 BMJ **i** 1645

Antenatal care

The aims of antenatal care are to: •Detect any disease in the mother •Ameliorate the discomforts of pregnancy •Monitor and promote fetal wellbeing •Prepare mothers for birth •Monitor trends to prevent or detect early any complications of pregnancy: BP is the most important variable (eclampsia, p 96). Whenever the utility of other variables (weight, fundal height, urine analysis) is scrutinized, they are found to be insensitive, and not to fulfil the criteria for a good screening test (p 430).[1]

Who should give antenatal care? Not *all* women *need* see a doctor at least once per pregnancy or labour: midwives do very well on their own (with fewer interventions), calling in doctors *only if a specific need arises.*◄2►

The first antenatal visit is very comprehensive. ►Find an interpreter if she does not speak your language. *History:*

- Usual cycle length; LMP (a normal period?); expected delivery date ≈ 1yr and 7 days after LMP minus 3 months—unreliable if her last period was a withdrawal bleed; to allow for a cycle which is, say, 2 days *shorter* than 28 days, subtract, eg 2; add 2 or whatever the cycle is *long* by, if it is long.
- Contraception; drugs; past history, eg surgery to abdomen or pelvis.
- Any fertility problems; outcome and complications of past pregnancies.
- Is there family history of diabetes, BP↑, fetal abnormality or twins?
- Any past or family history of DVT or embolism? If so, ask a haematologist if screening is indicated for thrombophilia, *OHCM* p 620).
- Is she *poor* (eg gas/electricity supply cut off)? *Unmarried? Unsupported? Subject to domestic violence?* (See p 455.) *A substance abuser?* (See p 362.)
- Is the diet nutritious? Advise on avoiding pâtés and soft cheese (*OHCM* p 223) and vitamin overdose, eg no vitamin tablets or liver (p 94).

Examination: Check heart, lungs, breasts, nipples, BP, and abdomen. Consider pelvic examination if dates uncertain (unless dates will be confirmed later by scan), or if a cervical smear is needed. Any varicose veins?

Tests: Blood: Hb, group (antibodies if Rh–ve, p 242), syphilis and rubella serology, sickle test if black, α-fetoprotein/triple test (p 166 & 228), Hb electrophoresis + HBsAg (p 100 & 154) if relevant. Offer HIV test, with counselling (*OHCM* p 213). MSU for protein, glucose and bacteria. If she is foreign or is a TB contact or is a hospital worker, consider CXR after 14 weeks.

Ultrasound: in many units an ultrasound scan is routine (and an event for the parents) at 18 weeks, to confirm dates, look for fetal abnormalities and exclude ovarian cysts. If the mother is over 35 years old, consider amniocentesis at 16–18 weeks to exclude Down's syndrome (p 166).

Suggest: Parentcraft/relaxation classes; dental visit. Enquire about problems and anxieties. Consider need for *iron and folate* (p 139, p154, and p94).

Advise on: Smoking, alcohol, a healthy diet (*OHCM* p 482), and taking adequate rest. Ensure knowledge of social security benefits. Accustomed exercise and travel are OK (not to malarious areas, p 159) up to 34 weeks on most airlines. Intercourse is fine if there is no vaginal bleeding.

Later visits Check weight, urine for albumin and glucose, BP, fundal height, fetal movements (primips feel them ~19 weeks, earlier if multip), fetal heart—and lie and presentation from 32 weeks. Do Hb, eg at 28 & 36 weeks; look for Rh antibodies. Visits are monthly from 16 to 32 weeks, every 2 weeks until 36 weeks; then weekly. There is evidence that this is *too* often for most tests, but not often enough for BP and albuminuria.[3]

The head is usually engaged (p 84) by 37 weeks in Caucasian primips (if not, consider: large (or malpositioned) head, small pelvis or obstruction, placenta praevia, or wrong estimation of dates). At 36 weeks some check the pelvis clinically in primips. For favourable pelvis see page 86.

1 P Steer 1993 *BMJ* ii 697 ◄2►M Rowley/J Tucker 1996 *E-BM* i 84 & 191 3 D Daniel 1993 *BMJ* ii 1214

Hypertension in pregnancy

Essential hypertension Commoner in older multips, and present before pregnancy. You may need to modify or start therapy to keep BP <140/90mmHg. Severity and any association with pre-eclampsia (eg BP rise ≥+30/+15mmHg from baseline, progressive hyperuricaemia, proteinuria, or clotting activation) determines fetal outcome. Those with essential hypertension are 5 × more likely to develop pre-eclampsia than normotensive women. ►*When symptoms are episodic, think of phaeochromocytoma.*

Pre-eclampsia Terminology: see p 76. This is pregnancy-induced hypertension (PIH) with proteinuria ± oedema. It is a multisystem disorder originating in the placenta. The primary defect is failure of trophoblastic invasion of spiral arteries, so the arterial wall does not distend enough to allow sufficient blood flow to the placenta in late pregnancy, and increasing BP is a mechanism which partially compensates for this.[1] Pre-eclampsia also affects hepatic, renal and coagulation systems. It develops after 20 weeks and usually resolves within 10 days of delivery. Eclampsia (1 in 2000 maternities) is a major cause of maternal death and fetal morbidity/mortality. Pre-eclampsia is asymptomatic, so frequent screening is vital. It may recur in a subsequent pregnancy.

Predisposing factors *Maternal:* Primiparity; previous severe pre-eclampsia, family history of pre-eclampsia or eclampsia; short stature (<155cm) or overweight; age <20 or >35yrs; pre-existing migraine, BP↑ or renal disease increase risk. The incidence is lower in smokers. *Fetal:* Hydatidiform mole (↑BP at 20 weeks); multiple pregnancy; placental hydrops (eg rhesus disease). All have increased placental bulk.

Effects of pre-eclampsia Plasma volume is decreased. There is increased peripheral resistance. There may be placental ischaemia. If the BP is >180/140mmHg microaneurysms develop in arteries. DIC may develop. Oedema may develop suddenly (eg sudden weight gain of 1kg). Proteinuria is a late sign, indicating renal involvement which may be detected earlier by monitoring urate levels (levels >0.29μmol/L at 28 weeks, >0.34μmol/L at 32 weeks, >0.39μmol/L at 36 weeks suggest pre-eclampsia). Initially glomerular filtration is normal and only serum urate is raised but later urea and creatinine both increase. The liver may be involved (contributing to DIC)—and HELLP syndrome may be present (p 158). The placenta may develop infarcts. Fetal asphyxia, abruption, and small babies (p 104 & 119) may also occur.

Prevention of eclampsia This is achieved by regular antenatal BP checks and urinalysis. Large trials have diminished initial hopes for the role of aspirin. Calcium supplementation reduces BP and rates of pre-eclampsia, but it has not yet been shown to benefit mothers or babies in UK settings.

Symptomatic pre-eclampsia may mimic viral illness with *headache, chest* or *epigastric pain, vomiting,* and *pulse*↑—but also *visual disturbance, shaking, hyperreflexia,* and *irritability.* The mother is now in danger of *generalized seizures* (eclampsia) and urgent admission and treatment must occur. Death may be imminent from *stroke* (commonest), *hepatic, renal* or *cardiac failure.*

Management: early phase Admit[2] if BP rises by >30/20mmHg over booking BP; if BP reaches 160/100; if ≥140/90 with proteinuria, or if there is growth retardation. In hospital, measure BP 2–4-hourly, weigh daily, test all urine for protein, monitor fluid balance, check U&E, LFTs, urate and placental function, and platelets (beware falls to <110 × 10^9/L) regularly. Also do regular antenatal cardiotocography with ultrasound to check growth, and biophysical profiles. In asymptomatic pre-eclampsia, raised BP may be treated with drugs, eg methyldopa[3] 250mg–1g/6h under supervision in hospital if BP rises to 170/110mmHg, in order to buy time for fetal maturation, and if all other variables are satisfactory. If signs worsen deliver the baby (liaise with paediatricians). Delivery is the only cure. All women with pre-eclampsia should be given H_2-blockers when they go into labour.[4]

►►Managing impending eclampsia It is almost impossible to foretell eclamptic convulsions—so focus on ensuring that the patient is in a specialist unit, and, if possible, delivered before this stage is reached. If BP needs reducing, hydralazine 10mg IM/IV slowly may be given. (Chewing a 10mg nifedipine capsule may be a fast-acting alternative.) Close and repeated monitoring of BP is essential, and hydralazine can be repeated in boluses of 5mg IV slowly or by continuous IVI (50mg in 500mL 5% dextrose gives a 1mg/10mL solution—give at 200–300μg/min). Labetalol is an alternative to hydralazine. Dose: 50–100mg IV every 20–30min or 20–160mg/h as IV infusion.[3]

Whatever the hour, summon your consultant (not just the registrar, and do not make do with telephone advice).[2] ►*Do not leave the bedside.*

Catheterize and watch urine output. If the mother fits, protect the airway and give magnesium sulfate, as below.

Using magnesium sulfate in eclampsia Magnesium sulfate is better than diazepam once a fit has occurred and makes further fits less likely.[5]
Loading dose example: 4g in 100mL normal saline IVI over at least 5 mins.
Maintenance dose: 25g in 500mL IVI over 24h (1g/h).
Recurrent fits: Give 2–4g in 100mL IVI over at least 5 mins (2g if <70kg)
Monitoring: Check •Respiratory rate (should be >16/min) and Patellar reflexes every 15 min (see below) •Urine output (should be >25mL/h).
►Magnesium sulfate can cause paralysis due to toxicity at the neuromuscular junction. Loss of patellar reflexes, slurred speech, diplopia, flushes, and nausea precede respiratory depression and respiratory arrest. Magnesium sulfate is cleared by the kidney and so doses should be reduced if renal impairment exists (if urine output <25mL/h halve the maintenence dose to 0.5mL/24h). ►If respiratory depression or arrest occurs, stop magnesium therapy and give antidote: calcium gluconate 1g in 10mL normal saline IVI.

Diazepam may still have a rôle in suppressing fits that do not spontaneously remit, or those recurring at short intervals. 5–10mg can be given by slow IV, repeated every 15–20mins to keep the patient drowsy but rousable. Once therapeutic levels of magnesium have been achieved, diazepam should not be needed. In status epilepticus, take to ITU to paralyse and ventilate.

Pitfalls in the management of eclampsia and pre-eclampsia
- Believing that the disease will behave predictably, and that blood pressure is a good marker of disease activity. It is not.
- Ignoring mild proteinuria (eg 1+). Once this is present in every sample the patient may be dead within 24h.
- Believing that antihypertensives stop pre-eclampsia's course. They don't. Delivery is the only cure. Diuretics may further deplete the already reduced plasma volume, and are especially contraindicated (except in the rare left ventricular failure or laryngeal oedema complicating pre-eclampsia).
- Believing that delivery removes risk. In the UK, half of eclamptic fits occur postpartum of which half are >48h postpartum. Continue vigilance until clinically and biochemically normal. Avoid early discharge.
- Ergometrine should not be used for the third stage (oxytocin may be used). Ergometrine further increases BP so would risk stroke.
- Replace significant blood loss meticulously. Risks are hypovolaemia or fatal fluid over-load (lung injury→adult respiratory distress syndrome). Have one person (the most experienced) in charge of all the IVIs.[2]
- Failure to inform anaesthetists early and use intensive care facilities.

1 DA Clark 1994 *Lancet* **344** 969 2 DoH 1998 *Confidential Enquiry into Maternal Deaths* HMSO
3 1993 *Drug Ther Bul* **31** 53 4 DoH 1994 *Confidential Enquiry into Maternal Deaths*, p95, HMSO
5 Collaborative Eclampsia Trial 1995 *Lancet* **345** 1455 & E-BM 1996 **1**(2) 39,44 6 R Fox 1995 *BMJ* **ii** 1433

Antenatal infection

Maternal infections, mostly viral, affecting the fetus were previously known as 'TORCH' infections: **t**oxoplasmosis, **o**ther (eg syphilis), **r**ubella, **c**MV, **h**erpes (and hepatitis). The first 4 are acquired antenatally—herpes and hepatitis usually perinatally. The term TORCH is now obsolete as other agents are important (chickenpox; HIV, p 216–7). *See also* Erythrovirus (=Parvovirus, p 214). Zoster reactivation in pregnancy is *not* a risk for the baby.

Rubella Childhood vaccination prevents rubella-susceptibility. ►Asymptomatic reinfection can occur making serology essential in all pregnant rubella contacts. Routine antenatal screening finds those needing puerperal vaccination (avoid pregnancy for 3 months: vaccine is live). Symptoms (p 214) are absent in 50%. The fetus is most at risk in the first 16 weeks' gestation. 50–60% of fetuses are affected if maternal primary infection is in the first month of gestation: <5% are affected if infection is at 16 weeks. Risk of fetal damage is much lower (<5%) with re-infection.[1] Cataract is associated with infection at 8–9 weeks, deafness at 5–7 weeks (can occur with second trimester infection), cardiac lesions at 5–10 weeks. Other features: purpura, jaundice, hepatosplenomegaly, thrombocytopenia, cerebral palsy, microcephaly, mental retardation, cerebral calcification, microphthalmia, retinitis, growth disorder. Abortion or stillbirth may occur. If suspected in the mother seek expert help. Compare serum antibody levels 10 days apart and look for IgM antibody 4–5 weeks from incubation period or date of contact.

Cytomegalovirus (CMV) In the UK, CMV is a commoner cause of congenital retardation than rubella. Maternal infection is usually mild or asymptomatic. Symptoms are fever ± lymphadenopathy and sometimes sore throat. Up to 5/1000 live births are infected, of whom 5% will develop early multiple handicaps, and have cytomegalic inclusion disease (with non-specific features resembling rubella syndrome, plus microcephaly, choroidoretinitis). Another 5% go on to develop cerebral calcification (IQ↓); sensorineural deafness and psychomotor retardation. Diagnosis (paired sera) may be difficult. Also test throat swab, urine culture and baby's serum after birth. Reducing women's exposure to toddlers' urine (the source of much infection) during pregnancy can limit spread. NB: reactivation of old CMV may occur in pregnancy; it is rare for this to affect the baby. One way to know that +ve serology does not reflect old infection is to do serology (or freeze a sample) in the pre-pregnancy clinic.

Toxoplasmosis 40% of fetuses are affected if the mother has the illness (2–7/1000 pregnancies); the earlier in pregnancy the more the damage. Symptoms are similar to glandular fever. Fever, rash, and eosinophilia also occur. If symptomatic, the CNS prognosis is poor. Diagnose by reference laboratory IgG and IgM tests. Start spiramycin promptly in infected mothers. In symptomatic non-immune women test every 10 weeks through pregnancy. In those infected consider fetal cord blood sampling, eg at 21 weeks for IgM to see if the fetus is infected. All affected babies (diagnose by serology) should have pyrimethamine, 21 days of 0.25mg/kg/6h PO + sulfadiazine 50mg/kg/12h PO with folic acid supplements to protect against pyrimethamine's folate antagonism. Prevention includes avoiding eating raw meat, washing hands after touching raw meat, wearing gloves when gardening or dealing with cat litter, and avoiding sheep during lambing time.

HIV Babies have a 15% chance of acquiring HIV if the mother is +ve (higher risk in Africa; but HIV-2 is less likely than HIV-1 to be passed on). Offer mothers tests for HIV, only after counselling (*OHCM* p 212). Serology depends on detecting IgG and IgM antibodies (false +ve in up to 1.6%). Those with +ve serology should not be given steroids to accelerate fetal lung maturity. ►Vertical transmission can occur during vaginal delivery (first twins are twice as commonly infected as second), and Caesarean section is protective, possibly cutting neonatal infection by almost half[2]—as does zidovudine 100mg 5 times a day PO antepartum, and, during labour (2mg/kg IVI over 1h, and then 1mg/kg IVI until delivery), and then 2m/kg/6h PO for the baby for 6 weeks. Premature babies are more at risk of vertical transmission. Bottle feeding reduces vertical transmission—possibly by up to 50% (but bottle feeding is hazardous in some communities). Intrauterine exposure to zidovudine appears safe.[3]

Serology is difficult as transferred maternal antibodies persist up to 18 months in uninfected infants—but gene amplification via a polymerase chain reaction can detect neonatal HIV proviral sequences. Culture is also possible—but not all infected children give +ve cultures at birth, and specialized investigations may need to be performed, eg the detection of IgA (which does not cross the placenta) by modified Western blotting.

Intrauterine HIV is associated with prematurity and growth retardation (in developing countries, but not in Europe). Clinical illness appears sooner than in adult AIDS (eg at aged 6 months)—with hepatosplenomegaly, failure to thrive, encephalopathy, recurrent fevers, respiratory diseases (interstitial lymphocytic pneumonitis), lymphadenopathy, salmonella septicaemia, pneumocystis and CMV infection. Death is usually from respiratory failure or overwhelming infection. Mortality: 20% at 18 months. ►For treatment and advice on how to prevent transmission in labour, see p 155.

Intrauterine syphilis Routine maternal screening occurs (in the UK, numbers needed to screen to prevent 1 case=55,700);[4] if active infection is found treat the mother with procaine penicillin, eg as half a 1.8g ampoule of Bicillin®, IM daily for 10 days. Neonatal signs: rhinitis, snuffles, rash, hepatosplenomegaly, lymphadenopathy, anaemia, jaundice, ascites, hydrops, nephrosis, meningitis, ± keratitis and nerve deafness. *Nasal discharge exam*: Spirochaetes; *x-rays:* Perichondritis; *CSF:* ↑Monocytes and protein with +ve serology. *Treatment:* Give procaine penicillin 37mg/kg/24h IM for 3 weeks.

Listeria This affects 6–15/100,000 pregnancies—more during epidemics. Maternal symptoms: Fever, shivering, myalgia, headache, sore throat, cough, vomiting, diarrhoea, vaginitis. Abortion (can be recurrent), premature labour, and stillbirth may occur. Infection is usually via infected food (eg milk, soft cheeses, pâté). ►Do blood cultures in any pregnant patient with unexplained fever for ≥48h. Serology, vaginal and rectal swabs do not help (it may be commensal there). See *OHCM* p 223.

Perinatal infection usually occurs in the second or third trimester. 20% of affected fetuses are stillborn. Fetal distress in labour is common. An early postnatal feature is respiratory distress from pneumonia. There may be convulsions, hepatosplenomegaly, pustular or petechial rashes, conjunctivitis, fever, leucopenia. Meningitis presents more commonly after perinatal infection. Diagnosis is from culture of blood, CSF, meconium, and placenta. Infant mortality: 30%. Isolate baby (nosocomial spread can occur). Treat with ampicillin 50mg/kg/6h IV and gentamicin 3mg/kg/12h IV until 1 week after fever subsides. Monitor gentamicin levels.

Sheep-borne conditions Listeriosis, toxoplasmosis and ovine chlamydia (*Chlamydia psittaci*) can be contracted from sheep. Ovine chlamydial infection is rare, can cause DIC, septicaemia and renal failure in pregnant women and abortion of the fetus. Diagnose by serology; treat with erythromycin or tetracycline. ►Pregnant women should not handle sheep or lambs.

1 G Gilbert 1991 *Infectious Diseases in Pregnancy & Newborn Infant* Harwood, Switzerland 2 European Collaborative Study 1994 *Lancet* **343** 1464 3 S Lee 1999 *JAMA* **281** 151 4 A-K Hurtig 1998 *BMJ* **ii** 1617

Perinatal infection

Hepatitis B virus (HBV) Although chronic carriers were uncommon in the UK, with the rise of drug addiction and a large immigrant population it is becoming more frequent, and some are now recommend that all mothers be screened. If the mother develops acute infection in the mid- or third trimester there is high risk of perinatal infection. Her risk of death is 0.5–3%. Most neonatal infection occurs at birth.

Hepatitis E Maternal morality is 20–40%.* Death is usually postpartum, preceded by coma and massive PPH. A vaccine is awaited.

Herpes hominis 80% is due to herpes simplex type II virus. 50% of babies will be infected during birth if the mother has active cervical lesions. Take viral cultures weekly (from 36 weeks) from the cervix of all women with a history of herpes. If virus is present, aim for elective Caesarean section. When membranes rupture spontaneously still perform Caesarean if within 4h of rupture. Neonatal infection usually appears at 5–21 days with vesicular pustular lesions, often at the presenting part or sites of minor trauma (eg scalp electrode). Periocular and conjunctival lesions may occur. With systemic infection encephalitis (focal fits or neurological signs), jaundice, hepatosplenomegaly, collapse and DIC may occur. Infected neonates should be isolated and treated with aciclovir (p 256). Seek expert help.

Chlamydia trachomatis Associations: low birth weight, premature membrane rupture, fetal death. ~⅓ of infected mothers have affected babies. Conjunctivitis develops 5–14 days after birth and may show minimal inflammation or purulent discharge. The cornea is not usually involved.
Complications: Chlamydia pneumonitis, pharyngitis or otitis media.
Tests: Immunofluorescence or culture. Giemsa smear: many inclusions.
Treatment: 1% tetracycline ointment or drops 6-hourly for 3 weeks, + erythromycin 10mg/kg/6h PO for ~3 weeks eliminates lung organisms. Give parents/partners erythromycin. *During* pregnancy, erythromycin is used, but amoxicillin 500mg/8h PO for 1 week works OK, and is better tolerated.[1]

Gonococcal conjunctivitis Occurs within ~4 days of birth, with purulent discharge and lid swelling, ± corneal hazing, corneal rupture and panophthalmitis. *Treatment:* Infants born to those with known gonorrhoea should have *benzylpenicillin* 30mg/kg IM stat or a *cefalosporin* (eg *cefotaxime*), and *chloramphenicol* 0.5% eye-drops within 1h of birth. For active gonococcal infection give *benzylpenicillin* 25mg/kg/12h IM and 3-hourly 0.5% chloramphenicol drops for 7 days. Isolate the baby.

Ophthalmia neonatorum This is purulent discharge from the eye of a neonate <21 days old. Originally referring to *Neisseria gonorrhoea* there are many causes: chlamydiae, herpes virus, staphylococci, streptococci and pneumococci, *E coli* and other Gram –ve organisms. *Tests:* In a baby with a sticky eye take swabs for bacterial and viral culture, microscopy (look for intracellular gonococci) and chlamydia (eg immunofluorescence).

Clostridium perfringens Suspect this in any complication of criminal abortion—and whenever intracellular encapsulated Gram +ve rods are seen on genital swabs. It may also complicate death *in utero*, and it may also infect haematomas, and other anaerobic sites. *Clinical features:* Endometritis → septicaemia/gangrene → myoglobinuria → renal failure → death.[1]
Management: •Surgically debride all devitalized tissue. •Hyperbaric O_2. •High-dose IV benzylpenicillin (erythromycin if serious penicillin allergy). The use of gas gangrene antitoxin is controversial. Seek expert help.

For perinatal **listeria** and **streptococcal infection**, see p 260.

*See OTM 3e 1996 **1** M Alary 1994 *Lancet* **344** 1461

Prevention of hepatocellular cancer

Chronic infection will occur in most HBV-infected neonates, and a significant number develop hepatocellular cancer by age 30–40yrs (and most will develop cirrhosis by 50–60yrs)—so immunization really is important. ►Give infants of known carriers hepatitis immune globulin 0.5mL IM within 12h of birth, and hepatitis B vaccine 0.5mL (eg Engerix B® 10μg) within 7 days of birth and at 1 and 6 months.

Prematurity

►This is a leading cause of perinatal mortality and morbidity.

Premature infants are those born before 37 weeks' gestation. Prevalence: ~6% singletons, 46% of twin, 79% of triplet or higher order deliveries.[1] About 2% are before 32 weeks—when neonatal problems are greatest. In 25%, delivery is elective (p 110). 10% are due to multiple pregnancy; 25% are due to APH, cervical incompetence, amnionitis, uterine abnormalities, diabetes, polyhydramnios, pyelonephritis or other infections. In 40% the cause is unknown, but abnormal genital tract colonization (bacterial vaginosis) with ureaplasma and *Mycoplasma hominis* is implicated, either as a risk factor or risk marker.[2]

Management of preterm rupture of membranes Admit; take MSU, and HVS—using a sterile bivalve speculum. If liquor is not obvious its presence is suggested if nitrazine sticks (which are pH-sensitive) turn black (false +ve with infected vaginal discharge, semen, blood and urine). In 80%, membrane rupture will be followed by onset of labour. The problem with the 20% who do not go into labour is balancing the advantages of remaining *in utero* for increasing maturity and surfactant production against the threat of infection (which accounts for 20% of neonatal deaths after premature rupture of membranes). Intrauterine infection supervenes after membranes have ruptured in 10% within 48h, 26% by 72h, 40% by >72h. Prophylactic antibiotics may delay labour.[3] If infection develops, take blood cultures and give IV antibiotics (eg ampicillin 500mg/6h IV + netilmicin 150mg/12h IV) and expedite labour (p 110). If labour supervenes it should be allowed to progress. In the few cases where liquor ceases to drain for more than 48h the mother can be gradually mobilized.

Management of preterm labour In 50% contractions cease spontaneously. Treating the cause (eg pyelonephritis) may make it cease. Attempts to suppress contractions (tocolysis) are unlikely to succeed if membranes are ruptured or the cervix >4cm dilated. Use between 24–34 weeks. Consider transfer to hospital with SCBU facilities. Call paediatrician to attend to the baby at birth. See cord-cutting recommendations p 82.

Tocolytic drugs Absolute CI: chorioamnionitis, fetal death or lethal abnormality, condition (fetal or maternal) needing immediate delivery. Relative CI: fetal growth retardation or distress, pre-eclampsia, placenta praevia, abruption, cervix >4cm. The ritodrine regimen (simpler than salbutamol): see opposite. Continue infusion for 12–48h after contractions cease. Oral β-agonists, eg ritodrine 80mg/8h for 7 days may reduce relapse rates.[4] Monitor: maternal pulse, BP, T°, contractions and FHR. Salbutamol is an alternative (SE similar). Nifedipine 30mg PO stat (+20mg PO 90min later if still contracting), then 20mg/8h PO is as effective. SE: ↓BP, headache, flushing, transient tachycardia; myocardial infarction has also been reported.[5]

Glucocorticoids Betamethasone or dexamethasone 12mg/12h IM twice promotes fetal surfactant production, lowering mortality and complications of RDS (p 240) by 40–50%; <6> they also help close patent ductuses. Use before 34 weeks only. Avoid if severe pre-eclampsia, infection, or if HIV+ve. Benefit is maximal after 24h; effects last a week (after which doses can be repeated).

1 A Macfarlane 1998 *BMJ* **i** 566 2 P Hay 1994 *BMJ* **i** 295 3 B Mercer 1995 *Lancet* **346** 1271 4 C Holleboom 1996 *Br J Obs Gyn* **103** 702 5 S Guid Oel 1999 *NEJM* **340** 154.. <6> PA Crowley 1996 *E-BM* **1** 92

Prematurity, survival, and disability—the figures[1]

►One major, landmark question is: *Is the baby over 28 weeks' gestation?*

- The disability rate is 25% if gestation is <28 weeks—but half this if gestation is 28–29 weeks).
- 10% of those who survive at gestations <28 weeks will never be independently mobile, or communicate intelligibly with others.
- Only 4% of babies born before 24 weeks will survive, and of survivors, >50% will be severely disabled.
- Use of surfactant (p 240) has not reduced the viability threshold, or rates of severe disability in babies born at <28 weeks' gestation.

Guidance for infusion rates of ritodrine

Syringe pump (Add 3×5mL ampoules of ritodrine to 35mL of 5% dextrose.)		Controlled infusion device (Add 3×5mL ampoules ritodrine to 500mL of 5% dextrose.)	
Dose	*Rate*	*Dose*	*Rate*
50 micrograms/min	1mL/hour	50 micrograms/min	10mL/hour
100 micrograms/min	2mL/hour	100 micrograms/min	20mL/hour
150 micrograms/min	3mL/hour	150 micrograms/min	30mL/hour
200 micrograms/min	4mL/hour	200 micrograms/min	40mL/hour
250 micrograms/min	5mL/hour	250 micrograms/min	50mL/hour
300 micrograms/min	6mL/hour	300 micrograms/min	60mL/hour
350*micrograms/min	7mL/hour	*350 micrograms/min	70mL/hour

*maximum recommended dose

Start with 50 micrograms/minute. Increase by 50 micrograms/minute every 15 minutes until contractions cease or side-effects (maternal pulse >140 beats/min, FHR↑ by >20 beats/min, maternal systolic BP falls by >20mmHg, tremor, nausea, vomiting, flushing). Usual dose: 150–350 micrograms per minute. Total daily intravenous dose should not exceed 120 milligrams. Continue infusion for 12–48 hours after contractions cease.

Problems with tocolytics The main problems are hyperglycaemia and pulmonary oedema from fluid overload. Use only on specialist advice in those with known heart disease.[2] Avoid in those prone to supraventricular tachycardia, eg with Wolff–Parkinson–White or Lown–Ganong–Levine syndromes.

Monitoring

- Maternal pulse and blood pressure every 15 minutes.
- Maternal temperature and blood glucose 4-hourly (eg BM-Test® sticks).
- Monitor contractions and fetal heart rate.
- Keep strict fluid records (input/output charts).
- Check U&E every 24 hours (to avoid hypokalaemia) or more often if indicated. Check ECG if hypokalaemic.
- Auscultate lung fields regularly. Monitor maternal O_2 saturation if equipment is available.

►Chest pain, dyspnoea or dry cough, should lead to immediate cessation of infusion.

1 W Tin 1997 BMJ i 107 2 M de Swiet 1995 in *Medical Disorders in Obstetric Practice* 3e, Blackwell p 160

Intrauterine growth retardation

►When talking to parents, avoid the term *retardation* as this may imply to them the inevitability of mental handicap—which is not the case.

Distinguish premature babies from those who are small-for-gestational age (SGA): they are at risk from different problems after birth.

Causes of growth retardation Growth retarded (SGA) neonates are those weighing < the 10th centile for their gestational age (Tables, p 294).

Predisposing factors: Multiple pregnancy; malformation; infection; maternal smoking, diabetes, hypertension (eg pre-eclampsia), severe anaemia, heart and renal disease. About 10% are to mothers who will only ever produce small babies. Where placental insufficiency has been the cause, head circumference is relatively spared (the baby has been starved). This is then called asymmetrical intrauterine growth retardation (IUGR).

Antenatal diagnosis 50% are not detected before birth, and many babies suspected of IUGR turn out not to have it. Measuring changes in fundal height from the symphysis pubis is a reasonable method of measuring fetal growth, especially if used with centile charts. Oligohydramnios (p 120) and poor fetal movements are other indications of placental insufficiency. If growth retardation is suspected, growth *in utero* can be monitored by serial ultrasound examinations of head circumference and abdominal circumference. If umbilical cord Doppler blood flows are normal the outcome of growth retarded pregnancies is better (fewer premature births and stillbirths). Those with abnormal Dopplers may benefit from maternal low-dose aspirin (p 119), eg 75mg/24h PO. Biophysical profile monitoring (p 118) and antenatal cardiotocography (p 116) are used to try to detect those babies who are becoming hypoxic *in utero* and who would benefit from delivery. Advise the mother to stop smoking, to use a fetal kick chart (p 116) and to take plenty of rest.

Labour and aftercare Growth retarded fetuses are more susceptible to hypoxia, so monitor in labour (p 116). After birth, temperature regulation may be a problem, so ensure a warm welcome; nurse those <2kg in an incubator. After being relatively hypoxic *in utero* the Hb at birth is high, so jaundice is more common. They have little stored glycogen so are prone to hypoglycaemia. Feed within 2h of birth and measure blood glucose before each 3-hourly feed. If hypoglycaemic despite regular feeds, transfer to a special care unit. They are more susceptible to infection. Birth reveals those for whom abnormality was the cause of growth retardation.

Distinguishing growth retardation from prematurity Before 34 weeks' gestation there is no breast bud tissue, from then it develops at 1mm diameter/week. Ear cartilage develops between 35 and 39 weeks so premature babies' ears do not spring back when folded. Testes lie in the inguinal canal at 35 weeks, in the scrotum from 37. Labia minora are exposed in premature girls. Skin creases on the anterior ⅓ of the foot appear by 35 weeks (on anterior ⅔ by 39, and all over from 39). 'Prems' have red, hairy skin. Vernix is made from 28 weeks and is maximal at 36 weeks. Prems do not lie with legs flexed until 32 weeks. All limbs are flexed from 36 weeks.

Effects of IUGR in adult life Many studies have confirmed ↑risk from:

- Hypertension
- Coronary artery disease
- Non-insulin-dependent diabetes mellitus
- Autoimmune thyroid disease

So fetal malnutrition casts a long shadow. *Specific* early deficiencies are important too (eg iodine, iron). Supplements in one Guatemalan group resulted in better cognition at 15yrs follow-up compared with the control group.[1]

1 N Scrimshaw 1997 *BMJ* ii 825

2. Obstetrics

►►Fetal distress

Fetal distress signifies hypoxia. Prolonged or repeated hypoxia causes fetal acidosis. An early sign may be the passage of meconium in labour (p 128). Other signs that the fetus may be hypoxic are a fetal tachycardia persisting above 160 beats per minute (tachycardia may also occur if the mother has a high temperature or is dehydrated). Hypoxia may also be reflected by loss of variability of the baseline in the fetal heart rate trace and slowing and irregularity of the heart rate (especially late decelerations—p 116). ►►If the heart rate falls below 100 beats per minute urgent assessment is required. Hypoxia may be confirmed by the use of fetal blood sampling (p 116). When significant hypoxia appears to be present (eg pH <7.24), deliver promptly (eg by the quickest route available, eg Caesarean section or vaginal extraction). In complete anoxia the pH falls by 0.1 unit per minute.

►►Obstetric shock

Most obstetric shock is associated with severe haemorrhage. It should be remembered that with abruption, actual bleeding may be far in excess of that revealed *per vaginam* (p 108). Other causes of shock may be: ruptured uterus (p 134), inverted uterus (p 140); amniotic fluid embolus (p 143), pulmonary embolism, adrenal haemorrhage and septicaemia.

Septicaemia may lack classical signs (eg pyrexia) and must be considered where profound persisting shock is present,[1] be appropriately investigated (eg blood cultures), and treated, eg amoxicillin/clavulanic acid 1g/6h IV + metronidazole 500mg/8h IVI (+ gentamicin 1.5mg/kg/8h IV given over >3min; do levels, but not needed acutely, see *OHCM* p 181). Prompt resuscitation is required (see individual pages for management). Renal function and urine output should always be measured after shock has occurred (p 160). A late complication can be Sheehan's syndrome (also called Simmonds' disease) whereby pituitary necrosis leads to lack of thyroid-stimulating hormone, adrenocorticotrophic hormone and the gonadotrophic hormones hence leading to hypothyroidism, Addisonian symptoms and genital atrophy.

1 DoH 1991 *Report on Confidential Enquiries into Maternal Deaths in the UK 1985-7* HMSO pp 67 & 146

Postmaturity (prolonged pregnancy)

Prolonged pregnancy is defined as that exceeding 42 completed weeks or more from the LMP. Affecting 5–10% of pregnancies it is associated with increased perinatal mortality (5/1000 if 37–42 weeks, 9.7/1000 if >42 weeks). The dangers are placental insufficiency, and problems during labour due to the fetus being larger (25% are >4000g), the fetal skull more ossified and less easily moulded, the passage of meconium more common (25–42% labours), and fetal distress more common. Stillbirth rate is ↑ × 4, neonatal deaths ↑ × 3, and neonatal seizures ↑ × 10 in pregnancies going beyond 42 weeks compared with birth between 37 and 42 weeks.

Antepartum monitoring with use of kick charts (p 116), cardiotocography, and biophysical profiles (p 118) can be used to try to detect fetuses who may be becoming hypoxic. Doppler studies of cord blood flow may be used to look for absent end diastolic flow as a predictor of fetal compromise. Without evidence to suggest problems, induction should be recommended from 41+ weeks[1] after which time there are higher rates of Caesarean section for those managed 'conservatively'. Use ultrasound dates not LMP for calculating gestation.[2] 'Membrane sweeps' remain a valid non-pharmacological prelude to induction; more women go into spontaneous labour if as much membrane as possible is swept from the lower segment at examination between 41–42 weeks than if examined unswept.[3] Induction with vaginal prostaglandins may be associated with lower rates of instrumental delivery than induction with oxytocin.[4] It is estimated that 500 inductions are needed to prevent 1 perinatal death.[1] After induction, monitor the fetus in labour (p 116).

Postnatal signs of postmaturity: Dry, cracked, peeling, loose skin; decreased subcutaneous tissue; meconium staining of nails and cord.

Prelabour rupture of membranes at term[5]

2–4% of term births are complicated by prelabour rupture of membranes without labour spontaneously starting within 24h. It is usual practice when labour does not ensue within a few hours of membrane rupture to start labour with an oxytocin IVI to reduce the possibility of ascending infection. It is helpful to give vaginal prostaglandins when the cervix appears unfavourable. Routine use of prostaglandins does not reduce the rate of Caesarean section (but does reduce time to delivery). Waiting 12h after the membranes rupture before instituting oxytocin is associated with lower rates of Caesarean section (rate ~11%) as opposed to early use of oxytocin (rate ~15–20%). When delay is intended maternal temperature must be monitored and oxytocin started should pyrexia develop.

1 J Grant 1994 *Br J Obs Gyn* **101** 99 **2** J Garlosi 1997 *Br J Obs Gyn* **104** 792 **3** H Allott 1993 *Br J Ob Gyn* **100** 898–903 & M El-Torkey 1992 *Ibid* **99** 543 & J Grant 1993 *Ibid* 100 889 & M Griffiths 1995 BMJ **ii** 257 **4** *Drug Ther Bul* 1997 **35** 17 **5** S Duncan 1992 *Br J Obs Gyn* **99** 543

►►Antepartum haemorrhage (APH)

Traditionally this has been defined as bleeding at >28 weeks' gestation. Any bleeding in pregnancy is associated with increased perinatal mortality. Severe bleeds can cause maternal death.

►Avoid vaginal examination: placenta praevias may bleed catastrophically.

Dangerous causes Abruption, placenta praevia, vasa praevia (here the baby may bleed to death).
Other uterine sources: Circumvallate placenta, placental sinuses.
Lower genital tract sources: Cervical polyps, erosions and carcinoma, cervicitis, vaginitis, vulval varicosities.

Placental abruption ('Accidental haemorrhage') Part of the placenta becomes detached from the uterus. The outcome depends on the amount of blood loss and degree of separation. The cause is unknown but it is associated with pre-eclampsia, may recur in a subsequent pregnancy (6%), is commoner in smokers and may complicate external cephalic version. Bleeding may be well localized to one placental area and there may be delay before bleeding is revealed.
Consequences: Placental insufficiency may cause fetal anoxia or death. Compression of uterine muscles by blood causes tenderness, and may prevent good contraction at all stages of labour, so beware a PPH (which occurs in ~25%). Posterior abruptions may present with backache. There may be uterine hypercontractility (>7 contractions per 15min). Thromboplastin release may cause DIC (10%). Concealed loss may cause maternal shock after which beware renal failure and Sheehan's syndrome (p 106).

Placenta praevia (For terminology and complications see p 78). The placenta lies in the lower uterine segment. Bleeding is always revealed.

Distinguishing *abruption* ——►	from *placenta praevia:*
Shock out of keeping with the visible loss	Shock in proportion to the visible loss
Pain constant	No pain
Tender, tense uterus	Uterus not tender
Normal lie and presentation	Both may be abnormal
Fetal heart: absent/distressed	Fetal heart usually normal
Coagulation problems	Coagulation problems rare
Beware pre-eclampsia, DIC, anuria	Small bleeds before large

Note: the risk of PPH is increased in both conditions. The lower segment may not contract well after a placenta praevia.

Management of APH Always admit. ►►If bleeding is severe call emergency ambulance, put up IVI, take bloods and raise legs. Give O_2 at 15L/min via mask with reservoir. On admission, if shocked give fresh ABO Rh compatible or O Rh–ve blood (eg 6U, 2 IVIs) fast until systolic BP >100mmHg. Send blood for clotting screen. Catheterize bladder; keep renal output >30mL/h. Call anaesthetist to monitor fluids (CVP lines help). *Summon expert help urgently.* If bleeding is severe, *deliver*—Caesarean section for placenta praevia (sometimes for abruption, or induction). Beware PPH.

For milder bleeding, set up IVI, do Hb, crossmatch, coagulation studies and U&E. Check pulse, BP and loss regularly. Establish diagnosis (ultrasound of placenta, speculum examination). If placenta praevia is the diagnosis, keep on the ward until delivery (usually by Caesarean section at 37–38 weeks). If pain and bleeding from a small abruption settles and the fetus is not compromised the woman may go home (after anti-D, if indicated), but treat as 'high-risk' pregnancy thereafter. Arrange follow-up.

Using anti-D immunoglobulin[1]

Dose 250u for gestations <20 weeks, 500u if >20 weeks. Give into deltoid (buttock absorption is too slow) as soon as possible after incident, at latest within 72h. After 20 weeks do Kleihauer test (FBC bottle of maternal blood; fetal RBCs therein are less susceptible to lysis, enabling them to be counted, so measuring the bleed's volume).

Postnatal use 500u is the normal dose after 20 weeks' gestation. 37% of Rh–ve women give birth to Rh–ve babies and these women do not need anti-D.

- Anti-D should be given to all Rh–ve women where the baby's group cannot be determined (eg macerated stillbirths), or if circumstances are such that the baby's group is unknown 72h post delivery.
- Do a Kleihauer test on all those eligible for anti-D. You cannot get round this requirement by giving everyone a double dose of anti-D, hoping that this will be enough. Such a policy would waste anti-D (volunteer donor-dependent) and would undertreat some patients.[2] 500u anti-D can suppress immunization by up to 4mL of fetal red cells (8mL of fetal blood), but 1% of women have transplacental haemorrhage (TPH) of >4mL, especially after manual removal of placenta, and with Caesarean section. A Kleihauer test is especially important in stillbirth, as massive spontaneous transplacental haemorrhage can be the cause of fetal death. Where >4mL TPH is suggested by the Kleihauer screen, a formal estimation of the TPH volume is required and 500u anti-D given for every 4mL fetal cells transfused (maximum 5000u anti-D at 2 IM sites/24h). Liaise with the Regional Transfusion Service in the UK. Check maternal blood every 48h to determine clearance of cells and need for continuing anti-D.
- Don't give prenatal anti-D if antibodies to anti-D are present.
- Any mother receiving anti-D prenatally (see below), should also receive it postnatally unless she delivers a Rh-negative baby.

Use of anti-D in abortion in rhesus negative mothers

1. Anti-D should be given to all having surgical terminations of pregnancy unless they are already known to have anti-D antibodies.
2. Anti-D should always be given where spontaneous abortion is followed by instrumentation.
3. Anti-D should be given where spontaneous complete abortion occurs after 12 weeks' gestation.
4. With threatened abortion after 12 weeks give anti-D; if bleeding continues intermittently give anti-D 6-weekly until delivery.
5. With threatened abortion before 12 weeks, determine the mother's group and give anti-D if she is negative, and the pregnancy seems viable. Give anti-D within 96h of bleed.

Use of anti-D in pregnancy in Rh–ve mothers

1. Significant TPH may occur: with chorionic villus sampling; external cephalic version; APH; uterine procedures (eg amniocentesis); abdominal trauma. Use 250u before 20 weeks' gestation, 500u after 20 weeks.
2. Anti-D should be given in cases of ectopic pregnancy.
3. For threatened abortion see above.

NB: giving additional anti-D to Rh–ve primips, eg 500IU at 28 and 34 weeks reduces risk of sensitization from 1.12% to 0.28%.[3] Ask your lab.

1 UK Blood Transf. Working P 1991 *Prescrib J* **31** 137 2 D Lee 1993 BMJ **ii** 1145
3 S Mayne 1997 BMJ **ii** 1588

Induction of labour

5–20% of UK labours are induced artificially, usually because it has been decided that to remain *in utero* is relatively more risky for the fetus than to be born, but in some it is because of risk to the mother. 75% of inductions are for hypertension, pre-eclampsia, prolonged pregnancy or rhesus disease. Other indications are diabetes, previous stillbirth, abruption, fetal death *in utero* and placental insufficiency.

►Inducing mothers at 41+ weeks reduces stillbirth rates.

Contraindications Cephalopelvic disproportion which is absolute, malpresentations other than breech or face presentation, fetal distress, placenta praevia, cord presentation, vasa praevia, pelvic tumour, previous repair to cervix. Cone biopsy requires caution.

Cervical ripeness When an induction is being planned the state of the cervix will be assessed. In 95% of women at term the cervix is ripe. If primips are induced with an unripe cervix (Bishop's score ≤3, see below) the rates of prolonged labour, fetal distress and Caesarean section are increased. This is less marked in multips.

Modified Bishop score	0	1	2
Cervical dilatation (cm)	0	1–2	3–4
Length of cervix (cm)	>2	1–2	<1
Station of head (cm above ischial spines)	−3	−2	−1
Cervical consistency	firm	medium	soft
Position of cervix	posterior	middle	anterior

A score of >5 is 'ripe'. An unripe cervix may be ripened using one prostaglandin (PGE2) vaginal tablet (3mg) the evening before or the morning of induction. If antenatal fetal heart rate monitoring is indicated, this should commence before prostaglandin insertion. If there is failure to ripen (occurs in 12%) PGE2 may be repeated 6–8h later. If the cervix still remains unripe consider Caesarean section. PGE2 may stimulate uterine contractions or precipitate labour.

Once the cervix is ripe, rupture the membranes (amniotomy) and start intrapartum fetal heart rate monitoring using a scalp clip or pulse oximetry (less invasive, see OHCM p 658). Oxytocin is given IV in 5% dextrose using a pump system (eg Ivac®). Infusions start at 2 milliunits (MU) per min, doubling every 20min until effective uterine contractions are produced (usually at a rate of 4–16MU/min: occasionally 32MU/min may be necessary). Beware uterine hyperstimulation and the use of large volumes of IV fluid (if >4 litres, there is risk of water intoxication—ie confusion, convulsions and coma). When the cervix is 5cm dilated the uterus is more sensitive to oxytocin and 8MU/min may be sufficient to maintain contractions. Note: the Dublin regimen (p 112) results in most women going into spontaneous labour.

Problems of induction •Iatrogenic prematurity. •Infection (use antibiotic cover (p 152) in women with heart lesions as risk of endocarditis). •Bleeding (vasa praevia). •Cord prolapse (eg with a high head at amniotomy). •Some will lead to Caesarean section.

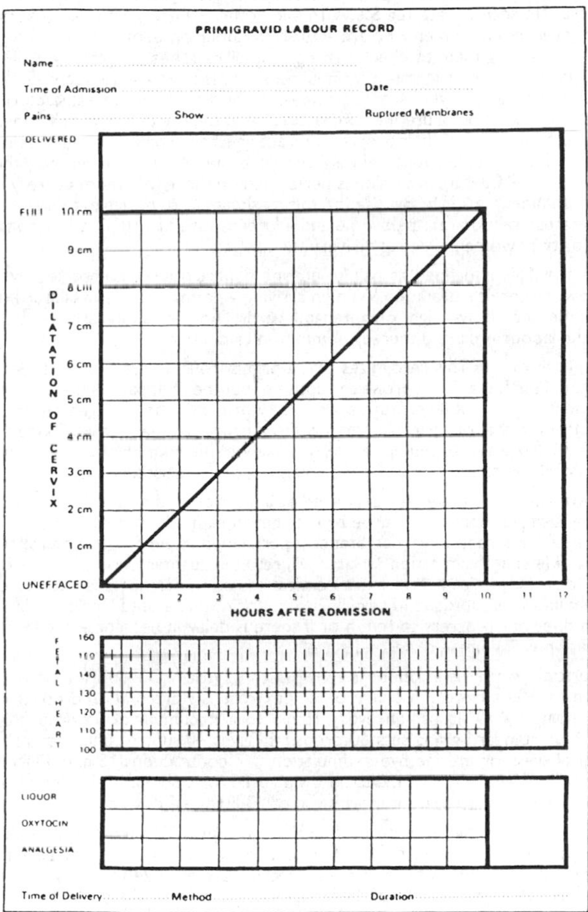

This graph shows the simple Dublin partogram ('simple' because it does not show 'latent' phase of labour). It has a steep *x/y* gradient of ratio 1:1.
Less steep ratios (eg 2:1) may predispose to premature intervention, as does inclusion of the 'latent' phase on the partogram.[1]

1 R Cartmill 1992 *Lancet* **339** 1520

The active management of labour[1]

Dublin is a centre of excellence for labouring mothers because of its coherent and very successful labour management plan, which leads to a low Caesarean section rate (eg 5% *vs* 14% for other centres). This depends on only ever having women who are actually in labour on labour ward, and regularly assessing them to check that cervical dilatation is progressing well—and taking action if it is not. Primiparous women with single, cephalically presenting babies, who are not achieving cervical dilatation satisfactorily have augmentation of uterine contractions with the use of oxytocin. Women are kept informed of their progress and are given an estimated time of delivery and are assured that delivery should be within 12h of entering the labour ward. Caesarean section is performed on those for whom delivery is not imminent at 12h. By use of this regimen it is possible to keep a Caesarean section rate below 5% and a forceps rate of ~10%, with the vast majority of women effecting delivery themselves.

Labour This is defined as painful uterine contractions accompanied by a 'show' or cervical dilatation. Women arriving who may not be in labour are accommodated overnight on antenatal wards. Those in labour are admitted to the labour ward and thereby committed to delivery.

Augmentation This recognizes that a primiparous uterus is an inefficient organ of birth that is *not* prone to rupture—but the multiparous uterus is an efficient organ but *is* rupture-prone. Oxytocin may be used to enhance efficiency in the primiparous uterus without danger to the mother. Oxytocin may be dangerous to multips as delay is likely to be from obstructed labour, so a decision to use it must only be made by senior obstetricians.

Examination Women are examined at admission and hourly for the first 3h by a single examiner (may be by rectal examination). Progress is assessed at 1h; artificial rupture of membranes is performed to aid progress and allow liquor viewing. Examination 1h later will result in augmentation of labour by oxytocin in primips if 1cm extra cervical dilatation has not been achieved. Examination is subsequently every 2h. Oxytocin will be used if primip dilatation does not progress at 1cm/h or if there is delay in descent in the involuntary pushing phase of second stage.

Oxytocin A uterus in labour is sensitive to oxytocin. Dublin uses a simple regimen. 10u oxytocin in 1 litre of 5% dextrose is started at 10 drops/min, increasing by 10 drops/min every 15min to a maximum of 60 drops/min (with UK standard giving sets 60 drops/min gives 40MU/min) unless there is fetal distress or uterine hyperstimulation (>7 contractions/15min). Only 1 bag is used ensuring that oxytocin is not used for >6h and water intoxication cannot occur (associated with use of >3 litres 5% dextrose).

Induction by artificial rupture of membranes (ARM). Women return to the antenatal ward to await onset of labour. Those 10% who do not go into labour spontaneously are returned to labour ward after 24h and oxytocin is used exactly as above. 90% of these women also deliver within 12h, thereby keeping Caesarean section rates low.

The partogram This graphs labour's progress (p 111). Dublin uses a simple partogram with time (on *x*-axis) plotted against cervical dilatation, and records fetal heart rate, state of liquor, analgesia, and oxytocin use. Many partograms are much more complicated.

Meconium in liquor At ARM this suggests placental insufficiency. Meconium other than light staining in good liquor volume prompts fetal blood sampling and scalp clip electronic monitoring, or prompt Caesarean section (fetal blood pH low, or very thick meconium).

1 K O'Driscoll 1986 *Active Management of Labour*, Baillière Tindall

The opposite page depicts Dublin practice for primiparous mothers with term babies of vertex presentation with a normal head. Its authors stress the benefit of their policies both to mothers and also from the financial management point of view as it allows them to have a personal midwife for each mother throughout the time that she is in labour, but with unit costs per delivery of only one-third of costs of UK hospitals.

Midwife monitoring is normally every 15min using a Pinard scope; electronic monitoring is used if there is meconium staining of liquor. Membranes are ruptured so that the liquor can be regularly inspected.

Many units in the UK often have quite different policies. For example, some would argue that artificially rupturing membranes may not be entirely beneficial as the liquor cannot cushion the fetal head and there is evidence that artificial rupture of membranes is associated with more fetal heart rate decelerations.[1] ARM may also facilitate spread of HIV from mother to baby (p 155). A review of current knowledge suggests that of early amniotomy, early use of oxytocin, and the provision of professional support throughout first labours, it is the latter which is the most important for reducing rates of operative delivery.[2] One large randomized USA trial did not find that active management of labour had any benefits, and it did not reduce rates of Caesarean section.[3] The debate as to whether to institute active management or to abandon it is being overtaken by women's views: many are rejecting intervention, even if it is offered.

1 J Barrett 1992 *Br J Obstet Gynae* **99** 5–9 2 J Thornton 1994 BMJ **ii** 366 (fig. 2 is captioned figure 3, and *vice versa*–a vital point in this paper!) ⟨3⟩ F Frigoletto 1995 NEJM 333 745 & E-BM 1996 **1** 174

Pain relief in labour

►Adequate pain relief in labour is the obstetrician's greatest gift to womankind. Not everyone wants natural birth—and do not make people feel guilty about requesting pain relief. A good anaesthetic agent in labour must be harmless to mother and baby, allow maintenance of maternal cooperation, and must not affect uterine contractility.

Education That given by the National Childbirth Trust meets all these criteria. Education about labour reduces fear; breathing exercises and relaxation techniques teach the mother ways to combat pain herself.

In the first stage, **narcotic injections** are often tried, eg pethidine 50–150mg IM (not if birth expected in <2–3h as neonatal respiratory depression may occur, reversible with naloxone 0.01mg/kg IV—this may be repeated after 3min if needed, or 0.1–0.2mg may be given as a single dose IM). Expect onset of analgesia to be within 20min and to last 3h. NB: doses of pethidine in the lower part of the range above will frequently produce vomiting, but no relief of pain.[1] Other SE: disorientation, ↓gastric emptying, neonatal respiratory depression. CI: mother on MAOIs (p 340).

Inhalational agents Nitrous oxide can be used throughout labour. Nitrous oxide 50% in oxygen (Entonox®) is self-administered using a demand valve. CI: those with a pneumothorax.

Pudendal block (sacral nerve roots 2, 3 and 4) uses 8–10mL of 1% lidocaine (=lignocaine) injected 1cm beyond a point just below and medial to the ischial spine each side. It is used with perineal infiltration for instrumental delivery, but analgesia is insufficient for rotational forceps.

Spinal block These may be used for rotational delivery or Caesarean section. For details and contraindications, see p 776.

Epidural anaesthesia See p 776. Pain relief is by anaesthetizing pain fibres carried by T11–S5. Epidurals must only be set up once labour is established (cervix >3cm). Set up IVI first, give 500mL Hartmann's solution to prevent ↓BP. Check pulse, BP, respirations, contractions and fetal heart every 15min after the epidural is set up. Top-ups are required ~2-hourly. Epidurals may be very helpful for the following: OP position (p 126), breech, multiple pregnancy, preterm delivery, pre-eclampsia, forceps delivery, inco-ordinate uterine contractions.

Problems: For those due to technique, see p 778. There may be postural hypotension (put up IVI, nurse 15° to left side), urinary retention (catheterize regularly), paralysis (pelvic floor muscle paralysis reduces rotation and voluntary effort in second stage, so increasing need for forceps). After delivery: urinary retention and headache (esp. after dural puncture).

Combined spinal epidural (CSE) anaesthesia gives quicker pain relief, with little or no motor blockade in most mothers, allowing standing, walking, sitting, and voiding urine. Using the intrathecal route (27G Whiteace needle) apparently does not cause a significant rise in the incidence of headache (only ~0.13%). The patient can control the amount dose, and this leads to a dose reduction of 35%, and reduces motor blockade. Women should inform their midwife if they notice light-headedness, nausea, or weak legs. Spontaneous delivery rates are not better than with traditional epidural.[2] ►Skilled anaesthetic help is vital.

Transcutaneous electrical nerve stimulation (TENS) Electrodes placed on the back, give pulses stimulating large nerve fibres to the brain, aiming to block pain impulses. It needs careful instruction but is under the mother's control. In 1 meta-analysis, 6 out of 9 trials showed no effect; those that did, showed only weak effects, eg ↑time before epidural use.[3]

1 F Reynolds 1997 *Lancet* **349** 4 2 A Shennan 1995 *Lancet* **345** 1514 3 *Bandolier* 1997 **4.3** 4

Pain: Yes or No?

Giving *prompt* and *generous* analgesia is the best way to ease a difficult labour: this way you *never give pain a chance*. This is exactly what most mothers want; but some, while not being masochists, want something different: explanation, dialogue, and the means to rise above pain—even, through pain, to register, for once, a maximum on their internal Richter scale of personal intensity. Pain is sometimes a form of energy, an opportunity, and a means of progressing from one mental state to another. People may fear pain just as they fear earthquakes, but they can also fear its opposite—total anaesthesia, the inability to be shocked, or a burnt-out unresponsiveness to life and the mysteries of its transmission—as illustrated by Monsieur Querry:*

'Who is she?'

'She was once my mistress...'

'You aren't afraid of her are you?'

'Perhaps. In a way.'

'Forgive me for saying it, M. Querry, but you do not strike me as a man who is afraid of women.'

'Have you never come across a leper, Father, who is afraid of striking his fingers because he knows they won't hurt any more?'

'I've known men rejoice when the feeling returns—even pain... You have to give pain a chance.' *Graham Greene *A Burnt-out Case,* 1960, Heinemann

Fetal monitoring

In high-risk pregnancy, antepartum cardiotocography and biophysical profiles by ultrasound (p 118) are used to monitor fetal activity and responsiveness. The aim is to detect intrauterine hypoxia prenatally.

Kick charts: In the last 10 weeks of pregnancy the mother can count the fetal movements daily and record the time at which the baby has made 10 movements. Although a poor predictor of fetal outcome, less than 10 movements in 12 hours may be a warning sign of problems and the mother should attend her obstetric unit for cardiotocography.

Cardiotocography: Doppler ultrasound detects fetal heart beats and a tocodynamometer over the uterine fundus records any contractions. A continuous trace is printed over ~30min (eg a paper speed of 1 or 2cm/min) with the mother lying semi-recumbent or in left lateral position or in the half-sitting position. A normal trace in an afebrile, mother at term who is not having drugs has a base rate of 110–150 beats/min, with a variability of 5–25 beats/min, and at least 2 accelerations (a common response to movement or noise) of an amplitude ≥15 beats/min over a 15–20min period. (Fetal heart rate falls by ~1 beat/min/week from 28 weeks.) An abnormal fetal heart rate is characterized by a baseline tachycardia of >170 beats/min or bradycardia (<100 beats/min), or a sinusoidal pattern. Loss of variability (<5 beats/min over a 40min period) and recurrent late or atypical decelerations are associated with fetal compromise and are the most important prognostic indicators of the test.[1]

Tests need to be done every 24h antenatally to identify the changing fetal heart rate pattern associated with hypoxia.

Intrapartum monitoring Death and disability due to complications of labour occur in <1:300 labours.[2] Intrapartum fetal heart rate monitoring aims to detect patterns known to be associated with fetal distress. The diagnosis of fetal distress may be supported by the passage of fresh meconium and fetal hypoxia on blood sampling.

The fetal heart rate is traditionally monitored by using a Pinard stethoscope between contractions, but with this method decelerations related to contractions may be missed.

Continuous fetal heart rate monitoring has poor predictive value, over-diagnosing fetal distress even if used with fetal blood sampling. Its value is uncertain even in high-risk labours—but it is widely used. Meta-analyses suggest that routine monitoring ↓rates of neonatal seizures, but increases operative deliveries.[3] Monitoring policies vary. Low-risk labours may be monitored intermittently. If high-risk, monitor throughout labour, ideally with scalp electrode or pulse oximetry. *Indications:* Abnormal admission trace; antenatal problems; use of oxytocin; fresh meconium (p 128). *Disadvantages:* Limited maternal mobility and discomfort.

►A combination of tachycardia, loss of baseline variability and shallow late decelerations is the best predictor of hypoxia.

Management of a poor trace: **1** Lie the mother on her left side and give O_2. Stop oxytocin. **2** Take fetal blood sample. If you do not have this facility, consider rapid delivery if the trace does not improve.

Fetal blood sampling: Fetal acidosis reflects hypoxia. Scalp blood pH of 7.3–7.4 is normal. If 7.25–7.29 repeat after 45min. If 7.2–7.24 consider Caesarean section. Levels <7.2 require immediate delivery unless in second stage when a level as low as 7.15 may be acceptable.

Fetal heart rate patterns and their clinical significance[4]

The normal pattern is described opposite. Accelerations suggest intact sympathetic activity and are rarely associated with hypoxia.

Loss of baseline variability Baseline variability of >5 beats/min shows response to vagal tone, sympathetic stimuli and catecholamines in a well oxygenated fetal brainstem. Loss of baseline variability may reflect a preterm fetus who is sleeping, drug effects (eg diazepam, morphine, phenothiazine) or hypoxia.

Baseline tachycardia Heart rate >170 beats/min is associated with maternal fever or β-sympathomimetic drug use, chorioamnionitis (loss of variation too), and acute/subacute hypoxia. Persistent rates >200 are associated with fetal cardiac arrythmia.

Baseline bradycardia Heart rates <110 beats/min is rarely associated with fetal hypoxia (except in placental abruption). It may reflect ↑ fetal vagal tone, fetal heart block, or, if spasmodic, cord compression.

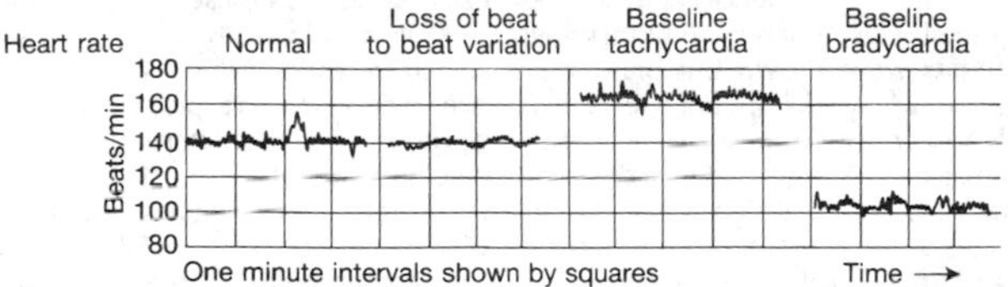

Early decelerations coinciding with uterine contractions reflect increased vagal tone as fetal intracranial pressure rises with the contraction. **Late decelerations**, when the nadir of the deceleration develops some 30sec after the peak of the uterine contraction, reflect fetal hypoxia, the degree and duration reflecting its severity. **Variable decelerations**, both in degree and relation to uterine contractions, may represent umbilical cord compression around the limbs or presenting part.

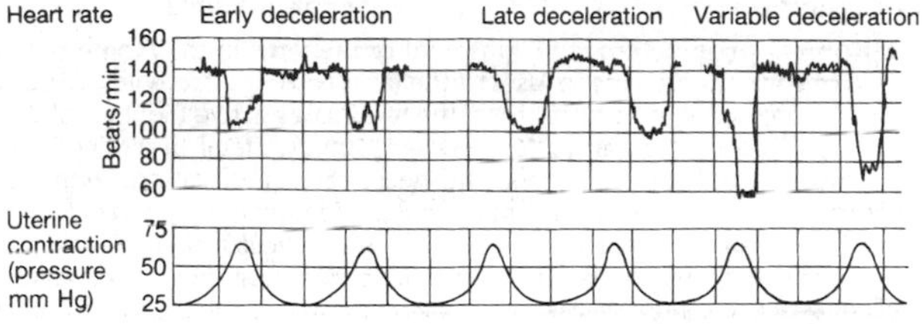

1 N Patel 1989 *Obstetrics* page 373–80, Churchill Livingstone 2 P Steer 1988 *Pregnancy and Risk*, John Wiley <3> SB Thaker 1996 E-BM 1 93 4 G Rooth 1987 *Int J Gyn Obs* **25** 159–67

Ultrasound

In each ultrasound examination, examine placental site and structure, assess liquor volume and fetal structure and wellbeing (see below).

Early in pregnancy If there is bleeding and pain, ultrasound can confirm intrauterine pregnancy (or ectopic) and the viability of the fetus. Where there is discrepancy between uterine size and dates, gestation can be estimated, a viable fetus ascertained (not missed abortion, p 22), or twins excluded—especially important after the use of fertility drugs or in the presence of hyperemesis gravidarum (also to exclude hydatidiform mole).

Estimation of gestational age Crown–rump length is measured from 6–12 weeks (~10mm at 7 weeks; ~55mm at 12 weeks). From 12 weeks the biparietal diameter can be measured (and femur length from 14 weeks so that there are 2 independent estimations with each procedure). Biparietal diameter measurements to estimate age are most accurate up to 20 weeks (unreliable from 34 weeks). Knowledge of gestational age is important in management of rhesus disease and in diabetic pregnancy (p 156)—and also helps if the date of the LMP is not known, or the cycle is irregular.

Fetal abnormality See *fetal nuchal translucency,* p 167. Many units offer routine scans to find abnormality at <18 weeks. Is the *routine* use of ultrasound justified? This depends on ultrasonography skill: in a USA study (*N*=15,151) no benefits were shown, but only 17% of structural abnormalities were found before 24 weeks; in Europe, benefits are greater as the pick-up rate is 21–84%. With the best machines and ultrasonographers, an increasing range of markers of fetal abnormality are discernible, eg nuchal thickness in Down's syndrome, but the sign is also +ve in ~6% of normal pregnancies. The more such markers, the greater the chance of abnormality (see p 167 for 'soft signs'). It is hard to know how to counsel women before these discerning scans: full informed consent is time-consuming, and itself causes psychopathology (p 168) and it seems odd to ask the mother what sort of informed consent she would like (but see p 169). Another problem is that many of chromosomal abnormalites suggested by early scans will spontaneously miscarry in subsequent weeks, and one will have overburdened the mother pointlessly.[1] Specific indications for scanning for abnormality include:

- Family history of neural tube defect
- Maternal diabetes or epilepsy
- AFP abnormal
- Oligohydramnios
- Twins
- Polyhydramnios

Biophysical profile scoring Ultrasound of the fetus in the womb over a period of up to 30min aims to assess if the fetus is being affected by acute or chronic asphyxia. With acute asphyxia the fetus loses active biophysical variables regulated by central nervous system outflow (fetal breathing, gross body movement, fetal flexor tone and heart rate accelerations with fetal body movement). Reduction in amniotic fluid demonstrated by pockets of fluid of less than 1cm depth measured in 2 perpendicular planes is taken to indicate chronic asphyxia. By use of specific criteria for these 5 variables a 'wellbeing' score can be reached. Management protocols according to score then help guide the obstetrician as to when intervention should take place.

Ultrasound is used as an adjunct to the diagnostic procedures of amniocentesis, fetoscopy, cordocentesis and chorionic villus biopsy.

In pregnancies where fetal growth is of concern (p 104) growth can be monitored by regular scans; the abdominal to skull circumference ratio being of interest. Fetal weight can be estimated when planning vaginal delivery of breech presentation (but less accurate for larger fetuses).

In later pregnancy, the lie and presentation of the fetus can be determined. If there is APH, placenta praevia can be excluded and the placenta visualized to look for abruption. With secondary postpartum haemorrhage, retained products of conception may be visualized.

Side-effects Ultrasound is one of the safest tests ever invented; nevertheless, over the years, fears have been expressed about inducing childhood cancers. There is now good evidence that this does not occur. There is one randomized trial indicating that *repeated* ultrasound with Doppler is associated with an increased risk (1.65) of birth weights below the third centile.[2]

Doppler ultrasound and fetal wellbeing[3]

Doppler ultrasound is a technique which can be used to assess circulation on both sides of the placenta. It has not been shown to be of use as a screening tool in routine antenatal care[4] but it has been shown to be of use in high-risk pregnancies. Waveform outlines (velocimetry) have been seen to be abnormal in small babies who ultimately died or were severely ill perinatally, and babies known to be small from real-time ultrasound have been shown not to be at risk if umbilical artery waveforms were normal, but if end-diastolic frequencies are absent the baby is likely to be hypoxic and acidotic. In management of growth-retarded babies uncomplicated by other obstetric problems surveillance using Doppler velocimetry is more cost-effective than use of cardiotocography, and may be sufficient as the sole extra means of surveillance (in addition to ultrasound examination of biophysical parameters).[5] ►Consider Caesarean section if umbilical artery Doppler velocimetry shows absent or reversed end diastolic velocities in pregnancies complicated by IUGR and hypertension—to prevent postnatal problems such as cerebral haemorrhage, anaemia, and hypoglycaemia.[6] These changes correlate with placental intervillous space ischaemia and spasm or occlusion of tertiary stem arterioles on the fetal side of the circulation. Placental intervillous ischaemia leads to centralization of fetal circulation so that blood returning from the placenta is shunted to fetal brain, coronary arteries and adrenals. Intervention studies based on knowledge of abnormal umbilical waveform patterns have resulted in babies small-for-gestational age (SGA) with abnormal waveform patterns being ~500g larger than expected when the mothers were given low-dose aspirin rather than placebo from the time of diagnosis. It is also the case that low-dose aspirin delays the onset of hypertension and reduces its severity in primiparous mothers whose babies had abnormal umbilical waveforms. However, aspirin has not been shown to be of benefit in low-risk pregnancies, where it has been shown to increase abruption rates.[7]

1 M Whittle 1997 *BMJ* **i** 918 2 B Ewigman 1993 *NEJM* **239** 821 3 Ed 1992 *Lancet* **339** 1083
4 J Davies 1992 *Lancet* **340** 1299 5 H Alstrom 1992 *Lancet* **340** 936 6 V Karsdorp 1994 *Lancet* **344** 1664
7 B Sibai 1993 *NEJM* **329** 1213

Amniotic fluid

Amniotic fluid (liquor) Made by amniotic cell secretion and maternal plasma filtrate, volumes are abnormal if the fetus cannot swallow it or contribute to it as urine. By 10 weeks the volume is 30mL, by 20 weeks 300mL, by 30 weeks 600mL. Maximal between 34 and 38 weeks (800–1000mL) it reduces thereafter by 150mL per week.

Oligohydramnios Liquor volume is <200mL. It is rare.
Associations: Prolonged pregnancy, prolonged membrane rupture, placental insufficiency, fetal urethral aplasia or renal agenesis. The (fatal) Potter's syndrome comprises fetal low-set ears, renal agenesis, hypoplastic lungs and amnion nodosum (clumps of fetal squames).

Polyhydramnios (hydramnios) Amniotic fluid exceeds 2–3 litres in 1 in 250 pregnancies. 50% of cases are associated with fetal abnormality, 20% with maternal diabetes. In 30% no cause is found.
Fetal causes: Anencephaly (no swallowing reflex), spina bifida, umbilical hernia, ectopia vesicae, oesophageal or duodenal atresia, hydrops fetalis, hyperextended attitude.
Maternal causes: Diabetes mellitus, multiple pregnancy. Presenting early in the third trimester, the mother may develop breathlessness and oedema. An abdominal girth of >100cm is suggestive. Ultrasound (p 118) is used to exclude multiple pregnancy and abnormalities. Polyhydramnios predisposes to premature labour, malpresentation, cord prolapse, placental abruption when membranes rupture, and PPH (the uterus does not contract well). As indomethacin given to the mother reduces fetal urine production it can be used to treat polyhydramnios (eg 25mg/6h PO). Fetal urine production returns to normal 24h after treatment stops. During labour, check early for cord prolapse. After delivery pass a nasogastric tube in the baby to check the oesophagus is patent.

Amniocentesis Amniocentesis is the sampling of amniotic fluid. It is used for prenatal diagnosis of abnormality; in the management of rhesus disease (p 242); and for estimation of fetal lung maturity (rarely performed now). Lung maturity is assessed from lecithin/sphingomyelin ratio of amniotic fluid. If >2, lungs mature; if <1.5, very immature. Amniocentesis for abnormality diagnosis is carried out at 16 weeks' gestation, when there is enough liquor to give reliable fetal cell culture and time to terminate the pregnancy in the light of results if this is desired. Early amniocentesis at 10–13 weeks can provide satisfactory samples, but has high rates of fetal loss (eg ~5%),[1] and may be associated with talipes equinovarus.[2] Chromosome results take 3–4 weeks to be ready. Ultrasound enables sampling from a good pool of liquor avoiding placental penetration. Using a sterile technique remove 15mL of fluid with a 21G needle. Give anti-D 250U IM to Rh–ve women afterwards. Counsel the woman beforehand.

Indications for amniocentesis: Advanced maternal age (≥35–37yrs for Down's syndrome); a previous child with a neural tube defect (1:20 subsequently affected) or raised maternal serum α-fetoprotein (p 168 & p 228)—though ultrasound is often now used instead to look for neural tube defects; when a parent carries a balanced chromosomal translocation (1 in 4–10 chance fetus affected); risk of recessively inherited metabolic disorder (p 210); when the mother carries an X-linked disorder (to determine fetal sex). Chorionic villus sampling (p 166) can provide earlier results for many of the above, allowing earlier termination of pregnancy in the light of results. The miscarriage rate after amniocentesis later, ie 16 week amnocentesis is ~1%. See p 166.

1 A Nicolaides 1994 *Lancet* **344** 435 2 K Sundberg 1997 *Lancet* **350** 697

Multiple pregnancy

Incidence[uk] Twins: 1/105 pregnancies (33% monozygotic); triplets: 1/10,000.

Predisposing factors Previous twins; family history of twins (dizygotic only); increasing maternal age (<20yrs 6.4/1000, >25yrs 16.8/1000); induced ovulation and *in vitro* fertilization (1430 babies born from multiple births due to *in vitro* fertilization in 1992 (UK);[1] race origin (1/150 pregnancies for Japanese, 1/36 in Nigerian Igbo women). The worldwide rate for monozygotic twins is constant at 3–5/1000.[2]

Diagnosis Early in pregnancy the uterus may be felt to be large for dates and there may be hyperemesis. Later there may be polyhydramnios. The signs are that >2 poles may be felt; there is a multiplicity of fetal parts; 2 fetal heart rates may be heard (reliable if beating at rates different by >10 beats/min). Diagnosis may be made or confirmed by ultrasound.

Complications during pregnancy Polyhydramnios (p 120); pre-eclampsia is more common (30% twin pregnancies, 10% singleton); anaemia is more common (iron and folate requirements are increased). There is an increased incidence of APH (6% for twins, *vs* 4.7% for singletons) due to both abruption and placenta praevia (large placenta).

Fetal complications Perinatal mortality for twins is 36.7/1000 (8/1000 if single; 73/1000 for triplets; and 204 for higher multiples—in 1993). The main problem is prematurity. Mean gestation for twins is 37 weeks, for triplets 33 weeks. Light-for-dates babies (p 104) are more common (growth rate the same as for singletons up to 24 weeks but may be slower thereafter). Malformation rates are increased 2–4 times, especially in monozygotic twins. Ultrasound is the main diagnostic test. Selective fetocide (eg with intracardiac potassium chloride) is best used before 20 weeks if indicated.[2] With monozygotic twins, intermingling blood supply may result in disparate twin size and one being born plethoric (hence jaundiced later), the other anaemic. If one fetus dies *in utero* it may become a fetus papyraceous which may be aborted later or delivered prematurely.

Complications of labour PPH is more common (4–6% in singletons, 10% in twins). Malpresentation is common (cephalic/cephalic 40%, cephalic/breech 40%, breech/breech 10%, cephalic/transverse (Tv) 5%, breech/Tv 4%, Tv/Tv 1%). Rupturing of vasa praevia, increased rates of cord prolapse (0.6% singleton, 2.3% twins), premature separation of the placenta and cord entanglement (especially monozygous) may all present difficulties at labour. Despite modern technology some twins remain undiagnosed, staff are unprepared, and syntometrine may be used inappropriately, so delaying delivery of the second twin. Epidural anaesthesia is helpful for versions.

Management •Ensure adequate rest (need not entail admission).
- Use ultrasound for diagnosis and monthly checks on fetal growth.
- Give additional iron and folate to the mother during pregnancy.
- More antenatal visits, eg weekly from 30 weeks (risk of eclampsia↑).
- Tell the mother how to identify preterm labour, and what to do.
- Consider induction at 40 weeks. Have an IVI running in labour and an anaesthetist available at delivery. Paediatricians (preferably one for each baby) should be present at delivery for resuscitation should this be necessary (second twins have a higher risk of asphyxia).

Monozygous or dizygous? Monozygous twins are always same-sex and the membrane consists of 2 amnions and 1 chorion (if in doubt send for histology).

1 DoH 1996 *Report on Confidential Enquiry into Maternal Deaths in the United Kingdom 1991-93* HMSO p9
2 B Magowan 1998 *The Diplomate* **5** 11

Triplets are difficult . . . more than simply difficult

Bringing up one child is difficult: bringing up twins is often very very difficult—but bringing up triplets is more than very very very difficult: it is frequently a source of significant psychopathology. During infertility consultations, eager couples may say in one breath: "We wouldn't worry about twins. . . delighted—even triplets would be OK. . ." But how do they know, and would they find the following information chastening?

Even 4 years after their birth, all mothers in one study[1] suffered from exhaustion and emotional distress. The relationships with the children was often difficult (aggression and conflicts). One-third of mothers had sufficient depression to require psychotropic medication, and one-third spontaneously expressed regrets about having triplets. But do not conclude from this that it will necessarily be right to offer mothers selective termination. After triplets have been reduced to twins *in utero*, subsequently one-third of mothers will suffer emotional problems (persistent sadness and guilt) up to one year. However, adjustment had occurred in ~90% by 2 postnatal years.[2]

1 M Garel 1997 *Furtil Steril* **67** 1162 **2** M Garl 1997 *Human Reprod* **12** 617

Breech presentations

Breech presentation is the commonest malpresentation. Although 40% of babies are breech at 20 weeks, 25% will be at 32 weeks, and only 3% by term. It is normal in pregnancy for the buttocks to come to lie in the fundus. Conditions predisposing towards breech presentation: contracted pelvis, bicornuate uterus, fibroid uterus, placenta praevia, oligohydramnios, spina bifida or a hydrocephalic fetus. Ultrasound may show the cause and influence the management.

Extended breech presentation is commonest—ie flexed at the hips but extended at the knees. **Flexed breeches** sit with hips and knees both flexed so that the presenting part is a mixture of buttocks, external genitalia and feet. **Footling breeches** are the least common. The feet are the presenting part and this type has the greatest risk (5–20%) of cord prolapse.

Diagnosis of breech presentation should be made antenatally. The mother may complain of pain under the ribs. On palpation the lie is longitudinal, no head is felt in the pelvis and in the fundus there is a smooth round mass (the head) which can be ballotted, a sensation akin to quickly sinking an apple in a bowl of water.

External cephalic version (ECV)—turning the breech by manoeuvring it through a forward, less commonly backward,[1] somersault. Turn the baby only if vaginal delivery planned. Traditionally carried out at 34–36 weeks' gestation, it can be used from 37 weeks using tocolysis. Success rate ~53%.[1] Version contraindications: placenta praevia, multiple pregnancy, APH, small-for-dates babies, in mothers with uterine scars, pre-eclampsia or hypertension (the risk of abruption is increased), who have a bad obstetric history. Give anti-D (500u) to rhesus-negative patients and take Kleihauer test to detect the 1% who may need additional anti-D.[1]

Mode of delivery Caesarean section is often advocated on the unproven[2] grounds of safety. Aim to discuss all the options with the mother. Consider breech delivery if:[2]

- Experienced obstetrician available
- Estimated fetal wt 2500–3500g by scan
- No evidence of growth retardation
- Good shape/size pelvis on CT pelvimetry
- Labour augmentation/induction avoided
- Good progress in labour stage 1 and 2
- Extended breech presentation (or well flexed if multip)
- No neck hyperextension
- Normal volume of liquor
- No placenta praevia
- No pre-eclampsia; no distress

If all criteria are met fetal loss may be < 1% (possibly much less).[3]

Assisted breech delivery The breech engages in the pelvis with the bitrochanteric diameter (9.5cm) transverse. With further descent through the pelvis, rotation occurs so the bitrochanteric diameter lies antero-posteriorly as it emerges from the birth canal, being born by lateral flexion of the trunk. External rotation then occurs so that this diameter is again transverse. The shoulders enter the pelvis with the bisacromial diameter transverse, rotate through 90° emerging in the AP diameter. The head enters the pelvis with the sagittal suture transverse and rotates 90°. When the baby is completely born it is allowed to hang for about 1–2 minutes until the nape of the neck is well seen. The body is then lifted above the vulva by an assistant, the head being delivered with forceps.

►Check baby for hip dislocation (↑incidence): also, if vaginal delivery, for Klumpke's paralysis (p 724) and signs of CNS injury.

1 G Hughes 1997 *J Obs Gynae* **17** 127 2 J Kingdom 1992 BMJ **ii** 1090 3 J Thorpe-Beeston 1992 BMJ **ii** 749 & 1090

Other malpresentations

Occipitoposterior presentation (OP) In 50% of patients the mothers have a long 'anthropoid' pelvis. Diagnosis may be made antenatally by palpation (p 85). On vaginal examination the posterior fontanelle will be found to lie in the posterior quadrant of the pelvis. Labour tends to be prolonged because of the degree of rotation needed, so adequate hydration and analgesia (consider epidural) are important. During labour 65% rotate 130° so that the head is occipitoanterior at the time of birth, 20% rotate to the transverse and then arrest ('deep transverse arrest'), 15% rotate so that the occiput lies truly posterior and birth is by flexion of the head from the perineum. Although in 73% delivery will be a spontaneous vaginal delivery, 22% will require forceps and 5% a Caesarean section.

Face presentation Incidence 1:500. 15% are due to congenital abnormality such as anencephaly, tumour of or shortened fetal neck muscles. Most occur by chance as the head extends rather than flexes as it engages. Antenatal diagnosis: the fetal spine feels S-shaped, the uterus is ovoid without fullness in the flanks and there is a deep groove between the occiput and the back. On early vaginal examination, the nose and eyes may be felt but later this will not be possible because of oedema. Most engage in the transverse (mentobregmatic diameter ≈9.5cm). 90% rotate so that the chin lies behind the symphysis (mentoanterior) and the head can be born by flexion. If the chin rotates to the sacrum (mentoposterior), Caesarean section is indicated.

Brow presentation This occurs in 1:2000 deliveries and is often associated with a contracted pelvis or a very large fetus. Antenatal diagnosis: the head does not engage (mentovertical diameter ≈13cm) and a sulcus may be felt between the occiput and the back. On vaginal examination the anterior fontanelle and supraorbital ridges may be felt. Deliver by Caesarean section.

Transverse lie (compound shoulder presentation) This occurs in 1 in 400 deliveries and is usually in multiparous women. Other predisposing factors: multiple pregnancy, polyhydramnios; in primips: arcuate or septate uterus, placenta praevia, contracted pelvis. Antenatal diagnosis: ovoid uterus wider at the sides, the lower pole is empty, the head lies in one flank, the fetal heart is heard in variable positions. On vaginal examination with membranes intact no distinguishing features may be felt, but if ruptured and the cervix dilated, ribs, shoulder or a prolapsed hand may be felt. The risk of cord prolapse is high. External cephalic version (p 124) may be attempted from 32 weeks. If malpresentation persists or recurs Caesarean section will be necessary. Those with persistent instability of lie need hospital admission from 37 weeks (to prevent cord prolapse at home when the membranes rupture) and decision as to elective Caesarean section or induction just after external version (called a stabilizing induction).

►►Prolapsed cord

Cord prolapse is an emergency because of the risk of cord compression causing fetal asphyxia. There is an increased incidence at twin deliveries, footling breech delivery and with shoulder presentations. If a cord presentation is noted prior to membrane rupture, carry out Caesarean section. Always be aware when artificially rupturing membranes, when the presenting part is poorly applied, that cord prolapse is a possible risk.

Management The aim is to prevent the presenting part from occluding the cord. ►►This may be effected by:

- Displacing the presenting part by putting a hand in the vagina; push it back up (towards mother's head) during contractions.
- Using gravity, either place the woman head down or get her into knee–elbow position (kneeling so rump higher than head).
- Infuse 500mL saline into bladder through size 16 catheter.
- Keep cord in vagina: do not handle it (to prevent spasm).

If the cervix is fully dilated and the presenting part is sufficiently low in pelvis, deliver by forceps (if cephalic) or by breech extraction (by a suitably experienced obstetrician). Otherwise arrange immediate Caesarean section, if the fetus is still alive. There are few other emergencies where speed is so vital.

►►Impacted shoulders

Also called shoulder dystocia, this refers to an inability to deliver the shoulders after the head has been delivered.

Associations: Large fetus; postmature fetus; abnormality; short cord. The danger is death from asphyxia.

Management

- Place the mother in lithotomy with buttocks supported on a pillow over the edge of the bed. Lithotomy position increases the pelvic outlet. Give a large episiotomy.
- As an assistant gives firm suprapubic pressure apply firm pressure to the fetal head towards the floor. If this fails, check anterior shoulder is under the symphysis (where the diameter of the outlet is widest); if not rotate it to be so and repeat traction. If this fails, rotation by 180° (so posterior shoulder now lies anteriorly) may work. If the baby dies prior to delivery, cutting through both clavicles (cleidotomy) with strong scissors assists delivery.
- Check the baby for damage, eg Erb's palsy or fractured clavicle.

Meconium-stained liquor

In late pregnancy, it is normal for some babies to pass meconium (bowel contents) which stains the amniotic fluid a dull green. This is not significant. During labour, fresh meconium, which is dark green, sticky and lumpy, may be passed. This may be a response to the stress of a normal labour, or a sign of distress, so transfer to a consultant unit (if in a GP unit) and commence continuous fetal heart rate monitoring (p 116). Aspiration of fresh meconium can cause severe pneumonitis. As the head is born, suck out the oropharynx and nose. Have a paediatrician in attendance (p 244) to suck out pharynx and trachea under direct vision using a laryngoscope.

2. Obstetrics

Forceps

Forceps are designed with a cephalic curve, which fits around the fetal head, and a pelvic curve which fits the pelvis. Short-shanked (eg Wrigley's) forceps are used for 'lift out' deliveries, when the head is on the perineum; long-shanked (eg Neville Barnes) for higher deliveries, when the sagittal suture lies in the AP diameter. Kielland's forceps have a reduced pelvic curve, making them suitable for rotation (only in experienced hands).

Conditions of use The head must be engaged; the membranes ruptured; the position of the head known and the presentation suitable, ie vertex or face (mentoanterior); there must not be cephalo-pelvic disproportion (moulding not excessive); the cervix must be fully dilated and the uterus contracting, and analgesia adequate (perineal infiltration for the episiotomy; pudendal blocks may be sufficient for mid-cavity forceps and ventouse deliveries but not for Kielland's). The bladder must be empty.

Indications for use Forceps may be used when there is delay in the second stage: this is frequently due to failure of maternal effort (uterine inertia or just tiredness), epidural analgesia, or malpositions of the fetal head. They may be used when there is fetal distress or a prolapsed cord or eclampsia—all occurring only in the second stage. They are also used to prevent undue maternal effort, eg in cardiac disease, respiratory disease, pre-eclampsia. They are used for the after-coming head in breech deliveries.

Technique This should be learnt from demonstration. The following is an *aide-mémoire* for non-rotational forceps. Place the mother in lithotomy position with her bottom just over the edge of the delivery bed. Use sterilizing fluid to clean the vulva and pernieum; catheterize; check the position of the head. Insert pudendal block and infiltrate the site of the episiotomy (not necessary if she has an epidural). Assemble the blades to check they fit, with the pelvic curve pointing upwards. The handle which lies in the left hand is the left blade and is inserted first (to the mother's left side) and then the right: the handles should lock easily. Traction must not be excessive (the end of bed is not for extra leverage!). Synchronize traction with contractions, guiding the head downwards initially. Do a large episiotomy when the head is at the vulva. Change the direction of traction to up and out as the head passes out of the vulva. If the baby needs resuscitation, hand it to the paediatrician. Give vitamin K (p 244).
Complications of forceps: Maternal trauma; fetal facial bruising and VII paralysis (usually resolves).

Ventouse The ventouse, or vacuum extractor, is associated with less maternal trauma than forceps[1] and is preferred worldwide but not in the UK (4.8% of deliveries in 1994–5 *vs* 5.8% by forceps).[2] It may be used in preference to rotational forceps because, as traction is applied, with the cup over the posterior fontanelle, rotation during delivery will occur. It can be used through a partially dilated cervix (primips should be almost fully dilated, multips >6cm), but should not be used if the head is above the ischial spines. A cup is applied with a suction force of 0.8kg/cm^2. The baby's scalp is sucked up to form a 'chignon' which resolves in 2 days. There is increased rate of fetal cephalhaematoma (p 144) and neonatal jaundice so give vitamin K (p 244). Maternal trauma still occurs in ~11%.[3]

Follow-up in surviving adults shows no consistent trend to physical or cognitive impairment from low-outlet instrumental deliveries.[4]

1 AH Sultan 1994 BMJ **i** 887 2 A Macfarlane 1998 BMJ **316** 566 3 J Drife 1996 *Br J Obs Gynae* **103** 619
4 D Seidman 1991 *Lancet* **i** 1583

2. Obstetrics

Caesarean section

Incidence 5–13% of all labours. Maternal mortality: 0.33/1000. Morbidity is higher—from infection, ileus, thromboembolism, and delay in bonding—unless done under epidural anaesthesia. Factors contributing to this high section rate include over-diagnosis of fetal distress by cardiotocography, fear of litigation should brain damage follow difficult vaginal delivery, and more induced labours (oxytocin may promote fetal distress).

Lower uterine segment incision The almost universal use of this incision makes uterine rupture (p 134) in subsequent pregnancy much less common, allows better puerperal healing, reduces infection as the wound is extraperitoneal, and has lower post-operative complication rates.

Classical Caesarean section (vertical incision) Rarely used. Indications: •Fetus lies transverse, with ruptured membranes and liquor draining •Structural abnormality makes lower segment use impossible •Constriction ring present •Fibroids (some) •Some anterior placenta praevia when lower segment abnormally vascular •Mother dead and rapid birth desired •Very premature fetus, lower segment poorly formed.

Before an emergency section ►*Explain to the mother what is to happen.*

- Activate the anaesthetist, theatre staff, porters and paediatrician.
- Have the mother breathe 100% O_2 if there is fetal distress.
- Neutralize gastric contents with 20mL of 0.3 molar sodium citrate, and promote gastric emptying with metoclopramide 10mg IV. (NB: there is no time for H_2 agonists to work; ranitidine is kept for elective sections, eg 150mg PO 2h before surgery.) Consider pre-operative emptying of stomach (eg if prolonged labour or opiate given). The stomach should be routinely emptied prior to extubation to minimize risk of postoperative aspiration.[1] See Mendelson's syndrome, p 134.
- Take to theatre (awake); set up IVI. Take blood for crossmatch, eg 2u; (6u and 2 IVIs if previous section + anterior placenta praevia—see below).
- Catheterize the bladder. Tilt 15° to her left side on operating table.
- Use pulse oximetry peri- and post-operatively in those with dark skins (cyanosis is difficult to detect).[3a]
- Tell the paediatrician if the mother has had opiates in the last 4h.

Note: halothane should not be used for obstetric procedures because uterine muscle relaxation increases bleeding. Other anaesthetic problems include vomiting on induction (see rapid sequence induction, p 770), and light anaesthesia (out of consideration for the baby) causing paralysed awareness. ►In reducing maternal mortality, the importance of having an experienced anaesthetist cannot be overemphasized.

Indications for *elective* Caesarean sections Known cephalo-pelvic disproportion; placenta praevia; some malpresentations (p 126); after vaginal surgery (suburethral repair; vesico-vaginal fistula repair); with some maternal infections, eg herpes, HIV (p 98). If a repeat section is planned, arrange ultrasound placental localization to exclude placenta praevia as this is more common and more likely to be complicated by placenta accreta (hence risk of massive haemorrhage) in the presence of a uterine scar.

Emergency section may be needed because of antenatal complications, eg severe pre-eclampsia, abruptio placentae (baby still alive). In others, the need becomes apparent during labour: fetal distress; prolapsed cord (if fetus alive); after failed induction; or failure to progress.

Trial of scar in labour: See p 134. Beware oxytocin. *Antibiotic prophylaxis* is recommended.[3b] Infection (wound, endometritis and UTI) is reduced by IV antibiotics (eg 2g cefradine at induction, 1g at 6h and 12h post-op) for both emergency and elective sections.[2] Longer courses do not appear to be superior, nor is use of more expensive second generation cefalosporins.

After Caesarean section In Rh–ve mothers, remove all excess blood from peritoneal cavity. Use a Kleihauer test (p 109) to determine dose of anti-D. Mobilize the mother early. If purported cephalo-pelvic disproportion led to section, consider pre-discharge radiographic pelvimetry.

Complications •PPH •Retained placental tissue •Ureter trauma •Vesico-uterine fistula •Fetal injury (eg fracture) •Colon injury

Prophylaxis against thromboembolism[3c] *Low-risk:* Women with no risk factors undergoing elective Caesarean section in an uncomplicated pregnancy require only early mobilization and good hydration.

Moderate risk:
- Age >35 years
- Obesity (>80kg)
- Para 4+
- Pre-eclampsia
- Emergency section in labour
- Gross varicose veins
- Current infection
- >4 days prior immobility
- Major current illness

These women require heparin prophylaxis or mechanical methods.

High-risk: These women should all receive heparin until 5 days post-operatively or until fully mobilized and use of leg stockings confers additional benefit.
- Any woman with 3 risk factors above
- Extended surgery, eg Caesarean hysterectomy
- FH or past history of thromboembolism or thrombophilia
- Paralysed lower limbs
- Women with antiphospholipid antibody (cardiolipin antibody or lupus anticoagulant)

Women who have had thromboembolism in pregnancy should receive thromboprophylaxis for 6 weeks postpartum.

1 DoH 1994 *Report on Confidential Enquiry into Maternal Deaths in the United Kingdom 1988-90* HMSO
2 M Turner 1992 *J Obs Gynae* **12** (sup 1) 520 **3** DoH 1996 *Report on Confidential Enquiry into Maternal Deaths in the United Kingdom 1991-93* HMSO (a) p200, (b) p83, (c) p58

►►Uterine rupture

Ruptured uterus is rare in the UK (1:1500 deliveries—but 1:100 in parts of Africa). Associated maternal mortality is 5%, and the fetal mortality 30%. ~70% of UK ruptures are due to dehiscence of Caesarean section scars. Lower segment scars are far less likely to rupture (1.4%) than the classical scars (6.4%)—see p 132. Other risk factors: •Obstructed labour in the multiparous, especially if oxytocin is used •Previous cervical surgery •High forceps delivery •Internal version •Breech extraction. Rupture is usually during the third trimester or in labour. ***Trial of scar:*** a frequent question is: *Is it safer to do a repeat Caesar or to allow a scarred uterus (past Caesar) to labour?* In general, a trial of labour is safer than automatic repeat Caesars—particularly if the thickness of the lower uterine segment is >3.5mm on ultrasound at 36–38 weeks, according to a careful prospective study (*N* = 642).[1]

Signs and symptoms Rupture is usually in labour. In a few (usually a Caesarean scar dehiscence) rupture precedes labour. Pain is variable, some only having slight pain and tenderness over the uterus. In others pain is severe. Vaginal bleeding is variable and may be slight (bleeding is intraperitoneal). Unexplained maternal tachycardia, sudden maternal shock, cessation of contractions, disappearance of the presenting part from the pelvis, and fetal distress are other presentations. postpartum indicators of rupture: continuous PPH with a well-contracted uterus; if bleeding continues postpartum after cervical repair; and whenever shock is present.

Management If suspected in labour, laparotomy should be carried out, the baby delivered by Caesarean section and the uterus explored at operation. ►►•Give O_2 at 15L/min via a tight-fitting mask with reservoir •Set up IVI •Crossmatch 6u of blood and correct shock by fast transfusion. •Arrange laparotomy. The type of operation performed should be decided by a senior obstetrician; if the rupture is small, repair may be carried out (possibly with tubal ligation); if the cervix or vagina are involved in the tear, hysterectomy may be necessary. Care is needed to identify the ureters and exclude them from sutures. Give post-operative antibiotic cover, eg ampicillin 500mg/6h IV and netilmicin 150mg/12h IV (unless there is renal impairment). 85% of spontaneous ruptures require hysterectomy, but >66% of ruptured scars are repairable.

►►Mendelson's syndrome

This is the name given to the cyanosis, bronchospasm, pulmonary oedema, and tachycardia which develops due to inhalation of acid gastric contents during general anaesthesia. Clinically it may be difficult to distinguish from cardiac failure or amniotic fluid embolus. Pre-operative H_2 antagonists, sodium citrate, gastric emtying, cricoid pressure (p 770), the use of cuffed endotracheal tubes during anaesthesia and pre-extubation emptying of stomach aim to prevent it (p 132).

Management ►►Tilt the patient head down. Turn her to one side and aspirate the pharynx. Give 100% oxygen. Give aminophylline 5mg/kg by slow IVI and hydrocortisone 1000mg IV stat. The bronchial tree should be sucked out using a bronchoscope under general anaesthesia. Antibiotics, eg ampicillin and netilmicin (as above), should be given to prevent secondary pneumonia. Ventilation on intensive care may be needed. Physiotherapy should be given during convalescence

1 P Rozenberg 1996 *Lancet* **347** 281

Abdominal pain in pregnancy

►With any pain in pregnancy think, could this be the onset of labour?

Abdominal pain in pregnancy may be from ligament stretching or from symphysis pubis strain. Some other causes are given here. In early pregnancy remember abortion (p 22) and ectopic pregnancy (p 24).

Abruption The triad of abdominal pain, uterine rigidity and vaginal bleeding suggests this. It occurs in between 1 in 80 and 1 in 200 pregnancies. Fetal loss is high (up to 60%). A tender uterus is highly suggestive. Ultrasound may be diagnostic (but not necessarily so). A live viable fetus merits rapid delivery as demise can be sudden. Prepare for DIC which complicates 33–50% of severe cases, and beware PPH which is also common. See p 108.

Uterine rupture See opposite, p 134.

Uterine fibroids For torsion and red degeneration, see p 150.

Uterine torsion The uterus rotates axially 30–40° to the right in 80% of normal pregnancies. Rarely, it rotates >90° causing acute uterine torsion in mid or late pregnancy with abdominal pain, shock, a tense uterus and urinary retention (catheterization may reveal a displaced urethra in twisted vagina). Fibroids, adnexal masses, or congenital asymmetrical uterine anomalies are present in 90%. Diagnosis is usually at laparotomy. Delivery is by Caesarean section.

Ovarian tumours For torsion and rupture, see page 150.

Pyelonephritis See p 160.

Appendicitis Incidence: ~1/1000 pregnancies. This is not commoner in pregnancy but mortality is higher (especially from 20 weeks). Perforation is commoner (15–20%). Fetal mortality is ~5–10% for simple appendicitis; ~30% when there is perforation. The appendix migrates upwards, outwards and posteriorly as pregnancy progresses, so pain is less well localized (often paraumbilical or subcostal) and tenderness, rebound and guarding less obvious. Peritonitis can make the uterus tense and woody-hard. Operative delay is dangerous. Laparotomy over site of maximal tenderness with patient tilted 30° to the left should be performed by an experienced obstetric surgeon.

Cholecystitis Incidence 1–6 per 10,000 pregnancies. Pregnancy encourages gallstone formation due to biliary stasis and increased cholesterol in bile. Symptoms are similar to the non-pregnant with subcostal pain, nausea and vomiting. Jaundice is uncommon (5%). Ultrasound confirms the presence of stones. The main differential diagnosis is appendicitis and laparotomy is mandatory if this cannot be excluded. Treatment is similar to the non-pregnant aiming for interval cholecystectomy after the puerperium.

Rectus sheath haematoma Very rarely, bleeding into the rectus sheath and haematoma formation can occur with coughing (or spontaneously) in late pregnancy causing swelling and tenderness. Ultrasound is helpful.[1] Laparotomy is indicated if the diagnosis is in doubt.

Abdominal pain may complicate pre-eclampsia by liver congestion. Rarely, in severe pre-eclampsia the liver perforates.

1 G Chamberlain 1991 *BMJ* i 1390

Stillbirth

Stillbirths are those babies born dead after 24 weeks completed gestation. Death *in utero* may take place at any stage in pregnancy or in labour. Delivery of these babies presents an emotional strain for both mother and attendant staff as the pain and process of labour may seem so futile and mothers may feel guilty—and that this is in some way a punishment.

Some hours after a fetus has died *in utero* the skin begins to peel. On delivery such fetuses are described as *macerated*, as opposed to *fresh* stillbirths. If left, spontaneous labour usually occurs (80% within 2 weeks, 90% within 3 weeks), but it is common practice to induce labour once death is diagnosed, to prevent a long wait for labour for the mother, and minimize risk of coagulopathy. DIC (p 142) is rare unless a dead fetus of more than 20 weeks' gestation has been retained for >3 weeks, but if tests indicate a clotting disorder is present, some authorities recommend heparin (1000u IV/h for up to 48 hours prior to onset of labour)—but get expert advice. Stop any heparin prior to labour, or if it supervenes. Ensure excellent supply of freshest possible blood and fresh frozen plasma are available at delivery.

Causes of stillbirth Pre-eclampsia, chronic hypertension or renal disease, diabetes, infection, hyperpyrexia (T° >39.4°C), malformation (11% of macerated stillbirths and 4% of fresh have chromosomal anomalies), haemolytic disease, postmaturity. Abruption and knots in the cord may cause death in labour. In 20% no cause is found.

Diagnosis The mother usually reports absent fetal movements. No heart sounds (using Pinard's stethoscope, Doppler or cardiotocography). There is no fetal movement (eg heart beat) on ultrasound. It may help the mother to see lack of heart beat.

Management The mother may want to go home after diagnosis to reflect, collect things and make arrangements. Check maternal T°, BP, urine for protein, and blood clotting screen if fetus not thought recently demised. Labour is induced using prostaglandin vaginally; or extra-amniotically (dose varied with uterine response). Oxytocin IV used concomitantly risks uterine or cervical trauma so use *after* prostaglandin extra-amniotic infusion ceases. Oxytocin infusion alone (p 110) may be used for induction if the cervix is ripe (Bishop's score ≥4, gestation ≥35 weeks). Amniotomy is traditionally contraindicated as it risks infection. Some use mifepristone orally before using prostaglandins to induce abortion.

Ensure good pain relief in labour (if epidural, check clotting tests all normal). Do not leave the mother unattended. When the baby is born wrap it (as with any other baby) and offer to the mother to see and to hold—if the mother so desires. A photograph may be taken for her to take home, a lock of the baby's hair and palm-print given (keep in notes for later if she does not want them then). Unseen babies are difficult to grieve for. Naming the baby and holding a funeral service may help with grief.

Labour ward procedure (to try to establish cause) Thorough examination of the stillbirth, clinical photographs. Take time to talk to parents about how helpful a postmortem may be to them, in understanding what happened, and planning further pregnancies. If consent is refused, MRI and cytogenetics (± small volumes of tissue for metabolic studies) may be acceptable but are less informative.[1] Do placental histology. High vaginal swab for bacteriology. Maternal and fetal blood for TORCH[etc] screen (p 98). Mother's blood for Kleihauer acid test, p 109 (detects fetomaternal transfusion—a cause of unexplained stillbirth), and lupus anticoagulant. Examination of fetal blood and skin for chromosomes.

1 P Perry 1997 *Lancet* **349** 55 (MRI may miss significant pathologies)

Helping parents after stillbirth

- Offer lactation suppression (bromocriptine 2.5mg PO on day 1, then 2.5mg/12h PO for 14 days), but beware if pre-eclampsia. Give parents a follow-up appointment to discuss causes found by the above tests. Consider a domiciliary visit if parents prefer. Refer for genetic counselling if appropriate.
- In England, a *Certificate of Stillbirth* is required (issued by an obstetrician), which the parents are required to take to the Registrar of Births and Deaths within 42 days of birth. The father's name only appears in the register if the parents are married, or if both parents make the registration.
- The Registrar then issues a Certificate of Burial or Cremation which the parents then give to the undertaker (if they have chosen a private funeral—in which case they bear the cost of the funeral), or to the hospital administrators if they have chosen a hospital funeral—for which the hospital bears the cost. Parents are issued with a Certificate of Registration to keep which has the name of the stillborn baby (if named), the name of the informant who made the registration, and the date of stillbirth.
- UK hospitals are directed by the Department of Social Security to offer 'hospital' funerals for stillbirths (arranged through an undertaker). If the parents offer to pay for this, the hospital may accept. The hospital should notify the parents of the time of funeral so that they may attend, if they wish. With hospital funerals a coffin is provided and burial is often in a multiple-occupancy grave in a part of the graveyard set aside for babies. The hospital should inform parents of the site of the grave. Graves are unmarked, so should the parents not attend the funeral and wish to visit later it is recommended that they contact the graveyard attendants for the grave to be temporarily marked. Parents may buy a single occupancy grave, if they wish, on which they can later erect a headstone. Hospitals can arrange cremations, but the parents pay for this and parents should be told that there are unlikely to be any ashes after cremation.[1]
- In addition to arranging a follow-up appointment with the obstetrician to discuss implications for future pregnancy, and the cause (if known) of the stillbirth, it is helpful to give parents the address of a local branch of an organization for bereavement counselling, eg SANDS.[2] Grief may take a long time to resolve (p 442) and parents may find it difficult to contact ordinary medical staff without the 'excuse' provided by asking about the baby's ailments.

Each maternity unit should have a bereavement counsellor to support the mother and father, and help guide them through the formalities.

Note: in the UK statutory maternity pay and the maternity allowance and social fund maternity payments are payable after stillbirth.

1 Guidelines for professionals on pregnancy loss and the death of a baby (Royal College of Obstetricians and Gynaecologists) **2** SANDS (*Stillbirth & Neonatal Death* Society), 28 Portland Place, London WIN 4DE, UK (tel. 0171 436 5881)

Post-partum haemorrhage (PPH)

Primary PPH is the loss of greater than 500mL (definitions vary) in the first 24h after delivery. This occurs after ~6% of deliveries; major PPH (>1 litre) in 1.3%. Causes: uterine atony (90%), genital tract trauma (7%), clotting disorders—p 142 (3%). Death rate: 2/yr in the UK; 125 000/yr worldwide.[1]

Factors predisposing to poor uterine contractions •Past history of atony with PPH. •Retained placenta or cotyledon. •Ether or halothane anaesthesia. •A large placental site (twins, severe rhesus disease, large baby), low placenta, overdistended uterus (polyhydramnios, twins). •Extravasated blood in the myometrum (abruption). •Uterine malformation or fibroids. •Prolonged labour. •Poor second stage uterine contractions. •Trauma to uterus or cervix. •Older mothers.

Management •Give ergometrine 0.5mg IV. •Call emergency ambulance unit (p 92)—if not in hospital. Give high-flow O_2 as soon as available. •Set up IVI (2 large-bore cannulae). •Call anaesthetist[1] (a CVP line may help guide fluid replacement, but not if it causes delay). •If shocked give Haemaccel® or fresh blood of the patient's ABO and Rh group (uncrossmatched in emergency) *fast* until systolic BP >100mmHg and urine flows at >30mL/h (catheterize the bladder). •Is the the placenta delivered? If it is, is it complete? If not, explore the uterus. •If the placenta is complete, put the patient in the lithotomy position with adequate analgesia and good lighting. Check for and repair trauma. •If the placenta has not been delivered but has separated, attempt to deliver it by controlled cord traction after rubbing up a uterine contraction. If this fails, ask an experienced obstetrician to remove it under general anaesthesia. Beware renal shut-down.

If bleeding continues despite all the above, give 10 units of oxytocin in 500mL dextrose saline, eg at a rate of 15 drops/min. Bimanual pressure on the uterus may decrease immediate loss. Inform consultant. Check that blood is clotting (5mL should clot in a 10mL round-bottomed glass tube in 6min; formal tests: platelets, prothrombin ratio, kaolin–cephalin clotting time, fibrin degradation products). Explore the uterus for possible rupture. If uterine atony is the cause, and the circulation is still compromised, give carboprost 250µg (15-methyl prostaglandin F2α) eg as Hemabate® 1mL deep IM (max 8 doses, each >15min (usually 90 minutes) apart). SE: nausea, vomiting, diarrhoea, T°↑; (less commonly—asthma, BP↑, pulmonary oedema).[2] It controls bleeding in ~88%. Rarely, uterine packing, internal iliac artery or uterine vessel ligation or hysterectomy (possibly safest) is needed to stop bleeding. Ask a haematologist's advice on clotting factor replacement (fresh frozen plasma contains all of them; the cryoprecipitate has more fibrinogen, but lacks antithrombin III).

Secondary PPH This is excessive blood loss from the genital tract after 24h from delivery. It usually occurs between 5 and 12 days and is due to retained placental tissue or clot. Secondary infection is common. Uterine involution may be incomplete. If bleeding is slight and there is no sign of infection it may be managed conservatively—but heavier loss, the suggestion of retained products on ultrasound, or a tender uterus with an open os, requires exploration. Crossmatch 2 units of blood pre-operatively. Give antibiotics (eg ampicillin 500mg/6h IV, metronidazole 1g/12h PR) if there are signs of infection. Carefully curette the uterus (it is easily perforated at this stage). Send currettings for histology (excludes choriocarcinoma).

1 J Drife 1997 *Br J Obs Gyn* **104** 274 2 *Drug Ther Bul* 1992 **30** 89

Managing those refusing blood transfusion in pregnancy[1]

- Know maternal attitude to transfusion at booking.
- Give oral iron and folate to mother to maximize haemoglobin stores.
- Book for delivery where good facilities to deal with haemorrhage promptly (including facilities for hysterectomy).
- Arrange ultrasound to know placental site.
- Inform consultant when admitted in labour. Ensure experienced staff conduct labour. Give oxytocin as soon as the baby is delivered. Do not leave the mother alone for first hour post-delivery.
- Consultants should perform Caesarean section if required.
- Haemorrhage should be dealt with promptly, and clotting disorders excluded early. Involve a consultant obstetrician early (to decide if hysterectomy may be needed), and a consultant anaesthetist (for help with fluid replacement and for use of intensive care facilities). Liaise with a consultant haematologist. Avoid dextran (adversely affects haemostasis), but Haemacel® is useful.
- Ensure the woman does not want to change her mind and receive a tranfusion.
- Should the woman die of exsanguination both bereaved relatives and distressed staff should be offered support.

1 DoH 1996 *Report on Confidential Enquiry into Maternal Deaths in the United Kingdom 1991-93* HMSO p44-7.

Retained placenta

Physiological third stage takes 30min. With the use of oxytocic drugs at delivery and controlled cord traction, ie active management, the third stage is complete in 10min in 97% of labours, and a placenta not delivered in 30min will probably not be expelled spontaneously. The danger with retained placenta is haemorrhage. *Associations:* Previous retained placenta; previous uterine surgery; preterm delivery; maternal age >35 years; placental weight <600g; petihidine use in labour; induced labour; parity >5.[1]

Management If the placenta does not separate readily, avoid excessive cord traction—the cord may snap or the uterus invert. Check that the placenta is not in the vagina. Palpate the abdomen. If the uterus is well contracted, the placenta is probably separated but trapped by the cervix. Wait for the cervix to relax and release it. If the uterus is bulky, the placenta may have failed to separate. Rub up a contraction, put the baby to the breast (stimulates oxytocin production) or give more Syntometrine®, and empty the bladder (a full bladder causes atony). If the placenta still will not deliver, prepare to remove it manually (delay may precipitate a PPH).

Manual removal Set up IVI and crossmatch blood (eg 2u). Call the anaesthetist. The procedure can be done under epidural if *in situ*; halothane assists by relaxing the uterus. Obtain consent. With the mother in lithotomy position, using aseptic technique, place one hand on the abdomen to stabilize the uterus. Insert the other hand through the cervix into the uterus. Following the cord assists finding the placenta. Gently work round the placenta, separating it from the uterus using the ulnar border of the hand. When separated it should be possible to remove it by cord traction. Check that it is complete. Give oxytocic drugs and start antibiotics, eg doxycycline 200mg stat, 100mg/24h and metronidazole 400mg/8h PO.
Rarely, the placenta will not separate (placenta accreta) and hysterectomy may be necessary—by a senior obstetrician.

►►Uterine inversion

Inversion of the uterus is rare. It may be due to mismanagement of the third stage, eg with cord traction in an atonic uterus and a fundal insertion of the placenta. It may be completely revealed, or partial when the uterus remains within the vagina. Even without haemorrhage the mother may become profoundly shocked.

Management The ease with which the uterus is replaced depends on the amount of time elapsed since inversion, as a tight ring forms at the neck of the inversion. With an inversion noted early before shock sets in, replacement by hand may be possible. If shock has ensued, set up a fast IVI and infuse colloid or blood. Summon expert help. Under halothane anaesthesia to relax the uterus, hold the uterus in the vagina with one hand. Run two litres of warm 0.9% saline fast into the vagina through cystoscopy tubing (or with a funnel and tube) with an assistant holding the labia encircled tightly around the operator's arm to prevent the fluid running away. Running the fluid through a silastic ventouse cap held in the vagina improves the 'vaginal seal'.[2] The hydrostatic pressure of the water should reduce the uterus. Once the inversion has been corrected, give ergometrine to contract the uterus and prevent recurrence.

1 M Soltan 1997 *J Obs Gynae* **17** 245 2 O Ogueh 1997 *Br J Obs Gyn* **104** 792

►►DIC and coagulation defects

DIC in pregnancy is always secondary to stimulation of coagulation by procoagulant substance release in the maternal circulation. Known triggers are: retention of a dead fetus (of greater than 20 weeks' gestation which has been dead for >3 weeks); pre-eclampsia; placental abruption; endotoxic shock; amniotic fluid embolism; placenta accreta; hydatidiform mole; prolonged shock from any cause; acute fatty liver of pregnancy (p 158).

Pathogenesis of DIC: Thromboplastins are released into the circulation, fibrin and platelets are consumed as intravascular clotting occurs. *Tests:* Kaolin-cephalin clotting time↑ (↓ factors II, V, VII), fibrinogen↓, fibrin degradation products↑. In situations where DIC is a possibility send blood for cross-match, platelets, partial thromboplastin time or accelerated whole blood clotting time, prothrombin time, fibrinogen estimation and fibrin degradation products. Preliminary results should be available in 30min.

Management: Presentation may be as heavy bleeding and shock, and the first measures must be the correction of shock. ►►Give O_2 at 15 litres/min via a tight fitting mask with reservoir. Set up at least 1, preferably 2, wide-gauge IVIs, take bloods as above, and give blood fast (group-compatible blood—available in 5–10min or O Rh–ve blood if desperate). Stored blood is deficient in clotting factors. Give fresh frozen plasma to normalize the kaolin-cephalin clotting time and the prothrombin time. Platelets are indicated with prolonged bleeding and low platelet count. Calcium is sometimes needed to counteract citrate in stored blood (eg 10mL of 10% calcium gluconate IVI, eg after 6u of blood. Seek expert help from a haematologist. The condition is usually self-limiting if the stimulus can be removed. In the case of intrauterine death and abruption (p 108) removal of the uterine contents is the way to correct the the stimulus, and this should be done as promptly as possible. *Mortality:* <1% if placental abruption; 50–80% if infection/shock.

Autoimmune thrombocytopenic purpura (AITP) Incidence 1–2; 10,000 pregnancies. IgG antibodies cause thrombocytopenia (associated with increased bone marrow megakaryocytes) in the mother, and being able to cross the placenta, they cause thrombocytopenia in ~10% of fetuses. Exclude systemic lupus erythematosus in the mother (thrombocytopenia may be an early presentation; do DNA binding, *OHCM* p 672). Consider maternal HIV. If maternal platelets fall below 20×10^9/L or 50×10^9/L near delivery,[1] give steroids. Rarely, splenectomy is necessary during pregnancy (ideally in the second trimester). Immunoglobulin IgG 0.4g/kg IV for 5 days is sometimes used near expected date of delivery, inducing maternal and fetal remission for up to 3 weeks but it is extremely expensive. Aim for non-traumatic delivery for both mother and baby. Neonatal platelet count may fall further in the first days of life, then gradually rise to normal over 4–16 weeks. Treatment is not needed unless surgery is contemplated. Maternal mortality due to AITP is now negligible, but fetal mortality remains (due to intracranial bleeding). Take cord blood at delivery. If platelets $<20 \times 10^9$/L give baby IgG 1g/kg IVI at birth. If platelets low at birth observe baby for 2–5 days as further falls likely.

Thrombocytopenia in pregnancy[1] **1** Spurious (try citrated bottle).
2 Pregnancy-associated thrombocytopenia[2] (benign gestational thrombocytopenia)—mild and self-limiting (platelets stay above 100×10^9/L).
3 Autoimmune thrombocytopenia.
4 Pre-eclampsia (platelets may fall early, preceding clotting abnormality).
5 Disseminated intravascular coagulation (DIC, see above).
6 Haemolytic uraemic syndrome (p 280), and thrombotic thrombocytopenic purpura (2 ends of a microangiopathic spectrum, *OHCM* p 397).
7 Folate deficiency.
8 Congenital (May–Heggin anomaly, hereditary macrothrombocytopenia).
9 Marrow disease; hypersplenism.

1 E Letsky 1996 *Br J Haematol* **95** 21 **2** M Pillai 1993 *Br J Obstet Gynae* **100** 201

Amniotic fluid embolism[1]

This condition, with a mortality up to 80% presents with sudden dyspnoea and hypotension, heralded, in 20%, by seizures. 40% also develop DIC, and of those who survive the initial collapse 70% go on to develop pulmonary oedema (acute respiratory distress syndrome, ARDS, *OHCM* p 350). An anaphylactic type of response occurs to (possibly abnormal) amniotic fluid in the maternal circulation. *Presentation* is often at the end of the first stage of labour or shortly after delivery but can complicate amniocentesis, or termination of pregnancy, and has even occurred up to 48h postpartum. Previously it was said to be related to uterine hyperstimulation (multiparous short labour and use of oxytocin). This may be anecdotal. Risk increases with increasing maternal age.

Management ►►The first priority is to prevent death from respiratory failure. Give mask oxygen and call an anaesthetist urgently. Endotracheal intubation and ventilation may be necessary. Set up IVI lest DIC should supervene. Treatment is essentially supportive—important steps are detailed below. Diagnosis may be difficult: exclude other causes of obstetric shock (p 106).

- Cardiopulmonary resuscitation if indicated.
- Give highest available O_2 concentration. If unconscious ventilate and use 100% inspired O_2.
- Monitor for fetal distress.
- If hypotensive, give fluids rapidly IVI to increase preload. If still hypotensive consider inotropes: dobutamine (a better inotrope than dopamine), eg in a dose range of 2.5–10μg/kg/min IVI may help.
- Pulmonary artery catheterization (Swan–Ganz catheter if available) helps guide haemodynamic management.
- After initial hypotension is corrected, give only maintenance requirements of fluid to avoid pulmonary oedema from acute respiratory distress syndrome. Transfer to intensive care unit as soon as possible.
- Treat DIC with fresh whole blood or packed cells and fresh frozen plasma. Use of heparin is controversial,[2] there is insufficient data to warrant routine heparinization.[1]

Should the woman die, specifically request that the lungs be examined for the presence of amniotic squames (to confirm the diagnosis).[3]

1 S Clark 1990 *Obstetrical Gynecological Survey* **45** 360 **2** DoH 1994 *Report on Confidential Enquiries into Maternal Deaths in the United Kingdom 1988-90*, London, HMSO **3** DoH 1996 *Report on Confidential Enquiries into Maternal Deaths in the United Kingdom 1991-3* HMSO page 66

Birth injuries to the baby

Moulding This is a natural phenomenon rather than an injury. The skull bones are able to override each other (p 86) to reduce the diameter of the head. Moulding is assessed by the degree of overlap of the overriding at the sutures. If moulding is absent, the cranial bones are felt separately. With slight moulding, the bones just touch, then they override but can be reduced; finally they override so much that they cannot be reduced. Excessive moulding during labour indicates cephalo-pelvic disproportion, and can result in intracranial damage.

Cephalhaematoma This is a *subperiostial* swelling on the fetal head, and its boundaries are therefore limited by the individual bone margins (commonest over parietal bones). It is fluctuant. Spontaneous absorption occurs but may take weeks and may cause or contribute to jaundice.

Caput succadaneum This is an oedematous swelling of the scalp, superficial to the cranial periosteum (which does not, therefore, limit its extent) and is the result of venous congestion and exuded serum caused by pressure against the cervix and lower segment during labour. The presenting part of the head therefore has the swelling over it. It gradually disappears in the first days after birth. When ventouse extraction is used in labour a particularly large caput (called a chignon) is formed under the ventouse cup.

Erb 's palsy This may result from a difficult assisted delivery, eg shoulder dystocia. The baby's arm is flaccid and the hand is in the 'porter's tip' posture (p 724). Exclude a fractured clavicle and arrange physiotherapy. If it has not resolved by 6 months, the outlook is poor.

Subaponeurotic haematoma Blood lies between the aponeurosis and the periosteum. As haematoma is not confined to the boundaries of one bone, collections of blood may be large enough to result in anaemia or jaundice. They are associated with vacuum extractions.

Skull fractures These are associated with difficult forceps extractions. They are commonest over parietal or frontal bones. If depressed fractures are associated with neurological signs, ask a neurosurgeon if the bone should be elevated.

Intracranial injuries Intracranial haemorrhage is especially associated with difficult or fast labour, instrumental labour, and breech delivery. Premature babies are especially vulnerable. Normally a degree of motility of intracranial contents is buffered by cerebrospinal fluid. Excessive moulding and sudden changes in pressure reduce this effect and are associated with trauma. In all cases of intracranial haemorrhage check babies' platelets. If low, check mother's blood for platelet alloantibodies (PLA1 system). Subsequent babies are at equal risk. IV maternal immunoglobulin treatment is being evaluated.

Anoxia may cause intraventricular haemorrhage (p 232). Asphyxia causes intracerebral haemorrhage (often petechial) and may result in cerebral palsy. Extradural, subdural and subarachnoid haemorrhages can all occur. Babies affected may have convulsions, apnoea, cyanosis, abnormal pallor, low heart rate, alterations in muscle tone, restlessness, somnolence or abnormal movements. Treatment is supportive and expectant. See p 232 & p 234.

2. Obstetrics

Episiotomy and tears

Perineal tears These are classified by the degree of damage caused. Tears are most likely to occur with big babies, precipitant labours, babies with poorly flexed heads, shoulder dystocia, when forceps are used, or if there is a narrow suprapubic arch.

Labial tears These are common and can be very uncomfortable, but heal quickly and suturing is rarely helpful.

First degree tears These tears are superficial and do not damage muscle. They may not need suturing unless blood loss is marked.

Second degree tears These lacerations involve perineal muscle and if severe may involve the anal sphincter. They are repaired in a similar fashion to repair of episiotomy (see below).

Third degree tears Damage extends through the anal mucosa and can extend into the rectum. Repair is carried out, by an experienced surgeon, under epidural or general anaesthesia. Rectal mucosa is repaired first using catgut from above the tear's apex to the mucocutaneous junction. Muscle is interposed. Vaginal mucosa is then sutured. Severed ends of the anal sphincter are apposed using figure-of-eight stitches. Finally skin is repaired. Avoid constipation post-operatively by using a high-fibre diet and faecal softeners.

Episiotomy This is performed to enlarge the outlet, eg to hasten delivery of a distressed baby, for instrumental or breech delivery, to protect a premature head, and to try to prevent 3° tears (but anal tears are not reduced by more episiotomies in normal deliveries).[1]

The tissues which are incised are vaginal epithelium, perineal skin, bulbocavernous muscle, superficial and deep transverse perineal muscles. With large episiotomies, the external anal sphincter or levator ani may be partially cut, and ischiorectal fat exposed.

Technique: Hold the perineal skin away from the presenting part of the fetus (2 fingers in vagina). Infiltrate area to be cut with local anaesthetic, eg 1% lidocaine (=lignocaine). Still keeping the fingers in the introitus, cut mediolaterally towards the ischial tuberosity, starting medially (6 o'clock), so avoiding the Bartholin's glands.

Repair: (See diagrams opposite.) NB: use resorbable sutures, but not glycerol-impregnated cat-gut (risks long-term dyspareunia). In lithotomy, and using good illumination, repair the vaginal mucosa first. Start above the apex using interlocking stitches 1cm apart, 1cm from wound edges. Tie off at mucocutaneous junction of fourchette. Then repair muscles with interrupted stitches to obliterate any dead spaces. Finally close the skin (subcutaneous stitch is more comfortable than interrupted stitches).

Problems with episiotomy: Bleeding (so may increase chance of spread of HIV from mother to baby); infection and breakdown; haematoma formation. For comfort some suggest ice packs, salt baths, hair dryer to dry perineum. 60% of women suffer perineal damage (episiotomy or tear) with spontaneous vaginal delivery; rectal diclofenac can provide effective analgesia.[2] Superficial dyspareunia: see p 74. If labia minora are involved in the skin bridge, the introitus is left too small. If the deep layers are inadequately sutured, the introitus becomes rather rounded exposing the bladder to coital thrusts.

1 T Henriksen 1992 *Br J Obst Gynae* **99** 950 2 J Searles 1998 *Br J Obs Gyn* **105** 627

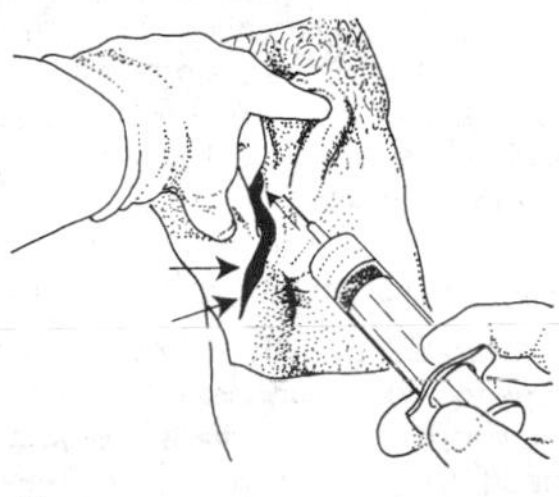

(1)
Swab the vulva towards the perineum. Infiltrate with 1% lignocaine → (*arrows*).

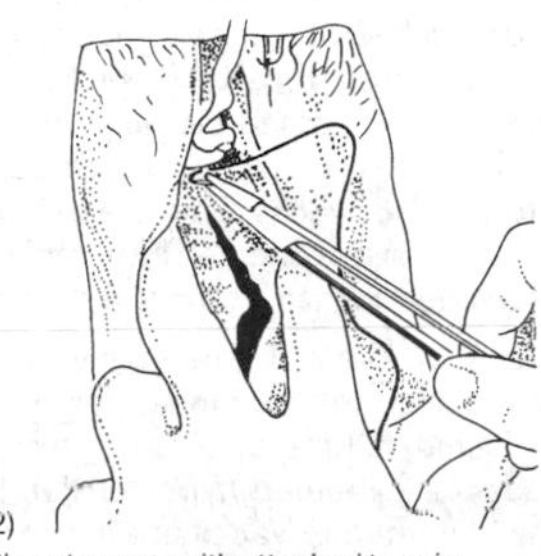

(2)
Place tampon with attached tape in upper vagina. Insert 1st suture above apex of vaginal cut (not too deep as underlying rectal mucosa nearby).

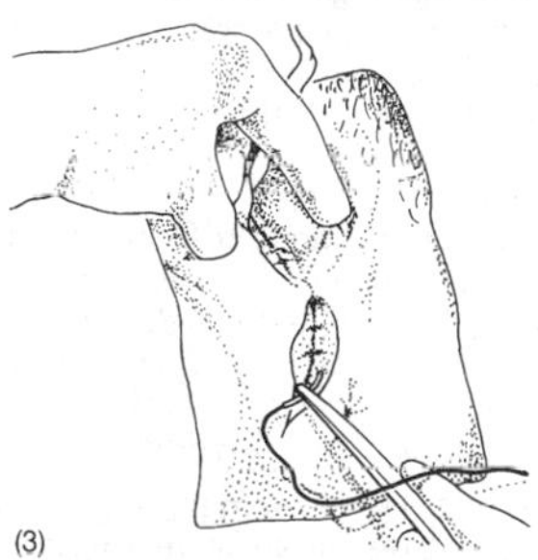

(3)
Bring together vaginal edges with continuous stitches placed 1 cm apart. Knot at introitus under the skin. Appose divided levator ani muscles with 2 or 3 interrupted sutures.

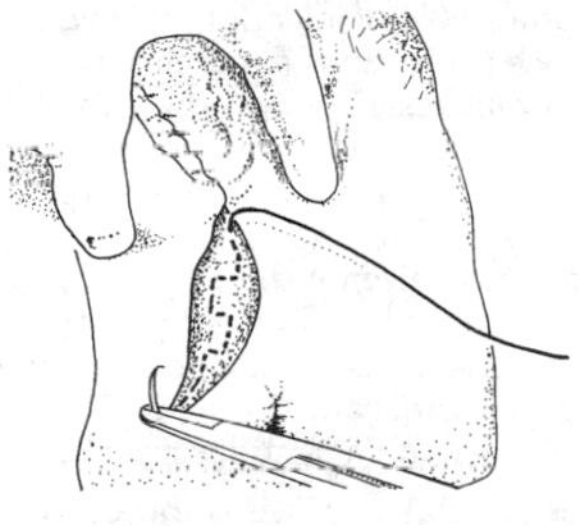

(4)
Close perineal skin (subcuticular continuous stitch is shown here).

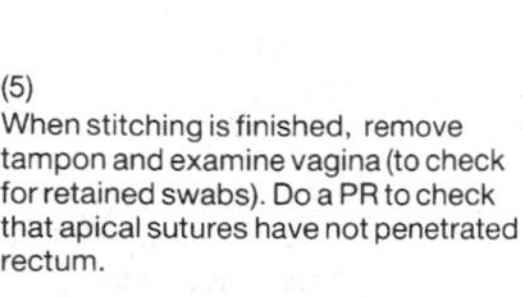

(5)
When stitching is finished, remove tampon and examine vagina (to check for retained swabs). Do a PR to check that apical sutures have not penetrated rectum.

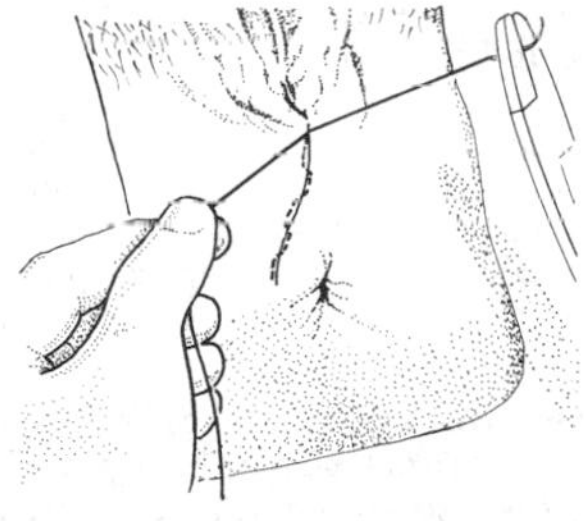

The puerperium[1]

The puerperium is the 6 weeks after delivery. The uterus involutes, from 1kg weight at delivery to 100g. Felt at the umbilicus after delivery, it is a pelvic organ at 10 days. Afterpains are felt (especially while suckling) as it contracts. The cervix becomes firm over 3 days. The internal os closes by 3 days, the external os by 3 weeks. Lochia (endometrial slough, red cells and white cells) is passed *per vaginam*. It is red (*lochia rubra*) for the 1st 3 days, then becomes yellow (*lochia serosa*) then white over the next 10 days (*lochia alba*), until 6 weeks. The breasts produce milky discharge and colostrum during the last trimester. Milk replaces colostrum 3 days after birth. Breasts are swollen, red and tender with physiological engorgement at 3 to 4 days.

The first days If Rh–ve, give anti-D, within 72h, p 109. Check T°, BP, breasts, legs, lochia, fundal height. Teach pelvic floor exercises. Persistent *red lochia*, failure of *uterine involution* or *PPH* (p 138) suggest retained products. *Sustained hypertension* may need drugs (*OHCM* p 302). ►Check *rubella immunity*. Vaccinate if non-immune but delay until postnatal exam if anti-D given. *Check Hb* on postnatal day 1 or ≥day 7: postpartum physiological haemodilution occurs from days 2–6.

Puerperal pyrexia is a temperature >38°C in the first 14 days after delivery or miscarriage. Examine fully (chest, breasts, legs, lochia and bimanual vaginal examination). Culture MSU, high vaginal swabs, blood and sputum. 90% of infections will be urinary or of the genital tract. Superficial perineal infections occur around the second day. *Endometritis* gives lower abdominal pain, offensive lochia and a tender uterus (on bimanual vaginal exam). Endometritis requires IV antibiotics (see below) and uterine curettage. For breast infection give flucloxacillin 250mg/6h PO early, to prevent abscesses. Suckling or breast expression should continue to prevent milk stagnation. Even if the cause of pyrexia is not apparent, it is wise to treat with amoxicillin 500mg/8h PO or IV and metronidazole 400mg/8h PO. NB: puerperal infection can be prevented by cleansing the birth canal at every vaginal examination with 0.25% chlorhexidine (if applied to the baby at birth, neonatal infections are also reduced, eg in labours in Africa).[2]

Superficial thrombophlebitis This affects 1% of women, presenting with a painful tender (usually varicose) vein. Give anti-inflammatories, eg ibuprofen 400mg/8h PO pc. Bandage and elevate the leg. Recovery is usual within 4 days. *Deep vein thrombosis:* See p 151.

Puerperal psychosis (1:500 births): This is distinguished from mild depression which often follows birth by a high suicidal drive, severe depression (p 336), mania, and more rarely schizophrenic symptoms (p 358) with delusions that the child is malformed. If an acute organic reaction (p 350) is present, suspect puerperal infection. It may be worthwhile explaining to mothers that the puerperium is not always a time of joy, and they may feel low—and should let the midwife, health visitor or GP know about negative feelings, persistent crying, sleeplessness, and feelings of inadequacy—as early recognition of the problem is the best way to avoid what can be an intensely destructive experience. *Treatment:* See p 408 for a fuller discussion.

The 6-week postnatal examination gives a chance to: •See how mother and baby relate. •Do BP & weight. •Do FBC if anaemic postnatally. •Arrange a cervical smear if not done antenatally. •Check contraceptive plans (p 68) are enacted (start Pills ~4 weeks postnatally). •Ask about depression, backache, incontinence.[1] Ask 'have you resumed intercourse?' Sexual problems are common, and prolonged: ~50% report that intercourse is less satisfactory than pre-pregnancy, with major loss of libido, and dyspareunia the chief complaints. Vaginal examination to check healing is *not* usually needed.[1]

1 C MacArthur 1999 *Lancet* 353 343   2 T Taha 1997 BMJ **ii** 216

Fibroids in pregnancy

Fibroids 5/1000 Caucasian women have fibroids in pregnancy. They are commoner in Afro-Caribbean women. They may cause abortion. They increase in size in pregnancy—especially in the second trimester. If pedunculated they may tort. Red degeneration is when thrombosis of capsular vessels is followed by venous engorgement and inflammation, causing abdominal pain (± vomiting and low grade fever), and localized peritoneal tenderness—usually in the second half of pregnancy or the puerperium. *Treatment* is expectant (bed rest, analgesia) with resolution over 4–7 days.

Most fibroids arise from the body of the uterus and do not therefore obstruct labour, as they tend to rise away from the pelvis throughout pregnancy. If large pelvic masses of fibroids are noted prior to labour Caesarean section should be planned. Obstruction of labour also needs Caesarean section.

Ovarian tumours in pregnancy

These are found in ~1/1000 pregnancies. It is easier to distinguish them (lying as they do in the rectovaginal pouch) with an anteverted uterus than with a gravid retroverted uterus. Suspicion of presence of a tumour can be confirmed by ultrasound. Torsion of ovarian cysts is more common in pregnancy and the puerperium than at other times. Cyst rupture and haemorrhage into cysts may also occur, but are not more common than at other times. Torsion may present with abdominal pain, nausea, vomiting, shock, local tenderness (usually at 8–16 weeks). 2–5% of tumours are malignant. Suspect malignancy with ruptures (then biopsy other ovary). ~25% of malignant tumours will be dysgerminomas.

Tumours can become necrotic due to pressure on them in labour. Tumours lying in the pelvis can obstruct labour so Caesarean section will be needed unless they are cysts which can be aspirated under ultrasound control before labour.

Asymptomatic simple cysts <5cm across can be left until after delivery if watched by ultrasound. Those 5–10cm may be aspirated under ultrasound control (and the aspirate examined cytologically).[1] Other tumours (those that are complex multilocular or with solid portions on ultrasound) should be removed at about 16 weeks' gestation (by which time the pregnancy is not dependent on the corpus luteum and miscarriage is less likely) to exclude carcinoma and prevent complications developing. If the diagnosis is made late in pregnancy and the tumour is not obstructing the pelvis, it is usual to let labour progress normally, and to remove the tumour in the early puerperium because of the risk of torsion then.

1 C Buckley 1989 *Br J Obstet Gynae* **96** 1021

Venous thromboembolism (VET) in pregnancy

►*Investigate any unexplained calf or chest symptoms* ***today***. Thromboembolism is the chief UK cause of maternal death.[1] VET risk rises 6-fold in pregnancy (~0.3–1.6% of pregnancies: 20–50% occur antenatally—in *any* trimester), and risk rises still further with immobility, weight (>80Kg), age, smoking, long (>3h) air travel, and surgery, eg Caesarean section. 50% of those with 1st VET have *thrombophilia* (below), so look for this.[1] Women with lupus anticoagulant risk arterial and venous thrombosis, eg in atypical veins, eg portal or arm.

Pulmonary embolism Small emboli may cause unexplained pyrexia, syncope, cough, chest pain, and breathlessness. Pleurisy should be considered due to embolism unless there is high fever or much purulent sputum. Large emboli present as collapse with chest pain, breathlessness and cyanosis. There will be a raised JVP, third heart sound and parasternal heave.

Tests: Chest x-ray and ECG may be normal (apart from showing a tachycardia, the most consistent finding). ECG changes of deep S-wave in lead I and Q-wave and inverted T-wave in lead III can be caused by pregnancy alone. Blood gases may be helpful ($P_aO_2\downarrow$; $P_aCO_2\downarrow$).

Ventilation/perfusion lung scans are safe in pregnancy and are recommended.

Treatment: Massive emboli may require prolonged cardiac massage and consideration of pulmonary embolectomy. Give heparin 5,000u IV, then ~1600u/h IVI in 0.9% saline by syringe pump. Monitor APPT (*OHCM* p 596). After 3–7 days on IV heparin maintain on long-term heparin (eg 10,000u/12h sc with careful monitoring. Keep level <0.2u/mL.) Heparin can cause maternal osteopenia (reversible after stopping) with prolonged use and can cause thrombocytopenia and alopecia. Warfarin is teratogenic (Conradi–Hünermann syndrome, p 744) and is used antenatally up to 36 weeks only in those with artificial heart valves. sc heparin is continued through labour with no increased risk of PPH, but epidural anaesthesia is contraindicated. Heparin postpartum is reduced to 7500u/12h sc. Continue for 6 weeks postpartum (or if postnatal thrombosis, for a minimum of 6 weeks). Some choose warfarin use after 7 days postnatally.

Deep vein thrombosis (DVT) DVTs typically present with calf pain. For other signs, see *OHCM* p 92. Often symptoms are not clear-cut. Tests: contrast or Ultrasound or radionuclide venography; (avoid ^{125}I fibrinogen in pregnancy). Treat with heparin throughout pregnancy—to double the activated partial thromboplastin time (APTT); after 7–9 days give sc unfractionated heparin 10,000u, or enoxaparin 40mg/day sc; monitor platelets (heparin-induced thrombocytopenia; NB: long-term monitoring of APTT is not usually done, as no one knows the value to aim for). After delivery warfarin may be used (breast feeding is OK). Monitor INR meticulously.

Prophylaxis Risks of heparin and warfarin antenatally (see above) reserves antenatal (eg all trimester) heparin use for higher-risk cases ie in recurrent thromboembolism or thromboembolism associated with thrombophilia (below). Lower risk women (previous single thromboembolic episode) receive heparin 7500u sc during labour, induction or Caesarean section (after taking plenty of blood in case crossmatch is needed) and then use heparin for 6 weeks post-delivery or heparin then warfarin (as above).

Recurrent thromboembolism (RTE) *Is thrombophilia present?* (*OHCM* p 620). Look for: •Factor V Leiden mutation: this ↓factor V breakdown by protein C (activated protein C (APC) resistance) •Protein C or S deficiency •Antithrombin III↓ •Lupus anticoagulant ± cardiolipin antibody—especially if arterial RTE, atypical site or associated with bad obstetric history (thrombophilia is associated with eclampsia, placental abruption,[2] growth retardation, and stillbirth, perhaps as these are related to intervillous or spiral artery thrombosis).

1 DoH 1998 *Confidential. Enq. into Maternal Deaths 1994-6*, HMSO (VET deaths ≈15/yr) 2 NEJM 1999 **340** 9

Cardiac disease in pregnancy

During pregnancy cardiac output increases to a maximum of 30–40% above non-pregnant levels. This is effected by ↑ heart rate and stroke volume.

Heart disease affects 0.5–2% of pregnant women. Examine the heart carefully early in all pregnancies. Ask the opinion of a cardiologist if there is doubt: •Past history (eg congenital heart disease, rheumatic fever). •Previous Kawasaki disease (now a more common cause of acquired heart disease than rheumatic fever). •Murmurs (other than those below).

60% of maternal cardiac deaths occur after delivery. Cardiac failure can occur at any stage in pregnancy but risk increases as pregnancy advances and is most in the early puerperium. Marfan's and Eisenmenger's syndrome (p 748—monitor Hb and pulse oximetry; admit from second trimester), 1° pulmonary hypertension, coarctation of the aorta (surges of BP↑ in the proximal segment), severe aortic or mitral stenosis and inoperable cyanotic heart disease are associated with ↑ maternal mortality, so advise against pregnancy—or arrange the most meticulous care. Termination may be medically advised.

Seek specialist advice when managing patients with prosthetic valves requiring anticoagulation. Heparin from 7–16 weeks IV via a Hickman line and from 36 weeks IV as an inpatient may be used.

Antenatal management Regular visits to cardiologist/obstetric combined clinic. Prevent anaemia, obesity and smoking. Ensure sufficient rest. Treat hypertension. Treat infections early. Give antibiotic cover for dental treatment (*OHCM* p 314). Examine carefully to exclude pulmonary oedema and arrhythmias at all visits. Heart failure requires admission.

Labour If cardiac reserves are good before labour, risks during labour are low. Have oxygen and drugs to treat cardiac failure to hand. Avoid lithotomy position (dangerous ↑venous return after labour—the best position is semi-sitting). Aim for vaginal delivery at term with a short second stage (lift out forceps or ventouse). Give antibiotic cover, eg ampicillin 500mg IV and gentamicin 80mg IV repeated twice at 8-hourly intervals, if valve or septal defect. Pain relief should be good. Epidurals are safe if hypotension is avoided. Beware large volumes of IV fluids. Avoid ergometrine. Caesarean section should not be attempted (except during eclampsia) if the patient is in failure. Cardiac failure is most likely within the first 24h after delivery, so ensure very careful observations at this time.

Cardiac failure If symptoms or signs detected, admit the mother for bed rest, and treatment with diuretics ± digoxin. If acute failure develops, give 100% oxygen, nurse semi-recumbent, and give furosemide (=frusemide) 40mg IV slowly (<4mg/min), morphine 10mg IV, and aminophylline 5mg/kg by slow IVI (over >15min). If there is no improvement, consider ventilation. (There is no specific information on the use of nitrates in labour.)

Arrhythmias *Atrial fibrillation:* Is there mitral stenosis too?—admit to hospital. Treatment is as for the non-pregnant and may include digitalization or cardioversion. *Supraventricular tachycardia:* This may precipitate cardiac failure. If Valsalva manoeuvre and carotid massage fail, anaesthetize and cardiovert.

These signs may be normal in pregnancy •Pulses are ↑ in volume.
- Neck veins pulsate more vigorously (but JVP should not be ↑).
- The apex beat is forceful (but <2cm lateral to midclavicular line).
- Oedema.
- The first heart sound is loud and a third heart sound can be heard in 84%.
- An ejection systolic murmur is heard in 96% of women.
- Systolic or continuous murmurs over right and left second intercostal spaces 2cm from sternal edge, modified by stethoscope pressure, are thought to be due to blood flow in mammary vessels.
- Venous hums may be heard in the neck (modified by posture).
- CXR may show slight cardiomegaly, ↑pulmonary vascular markings, distension of pulmonary veins due to ↑ cardiac output.

Psychopharmacology in pregnancy

For puerperal depression, see p 408.

We always try to avoid drugs in pregnancy, but sometimes psychotropics are essential, eg if the mother is neglecting herself or her pregnancy. When psychotropic drugs are used, they must be combined with well-planned psychosocial support from a trusted confidant of the patient.

Depression in pregnancy—*Unipolar:* For diagnosis, see p 324. Try to wait until the second trimester before prescribing, and avoid SSRIs (p 341) as there is little experience with their use. Most experience is with tricyclics (p 340) such as amitriptyline—which are therefore the first choice when drugs are essential, despite warnings in naturally cautious *Data sheets* which read '...*The safety of amitriptyline has not been established in pregnancy. It is not recommended during pregnancy, especially during the first and third trimesters unless there are compelling reasons, and, in these patients, the benefits should be weighed against the possible hazards to mother, fetus, and child... Animal experiments have shown harmful effects at exceptionally high doses...*' For these reasons, it is wise to discuss decisions with another doctor, or your local drug information service. Problems are unlikely, but the exact risk of teratogenesis cannot be stated. Withdrawal effects have been noted in neonates, eg agitation and respiratory depression with amitriptyline, and colic, spasms, and hyper- or hypotension with imipramine.[2] Get a second opinion if ECT may be indicated. In general, breast feeding is contraindicated, as metabolites pass to the baby.

Bipolar: Lithium (see p 354) *is* linked with teratogenicity (eg displacement of the tricuspid valve into the right ventricle). Offer specialist fetal echocardiography at 16 weeks in those women electing to remain on lithium. Used outside the first trimester, lithium can still cause problems with the fetal renal and thyroid function. Monitor drug levels frequently (exactly 12h post-dose), and keep the dose as low as possible, and, in general, aim for a level of <0.4mmol/l.[1] Do not change brands, as bioavailability varies. Do extra monitoring during intercurrent illness, D&V, and when poor compliance or toxicity is suspected (tremor, drowsiness, visual disturbance).

If lithium is stopped for a pregnancy or labour, restart it within a few days of birth. It is excreted in breast milk, so breast feeding is contraindicated.

Phenothiazines in pregnant schizophrenics There is conflicting data on safety—but there is agreement that most pregnancies will be unaffected. Pre-birth exposure may result in a syndrome of hyperreflexia, hypertonia, and tremor which may persist for the first months of life. NB: rates of fetal abnormality are increased in schizophrenia, even in those taking no drugs.[1] The *Data sheet* for chlorpromazine reads '... *There is inadequate evidence of safety in human pregnancy but it has been widely used for many years without apparent ill consequence. There is evidence of harmful effects in animals... It should be avoided in pregnancy unless the physician considers it essential. It may occasionally prolong labour, and at such a time should be withheld until the cervix is dilated 3–4cm. Possible adverse effects on the neonate include lethargy or paradoxical excitability, tremor, and low Apgar score... Being excreted in milk, breast feeding during treatment should be suspended...*'

Anxiety in pregnancy Temazepam has been used successfully in those where insomnia has been a real problem. Avoid diazepam around the time of delivery, as withdrawal may occur in the baby (floppy baby syndrome). Avoid β-blockers, as these retard fetal growth.[1] Relaxation techniques (p 344) and supportive psychotherapy (p 376) are far more appropriate.

1 JL Cox & K Nicholls 1996 *Prescribers' Journal* **36** 192 **2** ABPI 1996 *Data-sheet Compendium:* 1996–7

Anaemia in pregnancy

►Even a small PPH may become life-threatening if the mother is anaemic. Anaemia predisposes to infection, and makes heart failure worse. Worn-out, anaemic mothers may not cope with their offspring. Anaemia is the main cause of perinatal problems associated with malaria; above all, anaemia is a leading mechanism by which poverty exacts its morbid toll in pregnancy.

WHO definition of anaemia of pregnancy Hb <11g/dL. By this standard 50% of women not on haematinics become anaemic. The fall in Hb is steepest around 20 weeks' gestation, and is physiological (p 80); indeed failure of Hb to fall below 10.5g/dL (but not further than ~9.5g/dL) indicates ↑risk of low birth weight or premature delivery.[1]

Who is prone to anaemia? Those who start pregnancy anaemic, eg from menorrhagia, hookworm, malaria, with haemoglobinopathies; those with frequent pregnancies, twin pregnancy, or a poor diet.

Antenatal screening includes Hb estimation at booking, at 28 and 36 weeks. In black patients do sickle-cell tests, in others of foreign descent consider Hb electrophoresis for other haemoglobinopathies. From malarious areas consider malaria, and thick films. See p 159.

Treatment Pregnancy ↑iron needs by 700–1400mg (per pregnancy), provided for by a pregnancy-induced 9-fold increase in iron absorption.[2] The routine use of daily oral iron has never been shown to offer any clinical benefit[3]—and harm is possible.[2] Offer iron to those likely to be iron deficient (see above) or who would refuse transfusion if haemorrhage (p 139). *Parenteral iron* may be given (to those with iron deficiency anaemia not tolerating oral iron) as iron sorbitol citric acid 1.5mg/kg IM daily (max 100mg/injection) as per *Data Sheet* >24h after stopping oral iron to prevent toxic reaction of headache, nausea and vomiting. Haemoglobin rises over 6 weeks, so late severe anaemia (Hb <9g/dL) may need blood transfusion. One unit of blood increases the Hb by ~0.7g/dL.

Thalassaemia These globin chain production disorders are found in Mediterranean, Indian and South-east Asian populations. Although anaemic, never give parenteral iron as iron levels are high. Seek expert advice as to use of oral iron and folate. β-Thalassaemia does not affect the fetus but in homozygotes regular transfusions sustain life only until young adulthood. There are α chains in fetal HbF, so in α-thalassaemias the fetus may be anaemic or, if severe, stillborn. Mothers carrying lethally affected hydropic fetuses risk severe pre-eclampsia, and delivery complications due to a large fetus and bulky placenta. Prenatal diagnosis is possible by chorionic villus sampling (p 166) for thalassaemias anticipated by parental blood studies.

Sickling disorders can affect blacks of African origin, Saudi Arabians, Indians and Mediterranean populations. **Sickle-cell trait** is not usually a problem. **Sickle-cell disease** predisposes to abortion, preterm labour, stillbirth, crisis. There is a chronic haemolysis (eg Hb 6–9g/dL). Regular 3–4u blood transfusions every 6 weeks (so a problem is development of atypical antibodies) prevents crises. Infection may induce crises, and dehydration exacerbate them; treat with exchange transfusions (*OHCM* p 588). **Sickle-cell haemoglobin C disease** is a milder variant of sickle-cell disease. Hb levels usually near normal so women may be unaware they are affected. They are still susceptible to sickling crises in pregnancy and the puerperium, so antenatal diagnosis is essential. Prenatal sickle-cell diagnosis is possible by chorionic villus sampling.

►Aim for diagnosis at birth (cord blood) *at the latest* so that penicillin pneumococcal prophylaxis may be started (*OHCM* p 588).

1 P Steer 1995 *BMJ* **i** 489 2 JF Barrett 1994 *BMJ* **ii** 79 3 US Prev. Task Force 1993 *JAMA* **270** 2846

HIV in pregnancy and labour[1,2]

In sub-Saharan Africa HIV is common (prevalence ~24% in apparently well antenatal patients—and there are millions of AIDS orphans). In Zimbabwe 120,000 HIV+ve mothers give birth each year. Many babies are not infected *in utero* but become so during parturition. Most mothers at risk of passing on HIV to the next generation (vertical transmission) do not want to know their HIV status, or cannot afford to find out. (If their husband is uninfected, what is the chance of him remaining loyal?) In our section on perinatal HIV (p 98) we comment that zidovudine (AZT) and Caesarean section can prevent vertical transmission—but this is not much help if the nearest hospital is 3 hours away by wheelbarrow, and has only basic drugs. What is needed is much more cost-effective advice.

- Only give blood transfusions if absolutely necessary.
- Avoid any procedure likely to lead to maternal cells contacting fetal blood—eg external cephalic version, and amniocentesis.
- In instrumental deliveries, try to avoid abrasions of the fetal skin. Vacuum extractors may be preferable to forceps.
- When you clamp the cord, ensure there is no maternal blood on it.
- Artificial rupture of membranes and episiotomies should be left to the last possible moment, or avoided altogether.
- Avoid fetal scalp electrodes, and doing fetal scalp blood samples.
- If the membranes have ruptured, and labour is delayed or slow, consider the use of oxytocin to decrease exposure of the fetus to HIV.
- During Caesarean sections, open the last layer by blunt dissection, to avoid minor cuts from to the baby from the scalpel.
- Rinse the baby after birth; wipe the face away from mouth, eyes and nostrils.
- Unless there is apnoea, avoid suction catheters to aspirate mucus from the nostrils. The baby's face is likely to be covered with the mother's blood at this stage, and you do not want to force HIV into nostrils.
- Health programmes are likely to end up encouraging breast feeding because there is no satisfactory alternative. Humanized milk is expensive, and immediately indicates to the mother's neighbours that she was HIV+ve. Using humanized milk might also compound problems by removing the one free method of contraception: lactational amenorrhoea.
- Offer advice on avoiding future pregnancies. This is not an easy area. Encouraging the use of condoms is fine, but many will want the added protection of the Pill. IUCDs promote bleeding, and may increase spread to men. This may also be a problem with the progestogen-only pill, but note that the latter may cause less ectropion than the combined pill, and this might be advantageous. Sterilization is the hardest choice, especially when the mother now has no living children because of HIV.

Traditionally, drug therapy for HIV in pregnant patients has consisted in monotherapy with zidovudine—in contrast to non-pregnant women who are best treated with combination therapy (other agents include ritonavir and ddi, see *OHCM* p 218). The reason is that there are no good trials of combination therapy in pregnancy. Zidovudine monotherapy *may* be appropriate as the sole treatment in HIV +ve women with undepleted CD4 counts and low viral loads. In other circumstances, such treatment is likely to be suboptimal.[1] Get expert advice. If a patient on triple therapy falls pregnant, most experts would continue treatment.[1]

1 C Fischer 1998 *Lancet* **351** 1029   2 D Verkuyl 1995 *Lancet* **346** 293

Diabetes mellitus in pregnancy

►Meticulous control around conception reduces malformation rates.

Diabetes may be pre-existing or appear in pregnancy; glycosuria is common (glomerular filtration ↑ and tubular glucose reabsorption↓). Maternal glucose levels in pregnancy are normally very constant (4–4.5mmol/L) except after meals. Some screen at first antenatal visit with a blood sample 1h after a 50g glucose loaded fruit flavoured drink and do a full 75g oral glucose tolerance test (*OHCM* p 474) and glycated Hb (HbA_{1c}) if the blood glucose is ≥ 7.8mmol/L (or ≥ 7.0 according to new, untried WHO definitions)

Complications *Maternal:* Polyhydramnios (25%—possibly due to fetal polyuria), preterm labour (17%—associated with polyhydramnios). Stillbirth near term was common.

Fetal: Malformation rates increase 3–4-fold. Sacral agenesis, almost exclusive to diabetic offspring, is rare (CNS and CVS malformations are much commoner). Babies may be macrosomic (too large) or sometimes growth retarded and are postnatally prone to hypoglycaemia, hypocalcaemia, Mg^{2+}↓ and respiratory distress (surfactant production is delayed). They may be polycythaemic (so more neonatal jaundice).

Antenatal care Liaise with diabetologist. Confirm gestation with early ultrasound. Detailed abnormality scan at 18–20 weeks. Fetal echo at 24 weeks. Educate about benefits of normoglycaemia and home glucose monitoring: regular postprandial monitoring *does* prevent harm to the baby.[1] Insulin needs increase by 50–100%. One approach to normoglycaemia uses Actrapid® 20 minutes before meals with a Novopen® as described on p 262) with a single daily dose of Human Ultratard®. Admit unless there is good control at home. Avoid oral hypoglycaemics. Monitor fetal growth and wellbeing by ultrasound and cardiotocography.

Delivery Timing takes into account the control of diabetes, any pre-eclampsia, maturity and size of the baby, and with attention to fetal wellbeing. Delivery before 38 weeks may result in neonatal respiratory distress. Deliver the baby where there are good neonatal facilities. Traditionally, delivery was at 36–38 weeks to avoid stillbirth; but with close supervision pregnancies may go nearer to (but not beyond) term.

Labour Avoid acidosis and monitor the fetus (p 116). Avoid maternal hyperglycaemia (causes fetal hypoglycaemia). Monitor glucose; prevent hyperglycaemia with extra insulin (may need 5u/h) if β-sympathomimetics or glucocorticoids are used in preterm labour. Aim for vaginal delivery with a labour of less than 12h. Beware shoulder dystocia with macrosomic babies. With elective delivery, give normal insulin the evening before induction. During labour give 1 litre 10% glucose/8h IVI with 1–2u insulin/h via a syringe pump. Aim for a blood glucose of 4.5–5.5mmol/L. Check glucose hourly. Insulin needs fall during labour (and immediately postpartum). Halve insulin infusion rate post-delivery until a good meal has been eaten; then return to pre-pregnancy regimen. Do a Caesarean section if labour is prolonged.

Postnatal •Oral hypoglycaemics are contraindicated if breast feeding. •Encourage pre-pregnancy counselling *before* next pregnancy (p 94) to transfer to insulin. •Do a postpartum glucose tolerance test at 6 weeks. ~5% of those with gestational diabetes will be insulin dependent in <5yrs (higher risk if aged <30, non-obese, no family history, and for first pregnancies).[2] 50% develop non-insulin dependent diabetes in <10yrs.

►Advising exercise and avoiding obesity and smoking lowers this risk.

[1] M De Veciana 1996 E-BM **1**(4) 115 2 A Dornhorst 1994 *Br J Obs Gyn* **101** 286

Thyroid disease in pregnancy[1,2,3] (see also p 81)

►Whenever a mother isn't quite right postpartum, check her TSH & free T_4—but note that any apparent hypothyroidism may be transitory.

Biochemical changes in normal pregnancy NB: normal pregnancy mimics hyperthyroidism (pulse↑, warm moist skin, slight goitre, anxiety).

- Thyroid binding globulin & T_4 output rise to maintain free T_4 levels, p 81.
- High levels of HCG (p 78) mimic thyroid stimulating hormone (TSH).
- There is reduced availability of iodine (in iodine limited localities).
- TSH may fall below normal in the first trimester (suppressed by HCG).
- The best thyroid tests in pregnancy are free T_4, free T_3 and TSH.

Pre-pregnancy hyperthyroidism Treatment options include antithyroid drugs (but 60% relapse on stopping treatment), radioactive iodine (contraindicated in pregnancy or breast feeding: avoid pregnancy for 4 months after use), or surgery. Fertility is reduced by hyperthyroidism.

Hyperthyroidism in pregnancy[1] This is usually Graves' disease. There is increased risk of prematurity, fetal loss, and possibly, of malformations.[2] Severity of hyperthyroidism often falls during pregnancy. Transient exacerbations may occur in the first trimester and postpartum. Treat with carbimazole or propylthiouracil (may cross placenta less). Keep dose as low as possible (reports of neonatal scalp defects are unreplicated in systematic studies, and antithyroid drugs are said to be relatively safe).[1] Once under control, keep dose at ≤10mg/24h PO, keeping T_4 at the top of the normal range. Monitor at least monthly. Some advocate stopping antithyroid drugs in the last month of pregnancy.[2] Propylthiouracil is preferred postpartum if breast feeding (less concentrated in breast milk). If hyperthyroidism cannot be controlled by drugs, partial thyroidectomy can be done in the second trimester. Screen all women with a history of Hashimoto's or Graves' disease for TRAb (TSH-receptor stimulating antibodies); high levels can cause fetal and neonatal hyperthyroidism: blocking them causes hypothyroidism.

Hypothyroidism Relatively rare, it is associated with relative infertility. In untreated hypothyroidism there are increased rates of miscarriage, stillbirth, premature labour[1] and abnormality.[2] T_4 requirements may increase up to 50%. Monitor adequate replacement by T_4 and TSH measurements each trimester.[1] Requirements return to pre-pregnancy levels postpartum.

Postpartum thyroiditis Prevalence: ~5%. There is transient hyperthyroidism initially followed by hypothyroidism (manifesting 4–5 months postpartum). 40% of those affected develop permanent thyroid failure and 25% of those with transient disease become hypothyroid 3–4 years later. TRAb antibodies are absent. The hyperthyroid phase does not usually need treatment as it is self-limiting. If treatment is required β-blockers are usually sufficient. Antithyroid drugs are ineffective because thyrotoxicosis results from thyroid destruction causing increased thyroxine release, rather than increased synthesis. The hypothyroid phase is monitored for >6 months, and the woman treated if she becomes symptomatic. Withdraw treatment after 6–12 months for 4 weeks to see if long-term therapy is required.[2] Hypothyroidism may be associated with postpartum depression, so check thyroid status of women with postpartum depression.

Neonatal thyrotoxicosis Seen in 1% of babies of women with past Graves' disease, even if now controlled, and off drugs, due to TSH-receptor stimulating antibodies crossing the placenta. Fetal tachycardia (rate >160/min) in late pregnancy and intrauterine growth retardation may indicate fetal thyrotoxicosis. In those born to mothers taking antithyroid drugs it may not be manifest until the baby has metabolized the drug (7–10 days postpartum). Test thyroid function in affected babies frequently. Antithyroid drugs may be needed. It resolves spontaneously at 2-3 months, but perceptual motor difficulties, and hyperactivity can occur later in childhood.[2]

1 M O'Doherty 1999 BMJ i 5 2 1995 *Drug Ther Bul* **33** 75 3 R Hall 1993 *Br J Obs Gyn* **100** 512

Jaundice in pregnancy

►Get expert help *promptly*. Jaundice in pregnancy may be lethal. Know exactly what drugs were taken and when (*prescribed* or *over-the-counter*). Where has she travelled to? What life-style or occupational risks are there?

Jaundice occurs in 1 in 1500 pregnancies. Viral hepatitis and gallstones may cause jaundice in pregnancy and investigation is similar in the non-pregnant. Those with Gilbert's and Dubin–Johnson syndrome (*OHCM* p 696–8) do well in pregnancy (jaundice may be exacerbated with the latter).

Intrahepatic cholestasis of pregnancy Pruritus, eg over limbs and trunk, and mild jaundice (bilirubin <100μmol/L) occurs in the second half of pregnancy—and may be associated with mild epigastric pain, anorexia, and malaise, with a bleeding tendency—if malabsorption leads to lack of vitamin K. Plasma aspartate aminotransferase is mildly raised (<300u/L). Exclude viral hepatitis. There is risk of preterm labour, fetal distress, and perinatal death, so monitor fetal wellbeing and consider delivery, at ~37 weeks, eg if any sign of fetal compromise. Monitor prothrombin time and give vitamin K if prolonged. Give vitamin K to the baby at birth. Jaundice clears within 4 weeks of delivery. It is a contraindication to oestrogen-containing contraceptive Pills and recurs in 40% pregnancies.

Acute fatty liver of pregnancy Incidence: 1:9000–13,000 deliveries—so it is rare but grave. The mother develops abdominal pain, jaundice, headache, and vomiting, ± thrombocytopenia and pancreatitis. There is associate pre-eclampsia in 30–60%. It usually occurs after 30 weeks. There is hepatic steatosis with microdroplets of fat in liver cells. Deep jaundice, uraemia, severe hypoglycaemia and clotting disorder may develop causing coma and death. Give supportive treatment for liver and renal failure and treat hypoglycaemia vigorously (CVP line). Correct clotting disorder with vitamin K, fresh frozen plasma and antithrombin III. Expedite delivery. Epidural anaesthesia is contraindicated. Beware PPH and neonatal hypoglycaemia. Mortality can be as low as 18% maternal and 23% fetal. Other causes of fatty liver (steatosis): yellow fever, tetracycline, sodium valproate, Reye's syndrome (p 756).

Some other causes of jaundice in pregnancy

- Viral hepatitis; ALT, eg >200u/L; maternal mortality↑ in E virus, *OHCM* p 211.
- The jaundice of severe pre-eclampsia (hepatic rupture and infarction can occur); ALT <500u/L; bilirubin <86μmol/L.[1]
- Rarely complicating hyperemesis gravidarum (can be fatal); ALT <200u/L.
- Hepatitis may occur if halothane is used for anaesthesia (so avoid it).
- HELLP syndrome (haemolysis, elevated liver enzymes, and low platelet count). Incidence in pregnancy: 0.1–0.6%; in pre-eclampsia: 4–12%. It causes: right upper quadrant/epigastric pain, malaise, nausea, vomiting, headache, jaundice, microangiopathic haemolytic anaemia, DIC, LDH↑, ALT↑ <500u/L, bilirubin <86μmol/L.[1] It recurs in 20%.[2] Treatment: get expert help. Admit to hospital. Deliver if severe.

Hepatitis B Check HBsAg in all women with jaundice. Staff should be careful to avoid contact with blood during delivery of those who are positive, and be especially careful with disposal of 'sharps'. Give 200u specific hepatitis B immune globulin (HBIG) IM to the anterolateral thigh to babies of affected mothers at birth—*plus* hepatitis B vaccine (0.5mL H-B-Vax II® into the other anterolateral thigh) at birth, 1 month and 6 months. Offer vaccination to *all* the family. Do serology at 12–15 months old. If HBsAg –ve and anti-HBs is present, the child has been protected.

Tests Do all the usual tests (*OHCM* p 484), eg urine tests for bile, serology, LFTs, and ultrasound. Special tests may be needed to show fat, eg oil red O, to fresh-frozen biopsy samples—if coagulation status allows biopsy.

1 TA Knox 1996 NEJM **335** 569 2 M Geary 1997 *Br J Obst Gynae* **104** 887

Malaria in pregnancy

In any woman who presents with odd behaviour, fever, jaundice, sweating, DIC, fetal distress, premature labour, seizures, or loss of consciousness, always ask yourself: ►*Could this be malaria?* If so, do thick and thin films. Confirm (or exclude) pregnancy. Seek expert help (eg from Liverpool, below).

Malaria can be particularly dangerous in pregnancy, with serious complications being more common, particularly in those with no malaria immunity. In some places, such as Thailand, malaria is the leading cause of maternal mortality. Cerebral malaria has a 50% mortality in pregnancy. Third stage placental autotransfusion may lead to fatal pulmonary oedema. Hypoglycaemia may be a feature of malaria in pregnancy (irrespective of whether quinine has been given).[1]

Other associations between malaria and pregnancy are anaemia, abortion, stillbirth, and low birth weight and prematurity. PPH is also more common. Hyperreactive malaria splenomegaly (occurs typically where malaria is holoendemic) may contribute to anaemia via increased haemolysis.[2]

Treatment of malaria is as described in *OHCM* p 196. Chloroquine and quinine (in full dosage) appear to be safe in pregnancy, but beware hypoglycaemia. For *falciparum* malaria, expect to use quinine as chloroquine resistance is widespread. Mefloquine can be used in the second and third trimesters for the treatment of uncomplicated falciparum malaria.

Transfer earlier rather than later to ITU. Women with a haematocrit <20% should get a slow transfusion of packed cells, if compatible, fresh, pathogen-free blood is available. Remember to include the volume of packed cells in calculations of fluid balance. Exchange transfusions may be needed—if facilities are available.

During labour, anticipate fetal distress, fluid-balance problems, and hypoglycaemia. Monitor appropriately. Send placenta for microscopy for malarial parasites. If they are present the baby may be infected (the parasites can cross the placenta—especially in non-immune mothers) and should be treated.[3]

Prevention in UK women Advise against visiting malarious areas. If is unavoidable, give prophylaxis (*OHCM* p 196). Emphasize importance of preventive measures such as mosquito nets and insect repellents. Chloroquine and proguanil are used in normal doses, if *P falciparum* strains are sensitive—but with proguanil, concurrent folate supplements should be given.

Maloprim® (dapsone+pyrimethamine) is contraindicated in first trimester; if given in second or third trimesters, give folate supplements too.

Mefloquine should be avoided as prophylaxis (exclude pregnancy before use, and avoid pregnancy for 3 months after use).

Trials of chemoprophylaxis in mothers living in endemic areas These show that chemoprophylaxis improves birth weight (↑by ~250g—and there are fewer very low birth weight babies). Red cell mass also improves. The effect of universal maternal chemoprophylaxis on the emergence of drug-resistant strains of malaria has not been quantified—and neither have sophisticated outcome studies been done on general neonatal wellbeing with maternal prophylaxis. Coarse analysis of the figures suggests that there is no adverse effect on either maternal or fetal mortality.[4]

►When in doubt, it is best to telephone an expert, eg, in the UK, from Liverpool (tel. 0151 708 9393).

1 H Gilles 1992 *Management of Severe and Complicated Malaria*, WHO, Geneva 2 I Bates 1994 *Trans Roy Soc Trop Med Hyg* **88** 277 **3** R Hurley 1995 in *Medical disorders in Obstetric Practise* 3e Blackwell p562 ◄4► P Garner 1997 E-BM **2** 15

Renal disease in pregnancy

Note: values considered normal in non-pregnancy may reflect decreased renal function in pregnancy. Creatinine >75μmol/L and urea >4.5mmol/L merit further investigation. See p 81. Glycosuria in pregnancy may reflect altered renal physiology and not necessarily imply hyperglycaemia.

►Treat asymptomatic bacteriuria in pregnancy. Check that infection and bacteriuria clear with treatment.

Asymptomatic bacteriuria This is found in 2% of sexually active women, and is more common (up to 7%) during pregnancy. With the dilatation of the calyces and ureters that occurs in pregnancy, 25% will go on to develop pyelonephritis, which can cause fetal growth retardation, fetal death and premature labour. This is the argument for screening all women for bacteriuria at booking. If present on 2 MSUs treatment is given (eg amoxicillin 250mg/8h PO with a high fluid intake). Test for cure after 1 and 2 weeks. If the organism is not sensitive to amoxicillin, consider nitrofurantoin 50mg/6h PO with food.

Pyelonephritis This may present as malaise with urinary frequency or as a more florid picture with raised temperature, tachycardia, vomiting and loin pain. It is common at around 20 weeks and in the puerperium. Urinary infections should always be carefully excluded in those with hyperemesis gravidarum and in those admitted with premature labour. Treatment is with bed rest and plenty of fluids. After blood and urine culture give IV antibiotics (eg ampicillin 500mg/6h IV, according to sensitivities) if oral drugs cannot be used (eg if vomiting). Treat for 2–3 weeks. MSUs should be checked every fortnight for the rest of the pregnancy. 20% of women having pyelonephritis in pregnancy have underlying renal tract abnormalities and an IVU or ultrasound at 12 weeks' postpartum should be considered. In those who suffer repeated infection, nitrofurantoin (100mg/12–24h PO with food) may prevent recurrences. Avoid if the glomerular filtration rate is <50mL/min. SE: vomiting, peripheral neuropathy, pulmonary infiltration and liver damage.

Chronic renal disease With mild renal impairment without hypertension there is little evidence that pregnancy accelerates renal disorders. Patients with marked anaemia, hypertension, retinopathy, or heavy proteinuria should avoid pregnancy as further deterioration in renal function may be expected and fetal loss is considerable (up to 60%). Close collaboration between physicians and obstetricians during pregnancy in those with renal disease is the aim. Induction of labour may become advisable in those with hypertension and proteinuria, or if fetal growth is retarded.

Pregnancy for those on dialysis is fraught with problems (fluid overload, hypertension, pre-eclampsia, polyhydramnios). A 50% increase in dialysis is needed. Live birth outcome is 50%, at best. Outcome is better for those with renal transplants.[1]

Obstetric causes of acute tubular necrosis Acute tubular necrosis may be a complication of any of the following situations:

- Septicaemia (eg from septic abortion or pyelonephritis).
- Haemolysis (eg sickling crisis, malaria).
- Hypovolaemia, eg in pre-eclampsia; haemorrhage (APH, eg abruption, PPH, or intrapartum); DIC; abortion—or adrenal failure in those on steroids not receiving booster doses to cover labour.

Whenever these situations occur, monitor urine output carefully (catheterize the bladder). Aim for >30mL/h output. Monitor renal function (U&E, creatinine). Dialysis may be needed (*OHCM* p 390).

1 J Davidson 1997 *Prescribers' J* 37 46

Epilepsy in pregnancy

►If seizures occur in pregnancy, think *could this be eclampsia?*

Epilepsy *de novo* is rare in pregnancy. Epilepsy affects ~0.5% of women of childbearing age so a unit with 3000 deliveries per year has ~15 pregnant epileptic women at any one time. Seizure rate during pregnancy increases in ~25% of epileptic women, reduces in ~22% and is unchanged in the remainder. Where seizure rate increases this is often associated with lack of compliance with medication, or sleep deprivation. It is unusual for seizures to recur in pregnancy when preceded by a long seizure-free period.

Complications—*Maternal:*[1] Increased risk of third trimester vaginal bleeding. 1% convulse in labour. *Fetal:*[2] Increased risk of: prematurity; stillbirth; neonatal and perinatal death; haemorrhagic disease of the newborn. Epilepsy affects 3% of offspring when the mother has partial epilepsy, 5–10% if she has idiopathic generalized epilepsy.[3]

Abnormality Epilepsy in the mother (but not the father) is associated with fetal abnormality, particularly cleft lip and palate. Relative risk for a fetus having clefts compared to the non-epileptic population is 1.0 if the mother develops epilepsy after the pregnancy; 2.4 if she develops it after conception but is not treated with medication; and 4.7 if the fetus has been exposed to anticonvulsant drugs. Children of epileptic mothers taking medication are twice as likely to have some form of significant malformation, giving a malformation rate of 6%; (a 94% chance of the mother having a normal baby). Malformation is commoner if more than one anticonvulsant is taken, with high doses and if a sibling is already malformed.[3] Neural tube defects are commoner with carbamazepine and sodium valproate so screen for these (p 166). Phenytoin and phenobarbitone cause congenital heart disease and cleft lip.[2]

Management Avoid trimethadione and paramethadione (they are very teratogenic). Where anticonvulsants are needed the dose of the chosen drug should be kept as low as possible. Aim for 1 drug only. Be careful interpreting plasma phenytoin levels as free levels may remain the same despite a reduced bound level. Give folic acid supplements, eg 5mg/24h PO from prior to conception[3] and vitamin K_1 20mg/24h to the mother from 36 weeks if she is taking phenytoin, primidone, or phenobarbitone. Treat status epilepticus as in the non-pregnant except that the fetus should be monitored. It is associated with significant fetal and maternal mortality.[3] Deliver in hospital (1–2% epileptic women convulse during labour and the subsequent 48 hours). Give vitamin K to the baby at birth (p 244).

Neonates can suffer barbiturate withdrawal with hyperexcitability, tremulousness, impaired suckling and, occasionally, seizures at ~1 week if not breastfed. Usually, babies only require supervision, but if very tremulous, or if there are seizures, they may be given 3–5mg/kg/day phenobarbitone.

Puerperal readjustment of medication may be needed. There may be increased susceptibility to seizures while taking baths postnatally.[4] Mothers may safely breast feed but phenobarbitone can cause drowsiness in the baby.

1 J Donaldson 1995 *Medical Disorders in Obstetric Practice*, 3e, 536–40, Blackwell 2 *Drug Ther Bul* 1994 **32** 49
3 P Cleland 1996 *Prescribers' J* **36** 102 4 DoH 1996 *Confidential Enquiry into Maternal Deaths 1991-3*, HMSO

Connective tissue diseases in pregnancy[1]

Rheumatoid arthritis Symptoms are usually alleviated by pregnancy (but exacerbations may occur in the puerperium). Methotrexate use is contraindicated (teratogenic); sulfasalazine may be used (with folate supplementation). Azathioprine use may cause intrauterine growth retardation and penicillamine may weaken fetal collagen. Non-steroidal anti-inflammatories can be used in the first and second trimesters but are not recommended in the third as they can cause premature closure of the ductus arteriosus and late in pregnancy have been associated with renal impairment in the newborn. Congenital heart block is a rare fetal feature.

Systemic lupus erythematosus SLE exacerbations are commoner in pregnancy and the puerperium. Most are mild to moderate involving skin, but those with renal involvement and hypertension may deteriorate and are prone to pre-eclampsia. Of those with SLE glomerulonephritis and a creatinine >130μmol prior to conception only 50% achieve a live birth. Pre-eclampsia, oligohydramnios, and intrauterine growth retardation may occur. Both hydrallazine and methyldopa can be used in pre-eclampsia.

Planned pregnancy should be embarked on after 6 months stable disease without requiring cytotoxic suppression. Disease suppression may be maintained with azathioprine and hydroxychloroquine. Aspirin 75mg daily should be started prior to conception and continued throughout pregnancy and the fetus should be carefully monitored.

Rarely the fetus is affected by passively acquired maternal anti-Ro antibodies which can cause a self-limiting sunlight sensitive rash (usually face and scalp) for which no treatment is required, but more rarely can cause irreversible damage to the fetal heart conduction system causing congenital heart block (~65% of surviving neonates require a pacemaker).

Mothers requiring ≥7.5mg daily prednisolone in the 2 weeks before delivery should receive hydrocortisone 100mg/6h IV in labour.

The antiphospholipid sydrome Those affected have antiphospholipid antibodies (lupus anticoagulant and/or anticardiolipin antibodies) and a history of arterial thrombosis, venous thrombosis, or recurrent pregnancy loss (typically second trimester). It may be primary, or secondary to another connective tissue disorder (usually SLE in which it occurs in 10%). *Outcome:* Untreated, <20% of pregnancies proceed to a live birth due to:
- First trimester loss.
- Placental thrombosis causing placental insufficiency, leading to:
- Intrauterine growth retardation and •Fetal death.

Careful regular fetal assessment (Doppler flow studies and ultrasound for growth are required from 20 weeks) as appropriate obstetric intervention can substantially increase the number of live-born babies.

Management: Affected women are treated from conception with aspirin 75mg daily (heparin sc/12h until 34 weeks improves outcome).[2] Those who have suffered prior thromboses receive warfarin (may cause abnormal fetal cartilage development) or heparin (causes maternal osteoporosis; if unfractionated type used can cause thrombocytopenia). Some recommend heparin for first trimester and warfarin thereafter until near time of delivery. Heparin is used to cover labour (epidurals contraindicated).

Postpartum use either heparin or warfarin (breastfeeding contraindicated with neither) as risk of thrombosis is high.

Pregnancies in those with SLE (especially with renal disease) and antiphospholipid syndrome require specialist management.

1 BJ Hunt 1997 *Prescribers' J* **37** 54   2 R Rai 1997 BMJ **314** 253

2. Obstetrics

Maternal mortality

Maternal mortality is defined in the UK as the death of a mother while pregnant or within 42 days of termination of pregnancy, from any cause related to or aggravated by the pregnancy or its management, but not

from accidental or incidental causes. Deaths are subdivided into those from 'direct causes'—those in which the cause of death is directly attributable to pregnancy (eg abortion, eclampsia, haemorrhage)—and indirect deaths—those resulting from previous existing disease or disease developed during pregnancy, and which were not due to direct obstetric causes but were aggravated by pregnancy (eg heart disease). Late deaths are those occurring between 42 days and 1 year after termination, miscarriage or delivery that are due to direct or indirect maternal causes.

Since 1952 there have been confidential enquiries into maternal deaths. Reports on these are brought out 3-yearly. Since 1979 late deaths have been put into a separate group. Prior to 1979, as a result of the enquiries a certain proportion of deaths were considered to have had 'avoidable factors' (this term was used to denote departures from acceptable standards of care by individuals, including patients) but since 1979 the wider term of 'substandard care' has been used to cover failures in clinical care and other factors, such as shortage of resources and back-up facilities.

Maternal mortality has almost halved every decade since reports have been issued (deaths per 100,000 maternities have been 67.1 in 1955–7, 33.3 in 1964–6, 11 in 1973–5, and 12.2 in 1994–6 of which direct deaths were 6.1 per 100,000).[1] Rates are lowest for women <20 years (4.2 deaths/100,000 maternities *vs* 20.6 for women >40 years) and for second pregnancies (7.4 for para 1 *vs* 25.59 for para 4+).[2] It has been estimated that maternal deaths rates/100,000 births are 640 in Africa; 420 in Asia; 270 in Latin America; 30 in all developed countries and < 10 in Northern and Central Europe.[3]

In 1994–6, 443 deaths were recorded including 89 late deaths. Of these 144 were direct obstetric deaths; 174 were indirect obstetric deaths and 36 were fortuitous (in no way related to pregnancy, eg car accident). Rates vary considerably by region, direct obstetric mortality rate being 1.7/100,000 births in Northern Ireland in 1991–93 to 8.6/100,000 births in North West Thames Regional Health Authority.[2] Risk is increased for immigrant women, especially those from West Africa, Southern Africa and the Caribbean.[4]

In 1994–96 thromboembolism was the commonest cause of direct death in the UK (33% of deaths). Other direct causes: hypertensive disorders of pregnancy (13.8%); amniotic fluid embolism (11.8%); early pregnancy (10.4%)—(mainly ectopic pregnancy at 8.3%); genital tract sepsis (9.7%); haemorrhage (8.3%); uterine rupture (2%); fatty liver of pregnancy (1.4%).

Death rate from Caesarean section for the 1985–90 period was 0.33 per 1000 operations. No figure is available for 1994–6.

The maternal mortality rate was similar to the previous triennium for direct deaths, although more deaths were detected due to extra cases being collected through the Office of National Statistics. Care was considered substandard in 40% of cases of direct death showing in 1991–3, although in 11% of these the 'substandardness' consisted in the pregnant woman refusal of medical advice).

1 DoH 1998 *Report on Confidential Enquiries into Maternal Deaths in the United Kingdom 1994-6*, London, HMSO 2 DoH 1996 *Report on Confidential Enquiries into Maternal Deaths in the United Kingdom 1991-3*, London, HMSO 3 DoH 1994 *Report on Confidential Enquiries into Maternal Deaths in the United Kingdom 1988-90*, London, HMSO 4 J Ibison 1996 *Br J Obst Gynae* **103** 973

Perinatal mortality

This is the number of stillbirths and deaths in the first week of life/1000 total births. Stillbirths only include those fetuses of >24 weeks' gestation, but if a fetus of <24 weeks' gestation is born and then shows signs of life it is counted as a neonatal death in the UK and is therefore expressed in the figures (if dying within the first 7 days). Other countries use different criteria—including stillbirths from 20 weeks and neonatal deaths up to 28 days after birth, so it is not always easy to compare statistics.

Perinatal mortality is affected by many factors. Rates are high for *small* (61% of deaths are in babies <2500g) and *preterm* babies (70% of deaths occur in the 5% who are preterm). See p 102 & p 180. *Regional variation* in the UK is quite marked with rates for the Oxford region being considerably lower than for Merseyside. There is a *social class variation* with rates being less for social classes 1 and 2 than for classes 4 and 5. *Teenage mothers* have higher rates than mothers aged 20–29. From 30yrs rates rise until they are 3-fold higher than the low-risk group (20–29 years) by the age of 40–45. *Second babies* have the lowest mortality rates. Mortality rates are doubled for fourth and fifth children, trebled by sixth and seventh (this effect is not independent of social class as more lower social class women have many children). Rates are lower for *singleton births* than for multiple. Rates are higher for the offspring of mothers of *Bangladeshi* or *West Indian extraction* living in the UK, but are the same for those of Pakistani and UK extraction.

Perinatal mortality rates in the UK have fallen over the years from rates of 62.5/1000 in 1930–5 to 12–14/1000 in the 1990s. Declining mortality reflects improvement in standards of living, improved maternal health and declining parity, as well as improvements in medical care. The main causes of death are congenital abnormalities (22%), unclassified hypoxia (18%), placental conditions (16%), birth problems including cord problems (11%), maternal conditions and toxaemia (8%).

Examples of how changed medical care may reduce mortality are:
- Antenatal detection and termination of malformed fetuses.
- Reduction of mid-cavity procedures and vaginal breech delivery.
- Detection of placenta praevia antenatally.
- Prevention of rhesus incompatibility.
- Preventing progression of preterm labour.
- Better control of diabetes mellitus in affected mothers.
- Antenatal monitoring of 'at risk' pregnancies.

While we must try to reduce morbidity and mortality still further, this must not blind us to other problems that remain, such as the 'over-medicalization' of birth; the problem of reconciling maternal wishes to be in charge of her own delivery with the immediate needs of the baby; and the problem of explaining risks and benefits in terms that both parents understand, so that they can join in the decision-making process.

Prenatal diagnosis

'The first half of pregnancy can become a time of constant 'exams' to see if the baby can be allowed to graduate to the second half of pregnancy'.[1] Parents at high and, increasingly, those at low risk of having an abnormal baby are offered prenatal diagnosis if this might permit more effective treatment of the expected defect, or (more often) if they wish to terminate any abnormal pregnancy.

High-risk pregnancies (See p 210 for details of detectable problems.)
- Maternal age >35 (chromosome defects).
- Previous abnormal baby or family history of inherited condition.
- High-risk population (eg sickle cell in Afro-Caribbeans).

Problems ►*Anxiety while false +ve results are sorted out is a big problem.*
- Terminating normal fetuses, eg ♂ fetuses of carriers of X-linked conditions.
- Most abnormalities are in low-risk groups (∴ missable by selective screening).
- Services available, their quality, and the population made eligable, vary widely.
- Termination of female fetuses in cultures valuing males more highly.
- Devaluation of recent moves to promote a more positive view of handicapped or 'special needs' children.

Ultrasound At <18 weeks, skilled operators can detect an ever-increasing range of external and internal structural anomalies. See p 118, and opposite.

Ultrasound is best at detecting externally impinging structural abnormalities, eg anencephaly/spina bifida. Internal structural abnormality detection rate, eg for heart disease and diaphragmatic hernia, remains <50%. Fetuses with false +ve suggestion of abnormality are mostly associated with 'soft signs' on ultrasound, eg nuchal thickening (eg trisomy 21), choroid plexus cysts (trisomies 18 and 21), and echogenic bowel (trisomy 21 and cystic fibrosis). In one large study (*N*=33,376 fetuses; 725 abnormal; 55% of which detected prenatally) use of ultrasound 'soft signs' ↑total detection rate from 51% to 55% but ↑false +ves 12-fold from one in 2,332 to one in 188.[2]

α-Fetoprotein (AFP) AFP is a glycoprotein synthesized by the fetal liver and GI tract. Fetal levels fall after 13 weeks, but maternal (transplacental) serum AFP continues to rise to 30 weeks. Maternal AFP is measured at 17 weeks. In 10% with a high AFP there is a fetal malformation,[3] eg an open neural tube defect (but closed defects are missed), exomphalos, posterior urethral valves, nephrosis, GI obstruction, teratomas, Turner's syndrome (or normal twins). In ~30% of those with no malformation, there is an adverse outcome, eg placental abruption and third trimester deaths.[4] ►Monitor closely. 1 in 40 with a low AFP have a chromosomal abnormality (eg Down's). AFP is lower in diabetic mothers. NB: as this test is nonspecific on its own, it is of use for preliminary screening; those with abnormal values may be offered further tests (see below, and p 168 for the 'triple test').

Amniocentesis (p 120) is carried out under ultrasound guidance. Fetal loss rate is 0.5–1% at ~16 weeks' gestation, but ~5% for early amniocentesis at 10–13 weeks. Amniotic fluid AFP is measured (a more accurate screen for neural tube defects than maternal serum), and cells in the fluid are cultured for karyotyping and enzyme and gene probe analysis. Cell culture takes 3 weeks, so an abnormal pregnancy must be terminated at a late stage.

Chorionic villus biopsy At 10+ weeks, the developing placenta is sampled using a transcervical catheter or a transabdominal needle under ultrasound guidance. Karyotyping takes 2 days, enzyme and gene probe analysis 3 weeks, so termination of abnormal pregnancies is earlier, safer and less distressing than after amniocentesis. Fetal loss rate is ~4%. The procedure does not detect neural tube defects—and may itself cause fetal malformations.[5]

Fetoscopy This is carried out at ~18 weeks under ultrasound guidance. External malformations may be seen, fetal blood sampled and organs biopsied. The fetal loss rate is ~4%.

High resolution ultrasound and fetal nuchal translcency (FNT)

- Fluid accumulation in the neck at 10–14 weeks' gestation (↑FNT) reflects fetal heart failure, and is typically seen in any serious anomaly of the heart and great arteries.[6]
- There is a strong association between chromosomal abnormality and FNT. In one study, 84% of karyotypically proven trisomy 21 fetuses had a nuchal translucency >3mm at 10–13 weeks' gestation (as did 4.5% of chromosomally normal fetuses).[7]
- The greater the extent of FNT, the greater the risk of abnormality.[8]
- Nuchal translucency screening may be used to see who may benefit from more invasive chorionic villus sampling or amniocentesis, which may delineate the precise chomosomal abnormality (eg trisomies).
- It is useful for screening twins as early detection is best, for if selective fetocide is to be used risk of miscarriage is 3-fold higher if done after 16 weeks. Monochorionic twins have a higher false +ve rate for nuchal translucency thickness than dichorionic twins or singletons.[9]
- Note that the degree of neck flexion during the ultrasound examination may influence nuchal measurements.

1 J Dornan 1998 *Br J Obs Gyn* **105** 573 2 P Boyd 1998 *Lancet* **352** 1577 3 F Cunningham 1991 NEJM **325** 55 4 D Waller 1991 NEJM **325** 6 5 H Firth 1994 *Lancet* **343** 1069 6 B Mol & J Hyett 1999 BMJ **i** 70 & 81 7 K Nicolaides 1994 *Br J Obst Gynae* **101** 982 8 P Pandya 1995 *Br J Obst Gynae* **102** 957 9 N Sebire 1996 *Br J Obst Gynae* **103** 999

The triple blood test

Maternal serum AFP, unconjugated oestriol and total human chorionic gonadotrophin (HCG) are assessed in relation to maternal age, weight and gestation (determined by ultrasound) to estimate risk of Down's syndrome (and, in some places, of neural tube defects). If the test (and subsequent tests on those found to be at risk) were available to all mothers, detection of Down's syndrome would increase from 15% to about 50% (48% and 58% in two large studies, N=38,000).[1,2] See also screening by fetal nuchal translucency ultrasound (p 167).

Problems with the triple blood test—the triple conundrum

1 *It may not be the best test:* Some authorities say that adding unconjugated (o)estriol to the test could merely increase uncertainty. Also, there is evidence that *free* HCG is a better marker than total HCG.[3] A quadruple tests measures α and β HCG separately. Some centres are using Inhibin A measurements as well, and claim a 78% detection rate with 5% false +ves. It has also been pointed out that the wrong statistical test was used to demonstrate the test's benefits. Using Fisher's exact test to compare the 5 additional cases detected over and above what would have been detected by screening based on age alone, the Wald figures would not have been significant (P=0.24).[4] As the age at which mothers have their babies increases, any relative benefit of the triple test over age-related screening diminishes.

2 *The cost–benefit sums are hard to calculate*—as benefits depend on a high uptake of amniocentesis and termination. The detection rate is only 39% in those <37yrs. If you assume 100% uptake of amniocentesis and 100% uptake of abortion the cost per detected pregnancy is £36,256 (£28,000 if the detection rate is ~60%). This cost increases to £48,780 with 75% uptake of amniocentesis and 90% uptake of termination.[5] The position is further complicated by ethnic differences in reference intervals that have yet to be quantified. For example, the median value of HCG is too low for non-Caucasians (who will therefore have a higher false +ve rate).[6]

3 *The emotional cost to the mother is impossible to calculate:* From the parents' point of view, a telling statistic is that 56 out of every 57 women under 37yrs old who had a +ve test, proved, after amniocentesis, *not* to have an affected fetus. Amniocentesis causes fetal loss, and these losses will almost always be of normal babies. Newer screening regimens in the first trimester[2] will go some way to mitigating distress and anxiety.

We have no idea of the best way of counselling parents before the test. If you just hand out a leaflet, few will read it, and then when it comes to amniocentesis and termination, many will refuse—and the screening test wastes money, as well as laying health authorities open to litigation: 'I never understood that I might lose a normal baby ...' The alternative is to provide full details at the time of the initial blood test. The irony is that gaining informed consent is then the most expensive part of the test, and one which itself could cause much distress. Imagine an overjoyed expectant mother arriving in the clinic serenely happy in fulfilling her reproductive potential: the quintessence of health. She leaves only after being handed ethical conundrums of quite staggering proportions, involving death, disease, and human sacrifices, and a timetable for their resolution which would leave even the most fast-moving philosopher breathless and disorientated, and which may leave her forever bereft of one of Nature's most generous gifts: the fundamental belief in one's own wholeness.

1 J Haddow 1992 NEJM **327** 588 2 N Wald 1992 BMJ **ii** 391 & NEJM 1998 338 955–61 3 K Spencer 1992 BMJ **ii** 769 4 A Allman 1992 BMJ **ii** 768 5 V Macri 1992 BMJ **ii** 768 6 C Ford 1996 BMJ **i** 1040

Example of counselling before doing a less than perfect test, without distressing women with talk of having terminations for what may be a very much wanted pregnancy.

"We've got a package of tests we often use to see how the pregnancy is going on—would you like us to get on with what seems best (nothing is perfect!)—or are you the sort of person who would want to know in detail about each test? If so, we can arrange a time for you to come back for further discussions."

This allows the mother to pace her access to information in her own way—and each person's needs in this regard will be different.

3. Paediatrics

Subjects for students

Help for house officers

Relevant pages elsewhere: Infectious diseases (OHCM p170–250); perinatal infection p 100; anorexia nervosa p 348, play therapy p 384, autism p 402; squint p 486, retinoblastoma p 506; trauma (p 604–740); syndromes: p 742–60.

Introduction

The newcomer to paediatrics is presented with a double difficulty: not only are children in many important respects quite unlike adults, but they are themselves a very heterogeneous group: the neonate is unlike the toddler—who is unlike the school child or the adolescent. A whole book along the lines of this work could be written on each of these groups of children, and still give a rather sketchy account. But the newcomer should know, lest he becomes downhearted, that no one can say he has complete mastery of this subject. Rather than aiming for completeness, the aim is to be an effective paediatrician. This entails not endless hours in the library, but time on the wards (and in patients' homes, if the reader is lucky enough to have access to general practice patients)—to enlarge on those innate skills of listening and talking to mothers and children in language that each understands. Doctors who look after children have unrivalled opportunities to practise a holistic art, and it is possible that these doctors have a special skill here. We note with great interest that most patients between the ages of 15 and 20 who have acute leukaemia treated by paediatricians are cured—up to 63%, whereas only 32–42% of this age group survive if treated in adult units.

Time on the wards gives the embryo-paediatrician the opportunity to learn that great skill which no book can fully teach: how to recognize the seriously ill child. With the slow and painful accretion of many days and nights 'on call' the paediatrician's flair and instinctive judgment will develop in this regard. This flair can never be had from books alone, nor can it be had entirely without them, for as William Osler said: 'to study medicine without books is to sail an uncharted sea; to study medicine from books alone is not to go to sea at all'. With this metaphor in mind we offer the following set of charts with the warning that they do not all use the same scale, and that it has not been possible to mark every reef. The blank charts are included to encourage new voyages.

Child health, and the central facts dominating paediatrics

40% of the world's births are in countries with under-5s mortality ≥100/1000; ~10% of infants in these countries die before their 5th birthday.[1] Most of these deaths are preventable, not by applying the complicated measures described here, but by the provision of clean water, enough food, and simple vaccinations, along with the encouragement of breast feeding. Today's girl is tomorrow's (or this afternoon's) mother. If she is to have healthy, happy, well-nourished children, first and foremost she needs to love them—but love isn't all she needs. She need not be wealthy, but being poor is *so often* fatal. To escape from poverty she needs to be literate, know how to plan her family, find a midwife, a friendly doctor and a reasonable school for her children. Family support helps, as does a faithful husband who can provide a rôle-model which does not lead to alcohol, drug addiction, HIV, and preventable accidents—the chief threats to adolescent health.[2]

When parenting fails, eg in association with low maternal IQ, the cycle of poverty breeding poverty and disruptive behaviour *can* be broken by early intervention and family support. This can prevent mental retardation.[3,4]

1 J Wise 1998 BMJ **i** 1477 and www.who.ch NB: this gloomy statistic is not so gloomy as it was: in 1995 20% of these died before age 5. **2** L Jacobson 1994 *Br J Gen Prac* **44** 420 **3** M Hoghuhhi 1998 BMJ **i** 1545 **4** C Ramey 1998 *Am Psychol* **53** 109 and 1994 *Pediatrics* **94** 1064

Eliciting the history

The aim is not only to reach a diagnosis, but also to establish a good relationship with the parents and child, so that if there is nothing the matter with the child the parents feel able to accept this. Conversely, if there is serious or untreatable illness, the aim is to build up trust, so that the parents are able to accept the best advice, and the child feels that he or she is in safe, friendly hands. So if possible, avoid any hurry or distractions. Introduce yourself; explain your rôle in the ward or consulting room.

Presenting complaints Record the child's and mother's own words.

The present illness When and how did it start? Was the child quite well beforehand? How did it develop? What aggravates or alleviates it? Has there been contact with infections? Has the child been overseas recently?

Especially in infants, enquire about feeding, excretion, alertness, and weight gain. After ascertaining the presenting complaint further questioning is to test the various hypotheses of differential diagnosis.

Past health *In utero:* Toxaemia, rubella, Rh disease.
At birth: Prematurity, duration of labour, type of delivery, birth weight, resuscitation required, birth injury, malformations.

As a neonate: Jaundice, fits, fevers, bleeding, feeding problems.
Ask about later illnesses, operations, accidents, screening tests, drugs, allergies, immunization, travel and drug or solvent abuse.

Development (p 290) Does the mother remember milestones reliably? Consanguinity is common in some cultures and may be relevant to disease.

Drugs Prescribed and over-the-counter. Drug intolerances, and adverse drug reactions, and true allergies.

Family history Stillbirths, TB, diabetes mellitus, renal disease, seizures, jaundice, malformations, others. Are siblings and parents alive and well? Find out if a parent has had a myocardial infarction before 40 years old—if so, do serum lipids (>40% of these children will turn out to have hyperlipidaemia: the sooner it is treated, the better).

Social history It may be vital to know who the father is, but very damaging to ask the mother directly. Be prepared to allow information to surface slowly, after chats with friendly nurses. Ask about play, eating, sleeping (excessively wrapped or liable to cold?) and schooling. Who looks after the child if the parents work? What work do they do? Ask about their hopes, fears and expectations about the child's illness and his stay in hospital.

Privacy, dignity, and confidentiality These are easy to pay lip-service to, but very hard to ensure in busy paediatric wards, where space is at a premium. During an average stay in hospital most patients and their relatives will overhear confidential exchanges, and only a few will ever recall being offered a screen to preserve privacy during examinations.[1]

►*If the family does not speak your language, find an interpreter.*

1 G Rylance 1999 *BMJ* i 301

Systems review

	The neonate:	The toddler:	The older child:
Cardiorespiratory:	Tachypnoea; grunts Wheeze cyanosis	Cough Exertional dyspnoea	Cough; wheeze Sputum; chest pain
Gastrointestinal:	D&V; jaundice Stool frequency	D&V Stool frequency	D&V; abdominal pain Stool frequency
Genitourinary:	Wet nappies (how often?)	Wet nappies (how often?)	Haematuria; dysuria Sexual development
Neuromuscular:	Fits; odd attacks 'Jitters' Feeding ability	Fits Drowsiness Hyperactive? vision hearing gait	Headaches; fits; odd sensations; Drowsiness Academic ability vision; hearing co-ordination
ENT and teeth:	Noisy breathing	Ear discharge Teeth eruption	Earache/discharge Sore throat

General questions: Growth, weight, failure to thrive, fatigue, lumps, itch, fevers, bleeding tendency, family interaction questions.

►*If the family does not speak your language, find an interpreter.*

Physical examination: a method

No single routine will suffice for all children. If the child is very ill, examination must be limited (AVPU, p 175). Furthermore, points in the examination assume varying importance depending on age (for neonates, see p 231). But it is helpful to have some sort of standard—in this instance, a little boy of 3 years old whom you are seeing because of vomiting. Not everything on even this slimmed-down page will need to be done. The more experienced you are, the better you will be able to judge when and how to take short cuts. Do not mistake taking short cuts for being lazy. Use the time you save to be available to answer questions, and to address the fears and hopes of the parents and their child.

1 Wash and warm your hands. Encourage both parents be present.
2 Regard the child (eg while feeding). Is he ill or well? Restless, still or playing? If crying, is it high pitched or normal? Is he behaving normally? Any jaundice, cyanosis, rashes, anaemia or dehydration (p 250)?
3 Talk to the child. Explain what you are doing. This helps you both relax, and enjoy the occasion (*not* a trivial point: a happy doctor is an engaged doctor, and an engaged doctor is amenable to receiving subtle signs and covert communications). Feel free to take the child on to your lap. This is his or her natural environment. If he seems anxious, examine his teddy in a playful way, to allow him to build up trust.
4 If the child is quiet or asleep, now is the time to get any listening done, so examine his heart, lungs and abdomen. Start by using a warm stethoscope. Undress in stages.
5 Be methodical. For example, work up the arm to the neck; then up to the head and down through the rest of the body. Start with the finger nails, then the hands, radial pulse, BP, axillary and neck nodes, neck lumps. Is there neck stiffness?
6 Size and shape of head (p 294). Facial symmetry. Does the anterior fontanelle (between the parietal and frontal bones) feel tense (intracranial pressure ↑), or sunken (dehydration)?
7 Is there mucus in the nose? Leave the ears and throat alone.
8 Count the respirations. Is there intercostal recession (inspiratory indrawing of the lower costal area signifying respiratory obstruction)?
9 Percuss the chest and palpate the abdomen. Does it look distended (eg by spleen, liver, fluid, flatus, faeces)?
10 Undo the nappy, if worn. Have an MSU pot to hand. If urine is passed, make a clean catch (p 188). Inspect the nappy's contents. Examine the genitalia/anus. Find the testes. Rectal examination is rarely needed.
11 Note large inguinal nodes. Feel for any radiofemoral pulse delay.

Neurological examination After completing the above, much will have been learned about the nervous system; if in doubt, check:
Tone: Passively flex and extend the limbs.
Power and co-ordination: Watch him walk, run, and pick up a small toy and play with it, with each hand in turn. *Reflexes:* Look for symmetry.
Sensation: Light touch and pain testing are rarely rewarding. Fundi.

Ears/throat Leave to the end, as there may be a struggle. Mother holds the child on her lap, one hand on the forehead, holding his head against her chest, and the other round his waist, encircling his arms. Introduce a spatula and get one good look at mouth and tonsils. Inspect the teeth. Examine ear drums (p 528), using the same hold, but held laterally.

Growth Chart height, weight and head circumference (p 294).

TPR charts Pulse and respiratory rate; rectal T° is normally <37.8 °C.

Finally ask child and mother if there is anything else you should look at.

Is this child seriously ill?APLS

Recognizing that a child is seriously ill and in need of prompt help is a central skill of paediatrics.[1] It can be uncanny to watch the moment of transformation that this recognition brings to a normally reflective, relaxed-and-easy doctor who is now galvanized into an efficient, relentless device for delivering urgent care—'*omitting nothing necessary and adding nothing superfluous*': a frame of mind recommended by Graham Greene for murder, but equally well suited to the destruction of disease. If you are new to paediatrics, take every opportunity to observe such events, and, later, closely question the doctor about what made him act in the way he did, using this page to prepare your mind to receive and remember his or her answers.

Serious signs •Consciousness↓ (not engaging you; apathy; agitation; coma).
•Hyperventilation or using alae nasae/sternomastoids; wheeze; stridor; apnoea.
•Ashen, cyanosed or mottled complexion or signs of dehydration.
•Grunting ± chest retractions or head-nodding in time with respirations.[1]
•Weak/absent pulses, poor capillary refill. To elicit this, press on a digit for 5sec: capillary refill normally takes <2sec. *Don't rely on BP and pulse rate.*
•High core T°, but cold peripheries. Absence of fever may also be a bad sign.
•Unreactive or unequal pupils or decorticate (flexed arms, extended legs) or decerebrate (arms + legs extended) or rigid posture.
•Weak/high-pitched cry and no spontaneous movement during examination.

Age	Reference interval for: *Breathing rate*	*Pulse*	*Systolic BP mmHg*
<1yr	30–40/min	110–160/min	70–90
2–5yr	20–30/min	95–140/min	80–100
5–12yr	15–20/min	80–120/min	90–110
>12yr	12–16/min	60–100/min	100–120

Rapid assessment of the seriously ill child (Should take <1 minute.)

Airway: •Patency.
Breathing: •Work of breathing *Look:* Rate; recession; accessory muscle use; cyanosis *Listen:* Stridor; grunting; wheeze.
Circulation: •Pulse rate and volume; capillary refill; skin colour and T°
Level of response: •**A**=**A**lert •**V**=responds to **V**oice •**P**=responds to **P**ain; •**U**=**U**nresponsive (ie 'AVPU'). Also assess pupils & posture.

Causes Sepsis and trauma are common. The latter are may be non-accidental, so a false history may be offered. Others:
•Gastrointestinal: D&V; obstruction (volvulus)
•Hypoglycaemia; U&E↑; metabolic errors
•Congenital heart disease
•Intussusception (p 198)
•Gastrointestinal: D&V; obstruction (volvulus)
•Arrhythmias/myocarditis
•Haemolytic uraemic synd
•Cardiomyopathies
•DIC (p 244)
•Reye's syndrome (p 756)

Be alert to rare syndromes, eg toxic shock syndrome (*OHCM* p 222) or haemorrhagic shock encephalopathy syndrome (HSES; abrupt shock, with bloody diarrhoea, coma, convulsions, hepatomegaly, oliguria, and DIC).

►**Action—if very ill** •100% O_2 by tight-fitting mask with reservoir.
•Colloid: 20mL/kg bolus IV; repeat if no better. ≥60mL/kg may be needed.
•Do blood glucose (lab and ward test); U&E (ask specifically for HCO_3^-, and, if vomiting, Cl^-); FBC; thick film if tropical travel.
•Crossmatch blood if trauma is possible, or patient looks anaemic.
•Do swabs, blood culture (+suprapubic urine aspirate if >1yr, before starting blind treatment with IV antibiotics, eg ceftriaxone or cefotaxime, p 258).
•If worsening, insert CVP. Get expert help; do blood gases ± clotting screen.
•Ventilate mechanically, eg if bicarbonate is to be given (pH <7.15).
•Consider the need for CXR, MSU, and lumbar puncture.
•If perfusion is still poor (despite 60mL/kg colloid), or CVP >10cmH_2O, dopamine ± dobutamine may be needed. Vasodilatation with nitroprusside (p 304) may rarely be needed to promote cardiac output.

1 S Usen 1999 *BMJ* i 86 (this paper specifies the best signs of hypoxia, and relates these to mortality)

Learning to breast feed[1,2]

Reflexes Rooting (searching, with wide-open mouth) → suckling (jaw goes up and down while the tongue compresses the areola against the hard palate) → swallowing reflex (as milk reaches the oropharynx, the soft palate rises and shuts off the nasopharynx; the larynx rises, closing the trachea).

Skill Do not assume that this will come naturally. It's common to find learning to breast feed as hard as learning to drive—and as anxiety-provoking. The best way to learn is from an experienced person in comfortable surroundings—eg sitting in an upright chair, rather than inadequately propped-up in bed. Reassure that a few problematic feeds do not mean that the baby will starve, and that bottle feeding must be introduced. ►*Most term babies have plenty of spare capacity*—and perseverance will almost always be rewarded. Furthermore, 'top-up' bottle feeds may undermine confidence.

A good time to start breast feeding is immediately after the birth (good bonding; PPH risk↓), but delivery-room procedures may make this hard, eg intrapartum pethidine ± instrumental delivery, T° and BP measurements, washing, weighing, disposal to postnatal ward. ►It is never too late to put to the breast, provided lactation has been maintained.

Beware of intervening too quickly without observing the mother's efforts. Rather than saying 'that's completely wrong: do it like this. . .' it may be better to say 'good: you and your baby are going to get on fine. One extra tip you may find useful is. . .'

From the baby's point of view, breast feeding entails taking a large mouthful of breast-with-nipple, which he or she gets to work on with tongue and jaw. Ensure that the baby is close to the mother with head and shoulders facing the breast—which, if large, may need supporting (mother's fingers placed flat on the chest wall at the base of the breast: avoid the 'scissors' grip which stops the baby from drawing the lactiferous sinuses into his mouth).

- Avoid forcing the nipple into the mouth, eg by placing a hand over his occiput and pressing forwards. Cradle the head in the crook of the arm.
- Explain the signs of correct attachment:
  - Mouth wide open, and chin touching the breast (nose hardly touching).
  - The baby should be seen to be drawing in breast, not just nipple.
  - Lower lip curled back, maximally gobbling the areola (so angle between lips >100°). (Don't worry about how much areola can be seen above the top lip: this gives little indication of where the tongue and lower jaw are.)
  - Slow, rhythmic, and deep jaw movements, as well as sucking movements. (Note: the first few sucks may be fast, shallow, and non-nutrative: here the baby is inducing the mother's 'let-down' reflex, which promotes flow.)
- When helping with placing, it is quite appropriate to 'tease' the baby by brushing his lip over the nipple, and then away. This may induce a nice big gape. With one movement bring to the breast, aiming his tongue and lower jaw as far as possible from the base of the nipple—so his tongue can scoop in the nipple and a good mouthful of breast.
- Keeping on the postnatal ward for quite a few days, and having the mother learn with an experienced, friendly midwife is also of great benefit, but this facility is now rare in the UK.

1 D Henschel 1996 *Breast Feeding: A Guide for Midwives*, Books for Midwives Press ISBN 1 898507 12 0
2 Royal College of Midwives, 1988 *Successful Breast Feeding*, ISBN 1 870822 01 3

How to express breast milk

It is desirable for every breast feeding mother to learn this skill (access to teaching is *required* before the accolade of 'baby-friendly' can be granted to UK hospitals). There are at least 4 times when expressing is valuable:

- To relieve painful breast engorgement between feeds.
- To keep milk production going when it is necessary to give nipples a rest owing to soreness—which is quite a common problem.
- To aid nutrition if sucking is reduced for any reason (eg prematurity or cleft lip).
- If the mother is going to be separated from her baby for a few feeds, eg going out to work.

The best way to learn is from a midwife, and by watching a mother who is already successfully expressing milk. Pumps may be available. If not, wash hands, and dry on a clean towel, then, try to start flow by:

1. Briefly rolling the nipple: this may induce a let-down reflex, especially if the baby is nearby.
2. Stroke the breast gently towards the nipple.
3. With circular movements, massage the breast gently with the 3 middle fingers.

Applying warm flannels, or expressing in the bath may aid flow, eg while the mother is learning, and only a few drops are being expressed.

Teach the mother to find the 15 or so ampullae beneath the areola: they feel knotty once the milk comes in. Now with the thumb above the areola and the index finger below, and whole hand pressing the breast back on the chest wall, exert gentle pressure on the ampullae. With rhythmic pressure and release, milk should flow (have a sterile container to hand).

Take care that the fingers do not slip down on to the nipple, and damage the narrowing ducts. Fingers tire easily: practise is the key. Concentration is also needed to be sure to catch oddly angled jets.

If kept in a fridge, the milk lasts 24–48h. Frozen milk should be used within 3 months. It is thawed by standing it in a jug of warm water. Any unused should be discarded, not refrozen.

Breast feeding and social influences

Factors which make starting breast feeding harder •Family pressures, including partner's hostility (10% breast feed *vs* ~70% if he approves).[1]
•If mother and baby are separated at night in hospital.
•Urbanization, or whenever the mother is expected to work, and there is no convenient place for breast feeding.
•Cultural reframing of breasts as sex objects.
•Rôle-models: if mothers, grandmothers, and elder sisters are not breast feeding, younger sisters may feel embarrassed about starting.

Advantages of the breast ►The breast is the ideal place to learn to get to grips with the world, to watch one's mother from—as well as to sulk from.*
•Breastfeeding gives lower infant mortality rate (wherever there is poverty).
•Sucking promotes uterine contractions, so avoiding some PPHs.
•Bonding: eye-to-eye contact aids recognition, and stimulates further emotional input from the mother.
•Breast feeding is a total experience, stimulating all five senses.
•Breast feeding is cheap, and breast milk is clean.
•IgA, macrophages, lymphocytes (with interferon) and lysozyme protect from infection. Acids in breast milk promote growth of friendly lactobacillus in the baby's bowel. Gastro-enteritis may be less severe if the mother makes and transfers antibodies (an 'immune dialogue').
•Breast milk contains less Na^+, K^+ and Cl^- than other milk, so aiding homeostasis. If dehydration occurs, risk of fatal hypernatraemia is low.
•Breast feeding reduces the risk of juvenile-onset diabetes mellitus.
•Breast feeding protects against early-onset atopic eczema and other allergies.
•Breast feeding is contraceptive.
•There is (sometimes disputed) evidence that breast feeding raises IQ scores (possibly due to long chain fatty acids needed for neurodevelopment).
•Some protection in premenopausal years against maternal breast cancer.

Why is feeding on demand to be encouraged?
•It keeps the baby happy, and enhances milk production.
•Fewer breast problems (engorgement, abscesses).
Note: sleep is less disturbed if baby is kept in bed with mother.

Contraindications to breast feeding •An HBsAg +ve mother •An HIV +ve mother in developed countries •Amiodarone •Antimetabolites •Opiates.

Problems These include breast engorgement and breast abscess. Treat by using the breast more effectively (better latching-on); aim to keep breasts empty, eg by hourly feeds or milk expression (p 177).

If a breast abscess forms, discard the milk if it is pus-like. Give the mother flucloxacillin 250mg/6h PO (it is safe for her baby).

Treat sore nipples by ensuring optimal attachment (p 176), and moist wound healing (eg Jelonet® dressing) not by resting (except in emergencies).

Preterm breast milk is *probably* the best food for preterm infants. Give unheated, via a tube (p 246). Add vitamins D 1000u/day and K (p 246). Phosphate supplements may be needed. Note: even term babies may (rarely) develop rickets ± hypocalcaemia (eg with fits, recurrent 'colds' lethargy, or stridor), if exclusively breast fed, unless vitamin supplements are used (p 208).

***My mother groaned! My father wept,*
Into the dangerous world I lept:
Helpless, naked, piping loud:
Like a fiend hid in a cloud.

Struggling in my father's hands:
Striving against my swaddling bands:
Bound and weary I thought best
To sulk upon my mother's breast.

William Blake, *Infant sorrow*

Bottle feeding

There are few contraindications to breast feeding but many pressures not to (p 176–8). 64% of mothers start breast feeding, 52% are breast feeding at 2 weeks and 39% at 6 weeks. Most change to bottle because of lack of knowledge or no encouragement.

Advantages of bottle feeding Fathers can bottle feed. Many mothers are reassured to know how much milk the baby is taking. Babies can be fed in public without embarrassment. Some Asian mothers may follow traditional beliefs that colostrum is harmful and bottle feed until the milk comes in.

Infant formula (Cow's milk which has been 'humanized' by reducing the solute load and modifying fat, protein and vitamin content.) Whey-based formula is considered more suitable for infants than more protein-rich casein-based types, but brands are similar and shopping around for a brand which 'suits' the baby is rarely the answer to feeding problems.

Preparing feeds Hands must be clean, equipment sterilized and boiled water used—infective gastro-enteritis causes many deaths in poor countries and considerable morbidity in UK. Powder must be accurately measured. Understrength feeds lead to poor growth and overstrength feeds have, in the past, caused dangerous hypernatraemia, constipation and obesity.

Feeding Babies require ~150mL/kg/24h (30mL=1oz) divided over 4–6 feeds depending on age and temperament. Small-for-dates babies may need up to 200mL/kg/day, and large-for-dates babies <100mL/kg. Feeds are often warmed, but there is no evidence that cold milk is harmful. Flow should almost form a stream; check before each feed as teats silt up. The hole can be enlarged with a hot needle. Bottles are best angled so that air is not sucked in with milk.

Cow's milk allergy This develops in up to 1% of babies—with diarrhoea (may be bloody), vomiting, peri-oral rash, oedema and failure to thrive. Soya milk formula may be substituted. Cow's milk may be cautiously reintroduced at 1 year (can be risky so do in hospital). NB: allergies to soya are also a problem, so a protein hydrolysate may be needed.[1]

Soya milks These containing corn syrup or sucrose—but no lactose, are indicated in secondary lactose intolerance, galactosaemia and primary hypolactasia—as well as in vegan families, as they ban all cow's milk. Wysoy® is *not* the solution for infants with eczema: see p 589. Try a protein hydrolysate instead (eg Nutramigen®). Because of their high aluminium content, avoid soya milks if preterm, or if there is a renal problem.

Soya is *not* indicated in regrading after simple gastro-enteritis.[1]

Weaning Milk contains sufficient nourishment for the first 3 months. 'Solids' should be introduced at 3–6 months by offering cereal or puréed food on a spoon. Cereals should not be added to bottles. At 6 months 'follow-on' (protein-enriched) formula may be used and lumpy food should be started so that the baby can learn to chew. Doorstep/supermarket milk may be suitable after the first birthday, when it is no longer likely to provoke anaemia from microscopic gastrointestinal blood loss.

1 SG Mitton 1994 *BMJ* i 266

Preterm and light-for-dates babies

A neonate whose calculated gestational age from the last menstrual period is <37 completed weeks is preterm* (ie premature). Low-birth-weight babies fall into 3 groups:

1 < 2500g but appropriate for gestational age.
2 < 2500g term infants who are small for gestational age (ie weight below the 10th centile for gestation—see below).
3 Low-birth-weight preterm babies (weight is small for gestational age). 6% of UK infants are <2500g at birth, and 50% of these are preterm. 5% of pregnancies end in spontaneous preterm delivery, and 70% of all perinatal deaths occur in preterm infants (particularly if also growth-retarded).

	Tenth centile weight (grams)			
Weeks' gestation	*First born:* *boy*	*girl*	*Subsequent births:* *boy*	*girl*
32	1220	1260	1470	1340
33	1540	1540	1750	1620
34	1830	1790	2000	1880
35	2080	2020	2230	2100
36	2310	2210	2430	2310
37	2500	2380	2600	2480
38	2660	2530	2740	2620
39	2780	2640	2860	2730
40	2870	2730	2950	2810

Causes of prematurity These are mostly unknown. Smoking tobacco, poverty and malnutrition play a part. Others: past history of prematurity; genitourinary infection/chorioamnionitis (eg *Ureaplasma*)**; pre-eclampsia; polyhydramnios; closely separated pregnancies; multiple pregnancy; uterine malformation; placenta praevia; abruption; premature rupture of the membranes. Labour may be induced early on purpose or accidentally (p 110).

Estimating the gestational age Use the Dubowitz score (p 298).

Infants who are small for gestational age Causes and associations: malformations, multiple pregnancy, placental insufficiency (maternal heart disease, hypertension, smoking, diabetes, sickle-cell disease, pre-eclampsia). The incidence of live-born, very-low-birth-weight infants <1500g is ~0.6%. Neonatal mortality (within 28 days of birth) is ~25%. If the weight is 500–600g only about 10% survive, at best.

Gestational age (based on LMP and ultrasound) is more important for predicting survival than the birth weight alone.

Management If 32 weeks or less, transfer *in utero* to a special centre, if possible. Once born, protect from the cold. Measure blood glucose. Take to SCBU if glucose <2mmol/L. Measure blood glucose before each 3-hourly feed. Tube feed if oral feeds are not tolerated. If oral feeding is contraindicated (eg respiratory distress syndrome) IV feeding is needed (p 246).

Survival of very premature babies[1] (23–25 weeks' gestation) Survival is rising (1984–9=27%; 1990–4=42%, when 19% survived at 23 weeks, 40% at 24 weeks, and 54% at 25 weeks). Mortality is associated with the presence of cranial abnormalities on ultrasonography. ►16% of those born from 1984–9 survived without disability, but only 14% did so if born from 1990–4.

*Premature is now used as a synonym for preterm; beware older books, as premature once meant birth weight <5½lbs (2.5kg)—before the difference between light-for-dates and preterm was recognized.
**Also causes neonatal sepsis, respiratory distress & intraventricular haemorrhage (E-BM 1999 4 29).
1 H Emsley 1999 E-BM 4 25 (much of the disability relates to retinopathy, p 232).

3. Paediatrics

Common happenings in childhood[1]

Crying babies Crying peaks at ~8 weeks old (2–3h/day, especially in the evenings). The cries of hunger and thirst are indistinguishable. Feeding at adult-dictated intervals is apt to cause crying in many babies, so demand feeding is preferred.[2] Any thwarting of a baby's wishes may lead to crying, with bouts of screaming. No doubt there are good survival reasons for Nature making babies cry, but in the 20th century this provision may be counterproductive: prolonged crying (as well as lack of parental support) can even provoke child abuse in vulnerable families. Crying may be the last straw for a parent with few reserves. Aim to offer help *before* this stage (eg CRY-SIS self-help group, UK tel. 0171 404 5011). The key skill is not to make parents feel inadequate, and to foster a spirit of practical optimism with one or other parent sleeping and gaining rest whenever the child sleeps.

3-month colic Paroxysmal crying with pulling up of the legs, for >3h on ≥3 days/wk comprise the defining *rule of 3s*.[1] Studies have failed to show a GI cause. Cow's milk whey allergy, and parental discord and disappointment with pregnancy are implicated[2]—but it may be that such stressed parents may *report* more colic.[3] *Treatment:* Nothing helps for long. Try movement (eg carry-cot on wheels, or go for a drive). Trials[4] favour dimethicone (simethicone) drops (40mg/mL; 0.5–1mL PO before feeds; avoid if < 1 month). Few other drugs are licensed for this age group. Very occasionally, chloral is used. In breast fed babies, a cow's-milk-free diet for mother is unlikely to help, and a change to soya milk (p 179) in bottle fed babies is often tried in desperation, but often disappoints. Reassure strongly: but remember that a crying baby may be a sign of major family relationship problems.

Vomiting Effortless regurgitation of milk is very common during feeds. Vomiting between feeds is also common; if repeated, find the cause, eg gastro-enteritis; pyloric stenosis; hiatus hernia (p 272 mucus ± blood in vomit); pharyngeal pouch or duodenal obstruction (there is bile in the vomit). Observing feeding is helpful in deciding if the vomiting is projectile (eg over the end of the cot), suggesting pyloric stenosis.

Nappy rash or diaper dermatitis 4 types:

1 The common ammonia dermatitis—red, desquamating rash, sparing skin folds. The term is a misnomer, as moisture retention, not ammonia is the cause. It often responds to frequent changes of nappy (rinse them well), careful drying, and an emollient cream. Avoid tight-fitting rubber pants. 'One way' nappies may be helpful at night (eg Snugglers®).

2 Candida dermatitis (thrush): this may be isolated from ~½ of all nappy rashes. Its hallmark is satellite spots beyond the main rash. Mycology: see p 590. Treatment: as above, with nystatin or clotrimazole cream (± 1% hydrocortisone cream, eg as Nystaform HC® cream).

3 Seborrhoeic eczematous dermatitis: a diffuse, red, shiny rash extends into skin folds, often associated with other signs of a seborrhoeic skin, eg on occiput (cradle cap). Treatment: as for 1.

4 Isolated, psoriasis-like scaly plaques (p 586), which can be hard to treat.

Agents to avoid: Boric acid and fluorinated steroids (systemic absorption); oral antifungals (hepatotoxic); gentian violet (staining is unpopular).

Sleep problems See p 264.

1 G Still 1938 *Common Happenings in Childhood*, OUP and I St James-Roberts 1996 *Arch Dis Chi* **76** 356
3 P Rautava 1993 BMJ **ii** 600 & S Thacker 1993 BMJ **ii** 869 4 T Markestad 1997 *Practitioner* **232** 356–8

Chronic childhood illness, and family support

Diseases such as severe asthma, CNS disease, and neoplasia may cause disintegration of even the most apparently secure families: ►*consequent strife and marital breakdown may be more severe and have more far-reaching consequences than the illness itself.*

Remember that illness makes families poor, and movement down the social scale may lead to unpredictable consequences in the fields of housing and (un)employment.

Marital disharmony may seem to be beyond the scope of paediatrics, but any holistic view of child health *must* put the family at the centre of *all* attempts to foster child health and wellbeing.

In your practice you will see many families coping admirably with severe, prolonged illness in a child. But do not presume that because things are OK in clinic to day, you can afford to neglect the fostering of family life. Given a certain amount of stress almost *all* families will show psychopathology, in time. Your job is to delay this. Counselling skills are frequently needed (p 376)—but do they work? Various tools are helpful in answering this question:[1]

- Communication is vital in any family, and this can be measured by scales such as the Communication Skills Test (CST).
- The dyadic adjustment scale (DAS) looks at the emotional interaction within a marriage or any other pairing.
- The Miller Social Intimacy Scale (MSIS) looks at intimacy in relationships, and intimacy is, beyond doubt, a source of strength within a family experiencing illness in a child.
- Specific therapies which have been tried in randomized trials in families coping with severe chronic illness in a child include Emotionally Focused Marital Therapy (EMT), with these benefits:
  - Higher overall levels of marital adjustment (on the DAS scale). None of the couples receiving the active therapy deteriorated by >7 points, whereas one-third of couples in the control group had such a deterioration (which shows the stress these families were under, and supports the notion that family psychopathology in the face of chronic childhood illness is an evolving phenomenon—*reversible if you take certain steps*).
  - Better levels of intimacy as measured on MSIS scale, with effects persisting for at least 5 months.
  - Lower rates of negative communication (on the CST score).
  - Statistical analysis shows that only 2 couples would have to be treated for one additional couple to experience improvement.[2]

1 JG Walker 1996 *J Consult Clin Psychol* **64** 1029 2 W Linden 1997 *E-BM* **2** 46
NB: some couples were too stressed to participate, and others were excluded because of violence (ref 2)

Growth and failure to thrive

The capacity to grow and develop is the essence of childhood. If you want to find out if a child is healthy, the first question to ask is: *Is growth normal?* Take any opportunity to weigh and measure a child. A series of plots on centile charts (p 296) shows if growth is slow (growth curve crosses the centiles). NB: the growth rate in mid-childhood is 5–6cm/yr; this accelerates at puberty (peak height velocity), before epiphyses start to fuse.

Failure to thrive means poor weight gain in infancy (weight crosses centile lines in a downwards direction). Typically, head circumference is preserved relative to linear growth, which in turn is preserved relative to body weight.[1] In 95% this is due to not enough food being offered, or not enough food being taken. In developing countries, poverty is the chief cause; in the UK it is difficulty at home, emotional deprivation, or unskilled feeding techniques. Other causes: see below. NB: The diagnosis may simply be idiosyncratic growth pattern; normal child of short stature (prematurity, low birth weight, short siblings or parents)—particularly if he is happy and contented.

In the consultation:[2]

- Behaviour; activity level
- General health & happiness
- Signs of abuse (p 284)
- Family finances
- Chart family heights
- Feeding patterns
- Dysmorphic face
- Parental illness?

Be sceptical about reliability of data. Was the child clothed during weighings? Length measurements are particularly prone to error: growth velocity may be more useful than measurements taken at a single time.

Issues to address on the ward: •Feeding and maternal interaction. Is the child anorectic or ravenous (hyperphagic short stature syndrome)?
- If breast feeding, does he get a good mouthful of breast? If just the nipple, then his nose may be compressing the lactiferous ducts.
- If bottle feeding, does the teat's hole allow milk to flow through?
- Does weight gain return if the child is removed from the family?
- What is the minimum effective level of investigation?
- Is there ward evidence of relevance to child protection proceedings?

Tests: It is a great skill to know when and how to investigate. It is much better from the child's point of view (and cheaper!) to ask a trusted colleague's opinion before painful tests. In one study only 39 of 4880 tests were helpful.[2] MSU (expect false +ves if bags are used; suprapubic aspiration may be needed if <1yr old, but only if there are symptoms); U&E, plasma glucose, LFT, Ca^{2+}, proteins, immunoglobulins, CRP, T_4, TSH; FBC; sweat test; urinary amino and organic acid chromatography; stools for pathogens and sugar detection; CXR, renal or CNS ultrasound, skeletal survey for dwarfism and abuse; jejunal biopsy; echocardiogram and ECG.

Short stature

This is a height below the 3rd centile (p 296). If the parents are both small, their child will be likely to be small too (constitutional short stature accounts for ~80% of short children). Use the method shown on the charts to correct for mid-parental height. ►*Any chronic disease can cause short stature.* Hypopituitarism (an important cause of short stature) usually manifests after age 2yrs: look for relative obesity, without any other explanation for low growth velocity (ie <25th centile; measure for ≥1yr, see p 295). Deficiency of growth hormone (GH) is shown by an impaired rise (peak GH <15mu/L) after a stimulus (eg sleep or hypoglycaemia, induced by IV insulin, *OHCM* p 558). Pre-school screening for short stature is the aim. To be effective synthetic GH should be given early. Growth hormone dose example: 0.5–0.7u/kg/week SC, perhaps more during puberty. Daily doses are probably better than thrice weekly regimens.[3] Other pituitary hormones may also be deficient (*OHCM* p 558).

Other causes of short stature *Poverty:*	*Endocrine*	*Drugs:*	*Genetic:* Turner's
Poor or ineffective diet (also coeliac)	Hypothyroid	Steroids	Cystic fibrosis
Physical or psychological abuse	GH↓ (see above)		Noonan sy, p 754

Causes of height↑: Thyrotoxic, precocious puberty, Marfan's, homocystinuria.

Ethnospecific growth charts[4]

It is clear that some populations are inherently shorter than others, and this poses problems when using growth charts. Consider these facts:

- The Dutch are the tallest *nation* on earth (mean ♂ height = 1.84m): the tallest *population group* is the Masai people (eg in Tanzania and Kenya).[5] 185
- African and Afro-Caribbean 5–11yr-olds height is ~0.6 standard deviations scores (SDs) greater than white children living in England.
- Gujarati children and those from the Indian subcontinent (except those from Urdu- or Punjabi-speaking homes) have heights ~0.5 SDs less than white children living in England.
- Gujarati children's weight-for-height is ~0.9 SDs less than expected for Afro-Caribbeans, or white children in England—so Gujarati children's weight is ~1.5 SDs less than for white children living in England.
- Urdu and Punjabi children's weight is ~0.5 SDs less than expected for white children living in England.
- Published charts have centile lines 0.67 SDs apart; for height and weight shift the centile lines up by 1 centile line division for Afro-Caribbeans.
- Re-label Gujarati children's weight charts, so the 0.4th centile becomes the ~15th centile, and the 2nd weight centile becomes the ~30th centile.
- For most other Indian subcontinent groups, both height and weight should be shifted downwards: consider relabelling the 0.4th and 2nd centile lines 1.5th and 6th respectively.
- Body-mass index centiles are said to be appropriate for Afro-Caribbeans,[4] but recalculate as above for Indian subcontinent children, except for Gujarati speaking children (0.4th & 2nd centiles → 4th & 14th).

Trends towards increasing height with each generation occur at varying rates in all groups, so 3rd generation immigrants may be taller than expected using 2nd generation data. Intermarriage also confuses the issue.

Coeliac disease

Malabsorption typically presents with diarrhoea ± anaemia (folate or iron deficiency), possibly with abdomenal protrusion and eversion of the umbilicus. As subclinical/latent forms exist, investigate any unexplained anaemia, fatigue, 'irritable bowel' symptoms, diarrhoea, weight↓, arthralgia and eczema, and short stature.[6,7] Patients may present at *any* age.

Cause: Enteropathy induced by gluten (found in wheat and barley).

Diagnostic criteria:[6,7] IgA gliadin, anti-reticulin, and anti-endomysium antibodies are used as a screening test for diagnosis—the latter's specificity ≈100%.[7] Confirmation is by finding villous atrophy on small bowel biopsy: a swallowed Crosby capsule is guided to the small bowel under x-ray control, and fired by suction. Endoscopic distal duodenal biopsy is also possible. Villi return to normal on the special diet, and a gluten challenge is unnecessary, unless there is diagnostic doubt.

Treatment: Gluten-free diet: no wheat, barley, rye, oats, or any food containing them (eg bread, cake, pies). Rice, maize, soya, potatoes, sugar jam, syrup and treacle are allowed. Gluten-free biscuits, flour, bread and pasta are prescribable. Even minor dietary lapses may cause recurrence. After 5yrs a cautious reintroduction of gluten may be tried.

Other causes of malabsorption: Cystic fibrosis; post-enteritis enteropathy; giardia; rotaviruses; bacterial overgrowth; milk sensitivity.

1 M Donaldson 1994 BMJ i 596 2 H Marcovitch 1994 BMJ i 35 3 *Drug Ther Bul* 1989 **27** 97 4 S Chinn 1996 *Lancet* **347** 839 5 T Sheldon 1998 BMJ i 1929 6 J Walker-Smith 1990 *Arch Dis Chi* **65** 909 7 H Hin 1999 BMJ i 164

Diarrhoea

Worldwide, this kills more than 3×10^6 children/yr. Faeces are sometimes so liquid they are mistaken for urine. It is *normal* for breast fed babies to have liquid stools. Some cow's milks cause harmless green stools. Diarrhoea may be an early sign of *any* septic illness.

Gastro-enteritis The main danger from small intestine infection is dehydration ± U&E imbalance (p 250) brought on by D&V. Rotavirus is the most common cause. There is often associated otitis media or upper respiratory infection. Other enteric viruses: astrovirus, small round-structured viruses (SRSV, eg Norwalk agent), calicivirus. *Treatment:* ►If dehydrated, see p 250. Weighing the child (to monitor progress, and to quantify the level of dehydration, if a recent previous weight is available). Stop bottle milk (but if breast feeding, continue) and solids, and give oral rehydration mixture, eg Rehidrat® or Dioralyte®, which is 60mmol Na^+/L with an osmolarity of 240mmol/L, and is better in non-cholera diarrhoea than standard WHO solutions (90mmol and 311mmol/L respectively).[1] Milk is re-introduced after 24h (regrading is not required), or sooner if the child recovers and is hungry. Prolonged starvation delays recovery, and early use of full strength feeds is safe even in small babies.[2] NB: breast milk supplies antibodies and maintains milk production, but in some communities (eg if poor) breast milk is likely to be zinc-deficient, and zinc supplements help stop diarrhoea becoming chronic (eg 10mg zinc sulfate/day PO).[3]

Complications: Dehydration; malnutrition; temporary sugar intolerance after D&V with explosive watery acid stools. (Rare; manage with a lactose-free diet.) Post-enteritis enteropathy resolves spontaneously after 6–8 weeks.

Tests: Send stools for pathogens, including ova, cysts and parasites.

Prevention: Hygiene, good water and food, education, fly control.

Secretory diarrhoea *Causes:* Bacteria (campylobacter, staphylococcus, *E coli*, and, where sanitation is poor, salmonella, shigella and *Vibrio cholerae*); giardiasis; rotavirus; amoebiasis; cryptosporidium). Inflammatory bowel disease.

Toddler's diarrhoea 'Like peas & carrots'; due to intestinal hurry; resolves by 4yrs.

Other causes Food intolerance (coeliac disease; disaccharide, cows' milk or wheat intolerance, galactose, glucose or lactose intolerance: to find reducing substances mix 5 drops of stool with 10 drops H_2O + 1 Clinitest® tab); antibiotics; deficiencies (zinc, copper, Mg^{2+}, vitamins); kwashiorkor.

Causes of bloody diarrhoea Campylobacter; necrotizing enterocolitis (in neonates), intussusception (often <4 years old), pseudomembranous colitis; haemolytic uraemic syndrome (p 280); inflammatory bowel disease (rare, even in older children: look for weight↓; anaemia; WBC↑; platelets↑; ESR/CRP↑).

Malnutrition

This is not common in the UK, but, being a major cause of infant mortality and morbidity worldwide, it has a global importance to us all.

Kwashiorkor is due to dietary lack of protein and essential aminoacids. It is characterized by growth retardation, diarrhoea, apathy, anorexia, oedema, skin/hair depigmentation, anaemia and abdominal distension. Serum glucose, K^+, Mg^{2+}, cholesterol and albumin are low. *Treatment* depends on re-education (of child, family and politicians) as well as on offering a gradually increasing, high-protein diet with added vitamins. **Marasmus** is the deficiency of calories, with marked discrepancy between height and weight. *Presentation:* Abdominal distension, diarrhoea, constipation, infection. *Tests:* Serum albumin↓. In young children a mid-arm circumference <9.9cm (any age) predicts severe malnutrition better than being <60% of median weight for age, or 85% of median height for age and 70% of median weight for height. *Treatment:* Parenteral feeding may be needed to restore hydration and renal function. Next offer a balanced diet with vitamins. Despite this, stature and head circumference may remain reduced. NB: Kwashiorkor and marasmus may occur together.

Southern diarrhoea is only an excuse for Northern amnesia

As you read this page two events unfold: in Japan a child is born with a silver spoon in his mouth—his future assured thanks to incubators, ventilators, wealth and family planning; and, diametrically opposed to this birth another occurs somewhere in the Southern hemisphere where the silver was mined for that silver spoon. This child, according to our stereotype must 'Wait for his future like a horse that's gone lame—To lie in the gutter and die with no name.' We assume that this death is from diarrhoeal diseases which we are all working, more or less efficiently, towards controlling—and we are pleased to blame non-human agencies for these deaths. This model of our imperfect world does not stand up to scrutiny for two reasons: one is easy to understand (the diarrhoea was the mode of dying not the cause of death, which was poverty) and the other is impossible to understand—we didn't let him die. We wanted him to die: in fact we killed him: in some cases, literally. Watch this well-documented thought sequence: there are too many homeless children living in my back yard→This is a threat to health and hygiene→How do we deal with this?→Other threats to health and hygeine are vermin→Street children are a sort of vermin→vermin need eradicating→Let's shoot the vermin→Extrajudicial shooting of children—as is occurred in July 1993 in Rio de Janeiro. Most 'ordinary decent folk' approved of the killings when they phoned a local radio station,[5] as the events unfolded. . . 'I killed you because you had no future.'[6]

The point of all this is to illustrate that if we want to do something for children it is no good just doing something about the big killers—such as diarrhoea, and it's no good simply attacking poverty, for there is something dark in our human heart which needs addressing before purely statistical or biological interventions have a chance of success.

<1> T Rautanen 1997 *Arch Dis Chi* **76** 272 & ORS group *Lancet* **345** 282 <2> M Ruel E-BM 1998 **3** 13 **3** F Chew 1993 *Lancet* **341** 194 **4** R Beattie 1995 *Arch Dis Chi* 1995 **73** 354–5 **5** E Fernandes 1994 *Neth Q Hum Rights* **12** 117 **6** D Summerfield 1998 *Lancet* **351** 1955

Childhood urinary tract infection (UTI)

Presentation ►Often the child may be *non-specifically* ill. Infants may present with collapse and septicaemia, and toddlers as 'gastro-enteritis', failure to thrive, colic, or PUO. Many with dysuria and frequency have *no* identifiable UTI, and will often have vulvitis. The GU tract is normal in most with UTI, but ~35% have vesico-ureteric reflux, ~14% have renal scars (most will have reflux too), ~5% have stones, ~3% will develop hypertension. Each year in the UK, 10–20 children enter endstage renal failure programmes because of complications from reflux and chronic pyelonephritis.

Definitions *Bacteriuria:* Bacteria in urine uncontaminated by urethral flora. It may be *covert* (few, or unreported symptoms), and can lead to renal scarring; hypertension, and, very rarely, chronic renal failure. *UTI* denotes symptomatic bacteriuria, which may involve different GU sites (check for loin and suprapubic tenderness; ask about fever and dysuria). *Chronic pyelonephritis* is a histological/radiological diagnosis. Juxtaposition of a cortex scar and a dilated calyx is the key to its diagnosis. It is a major cause of hypertension and can result in renal failure, particularly if the kidneys are congenitally dysplastic.

During micturition, urine may *reflux* up ureters—identified by a micturating cystogram (requires catheterization) or MAG3 scan (catheterization not needed)—grading: I Incomplete filling of upper GU tract, without dilatation. II Complete filling ± slight dilatation. III Ballooned calyces.

Epidemiology Annual incidence of infection: boys: 0.17–0.23%; girls: 0.31–1%. (Sex ratios are reversed in neonates.) Recurrence: 35% if >2yrs old. Prevalence of covert bacteriuria in schoolgirls: ~3%. Prevalence of radiological abnormalities associated with UTI: 40% (½ have reflux; others: malpositions, duplications, megaureter, hydronephrosis). *Renal scars and age:* We used to concentrate on treating babies early, thinking new scars were rare after 4 years of age, but prospective ^{99m}Tc dimercaptosuccinate (DMSA) scintigraphy (the best test) shows new scars appearing on repeat scans in 43% of those <1yr old, 84% of those aged 1–5, and 80% of those >5yrs old.[1]

Tests[2] *Urine collection:* In infants, *suprapubic aspiration* is definitive (any organisms are significant) but invasive. An alternative is to wash genitals gently with water and tap repeatedly (in cycles of 1min) with 2 fingers just above the pubis, 1h after a feed, and wait for a *clean catch*, avoiding the first part of the stream. Do prompt microscopy and culture. >10^8 organisms/L of a pure growth signifies UTI. Ward ultrasound helps identify a full bladder. Method: clean skin over the bladder; insert a 21–23G needle in the midline 2.5cm above symphysis pubis. Aspirate as you advance the needle. Other devices: *dipslides* (go out of date rapidly), *culture pads* (Microstix®). *Urine bags* applied to the perineum cause many false +ves, and urine collection on *sanitary towels*, via a syringe, is much cheaper and perhaps preferable.

Ultrasound (U/S): As this is non-invasive, it is worthwhile even in first UTIs (specificity 99%; sensitivity 43%, but reflux and scarring may be missed). Almost all the significant lesions missed by U/S either occur in infants <2yrs, or occur with fever and vomiting, so if these are present and U/S is normal, proceed not to IVU, which is radiation-rich and unreliable, but to:

^{99}Technetium renography—static for scarring (^{99m}Tc DMSA scan, *OHCM* p 734), dynamic for obstructive uropathy—and *isotope cystography*.[3] *Micturating cystourethrography* is still the best way of excluding reflux (in general, it is *not* needed, if initial tests are normal, pyelonephritis is unlikely, there is no family history of reflux, and there are no *recurrent* UTIs; it is invasive and unpleasant, but careful preparation with play therapy (p 384) mitigates this.

1 D Benador 1997 *Lancet* 349 17 2 UTI Group 1991 *J Roy Col Phys* **25** 36 3 A Rickwood 1992 BMJ **i** 663

Treatment and prevention of urinary infections

Antibiotics: •Trimethoprim 50mg/5mL, 50mg/12h PO for 5 days (halve if <6mths; double if >6yrs), nalidixic acid, or co-amoxiclav •Encourage fluids •Avoid constipation •Encourage full voiding •Do repeat MSU.

Treatment of reflux: If prophylactic antibiotics fail, ureteric reimplantation can reduce reflux, but scarring remains. Keep on antibiotic prophylaxis.

Prevention Just one episode of reflux of infected urine may initiate renal scarring, so *screening* for bacteriuria is useless: damage happens too quickly. But once a UTI is suggested (eg by urine microscopy) treat it *at once*, whatever the age, before culture sensitivities are known, as renal damage may be about to happen—while at the same time doing all you can to ensure a high-quality urine sample is analysed. Consider trimethoprim prophylaxis while awaiting surgery or investigations. Screen siblings for reflux.

Acute lymphoblastic leukaemia (ALL)

ALL is the commonest childhood leukaemia; other forms: see *OHCM* p 602–5.

Causes One model invokes genetic predisposition with later exposure to triggers such as radiation, benzene, HTLV-1, or abnormal response to infection.[1,2]

Classification[3] *Common ALL* (75%): Blasts have characteristics of neither T (rosette) nor B lymphocytes, but have a characteristic surface polypeptide. Median age: 4yrs. Prognosis: good (86% 5yr survival).
B-cell ALL: Blasts look like those of Burkitt's lymphoma. Poorer prognosis (but now 70% disease-free survival). Subtypes: •*Early pre-B*, eg with cytoplasmic monoclonal antibodies (CD22+, CD79a+, CD19+) and surface immunoglobulins (sIg); •*Pre-B cell*; •*Transitional pre-B-cell*; •*B-cell* (sIg+, sIg_{κ}+, or sIg_{λ}).
T-cell ALL: Median age: 10yrs. Prognosis: ~40–50% disease-free survival.
Null-cell ALL: Blasts show none of the above features.
Classification by ploidy: Hypodiploid (7% of ALL patients), diploid (8%), pseudodiploid (42%), hyperdiploid with 47–50 chromosomes (27%) or hyperdiploid with >50 chromosomes (27%), or triploid/tetraploid (1%).

Worse prognosis in: Blacks, males, WCC >100 × 10^9/L; Philadelphia translocation [t(9;22)(q34:q11)] seen in 12% (0–15% disease-free at 5yrs).

The patient Presentation may be with pancytopenia (pallor, infection, bleeding), fatigue, anorexia, fever and bone pain (as blasts invade the marrow). The period before diagnosis is often brief (2–4 weeks).

Tests WCC↑, ↓ or ↔. Normochromic, normocytic anaemia ± platelets↓. Marrow: 50–98% of nucleated cells will be blasts. CSF: pleocytosis (with blast forms), protein ↑, glucose ↓. Biochemistry: urate↑, LDH↑.

Treatment[4] In the UK, almost all children are treated according to the MRC/UK-ALL protocol. This entails remission induction (± a brief period of intensified treatment to eradicate residual blast cells), CNS prophylaxis, and maintenance therapy. *Risk assessment* ensures only those most likely to relapse get the most aggressive 4-drug treatment with preventive meningeal irradiation (eg if presenting WCC >50 × 10^9/L; age >9yrs; T-cell immunophenotype; pre-B-cell with the t(1;19) translocation). Pneumocystosis is prevented by co-trimoxazole 10mg/kg/12h PO. While the WCC is <1.0 × 10^9/L use a neutropenic regimen.
Drugs used: High-dose cyclophosphamide, cytarabine, methotrexate (intrathecal), mercaptopurine, asparaginase, daunorubicin, etoposide, t(h)ioguanine, vincristine, prednisolone. NB: life-threatening myelosuppression occurs if deficient in thiopurine methyltransferase (so consider pre-R_x pharmacogenomic analysis).

Reinforce remission by use of non-cross-resistant drug pairs, to reduce the leukaemic clone, and lower the frequency of drug-resistant mutants and, therefore, relapse. Bone marrow transplants are not routinely used in ALL in children, but may be needed in those at highest risk, eg Philadelphia chromosome, WCC >200 × 10^9/L, MLL gene rearrangement, B-cell ALL with the t(8;14) translocation.

Much treatment, including IV cytotoxics, is now given at home.

Prognosis Many centres are reporting 75% 5-year event-free survival.

Pitfalls •Serious infection with no tell-tale fever or tachycardia—eg: zoster, measles, CMV, candidiasis, pneumocystosis. Sepsis management: p 191 & 248.

- Hyperuricaemia at induction after massive cell destruction. Prevent by pre-treating with a high fluid intake and allopurinol 10–20mg/kg/24h.
- Ignoring the patient's quality of life. Think of ingenious ways of entertaining the child while reverse barrier nursed.
- Omitting to examine the testes (a common site for recurrence).
- Inappropriate transfusion (leukostasis if WCC >100 × 10^9/L).
- Failing to treat side-effects of chemotherapy optimally—eg 5-HT_3 receptor antagonists such as ondansetron are better than other anti-emetics.[5]
- Failing to give support and encourage compliance. (Paediatricians may be better at avoiding this pitfall than adults' physicians, see p 171.)
- Drug-induced delayed cancer elsewhere (risk of CNS tumours or secondary acute myeloid leukaemia is ~3–4%). Risk assessment allows lower doses.

Febrile neutropenic patients who may be septicaemic (eg from an infected venous catheter)

Suspect infection when untoward events take place in a neutropenic patient (WCC <2 × 10⁹/L, or neutrophils <1 × 10⁹/L). Temperature should be monitored often. Transitory rises (≤38°C) *may* be ignored if lasting for <6h only if the child is well. The importance of parental (and child) education, and of swift routes to hospital need emphasizing.

Do blood cultures and MSU; swab all orifices. Do FBC and serology.
►Get expert advice from your senior, and a microbiologist.

Blind treatment will depend on local protocols, and may include imipenem, the broadest spectrum beta-lactam antibiotic, which may have advantages over cefalosporins if an anaerobe such as *Bacteroides* is suspected (NB: imipenem is not indicated in CNS infections).

Imipenem—*Dose in children <40kg:* 15mg/kg/6h max 2g/24h. Heavier children have the adult dose: 12.4mg/kg/6h IVI; max dose, eg 2g/24h. Do U&E. If creatine clearance <70mL/min, ↓dose frequency (see *Data sheet*). NB: do not use IM formulations IV, and the IM formulation is not to be used in children. If blood culture *does* prove +ve, either change imipenem after microbiological advice, or continue it for 5 days, provided he or she has been afebrile for >24h. If blood cultures are –ve, give for a few days and send home when well and afebrile for >24h.

Imipenem side-effects: (It is usually well-tolerated.) Thrombophlebitis, oliguria, anuria, polyuria, myoclonus, confusion, psychic disturbance, encephalopathy, vertigo, tinnitus, transient hearing loss, BP↓, pruritus, taste perversion, pseudomembranous colitis, arthralgia, eosinophilia, WCC↓, Hb↓, LFTs↑. There are no clinically important drug interactions.

If fever persists and blood cultures remain –ve ask: Is *aciclovir* indicated? Is a fungus possible (for *amphotericin* see *Data Sheet* & *OHCM* p 340).

Teicoplanin For blind treatment of the worst infections, consider adding this to imipenem. Dose: 6–10mg/kg/12h IV for 3 doses, then daily (neonates: 16mg/kg on day 1, then 8mg/kg/day). SE: (Usually none) Dizziness; headache, WCC↓, platelets ↓ or ↑, LFTs↑. Interactions: none.

1 F Greaves 1997 *Lancet* **349** 344 2 C Pui 1995 *NEJM* **332** 1618 3 D Hoelzer 1993 *NEJM* **329** 1343
4 G Rivera 1993 *NEJM* **329** 1289 ⑤ G Dick 1995 *Arch Dis Chi* **73** 243

Cystic fibrosis

This is one of the commonest autosomal recessive diseases (~1/2000; ~1/22 of Caucasians are carriers); it reflects mutations in the cystic fibrosis transmembrane conductance regulator gene (CFTR) on chromosome 7, which codes for a cyclic AMP-regulated chloride channel. There is a broad range of severity of exocrine gland function, leading to meconium ileus (neonates), lung disease akin to bronchiectasis, pancreatic exocrine insufficiency and a raised Na^+ sweat level—depending in part on the type of mutation (often ΔF_{508}; but other mutations, eg in intron 19 of CFTR, cause lung disease but no increased sweat Na^+).[1] Death may be from pneumonia or cor pulmonale. Most survive to adulthood (median survival is now 30yrs).

Antenatal (p 210) carrier-status testing is possible, as is pre-implantation analysis after *in vitro* fertilization: at the 8 cell stage, 1 cell is removed from the embryo, and its DNA analysed; only embryos without the cystic fibrosis gene are offered for implantation—this may be a more acceptable than terminating fully formed fetuses after chorionic villous sampling.

Diagnosis 10% present with *meconium ileus* as neonates. Most present later with *recurrent pneumonia* (±*clubbing*), steatorrhoea (if >7g/day/100g of ingested fat), or *slow growth*. *Sweat test*: Sweat Na^+ >60mmol/L (inaccurate if <100mg of sweat is collected or Na^+:Cl^- discrepancy >20mmol/L)—this test is difficult, so find experienced worker (false +ves in dehydration, endocrine diseases, if on certain antibiotics, and eczema[2]). *Other tests:* Genetic tests; CXR: shadowing suggestive of bronchiectasis, especially in upper lobes. Malabsorption screen. Glucose tolerance test. Lung function tests. Sputum culture. Mycobacterial colonization affects up to 20%—consider if rapid deterioration.

Treatment ►*Offer genetic counselling to every family* (p 212). Long survival depends on antibiotics and good nutrition. *Respiratory problems:* Physiotherapy (× 3/day) must start at diagnosis. Teach parents percussion + postural drainage. Older children learn the forced expiration technique. Organisms are usually *Staph aureus*, *H influenzae* (rarer), and *Streptococcus pneumoniae* in younger children. *Pseudomonas aeruginosa* acquisition is often late, but eventually > 90% are chronically infected.[3] *Berkholderia cepacia* (*Ps cepacea*) is associated with rapid progression of lung disease (prompt diagnosis using polymerase chain reaction on DNA samples may be available: isolate patient). Treat acute infection after sputum culture using higher doses, and for longer than normal. If very ill, ticarcillin (50–60 mg/kg/6h IV) + netilmicin (p 238), or ceftazidime (10– 30mg/kg/8h IV) alone may be needed before sputum results are known. Admissions may be reduced by using nebulized ticarcillin and tobramycin at home.[1] If reversible airways obstruction is a problem, give inhaled salbutamol (look for *Aspergillus* in sputum). Lung transplant (heart + lung, or double lung) works for some, with good results limited by donor availability (avoid raising hopes). Ensure pertussis, MMR, and pneumococcal vaccination.

Gastrointestinal problems and nutrition: Energy requirements are increased by 120–150% because of chronic lung inflammation. Most have steatorrhoea from pancreatic malabsorption and will need enzymes: Pancrex V® powder mixed with food for infants—and Pancrex V Forte® for older children, ≤10 tabs/meal—to give regular, formed, non-greasy bowel actions. Most older children have enzymes in microspheres (eg Pancrease®, Creon 25000®) so fewer tablets will be needed. Cimetidine 10mg/kg PO ½h before each meal may also be needed. If this controls steatorrhoea, a low-fat diet is not needed, but vitamin supplements are still required (A and D, eg as Abidec® 0.6mL/24h PO for infants or as multivitamin capsules 2/24h PO for older children). The diet should be high calorie/high protein. Fine-bore nasogastric feeding is needed only if weight cannot otherwise be maintained.

If GI obstruction occurs (eg if Pancrex® is omitted), urgent admission to a specialist hospital is needed for medical treatment (laparotomy is contraindicated unless perforation is imminent[1]).

Diabetes mellitus: Insulin may be needed. Adjust the dose to the (optimized) diet, not *vice-versa*. Only try oral hypoglycaemics if nutrition is satisfactory.

Psychological help: Parents and children need expert counselling. The Cystic Fibrosis Research Trust and regional centres may help here.[4]

Complications •Pneumonia (resistant organisms) •Haemoptysis •Nasal polyps •Pneumothorax (in 20%) •Diabetes ± cirrhosis •♂ infertility (stenotic or absent vas deferens) •Cholesterol gallstones •Pulmonary osteoarthropathy •IV therapy problems •Fibrosing colonopathy (thought to be related to enzyme dose).

Meconium ileus The baby usually presents with vomiting in the first 2 days of life. Distended loops of bowel may be seen through the abdominal wall, and if a firm mass is felt in one of the loops, this indicates that the cause is a hard plug of meconium. In most other causes of GI obstruction, lateral decubitus films will show fluid levels. This is not the case in meconium ileus. Tiny bubbles may be seen in the meconium. *Treatment:* Place a nasogastric tube. Seek expert advice. Surgical excision of the distal ileum (or whatever contains the most meconium) may be needed.

The future This may lie in agents to *reduce viscosity* of sputum with synthetic human DNA-ase which fragments viscous DNA from dead neutrophils in sputum (an example, with modest clinical effect, is Dornase alfa: it has been tried in a once-daily dose via an air compressor with a jet nebulizer).

Lung transplantation is getting safer; considered in those who are deteriorating (FEV_1 <30% of expected) despite maximum therapy, provided nutrition is good, and there is no active mycobacterial or aspergillus infection.

Gene therapy aims to deliver normal copies of the cystic fibrosis gene into patients, so allowing them to make CFTR protein. Viral vectors and liposomes have been used to get the gene into cells.

In a sense, the future is already here: but for most it's just too expensive.

1 W Zhou 1994 NEJM **331** 974 2 PL Brand 1996 *Lancet* **348** 932 3 S Fiel 1993 *Lancet* **341** 1070
4 5 Blythe Rd, Bromley, Kent, UK tel. 0181 464 7211

Rheumatic fever

This is a systemic febrile illness caused by a cross-sensitivity reaction to Group A β-haemolytic streptococcus, which, in the 2% of the population which is susceptible, may result in permanent damage to heart valves. It is common in the Third World, but is now rare in the West (incidence: ~5–10 per million children), although pockets of resurgence have been noted in the USA in areas of overcrowding[1]—which favours streptococcal spread. Some specific Group A streptococcal serotypes are known to be particularly rheumatogenic—eg type 5 of the M-protein serotypes. Other ubiquitous serotypes appear to be non-rheumatogenic (eg type 12).

Diagnosis The presence of 2 of Jones' major criteria or 1 major and 2 minor + evidence of preceding streptococcal infection: scarlet fever, a throat swab growing β-haemolytic streptococci or a serum ASO titre >333u/L (reference intervals vary) is strong evidence that rheumatic fever is present.

Major criteria (revised[2]):
Carditis (ie 1 of: changed murmur; cardiomegaly; CCF; friction rub)
Polyarthritis (often migratory)
Erythema marginatum (*OHCM* p 678)
Subcutaneous nodules
Sydenham's chorea (p 758)

Minor criteria (revised[2]):
Fever
ESR >20mm/h or C-reactive protein↑
Arthralgia, ie pain but no swelling
ECG: PR interval >0.2 sec.
Previous rheumatic fever or rheumatic heart disease

NB: do not count arthralgia if polyarthritis is being used as a major criterion—likewise for a long P–R interval if carditis is being used. Affected joints may be exquisitely tender. Those most commonly affected are the knees, ankles, elbows and wrists. There are no permanent sequelae. If the child seems to have rheumatic fever but little in the way of carditis, Doppler ultrasonography may reveal inaudible mitral regurgitation.[1] The classical lesion is the endocardial MacCullam patch seen at the base of the posterior mitral leaflet. Aortic, pulmonary and tricuspid valves are affected in descending order of frequency.

Treatment of rheumatic fever

- Bed rest and immobilization (to rest the heart and the joints).
- Relieve joint pain (aspirin, 80mg/kg/day, as in Still's disease, p 758).
- In severe carditis, enlist expert help. Prednisolone (eg 2mg/kg/24h PO) *may* reduce symptoms—but do not expect much impact on sequelae.[2]
- Penicillin for pharyngitis (eg 125mg/6h PO) preceded by one dose of benzylpenicillin (25mg/kg IM or IV).

Prophylaxis Rheumatic fever may be recurrent. Aim to prevent this by giving phenoxymethylpenicillin 250mg PO daily or sulfadimidine 250mg PO daily. Cover operations/dentistry with antibiotics (see below).

Infective endocarditis (IE)

Presenting signs Fever, splenomegaly, anaemia, rashes, heart failure, microscopic haematuria and murmurs. Further features: *OHCM* p 312.

Treating endocarditis before the organism is known (Do 3 blood cultures first.) Benzylpenicillin 25mg/kg/4h IV + netilmicin 2mg/kg/8h IV (p 238).

Preventing IE in those with heart lesions Ampicillin 30mg/kg IM/IV + gentamicin 2mg/kg IM at induction,[3] followed by ampicillin 30mg/kg IM/IV 6h later. Metronidazole 7.5mg/kg IV may also be added. This is recommended for any dentistry, colonic or GU procedure. ►See *OHCM* p 314.

1 L Veasy 1987 NEJM **316** 421 2 G Stollerman 1965 *Circulation* **32** 664–8 & *Lancet* 1995 **346** 391 3 Brit Soc for Antimicrob Chemoth 1992 *Lancet* i 1292 *See* D Albert 1995 *Medicine* 74 1–12 [meta-analysis]

Some metabolic diseases

Hypothyroidism *Congenital causes:* Genetically determined lack of thyroid-stimulating hormone (TSH); congenital goitrous hypothyroidism (eg defective enzymes for thyroxine synthesis or iodine lack); maternal antithyroid drugs (propylthiouracil). *Acquired:* Premature birth;[1] Hashimoto's thyroiditis; hypopituitarism; x-rays, Down's syndrome.

The patient: There may be no signs at birth: the first sign is often prolonged neonatal jaundice (p 236). Inactivity, excessive sleeping, slow feeding, little crying and constipation may occur. Look for coarse dry hair, a flat nasal bridge, a protruding tongue, hypotonia, umbilical hernia, slowly relaxing reflexes, slow pulse and delayed growth and mental development. Other later signs: IQ↓, delayed puberty (occasionally precocious), short stature, delayed dentition.

Universal neonatal screening: Filter paper blood spots (at 5–7 days old, from a heel prick) allow early diagnosis, and the prevention of serious sequelae.

Tests: T_4↓, TSH↑ (but undetectable in secondary hypothyroidism), ^{131}I uptake↓, Hb↓. Bone age is less than the chronological age. As it is undesirable to x-ray the whole skeleton, the wrist and hand are most commonly used. There are a large number of ossification centres. Each passes through a number of morphological stages, and using comparisons with key diagrams from 'normal' populations, a rough bone age may be determined. There is no hard-and-fast answer to the question of how much discrepancy (eg 2 years) between skeletal and chronological years is significant.[1]

Treatment with thyroxine: Infants need ~10μg/kg/day (≤50μg/day); this rises to ~100μg/day by aged 5yrs and to adult doses by 12yrs. Adjust according to growth rate and clinical response. Avoid high TSH levels.

Hyperthyroidism The typical child is a girl at puberty. Clinical and laboratory features are described in *OHCM* p 542. Treatment is with carbimazole, eg 15mg/24h PO for 18 months, with the dose adjusted according to response—or propylthiouracil 200mg/m^2/day PO. Relapses may occur.

Thyroid disease in pregnancy and neonates See p157.

The glycogenoses result from defects in the synthesis and degradation of glycogen. Abnormal stores may be deposited in liver, muscle, heart or kidney. Most types (there are at least 7) are inherited as an autosomal recessive. Types include: von Gierke disease (type I, p 759), Pompe's disease (type II, p 756), Cori disease (type III—hypoglycaemia, hepatomegaly, with failure to thrive), Anderson disease (type IV), McArdle disease (type V), Hers disease (type VI) and Tauri disease (type VII—phosphofructokinase↓—like McArdle's, with added haemolysis and gout: diagnose by muscle enzyme assay).

In McArdle's the cause is myophosphorylase deficiency (as shown on muscle biopsy). Inheritance: autosomal recessive. Stiffness and myalgia follow exercise (with electrically silent muscle contractions). During exercise, as circulating fatty acids become available, there may be some recovery ('second wind'[2]). Venous blood from exercised muscle shows low levels of lactate and pyruvate. Lack of phosphorylase staining in muscle biopsy confirms the diagnosis. There may be myoglobinuria (red urine ± renal failure). *Treatment:* Avoid extreme exercise. Oral glucose and fructose may help.

1 A Lucas 1996 *BMJ* i 1132 2 D Hilton-Jones 1996 *OTM* 3e 1465–6

Inborn errors of metabolism

These are very numerous, but some helpful generalizations about their acute presentations may be made. Signs include diarrhoea, lethargy, respiratory distress, metabolic acidosis (± odd body smells), jaundice, hypoglycaemia, U&E imbalance, fits and coma. Features may be intermittant, and provoked by crises (eg infection; dehydration). Look for:

Physical sign:	*Possible significance:*
Hepatosplenomegaly	eg amino acid and organic acid disorders, lysosomal storage diseases.
Coarse facies	Mucopolysaccharidoses, eg Hurler's syndrome, p 750, gangliosidoses, mannosidoses.
WCC↓, platelets↓	Organic acidurias.
Mental retardation	See p 204.
Failure to thrive	Aminoacidurias, organic aciduria, cystinuria, lactic acidosis, storage diseases.

A metabolic urine screen is helpful, but differs from laboratory to laboratory. It usually includes amino acids, organic acids, carbohydrates and mucopolysaccharides. Request expert laboratory help.

Acute surgical problems

Congenital hypertrophic pyloric stenosis This does not (contrary to its name) present at birth, but develops during the first month of life (♂/♀≈4). *Presentation:* Vomiting which occurs after feeds, and becomes projectile (eg vomiting over far end of cot). Congenital pyloric stenosis is distinguished from other causes of vomiting (eg gastric reflux) by 3 important negatives:

- The vomit does not contain bile, as the obstruction is so high.
- No diarrhoea: constipation is likely (occasionally 'starvation stools').
- Even though the patient is ill, he is rarely obtunded: he is alert, anxious, and hungry—and possibly malnourished, dehydrated, and always hungry.

Observe left-to-right LUQ (left upper quadrant) peristaltic waves during a feed (seen in late-presenting babies). Palpate the olive-sized pyloric mass: stand on the baby's left side and palpate with the left hand at the lateral border of the right rectus in the RUQ, during a milk feed—from a bottle or the left breast. The baby may be severely depleted of water and sodium chloride and this makes urinary output and plasma Cl^- (also K^+ and HCO_3^-) vital tests, which will guide the paediatrician in his resuscitative measures and will determine when it is safe to perform surgery (the chloride should be >90mmol/L). There is no rush.

Ultrasound detects early, hard-to-feel pyloric tumours (~14% of cases), but is only needed if examination is –ve.[1,2] Barium studies are 'never' needed.

Management: Before surgery (Ramstedt's pyloromyotomy) pass a wide-bore nasogastric tube.

Intussusception The small bowel telescopes, as if it were swallowing itself by invagination. Patients may be any age (usually 5–12 months) presenting with *episodic* intermittent inconsolable crying, with drawing the legs up (colic) ± vomiting. He may (but need not) pass blood PR (like red-currant jam or merely flecks: do a PR). A sausage-shaped abdominal mass may be felt. He may become shocked, and moribund. *Tests/Management:* The least invasive approach is ultrasound with reduction by air enema (preferred to barium). CT may be problematic, and is less available. Plain abdominal films may be reserved for when perforation is suspected. Doppler studies to show bowel viability have been used but are non-standard. If reduction by enema fails, reduction at laparoscopy or laparotomy is needed. Any necrotic bowel should be resected. *Pre-op care:* ►►Resuscitate, crossmatch blood, pass nasogastric tube. NB: children >4yrs present differently: rectal bleeding is less common, and they are more likely to have a long history (>3 weeks) and some sort of contributing pathology (Henoch–Schönlein purpura, Peutz–Jeghers' syndrome; cystic fibrosis, ascariasis, nephrotic syndrome or tumours such as lymphomas—in the latter obstructive symptoms caused by intussusception are the most frequent mode of presentation). Recurrence rate: ~5%.

Phimosis In this condition the foreskin is too tight (eg due to circumferential scarring) so that retraction over the glans is impossible. The flow of urine may be impeded, with ballooning of the foreskin. There may be recurrent balanitis. Time and trials of gentle retraction usually obviate the need for circumcision. Forced retraction may be causative, not therapeutic. Note: it is normal to have a simple non-retractile foreskin up to the age of 4yrs.

Post-operative pain relief Morphine IVI: child's loading dose: 100µg/kg in 30min, then 10–50µg/kg/h (neonates 5–7µg/kg/h, but same loading dose)—or diclofenac 0.5–1.5mg/kg/8–12h if over 1yr (eg a 12.5mg suppository every 8–12h if ~1yr old). Ibuprofen dose: 4–10mg/kg/6h PO (syrup is 100mg/5mL).

Other surgical problems: **appendicitis, hernias, volvulus, torsion of the testis, acute abdomen**: see p 272, p 218, OHCM p 132 and p 112.

1 J Langer 1997 E-BM 2 92 & P Godbole 1996 *Arch Dis Chi* **75** 335 2 M Rollins 1993 BMJ **i** 1065

Dyslexia

Reading ability usually goes hand-in-hand with intelligence, but when this is not the case, and someone with, say, an IQ of 130, finds reading difficult, the term dyslexia is often used. The term 'specific learning difficulty' is preferred by some people, as 'dyslexia' is often a term used by parents to help them cope with having a child whose general intellectual skills, including reading, are less than hoped for.

Essence There is a problem with appreciating phonemes, eg that 'cat' comprises /c/, /a/, and /t/. Breaking up unfamiliar words into phonemes and having a go at stringing them together is the central act of learning to read. This is what needs to be taught, educationalists now believe—and children should not be made to rely on unstructured guesswork that formed the basis of the 'look and say' approach to learning to read, which is now discredited as the sole means of equipping children for reading.

Children with dyslexia have difficulty in telling how many syllables there are in a word (don't we all?—'How many syllables are there in *strength*?' analytical dyslexics are prone to ask). They also have difficulty with verbal short-term memory—eg for meaningless strings such as telephone numbers. There is also a problem with telling if two words rhyme or not, and in distinguishing phonemes which sound similar (eg /k/ and /g/). There may also be left/right muddle. *Genetics:* Boys are more afflicted than girls, and show stronger genetic effects (up to 50% of boys are dyslexic if their fathers are too). Genes on chromosomes 1 and 15 are implicated, and linkage on chromosome 6 near the human leukocyte complex may explain associations between dyslexia and autoimmune diseases.[1]

Neurobiology Rarely, CNS examination reveals a left-sided cerebral lesion. Usually changes are only seen at *postmortem*, abnormalities in the perisylvanian regions, and unusual asymmetry of the plenum temporale (Wernicke's area), with cortical dysplasia and scarring.[2] Perhaps dyslexia reflects weak connectivity between the anterior and posterior parts of the language areas of the brain, and the angular gyrus.[3] Positron emission tomography shows that when dyslexic adults perform rhyme judgments and verbal short-term memory tasks they activate less than the full set of centres normally involved with these tasks.[4]

Management The first question to ask yourself is whether there is dyslexia because the person has not been taught the basic skills of phonemic segmentation. If this is the case, then what is needed is a good teacher, not a doctor. If teaching seems to make no difference to the level of skill attained, then the person may gain insight by discussing his or her problem with fellow sufferers, and by finding out about past dyslexics such as Leonardo da Vinci. Special educational programmes are available for addressing dyslexic problems, as the phonetic approach to learning to read usually presents problems. One famous study, forcefully questioning our standard 'wait-and-see' policy, found that good results could be obtained by identifying, *before* school starts, those children with phonological difficulties, and then giving them exercises in sound categorization using rhyme and alliteration activities, with special teaching of letter sounds.[5]

1 L Cardon 1994 *Science* **266** 276 2 AM Galaburda 1993 *Curr Opin Neurobiol* **5** 71 **3** http://www.shianet.org/~reneenew/hist.html **4** MJ Snowling 1996 BMJ 1096 **5** L Bradley 1983 *Nature* **310** 419

Precocious puberty

Sometimes, it may be quite normal for puberty to start as early as 8yrs old. The onset of puberty before this time warrants investigation.

Biology Each of the physical signs of puberty may be thought of as a bioassay for a separate endocrine event. Enlargement of the testes is the first sign of puberty in boys, and is due to pulses of pituitary gonadotrophin. Breast enlargement in girls and penis enlargement in boys is due to gonadal sex steroid secretion. Pubic hair is a manifestation of adrenal androgen production. The growth of boys accelerates when the volume of the testis reaches 10–12mL (as measured by comparison with the orchidometer's beads, p 752). Girls start to grow more quickly once their breasts have started to develop. Stage 4 breast development is a prerequisite for menarche (in most girls). The first clue to distinguish simple from pathological precosity is when this *consonance of puberty* goes awry: in Cushing's syndrome, pubic hair is 'too much' for the testicular volume; in hypothyroidism, the testes are large (FSH↑ because TSH↑↑) in the presence of a low growth velocity.

Precocious puberty is manifested in boys by a rapid growth of penis and testes, increasing frequency of erections, masturbation, the appearance of pubic hair, changing body odour, and acne. There will be corresponding changes in the secondary sexual characteristics of girls. The most important long-term consequence is short stature caused by early fusion of epiphyses. Enquire about symptoms of more general hypothalamic dysfunction: polyuria, polydipsia, obesity, sleep and temperature regulation disturbances. There may also be manifestations of raised intracranial pressure and visual disturbance.

Precocious puberty is at least 4 times as common in girls, compared with boys. In girls, often no cause is found, but in 80–90% of boys a cause is found. If onset is before 2yrs old the cause may well be a hamartoma in the hypothalamus. These may be revealed as non-enhancing, circumscribed lesions on computerized tomography. Other causes (mostly rare):

- CNS tumours and hydrocephalus
- Post encephalitis, meningitis, or cranial irradiation
- McCune–Albright syndrome (p 752)
- Craniopharyngioma
- Tuberous sclerosis
- Hepatoblastoma
- Choriocarcinoma
- Hypothyroidism

Investigations Skull x-ray, bone age by skeletal x-ray, CT scan of head, urinary 17-ketosteroids, pelvic ultrasound (girls), T_4.

Management: a physiological approach[1] ►Refer to a paediatric endocrinologist. Initiation of puberty depends on release from inhibition of neurones in the medial basal hypothalamus which secrete gonadotrophin-releasing hormone (GnRH), and on decreasing hypothalamic-pituitary sensitivity to –ve feedback from gonadal steroids. These changes are accompanied by a marked increase in frequency and magnitude of 'pulses' of luteinizing hormone (LH), and, to a lesser extent, follicle stimulating hormone (FSH). It is the ability to secrete GnRH pulses at a fast rate which leads to normal gonadal function. Continuous high levels of GnRH paradoxically suppress the secretion of pituitary gonadotrophins, and this forms the basis for treatment of precocious puberty with synthetic analogues of GnRH. After subcutaneous or nasal insufflation there is a reversal of gonadal maturation and all the clinical correlates of puberty (not for pubic hair, as there is no change in the secretion of androgens by the adrenal cortex). There is deceleration in skeletal maturation. Treatment is continued until the average age of puberty or of the menarche (eg ~11yrs old). Families need reassurance that the child will develop normally.

1 DP Merke 1996 *Arch Dis Chi* **75** 269–71

Primary antibody deficiency

Essence Synonyms for this condition include *hypogammaglobulinaemia*, ie not secondary to protein-losing enteropathy, chronic lymphatic leukaemia, or myeloma. Prevalence: ~4/100,000. The leading symptom is recurrent infections, needing repeated antibiotics, with the development of chronic infective states such as bronchiectasis and sinusitis. Other features:

•Failure to thrive •Nodular lymphoid hyperplasia (gut) •Absent tonsils
•Enteropathy •Hepatosplenomegaly •Anaemia.

Most diagnoses are in children >6yrs (presentation may also be in adulthood).

Classification *Common variable immune deficiency:* IgG↓, IgA↓, IgM variable. Typical age at referral: 6–10yrs old (with another peak at age 26–30yrs).[1]
X-linked antibody deficiency: Often ♂ >2yrs old and +ve family history. B-cell development may be abnormal.
IgG subclass deficiencies.
Specific antibody deficiency: Typically IgM, IgG, and IgA normal, but fails to respond to immunizations.
Selective IgA deficiency: Prevalence: 1:700. May be symptom-free.

Suspect antibody deficiency if •Failure to thrive •Recurrent infections •Severe infections needing surgery •Arthropathy •Hepatosplenomegaly

Laboratory clues include lymphopenia ± normal serum albumin but *low* total protein (low as immunoglobulins are missing—also making crossmatching hard as haemaglutinins are absent).[2]

When these signs are unexplained, refer to an immunologist, to assess antibody responses to protein and carbohydrate antigens, measure IgG subclasses, and count lymphocytes involved in antibody production (CD4, CD8, CD19, CD23 positive lymphocytes). Immunoglobulin levels are interpreted by age. There is a rôle for watching responses to test vaccinations.[1]

Management Aim to include the patient and the family in the process. Ensure prompt treatment of intercurrent infections. This may include postural physiotherapy, and bronchodilators as well as antibiotics.

Immunoglobulin replacement obviates most complications and is best delivered by a specialist immunologist, after detailed immunological assessment. Many patients can join a self-infusion programme. Before any infusion, active infection should be excluded (to minimize risk of adverse reactions), and a baseline check of transaminase enzymes, creatinine, and anti-IgA antibody titres should be done.[1]

The dose of IV immunoglobulin is determined by the severity and frequency of infections, and the plasma level of IgG. Most receive ~400mg/kg/month, usually as 2 doses, 2 weeks apart.[1] Hydrocortisone and an antihistamine should be to hand during an infusion. SE: headaches, abdominal pain, anaphylaxis.

Intramuscular immunoglobulins are not favoured, but the subcutaneous route is being investigated.[1]

Complications *Chest:* Bronchiectasis, granulomas, lymphomas.
Gut: Malabsorption, giardia, cholangitis, atrophic gastritis, colitis.
Liver: Acquired hepatitis, chronic active hepatitis, biliary cirrhosis.
Blood: Autoimmune haemolysis, ITP, anaemia of chronic disease, aplasia.
Eyes/CNS: Keratoconjunctivitis, uveitis, granulomas, encephalitis.
Others: Septic arthropathy, arthralgia, splenomegaly.

1 H Chapel 1994 BMJ i 581 & Roy Col Path 1995 *Consensus Document for Diagnosis and Management of Patients with Primary Antibody Deficiency* ISBN 0 9518574 5 2 2 D Unsworth 1997 *Lancet* **249** 435

Delay in walking

Babies usually learn to walk at ~1yr old. If this has not occurred by 20 months, ask yourself 2 questions: Is the child physically normal? Is development delayed in other areas too? The commonest causes reflect global delay, benign immaturity, and generalized joint hypermobility. In boys consider consider Duchenne muscular dystrophy early (genetic counselling *before* mother's next pregnancy). Note that congenital hip dislocation may present as 'walking delay' if the fact of limping is overlooked. The major reason for identifying late walkers is to exclude cerebral palsy.

Cerebral palsy comprises a range of chronic disorders of posture and movement caused by a non-progressive CNS lesion sustained before 2yrs old, resulting in poor motor development ± learning disability (35%) ± epilepsy.[1] Most are due to preterm delivery and 9–13% are thought to be due to intrapartum events such as fetal hypoxia (other causes: see below). *Prevalence:* 2/1000 (50% are of low birth weight). *Typical survival:* 20yrs if more or less quadriplegic (much longer if less affected).[2]

Prenatal factors:	*Perinatal factors:*	*Postnatal factors:*
APH (with hypoxia)	Birth trauma	Trauma; Intraventricular haemorrhage
X-rays; alcohol	Fetal distress	Meningoencephalitis
CMV; rubella; HIV	Hypoglycaemia	Cerebral vein thrombosis (from dehydration)
Toxoplasmosis	Hyperbilirubinaemia	
Rhesus disease	Failed resuscitation	

Clinical picture: Weakness, paralysis, delayed milestones, seizures, language and speech problems. *Spasticity* suggests a pyramidal lesion; unco-ordinated, involuntary movements and postures (dystonias) suggest basal ganglia involvement; ataxia suggests cerebellar involvement. Most children have either a hemiparesis or a spastic diplegia—eg both legs affected worse than the arms, so that the child looks normal until he is picked up, when the legs 'scissor' (hip flexion, adduction and internal rotation; with knee extension and feet plantar-flexed). Gait is broad based.

Type 1 Ataxic palsies (pure ataxia):
- Hypotonia ('floppy baby')
- Other defects rare
- Flexor plantars
- Associations: deafness; strabismus mental retardation (fits rare)
- Normal developmental milestones

Type 2 Ataxic diplegia:
- Hypertonia
- Other defects common
- Extensor plantars
- Associations: trauma hydrocephalus spina bifida; viruses

Dyskinetic cerebral palsy: Unwanted actions, breaks in movement flow, agonist/antagonist imbalance, poor posture control, hypotonia, hearing loss, dysarthria, poor visual fixation. Fits and IQ↓ are rare.

Assessment and management (p 290) Can he roll over (both ways)? Ability to come to the sitting position independently. Grasp. Transfer of objects from hand to hand. Effective head righting. Ability to shift weight (when prone) with forearm support. IQ. Treat epilepsy (p 268). Use calipers to prevent deformity (eg equinovarus, equinovalgus, hip dislocation due to excessive flexion and adduction). Attempts to show the benefits of neurodevelopmental physiotherapy (directed towards improving equilibrium and righting) have failed to show any benefit over simple stimulation of motor activity. Some parents prefer the Hungarian (Petö) approach[3] where one person (the 'conductor') devotes herself to the child and uses interaction with the child's peers to reinforce successes in all areas: manipulation, art, writing, fine movement, social interaction.

1 L Rosenbloom 1995 *Arch Dis Chi* **72** 350 2 F Palmer 1988 NEJM **318** 803 3 R Robinson 1989 BMJ **ii** 1145

Delay in talking

►When in doubt, ask the mother; test the hearing. *Ensure the result is reliable.*

Speech development After the first few months of life, language differentiation is already occurring. Chinese babbling babies can be distinguished from European ones. Before the first year babbling gives way to jargon—plausible-sounding 'words' which have little by way of fixed meaning.

- *At ~1 year* . . . .a few words may be used meaningfully.
- *At 1½ yrs old*. . .2-word utterances appear ("Daddy come").
- *At 2 years old*. . .subject–verb–object sentences appear ("I want a pudding").
- *At 3½ yrs old*. . .the child has mastered thought, language, abstraction and the elements of reason, having a 1000-word vocabulary at his or her disposal, enabling sentences such as: "I give her cake 'cos she's hungry".

Words exist to give ideas currency, and so often that currency proves counterfeit—a process which so often starts with *if*, eg "*If I hadn't thrown the cup on the ground, I might have got a pudding*". The uttering of "If. . .", linked with an emotional response, is the most human of all constructions, opening up worlds divorced from reality, providing for the exercise of imagination, the validation of dreams, the understanding of motives, and the control of events. The rest of life holds nothing to match the intellectual and linguistic pace of these few, first, baffling, years. Further linguistic development is devoted to seemingly conceptually minor tasks, such as learning the subjunctive, and expanding vocabulary.

There is much variation in speech timing: *what is clearly abnormal*?

Vocabulary size: If the child reaches 3 years old with <50 words, suspect:

- Deafness.
- Expressive dysphasia.
- Speech dyspraxia, particularly if there is a telegraphic quality to speech, poor clarity, and deterioration in behaviour (frustration).
- Audio-premotor syndrome (APM). The child cannot reflect the sounds correctly heard into motor control of larynx and respiration. Instead of babbling, the child is quiet, unable to hum or sing.
- Respiro-laryngeal (RL) dysfunction (dysphonia from incorrect vocal fold vibration/air flow regulation). The voice is loud and rough.
- Congenital aphonia (rare): the voice is thin, weak and effortful.

Speech clarity: By 2½years old, parents should understand their child's speech most of the time. If not, suspect deafness—or:

- Articulatory dyspraxia (easy consonants are *b* and *m* with the lips, and *d* with the tongue—the phonetic components of babbling. This is the commonest form of speech problem. ♂:♀ ≈3:1. Tongue-tie is a possible cause, and they will have trouble with sounds needing tongue elevation (*d* and *s*)—surgery to the frenum may be needed as well as speech therapy.
- APM or RL dysfunction, as described above.

Understanding: By 2½ years he should understand "Get your shoes", if not suspect: •Deafness—if the hearing is impaired (eg 25–40dB loss) secretory otitis media is likely to be the cause. Worse hearing loss is probably sensorineural. •Cognitive impairment. •Deprivation.

Some other causes of speech disorder For autism, see p 402. Others:

Acquired:	*Congenital:*
Post meningoencephalitis	Klinefelter's syndrome
Post head injury	Galactosaemia, histidinaemia
Landau–Kleffner syndrome (epilepsy + progressive loss of language)	Auditory agnosia
	Floating-harbo(u)r syndrome[1]

Speech therapy Refer early—and well before school starts.

1 Named after a boy seen at the Boston Floating Hospital, this syndrome comprises: short stature + delayed bone age + expressive language disorder (+ *normal* motor function) + triangular face with prominant nose ± hyperkinesis ± coeliac disease ± brachyphalangy (short hands and feet): *see* http://www3.ncbi.nlm.nih.gov/htbin-post/Omim/dispmim?136140

Impairment, disability, and handicap

WHO definitions *Impairment* entails a pathological process, eg spina bifida, which may cause certain *disabilities*, eg walking difficulty. Handicap is their social consequence (eg cannot walk to school).

Mental handicap ►*The mother often makes the first diagnosis*. An IQ <35 constitutes a severe learning disability (mental handicap, p 314).

►Beware conflating IQ with intellect: the latter implies more than problem-solving and memory: intellect entails the ability to speculate, to learn from mistakes, to have a view of oneself and others, to see relationships between events in different domains of experience—as well as the ability to use language either to map the world, or to weave ironic webs of deceit (and, on a good day, to do both simultaneously).

Causes: Severe mental impairment usually has a definable cause, whereas mild retardation is often familial, with no well-defined cause. Be prepared to refer to an expert, who may himself need to rely on an electronic database such as the *London Neurogenetics Database*.[1]
Congenital disorders are legion: chromosomal (eg Down's; fragile X, p 752); metabolic (eg PKU p 205). *Acquired:* Perinatal infection p 98–100, birth injury and cerebral palsy, and subsequent trauma, meningitis.

Lead exposure: This is a leading preventable cause of mildly impaired intellect. For example in 2-yr-olds for each 0.48μmol/L plasma increment there is an associated 5–8 point fall in IQ as measured on the Wechsler Intelligence Scale for children (revised[2]). This defect is long-lasting.
Biochemical defects associated with mental retardation—eg:
Homocystinuria: Paraplegia, fits, friable hair, emboli, cataracts; homocystine is found in the urine. Treat with a low methionine, cystine-supplemented diet, with large doses of pyridoxine.
Maple syrup urine disease: Hypoglycaemia, acidosis, fits, death. Urine smells of maple syrup, due to defective metabolism of branched chain keto acids. Treatment: high calorie amino-acid controlled diet. Thiamine has been tried.
Tryptophanuria: Rough, pigmented skin. Treat with nicotinic acid.

Management: Refer to an expert, so that no treatable cause is missed. Would the family like help from a self-help groups, such as MENCAP?[3] Other members of the family may need special support (eg normal siblings, who now feel neglected). If the IQ is >35, life in the community is the aim.

Physical handicap *Sensory:* Deafness,[4] see p 540.
Blindness: congenital defects are described on p 516. Principal acquired causes of blindness are: retinopathy of prematurity, vitamin A deficiency, onchocerciasis (p 512), eye injuries, cataract (eg Down's syndrome).[5]

CNS and musculoskeletal problems: (Congenital or acquired) Causes: accidents (eg near-drowning), cerebral palsy (p 202), spina bifida (p 228), after meningitis, polio, congenital infections (above), tumours, syndromes (p 742–58).

Wheelchairs:[6] Is it for indoors or outdoors? Patient-operated, motorized or pushed? What sort of restraints are needed to prevent the child falling out? If collapsable, how small must it be to get into the family car? Are the sides removable to aid transfer from chair to bed? Can the child control the brakes? Are there adjustable elevated leg rests? Liaise with the physiotherapist and the occupational therapist.

Calipers will allow some patients to stand and walk. Long-leg calipers are required for those with complete leg paralysis. The top should be constructed so that it does not induce pressure sores. A knee lock supports the knee in the standing position. An internal coil spring prevents foot drop.

1 M Baraitster 1993 *London Neurogenetics Database* OUP 2 D Bellinger 1992 *Paediatrics* **90** 855 3 123 Golden Lane, London (tel. 0171 454 0454) 4 VK Das 1996 *Arch Dis Chi* **74** 8 5 M Rogers 1996 *ibid* 299-303 6 Disabled Living Foundation, 380 Harrow Rd, London W9, tel 1071 289 6111

Check-list to guide management of handicap

Whether based in hospital or in the community the doctor should address each of these points:

- Screening and its documentation on local handicap registers.
- Communication with parents.
- Refer to and liaise with district handicap teams, and community paediatrician.
- Ensuring access to specialist services, including physiotherapy, orthopaedic surgery.
- Assessing special needs for schooling and housing.
- Co-ordinating neuropsychological/neurodevelopmental assessments.
- Co-ordinating measures of severity (eg electrophysiology ± CT/MRI).
- Liaison with dietitian on special foods.
- Promotion of long-term compliance with treatment or education programmes.
- Education about the consequences of the illness.
- Encourage contact with family support groups.
- Offering family planning *before* patients become unintentionally pregnant.
- Pre-conception counselling (with specialist in molecular genetics).
- Co-ordinating prenatal diagnostic tests and fetal assessment.

Phenylketonuria

Cause Absent or reduced activity of phenylalanine hydroxylase—inherited as an autosomal recessive (the gene—on chromosome 12—often mutates, and there is a full range of clinical manifestation from nearly symptom-free to severe mental impairment).

Clinical features Fair hair, fits, eczema, musty urine. The most important manifestations are impaired IQ and cognition.

Tests Hyperphenylalaninaemia (reference interval: 50–120μmol/L). 'Benign' phenylketonuria may be indicated by levels < 1000μmol/L.

Treatment See check-list above. Phenylalanine-low diet, to keep phenylalanine to <600μmol/L—by prescribing artificial food-substitutes (amino acid drinks) to give <300mg–8g natural protein/day (depending on age and severity of phenylalanine hydroxylase deficiency).[1]

There is much evidence to suggest that CNS damage (hypomyelination) is proportionate to the degree of phenylketonaemia, but some studies fail to show that stricter diets are associated with higher IQs.[2]

Prevention of manifestations Screen blood at 1 week (using a heel-prick and filter paper impregnation—the Guthrie test).

Maternal phenylketonuria However good the mother's control, subtle neurological impairment is likely.[1] The implication is that control during pregnancy should be even tighter than in childhood. Hence the need for pre-conception counselling.

1 MRC working party 1993 BMJ **i** 115   2 U Michel 1990 *Eur J Pediat* **149** (suppl 1) 34–8

Behavioural problems

►*Only enter battles you can win.* If the child can win, be more subtle (eg consistent rewards, not inconsistent punishments). Get health visitor's advice, and ensure that everyone is encouraging the same response from the child.

Entrances *Food refusal* and *food fads* are common. Reducing pressure on the child, discouraging parental over-reaction, and gradual enlarging of tiny portions of attractive food is usually all that is needed. Check Hb. *Overeating:* Eating comforts, and if the child is short on comfort, or if mother feels inadequate, the scene is set for overeating and life-long patterns are begun. Diets may fail until the child is hospitalized (p 348).

If obese, remember hypothalamic syndromes (eg Prader–Willi, p 756).

Pica is eating of things which are not food. There are likely to be other signs of disturbed behaviour, or ↓IQ.

Exits *Soiling* is the escape of stool into the underclothing.
Encopresis is the repeated passage of solid faeces in the wrong place in those >4yrs old. Faecal retention is the central event. *Constipation* is delay in defecation; it may lead to distress, abdominal pain, rectal bleeding, abdominal masses, overflow soiling ± 'lavatory-blocking' enormous stools (megarectum), and anorexia. Causes: often poor food, fluid or fibre intake. Fear—eg as a result of a fissure. Rarely Hirschprung's disease (think of this in infants if there is an explosive gush of faeces on withdrawing the finger after rectal exam, or if there is alternating diarrhoea with constipation and abdominal distension, and failure to thrive). *Action:* •Find out about pot refusal •Does defecation hurt? •Is there parental coercion? Try to break the vicious cycle of: large faeces→pain ± fissure→fear of the pot→rectum overstretched→call-to-stool sensation dulled→soiling→parental exasperation→coercion). Exonerate the child to boost confidence for the main task of obeying the call-to-stool to keep the rectum empty (eg by *docusate sodium*, then a dose of *sodium picosulfate* elixir or polyethylene glycol, followed by maintenance *methyl cellulose tablets* ± prolonged alternate-day *senna*). Psychological help (± family therapy, p 382) is very important. Give the family time to air feelings which encopresis engenders (anger, shame, ridicule).[1,2] Treat perianal cellulitis due to α-haemolytic streps with co-amoxiclav.

Enuresis: Bedwetting occurs on most nights in 15% of 5-yr-olds, and is still a problem in up to 3% of 15-yr-olds[3]—usually from delayed maturation of bladder control (there is often a +ve family history). Tests for diabetes, UTI and GU abnormality (p 188) can occasionally yield surprises. The term 'secondary enuresis' implies wetness after >6 months' dryness. *Treatment:* Avoiding acrimonious blame, fluid restricting before bed, and the passing of time may help. Reassure the child that he is neither infantile nor dirty. A system of rewards for dry nights as documented on a star chart above the child's bed may be effective. Alarms triggered by urine in the bed can provoke 65% to be dry after 3 weeks; the high relapse rate (30%) may be reduced by continuing training after dryness. In the UK, alarms may be loaned from Community Health/Child Guidance Services (see local phone directory) or Mini Drinite® (tel. UK 0181 441 9641). Imipramine 25–50mg/24h PO should not be used for >3 months, has side-effects, and high relapse rates on discontinuation.[2] Desmopressin 20–40µg (2–4 puffs) at night by nasal spray helps short-term. Oral dose (if >5yrs): 0.2mg at bedtime. Beware fluid overload, eg after gulping in swimming pool water, or going to rave parties; have 1 week 3-monthly with no drugs. CI: cystic fibrosis, uraemia, BP↑. Oxybutinin 2.5–5mg PO at night may help if bladder irritability diagnosed.

Hyperactivity The spectrum ranges from a level of activity > parents are happy with, to serious lack of concentration, impulsivity, and scholastic failure—known as *attention deficit disorder (ADD)* or *minimal brain dysfunction*. ADD is commoner in learning-disabled children. Parents say the child is never still, being 'on the go, as if driven by a motor', ± :

Squirming and fidgeting	Inconsiderate of others	Blurts out answers
Sustained attention↓	Interrupts continually	Behind with schoolwork
Speech↑	Instructions never obeyed	Butts in during games

Not *all* those with ADD are hyperactive. *There is no diagnostic test* (but positron emission tomography may show ↓function of frontal lobes and near connections). Most parents first note excessive activity at the toddler stage, but most locomotor hyperactivity at this stage abates with time, so the diagnosis is usually delayed until school entry or later. Signs generally attenuate during adolescence, but may persist into mid-adulthood. There is a familial tendency, and families with ADD are more likely to have other diagnoses too, such as learning difficulties, mood, anxiety and psychosocial disorders (DSM IV, p 312). *Treatment:* Take time to explain the condition. Offer a booklet.[4] Cognitive therapy may increase parental tolerance. Hypoallergenic diets (eg no tartrazine) are controversial and may cause obsessions in parents.

Psychostimulant (not depressant) drugs are an option if drugs are essential (confer with an expert): methylphenidate 0.08–0.25mg/kg/8h PO is said to offer the best benefit-to-hazard ratio,[5] but it is a controlled drug, only available on a named-patient basis (SE: insomnia, slowing of growth; monitor growth, BP, pulse). Other drugs: pemoline 0.5–2mg/kg/24h PO (effects are delayed for 6 weeks); haloperidol 0.01–0.04mg/kg/12h PO; imipramine 0.2–0.5mg/kg/ 8h, especially if co-existing anxiety or depression; clonidine (≤5mg/day PO in divided doses, particularly if tic disorder is also present).[5]

School phobia *Setting:* Emotional overprotection; high social class; neurotic parents; schoolwork of high standard. In truancy, the reverse is true. *Treatment:* Confer with headteacher, parents, and an educational psychologist. Escort by an education welfare officer aids the prompt return to school.

1 G Clayden 1992 *Arch Dis Chi* **67** 340 2 JM Smellie 1996 E-BM **2** 13 3 *Mayo Clinic Proc* 1996 **71** 857
4 See the ADD Family Support Group, tel +44 (0)1373 826045–or http://www.chadd.org/http://www.docnet.org, or http://www.familyinternet.com/peds/index/diseidxa.htm and E Taylor *The Hyperactive Child: a Parents' Guide*, M Dunitz 5 *Drug Ther Bul* 1995 **33** 57

Screening and child health promotion[1,2,3]

The main aims: •Encouraging breast feeding (p 176–8) •Monitoring development •Immunization •Overseeing growth (p 184) •Parental support •Education and reassurance about normal childhood events. •Talking to the child, and building up a good relationship to be used in later illnesses.

Monitoring The most cost-effective times to screen are unknown. A 'best buy' might be checks after birth (p 231), at 4–6 weeks—arrange vaccinations and DoH vitamin drops[1] (A, D & C, unless sure that diet/sunlight is adequate), then:

6–9 months:	Hips, testes descent, CVS examination.
18–24 months:	Educate on diet, dental care, accidents, walking (look for waddling), social and linguistic milestones; Hb if iron deficiency likely—may well be. Any parental depression?
4 years:	Testes descent, CVS examination. Nutrition, dental care.

At each visit: •Encourage airing of queries. •Ask about, and test for, squint, vision and deafness.[†] •Chart centiles. *Beware reading too much into a single test.* See Denver developmental test, p 288. Remember to correct age for prematurity. Note the milestones below. There is much individual variation.

1 month:	Lifts head when prone; responds to bell; regards face.
2 months:	Holds head at 45° when prone; vocalizes; smiles.
4 months:	Uses arm support when prone; holds head steady when sitting reaches out; rolls over; spontaneous smiling.
6 months:	Bears some weight on legs; on pulling to sitting, there is no head lag; resists your trying to take a toy from his grasp.
1 year:	Just stands; walks using a table's support; clashes cubes; pincer grip; can say 'Mummy' ± 'Daddy'. Plays 'pat a cake'.
18 months:	Can walk backwards; scribbles; 2-cube tower. 2–4 words. NB: drooling±throwing items on the floor is now abnormal.
2 years:	Kicks a ball; overarm 'bowling'; gets undressed.
3 years:	Jumps; can stand on one foot; copies; can build an 8-cube tower; knows his first and last name; dressing needs help.
4 years:	Stands on 1 foot for >4sec; picks the longer of 2 lines.

Immunization Offer the schedule given opposite, noting the items below.

*MMR vaccine:** Those aged 18 months to 5yrs who have not had the vaccine (even if they have had single measles vaccine) may have MMR with the pre-school booster of Diphtheria/Tetanus/Polio. There is no upper age limit. SE: Rash ± fever from day 5–10 for ~2 days (so give antipyretic advice); rare non-infectious parotid swelling, from week 3. *CI:* Fever, pregnancy (advise against this for 1 month), a previous live vaccine within 3 weeks or an injection of immunoglobulin within 3 months, primary immunodeficiency syndromes (not including HIV or AIDS), those receiving steroids (eg prednisolone ≥2mg/kg/day for >1 week in the last 3 months), leukaemia, lymphoma, recent radiotherapy, anaphylaxis induced by egg, neomycin or kanamycin (vaccine preservative). Non-anaphylactoid allergies are not contraindications, and nor is a past history of seizures or febrile convulsions.

Pertussis immunization SE: Pain and fever. Serious brain damage is so rare, that if it occurs at all, it is very hard to put a figure to. It is equivocally implicated in 1 in 2×10^6 injections.[3] *CI:* Past severe reaction to pertussis vaccine—ie indurated redness most of the way around the arm, or over most of the anterolateral thigh (depending on the site of the injection); or generalized reactions: fever >39.5°C within 48h of vaccination, anaphylaxis, prolonged inconsolable screaming, or other CNS signs (eg fits) occurring within 72h. *Special considerations: Most children with idiopathic epilepsy, or a family history of epilepsy (sibling or parent) should be vaccinated.* If in doubt, seek expert advice rather than withholding the vaccine. Those with stable CNS conditions (eg cerebral palsy, spina bifida) are *especially recommended* for vaccination. There is no upper age limit. Collapse (sudden loss of muscle tone, pallor, and unresponsiveness) is rare, and subsequent doses may be given without complication.[2] A single-antigen acellular vaccine is available (tel:[UK] 01708 379000).

Vacciation schedules

►An acute febrile illness is a contraindication to any vaccine.
Give live vaccines either together, or separated by ≥3 weeks. Do not give live vaccines if there is a primary immunodeficiency disorder, or if the child is taking steroids (equivalent to >2mg/kg/day of prednisolone).

Children with HIV ± AIDS: Give these all the usual immunizations (including live vaccines) except for BCG, in areas where TB prevalence is low.

Immunizations	The new suggested DoH schedule[2] (L=live vaccine)
3 days:	BCG[L] (if TB in family in last 6 months). See *OHCM* p 192.
2 months:	**'Triple'** (pertussis, tetanus, diphtheria) 0.5mL sc; **HiB** (eg in *single-dose vial* with triple, so just 1 prick); oral **polio**[L]. If premature still give at 2 postnatal months.
3 months:	Repeat **'triple'**, **HiB** and **polio**[L].
4 months:	Repeat **'triple'**, **HiB** and **polio**[L].
12–18 months:	First dose of **Measles/Mumps/Rubella**[L] (=MMR ɪ vaccine) for *both* sexes (0.5mL sc).
3–5yrs:	**Tetanus, diphtheria** & **polio**[L] booster; dose 2 of MMR ɪ.*
10–14yrs:	BCG[L]. (Also Rubella[L] for girls who have missed MMR ɪ.)
15–18yrs:	**Polio**[L] & **Tetanus+low-dose Diphtheria 'Td'** boosters.
Adult boosters:	**Tetanus, Polio, Rubella** (*OHCM* p 226, 234 & 214).

NB: haemophilus influenzae type B immunization (HiB) may be given in the same syringe as triple vaccine—which acts as the diluent for HiB (shake vigorously). Catch-up courses for those too old to have it with the triple may be given (eg with MMR ɪ, and on 2 other occasions). After this, 1 injection is all that is needed as immunity is very likely.

Hepatitis B vaccine: Give at birth, 1 and 6 months, if mother is HBsAg +ve (H-B-Vax ɪ®) 0.5mL IM—into the anterolateral thigh (the adult dose is 1mL into deltoid). (The first dose is accompanied by 200u hepatitis B immunoglobulin at a different IM site). Other risk groups: see *OHCM* p 512.

†A recent meta-analysis suggests that there is no value in these hearing tests: *BJGP* 1999 **49** 4
1 B Wharton 1999 *BMJ* i 2 (get from Health Visitor); dose of vit. D: 7μg/day; iron may also be needed (also 7μg/day). **2** J Labadie 1998 *BMJ* i 902 & D Hall 1995 *Health for all Children,* 3e **3** UK DoH 1996 *The aim of the 2nd measles dose is to eliminate measles (as in Finland). If we relied on a single dose, herd immunity would↓, and every 5yrs an epidemic could occur, as in the USA in 1990, when 135 children died (10% were older children who had been vaccinated). We are aware of a tenuous report of an association between vaccination and Crohn's disease. This has been fully considered by vaccination committees in many countries–none has changed its advice.

Genetic disease and prevention

►It is more important to be able to love the handicapped and to respect their carers than it is to prevent the handicap—for in doing the first we become more human. In the second, we risk our own inappropriate deification.

Gene probes These use recombinant DNA technology to link genetic diseases of unknown cause to DNA markers scattered throughout the human genome. Using fetal DNA from amniotic fluid cells (amniocentesis, p 166) in the second trimester, or from chorionic villus sampling (ChVS, p 166) in the first, it is possible to screen for many genetic diseases (opposite)—eg Huntington's chorea; muscular dystrophy; polycystic kidneys; cystic fibrosis; thalassaemias.

Enzyme defects Many of the inborn errors of metabolism can be diagnosed by incubation of fetal tissue with a specific substrate.

Chromosomal studies can be undertaken on cultured cells or on direct villus preparations. The most important abnormalities are aneuploidies (abnormalities in chromosome number)—eg trisomy 21, 18 and 13.

Screening for chromosomal abnormalities (eg the fragile X syndrome, p 752) may be performed on at-risk mothers who may be carriers.

Nondisjunction After meiosis one gamete contains two number 21 (say) chromosomes and the other gamete has no 21 chromosome. After union of the first gamete with a normal gamete the conceptus will have trisomy 21, and will develop Down's syndrome (but ~50% of such conceptuses suffer early miscarriage). This is the cause in about 95% of Down's babies, and is related to maternal age. Risk at 20yrs: 1 in 2000; 30yrs: 1 in 900; 35yrs: 1 in 365; 40yrs: 1 in 110; 45yrs: 1 in 30; 47yrs: 1 in 20.

Swapping chromosomal fragments Such a cell may end up with the correct amount of genetic material (a balanced translocation); but a gamete from such a cell may have one intact chromosome (say number 21), and another mixed chromosome (say number 14), which, because of the swap, contains material from chromosome 21. After union with a normal gamete, cells will have 3 parts of chromosome 21. This translocation trisomy 21 is the cause in ~2% of babies with Down's syndrome, and is not related to maternal age. If the father carries the translocation, the risk of Down's is 10%; if it is the mother, the risk is 50%. 0.3% of all mothers have this translocation.

Mosaicism A trisomy may develop during the early divisions of a normal conceptus, so that some cells are normal and others have trisomy 21. This accounts for 1–2% of Down's babies. They show variable clinical severity.

Other chromosomal abnormalities Turner's (p 758), Klinefelter's (p 750), Edward's (p 746), and Patau's (p 754) syndromes. In the *cri-du-chat* syndrome there is deletion of the short arm of chromosome 5, causing a high-pitched cry, CVS abnormalities, microcephaly, widely-spaced eyes, and a 'moon' face.

Down's syndrome[1] *Causes:* See above. *Recognition at birth:* Flat facial profile, abundant neck skin, dysplastic ears, muscle hypotonia and x-ray evidence of a dysplastic pelvis are the most constant features. Other features: a round head, protruding tongue, peripheral silver iris spots (Brushfield's), blunt inner eye angle, short, broad hands (eg with a single palmar crease), and an incurving 5th digit. Widely spaced first and second toes and a high-arched palate are more obvious later. If you are uncertain about the diagnosis, it is best to ask an expert's help, rather than baffle the mother by taking blood tests 'just in case it's Down's'. *Associated problems:* Duodenal atresia; VSD; patent ductus; ASD (foramen primum defects, p 224); and, later, a low IQ and a small stature. Helping the mother accept her (often very lovable) child may be aided by introducing her to a friendly mother of a Down's baby. *Prenatal diangosis:* p 166–8.

3. Paediatrics

Genetic counselling

Goal To provide patients with accurate, up-to-date information on their condition and its consequences for them and their relatives in such a manner as to allow them to make informed decisions.

►Genetic counselling is a specialty best conducted in regional centres to which you should refer affected families.[1] *Do not do blood tests on children lightly which might have long-term consequences, unless some form of treatment is available. The child may never forgive you for labelling him or her.*

In order to receive most benefit from referral:

- The affected person (proband) should come with family (spouse, parents, children, siblings); individuals can of course be seen alone as well.
- The family should be informed that a detailed pedigree (family tree) will be made, and medical details of distant relatives may be asked for.
- Irrational emotions (guilt, blame, anger) are common. Deal with these sensitively, and do not ignore. *Remember:* you do not choose your ancestors, and you cannot control what you pass on to your descendants.
- Warn patients that most tests give no absolute 'yes' or 'no' but merely 'likely' or 'unlikely'. In gene tracking, where a molecular fragment near the gene is followed through successive family members, the degree of certainty of the answer will depend on the distance between the marker and the gene (as crossing-over in meiosis may separate them).
- Accept that some people will not want testing, eg the offspring of a Huntington's chorea sufferer—or a mother of a boy who might have fragile X syndrome, but who understandably does not want her offspring labelled (employment, insurance and social reasons). Offer a genetic referral to ensure that her decision is fully informed (but remember: 'being fully informed' may itself be deleterious to health and wellbeing, p 169).

Chromosomal disorders include Down's (trisomy 21, p 210), Turner's (45, X0, p 758) and Klinefelter's (47, XXY, p 750) syndromes. Many genes are involved when the defect is large enough to be seen microscopically.

Autosomal-dominants Polycystic kidneys (16p), Huntington's chorea, (4p). A single copy of the defective gene is sufficient to cause damage, and so symptomless carriers do not usually occur.

Autosomal recessives Cystic fibrosis (7q), β-thalassaemia, sickle-cell (11p). In general, both genes must be defective before damage is seen, so carriers are common—and both parents must be carriers for offspring to be affected, so consanguinity (marrying relatives) increases risk.

X-linked Duchenne muscular dystrophy, Haemophilia A and B, fragile X (p 752). In female (XX) carriers a normal gene on the second X chromosome prevents the deleterious effects manifesting. The male (XY) has no such protection and so is affected by the disease.

Chromosome nomenclature Autosomes are numbered 1 to 22 roughly in order of size, 1 being the largest. The arms on each side of the centromere are designated 'p' (petite) for the short arm, and 'q' for the long arm. Thus 'the long arm of chromosome 6' is written '6q'.

NB: being pregnant and unwilling to consider termination does *not* exclude one from undergoing useful genetic counselling.

'Couple screening' A big problem with counselling is the unnecessary alarm caused by false +ve tests. In cystic fibrosis screening (analysis of cells in mouthwash samples) this is reducible by 97% (0.08% *vs* 3.2%) by screening mother and father together—who need only get alarmed if they *both* turn out to be screen-positive. The trouble with this is false reassurance. Many forget that they will need future tests if they have a different partner, and those who do not are left with some lingering anxieties.[2]

1 In UK, phone 0171 794 0500–to find nearest centre. 2 M Hall 1995 *BMJ* i 353

3. Paediatrics

Measles, rubella, mumps and erythroviruses

Measles *Cause:* RNA paramyxovirus. *Spread:* droplets. *Incubation:* 7–21 days. Infective from prodrome (catarrh, wretchedness, conjunctivitis, fever) until 5 days after rash starts. Conjunctivae look glassy; then the semilunar fold swells (Meyer's sign). *Koplik spots* are pathognomonic, grain-of-salt-like spots on buccal mucosa. They are often fading as the rash appears (starts behind ears, eg on days 3–5, then spreads down the body, becoming confluent).
Complications: Febrile fits, meningitis, D&V, keratoconjunctivitis; immunosuppression; subacute sclerosing panencephalitis, if immunosuppressed, giant cell pneumonitis. Intrauterine infection may cause malformations. The worst complication is the rare encephalitis (headache, lassitude, fits, coma)—≤15% may die; 25% develop fits, deafness or mental retardation.
Treatment: •Isolate—in hospital, if the patient is ill or immunocompromized or malnourished, or has pneumonitis, CNS signs, or dehydration.
- Ensure adequate nutrition (catabolism is very high). Continue breast feeding, even during diarrhoea. Pass a nasogastric feeding tube if intake is poor.
- Frequent mouth washes with water + 1% gentian violet to mouth lesions.
- Vitamin A needs rise;[1] 2 doses, + 1 more at 6 weeks later, (p 512) saves lives and prevents corneal ulceration. CI: pregnancy; known not to be deficient.
- Treat any 2° bacterial infection, antibiotics such as amoxicillin for otitis media and pneumonia. Prophylactic antibiotics have no clearly defined rôle. Paracetamol for fever.

Prognosis: Mostly excellent in rich countries—but it is a serious, mortal disease in poor countries (mortality >10%). *Immunization:* 2-dose regimen, p 208.

Rubella (known as german measles, german being *germane* ie closely akin to). *Cause:* RNA virus. *Incubation:* 14–21 days. The patient is infective 5 days before and 5 days after the day the rash starts. *Signs:* Usually mild; macular rash; suboccipital lymphadenopathy. *Treatment:* None is usually needed. *Immunization:* (live virus, p 208). Give at least 1000 TCID50 (tissue culture infective dose, 50) eg as 0.5mL Almevax® sc. CI: pregnancy. The best time to immunize girls who have not had the MMR vaccine is from 11 to 13yrs old.
Complications: Small joint arthritis. Malformations *in utero* (p 98).
Infection during the first 4 weeks: eye abnormalities in 70%; during weeks 4–8: cardiac abnormalities in 40%; weeks 8–12: deafness in 30%.

Mumps *Cause:* RNA paramyxovirus. *Spread:* Droplets and saliva.
Incubation: 14–21 days. *Immunity:* Lifelong, once infected. The patient is infective 7 days before and 9 days after parotid swelling starts.
Presentation: Prodromal symptoms (malaise, fever); painful swelling of the parotids, unilaterally at first, becoming bilateral in 70%.
Complications: Orchitis (± infertility), arthritis, meningitis, pancreatitis, myocarditis. Complete recovery is the rule.
Treatment: Rest; paracetamol syrup (120mg/5mL) for *high* fever or *severe* discomfort. Dose (per 6h PO): <3 months old: 5–10mg/kg (a loading dose of ≤40mg/kg PR may be needed[2]); 3 months–1yr: 60–120mg; 1–5yrs: 120–250mg; 6–12yrs 250–500mg. 60mg suppositories are available. Tepid (not cold) sponging augments paracetamol. Also unwrap and rehydrate (this avoids vasoconstriction). Usually antipyretics are *not* required, and there is evidence of increased mortality in severe sepsis.[3]

Erythrovirus (formerly parvovirus) Type B19 is the cause of the 'slapped cheek' syndrome, also known as 'fifth disease' and erythema infectiosum. This is usually a mild, acute infection of children, characterized by malar erythema (a raised, fiery flush on the cheeks) and a rash mainly on the limbs. Constitutional upset is mild. Arthralgia is commoner in adults—who may present with a glandular fever-like syndrome and a false +ve Paul–Bunnell test.[4] Spread is rapid in closed communities. It is also the cause of aplastic crises in sickle-cell disease. It is uncommon in pregnancy but risks fetal death in ~10% (especially mid-trimester),[5] and is a cause of hydrops fetalis by inhibition of multiplication and lysis of erythroid progenitor cells (monitor AFP for several weeks; if it rises abnormally, do ultrasound). Fetal/neonatal problems *do* occur: hydrops (occurs in ~3%, and is treated by intrauterine transfusion if severe), growth retardation, meconium peritonitis, myocarditis/infarction, glomerulonephritis, placentomegaly, hepatomegaly, oedema, rashes, anaemia, platelets/WCC↓, respiratory insufficiency, and deaths have been reported, but are rare. ~1 : 10 of those affected before 20 weeks will miscarry; in the remainder, the overall risk of congenital abnormality is ~1%.[6]

Hand, foot and mouth disease is caused by Coxsackievirus A16. The child is mildly unwell and develops vesicles on the palms and soles and in the mouth. They may cause discomfort until they heal, without crusting. *Incubation:* 5–7 days. *Treatment* is symptomatic.

Note Measles, rubella and mumps are notifiable diseases in the UK. MMR vaccine: see p 208–9. **Herpes infections** See OHCM p 202.

Roseola infantum This is a common, mild illness in infants (usually <1yr old), which causes a high fever, whose peak is followed by a macular (or maculopapular) rash. It is self-limiting. The cause is Herpes virus 6 (HHV-6), a double-stranded DNA virus, initially named Human B-cell lymphotropic virus. It morphogenetically related to the other five herpes viruses (HSV 1 and 2, Varicella zoster virus, EBV and CMV)—but is antigenically distinct.
Interaction between host immunities and other viruses may lead to increased cellular immunodeficiency and fatal illnesses. (Synonyms: exanthem subitum, fourth disease, three-day fever.)

Other causes of rashes in children See also skin diseases section (p 574).
- A transient maculopapular rash is a feature of many trivial viral illnesses (but a few macules may be a sign of early meningococcaemia).
- Purpuric rashes: meningococcaemia (p 258); Henoch–Schönlein purpura (p 275); idiopathic thrombocytopenic purpura (check FBC).
- Drug eruptions: maculopapular rashes in response to penicillins and to phenytoin are particularly common.
- Scabies (p 600); insect bites.
- Eczema (p 588); urticaria (p 578); psoriasis—guttate psoriasis may follow a respiratory tract infection in children (p 586); pityriasis rosea (p 594).
- Still's disease: transient maculopapular rash, fever and polyarthritis (p 758).

1 M Zacharias 1998 BMJ **i** 1552 2 G Hussey 1997 BMJ **i** 316 3 F Shann 1995 *Lancet* **345** 338
4 J Pether 1994 BMJ **i** 595 5 A Sanghi 1997 *B J Ob Gy* **104** 942 6 E Miller 1998 *B J Obs Gyn* **105** 174

Varicella (herpes) zoster

Chickenpox is a primary infection with varicella-zoster virus. Shingles is a reactivation of dormant virus in the posterior root ganglion.

Chickenpox *Presentation:* Crops of vesicles on the skin of different ages, typically starting on back. *Incubation:* 11–21 days. *Infectivity:* 4 days before the rash, until all lesions have scabbed (1 week). Spread is by droplets. It can be caught from someone with shingles. It is one of the most infectious diseases known. 95% of adults have been infected; immunity is life-long.
Tests: Fluorescent antibody tests and Tzanck smears are rarely needed.
Differential: Hand, foot and mouth disease; insect bites; scabies; rickettsia.
Course and dangers: Starts as fever. Rash appears ~2 days later, often starting on the back: macule→papule→vesicle with a red-surround→ulcers (eg oral, vaginal)→crusting. 2–4 crops of lesions occur during the illness. Lesions cluster round areas of pressure or hyperaemia. Chickenpox is dangerous if immunosuppressed, or in cystic fibrosis, severe eczema, and in neonates.
Treatment: Keeping cool may reduce the number of lesions. Trim nails to lessen damage from scratching. Daily antiseptic for spots may be tried (chlorhexidine). Flucloxacillin 125–250mg/6h PO if bacterial superinfection—treat for septicaemia if deteriorating. Antivaricella-zoster immunoglobulin (12.5u/kg IM max 625u) + aciclovir if immunosuppressed or on steroids and within 10 days of exposure (give as soon as possible, see *BNF*). Aciclovir is licensed as a 7-day course in chickenpox; begin within 24h of the rash. *Aciclovir child dose:* (20mg/kg/6h PO), eg <2yrs: 200mg/6h PO; 2–5yrs: 400mg/6h PO. ≥6yrs: 800mg/6h. Tablets are 200, 400 or 800mg; suspension: 200mg/5mL or 400mg/ 5mL. In renal failure, ↓ dose. There is *no* clear evidence on aciclovir ↓complications if immunocompetent, but it may help severe symptoms, eg in older patients, or 2nd or 3rd family contacts. If used, use at the first sign of infection. *Rare complications:* Pneumonia, meningitis, DIC, LFTs↑, Guillain–Barré, Henoch–Schönlein, nephritis, pancreatitis, myositis, myocarditis, orchitis, transverse myelitis, CNS thrombi, purpura fulminans, so, if susceptible, consider *live attenuated vaccine* before starting cytotoxics or high-dose steroids.

Shingles *Treatment:* Oral analgesia. Ophthalmic shingles: p 484. Aciclovir may reduce progression of zoster in the immunocompromised (may be rampant, with pneumonitis, hepatitis, and meningoencephalitis).[1] Aciclovir IVI dose: 10mg/kg/8h (over 1h), with concentration <10mg/mL.

Varicella in pregnancy In the UK chickenpox affects 3 per 1000 pregnancies. Complications (pneumonitis affecting 1 in 400, and encephalitis 1 per 1000 cases) are not commoner in pregnancy, despite pregnancy being an immunocompromised state.[2] Infection within the first 20 weeks (especially 13–20 weeks) may result in congenital varicella (cerebral cortical atrophy, cerebellar hypoplasia, manifested by microcephaly, convulsions and mental retardation; limb hypoplasia, rudimentary digits and pigmented scars). It is rare (~2%), can be mild, and does not occur with maternal shingles. If mother affected from 1 week before to 4 weeks after birth, babies may suffer severe chickenpox. Give the baby zoster immune globulin 250mg IM at birth; if affected, isolate from other babies, and give aciclovir.

Infection may be prevented by vaccination of susceptible women before pregnancy with live varicella vaccine, but testing for antibodies pre-conceptually is expensive, and cost-effectiveness depends on local rates of seronegativity. ~80% of those who cannot recall any previous chickenpox are, in fact, immune.[3] (Varicella zoster globulin can prevent infection in 50% when given to susceptible contacts—eg 1000mg IM). Evidence suggests that infected pregnant women should have aciclovir (above) to ameliorate the disease. The fetus does not appear to be adversely affected. Chickenpox at birth is a problem. Barrier nursing mother causes distress and is of unproven value—but the infant's mortality may be 20%.[2]

1 A Leung 1994 *Update* **49** 277 **2** D Seidman 1996 *BMJ* **ii** 701 **3** P Venkatesan 1996 *Practit* **240** 256

Childhood HIV infection

See *Prenatal HIV* (p 98), *HIV in labour* (p 155), *Adult HIV* (*OHCM* p 212–9).

Of the million or so[1] HIV+ve children, most live in Africa, where rates of transmission from mother to baby (vertical transmission) are twice as high as in the West. This may be due to concurrent infections, virulence differences, and frequencies of breast feeding (if an HIV +ve mother breast feeds, this ↑risk of vertical transmission by 14%).[2] Infection can occur from the first trimester; ~50% of infections occur around the time of delivery[1]—and is more likely if the mother has symptomatic HIV infection or a high viral load. In a cohort of 330 HIV +ve mothers, those with the p24 antigen had a 3-fold risk of transmission compared with those who were p24 –ve.[1] For the rôle of Caesarean section and zidovudine (AZT) in preventing vertical transmission, see p 98.

Diagnosing HIV-1 Standard tests cannot be used (placentally transferred IgG persists for ≤18 months). Virus culture and PCR (polymerase chain reaction) methods are reliable, and more sensitive than finding p23 antigen in the child's blood. HIV-specific IgA doesn't cross the placenta, but only occurs in 50% of infected infants <6 months old. Discuss these problems with a microbiologist. Monitoring CD4 cell count (*OHCM* p 212) has an important rôle in staging HIV infection. HIV-2 *can* pass vertically, but this is rare.[3]

Presentation Failure to thrive, feeding problems, fever, diarrhoea, repeated admissions for gastro-enteritis, hepatosplenomegaly, PUO, parotitis, lymphadenopathy, chest infections slow to clear, pneumonia, clubbing,[4] *pneumocystis carinii*, toxoplasmosis, tuberculosis, cryptococcosis, histoplasmosis, CMV infection, lymphoid interstitial pneumonitis.

Lymphoid interstitial pneumonitis (LIP): Signs: tachypnoea, hypoxia, clubbing, diffuse reticulonodular infiltrates on CXR, bilateral hilar lymphadenopathy. It is not an AIDS-defining illness, and it is 5-fold less serious than pneumocystosis.

Prognosis *Mean age at death:* 9.4yrs.[5] By 3yrs old, up to half with early-onset opportunistic infection have died, *vs* 3% of those with no such infection. Children with slow progression of HIV have persistent neutralizing antibodies. Transplacental passage of maternal neutralizing antibody may also have a rôle.[6]

Guidelines for preventing *pneumocystosis* (PCP) with co-trimoxazole[6]

Age / HIV status	*PCP prophylaxis*	*Do CD4 cell counts at:*
0–5wks, HIV exposed	No	1 month
5wks–4 months, HIV exposed	No	3 months
4–12 months: –HIV infected	Yes	6, 9, and 12 months
–Status unknown	Yes	6, 9, and 12 months
–No HIV infection	No	No monitoring needed
1–5 yrs, HIV infected	Yes, if CD4 <500 per μL or CD4 percentage <15%	At least 3–4 monthly
6–12yrs, HIV infected	Yes, if CD4 <200 per μL or CD4 percentage <15%	At least every 3–4 months

Ensure a full course of vaccines (include *Haemophilus* and *Pneumococcus*, but avoid live vaccines if seriously immunocompromised; avoid BCG in children with symptomatic HIV infection in areas where TB prevalence is low).

Treatment of HIV and of opportunistic infections Refer to a specialized HIV centre. Regimens are constantly being refined, and new drugs are under trial: see *Anti-HIV agents: OHCM* p 218: there is some evidence that children respond in a similar way to adults (eg didanosine is better than AZT).[7]

1 K Morris 1997 *Lancet* **350** 1683 2 D Dunn 1992 *Lancet* **340** 585 3 P Cavaco-Silva 1997 *Lancet* **249** 177
4 S Graham 1997 *Lancet* **349** 31 5 E-BM 1997 2 26 6 CDC 1995 *Morbid Mrtl Wkly Rep* **44** 1 7 E-BM 1998 **3** 15

Some gastrointestinal malformations

Oesophageal atresia (± tracheo-oesophageal fistula—TOF) At least 85% of these babies will have a tracheo-oesophageal fistula. 30% will have another abnormality. Signs: cough, airway obstruction (excessive secretions—'blowing bubbles'), abdominal distension, cyanosis and recurrent pneumonias. *Diagnosis:* Inability to pass a catheter into the stomach. X-rays will show it coiled in the oesophagus. Avoid contrast radiology. Use endoscopy instead. *Treatment:* Surgical correction of fistulae, using a cervical incision.

Diaphragmatic hernia *Signs:* Respiratory distress; bowel sounds in one hemithorax (usually left—so the heart is best heard on the right). Cyanosis augers badly (implying lung hypoplasia). It can present with difficult resuscitation at birth. It is associated with other malformations (in 50%, eg neural tube defects), trisomy 18, deletion of the small arm of chromosome 27, Pierre Robin (p 226) and Beckwith–Wiedmann (p 743) syndromes. Incidence 1:2200. *Diagnosis:* Prenatal: ultrasound; postnatal: CXR. *Treatment:*

- *Prenatal:* Refer to a fetal surgery centre (tracheal obstruction may be tried: it encourages lung growth, so pushing out other viscera).[1]
- *Postnatal:* Insert a large bore nasogastric tube as soon as you suspect the diagnosis. Face masks are contraindicated (so intubate and ventilate, if needed, with low pressures at a rate of 100/min and minimum positive end-expiratory pressure). Get urgent surgery in an appropriate centre.

Hirschsprung's disease Congenital absence of ganglia in a segment of colon leads to infrequent, narrow stools, GI obstruction and megacolon. Faeces may be felt *per abdomen*, and PR exam may disclose only a few pellet-like faeces. ♂/♀=3:1. *Complications:* GI perforation, bleeding, ulcers. Tests: barium enema or by sigmoidoscopy/biopsy of the aganglionic section, staining for for acetylcholinesterase-+ve nerve excess). Excision of the aganglionic segment is usually needed. This does not always lead to immediate recovery.

Hydroceles in infancy A processus vaginalis patent at birth, and allowing *only fluid* from the peritoneal cavity to pass down it, generally closes during the first year of life—so no action is usually needed. If the fluid-filled sac is adjacent to the spermatic cord, it is called an encysted hydrocele or a spermatic cord cyst. If the proximal opening of the processus vaginalis is wide, a true inguinal hernia is formed, and *action is always required*. . .

Inguinal hernias These are due to a patent processus vaginalis (the passage which ushers the descending testicle into the scrotum). They present as a bulge lateral to the pubic tubercle. They may be intermittent, appearing during crying. In 25% there are bilateral hernias. The aim is to repair these as soon as possible, before obstruction occurs. Note: there is often an associated hydrocele, and this may be difficult to distinguish from an incarcerated hernia—exploration is required if there is doubt.

Imperforate anus Most girls have a posterior fourchette fistula; most boys have a posterior urethral fistula (may pass meconium in urine). Absence of a perineal fistula in boys indicates communication with the urethran (∴ colostomy may be required). Do an IVU to reaveal commonly associated GU abnormalities. Posterior sagittal anorectoplasy (PSARP) is possible.[2]

Meckel's diverticulum See p 754.

Mid-gut malrotations Absent attachment of the mesentery of the small intestine may result in a volvulus of the mid-gut or obstruction of the third part of the duodenum by fibrotic bands. The child may not present for some years, until unexplained vomiting occurs. The passage of blood per rectum heralds mid-gut necrosis—and is an indication for emergency surgical decompression. See *OHCM* p 126 for acute gastric volvulus.

1 F Luks 1995 *BMJ* ii 1449 2 This repairs even high anorectal malformations, via an incision from the sacrum to the anal dimple; the rectum and urethra/vagina are likely to need careful teasing apart. Faecal continence is achievable in ~50%, failures typically occurring if there are associated sacral malformations. See J Martins 1997 *Rev Paul Med* **115** 1566 & C Chen 1998 *Paed Surg Int* **13** 133

Anterior abdominal wall defects[1,2]—*Gastroschisis:* A paraumbilical defect with evisceration (extrusion of viscera) of abdominal contents. Incidence: ~1.6/10,000—apparently rising, and possibly caused by a vascular event associated with cocaine use. The typical pregnancy is in a young, socially disadvantaged primip. There is usually *no* other defect, and corrective surgery has a good outcome in 90% (so deliver where there are good paediatric surgical facilities, if diagnosed prenatally—aim to diagnose at ultrasound).
Exomphalos: This is a ventral defect with herniation of the abdominal contents into the base of the umbilical cord. There is a covering with peritoneum. Incidence: ~4.3/10,000. Other abnormalities are frequently present.

1 L Chitty 1996 *BMJ* **ii** 891 2 KH Tan 1996 *BMJ* **ii** 903

Genitourinary diseases

Undescended testis—cryptorchidism (2–3% of neonates, 15–30% of prems; bilateral in 25% of these). On cold days retractile testes may hide in the inguinal pouch, eluding all but the most careful examination (eg while squatting, or with legs crossed, or in a warm bath). If it is truly undescended it will lie along the path of descent from the abdominal cavity. Early (eg at 1 year) fixing within the scrotum (orchidopexy) may prevent infertility and enables diagnosis of neoplasia[1] (otherwise risk ↑5–10-fold). Intranasal gonadotrophin-releasing hormone is unreliable. NB: biopsy may cause later malignancy.[2]

Urethral valves present with uraemia (p 280) and a palpable bladder after voiding; the flow is intermittent and feeble. Micturating cystogram studies show dilatation of the posterior urethra. Antenatal diagnosis: ultrasound.

Hypospadias The meatus is on the ventral side of the penis. It may be stenosed. ►Avoid circumcision: use foreskin for repair before school age.

Epispadias The meatus appears on the dorsal side of the penis.

Some congenital and genetic disorders *Horseshoe kidney:* The kidneys are fused in a midline hoop. Symptoms may be absent; or there may be obstructive uropathy and renal infections. IVU diagnosis: kidneys displaced medially; rotated collecting system.

Infantile polycystic kidneys may cause obstructed labour and respiratory difficulties, with later uraemia and BP↑. Radiology: collecting tubule cysts (<5mm across). The histology of the liver is always abnormal. Survivors risk UTIs and portal hypertension with haematemesis. Inheritance is recessive. The inheritance of adult polycystic disease (*OHCM* p 396) is dominant.

Ectopic kidney: This may reveal itself as a pelvic mass, or be seen on IVU. Associations: anorectal abnormalities, UTIs.

Renal agenesis causes oligohydramnios and Potter's facies (p 120) with early death if bilateral. Associations: unicornuate uterus.

Patent urachus: Urine leaks from the umbilicus.

Extrophy of the bladder: The bladder mucosa is exteriorized.

Double ureter: *Associations:* ureterocele, UTI, pyelonephritis; may be symptomless.

Renal tubular defects: There may be disturbance of any tubular function, eg renal glycosuria, cystinuria, or diabetes insipidus. In renal tubular acidosis conservation of fixed base is impaired, so that there is a metabolic acidosis with alkaline urine. *Symptoms:* Failure to thrive, polyuria and polydipsia.

Wilms' nephroblastoma This is the commonest intra-abdominal tumour of childhood (20% of all malignancies). It is an undifferentiated mesodermal tumour of the intermediate cell mass. It may be sporadic, or familial (2%), or associated with Beckwith–Wiedemann syndrome (BWS, p742), *a*niridia, GU malformations, and *r*etardation (WAGR). One of the Wilms' tumour gene (WT1 on chromosome 11) encodes a protein which is a transcriptional repressor downregulating IGF-II, an insulin-like growth factor.[3] Median age at presentation: 3.5yrs. 95% are unilateral. Staging:

- **I** Tumour confined to the kidney
- **II** Extrarenal spread, but resectable
- **III** Extensive abdominal disease.
- **IV** Distant metastases
- **V** Bilateral disease

The patient: Features include fever, flank pain, an abdominal mass. Haematuria is not common. Ultrasound: renal pelvis distortion; hydronephrosis.

Management: Avoid renal biopsy. Nephrectomy, chemotherapy (eg vincristine and doxorubicin) and radiotherapy can be curative.

1 UK testicular group. 1994 *BMJ* **i** 1393 & D Forman 1994 *BMJ* **ii** 666 2 AJ Swerdlow 1997 *BMJ* **i** 1507 3 G Skuse 1995 *Lancet* **345** 902

Ambiguous genitalia

►This is a rare phenomenon: refer promptly for expert help.

Gender determinants Distinguish between genetic, gonadal, phenotypic (eg affected by sex hormone secretion), and psychological sex.

History and examination Any exposure to progesterone, testosterone, phenytoin, aminoglutethamide? Previous neonatal deaths (the adrenogenital syndrome has recessive inheritance)? Note phallic size, and the position of the urethral orifice. Are the labia fused? Have the gonads descended?

Tests Buccal smear (Barr body present if ♀); white cell mustard stains to make Y chromosome fluoresce. These tests take <24h. Chromosome analysis takes 5–9 days. If there is a phallus and the buccal smear is 'female' the diagnosis is either true hermaphroditism, adrenogenital syndrome or maternal androgens (drugs, tumours). If there is a phallus and the buccal smear is 'male', tell mother that the baby is a boy.

Do not rely on appearances whenever babies have: bilateral cryptorchidism (at term), even if a phallus is present; unilateral cryptorchidism with hypospadias; penoscrotal or perineoscrotal hypospadias. These patients need examination by a paediatric endocrinologist to exclude androgen resistance (eg testicular feminization in which feminization will occur in adolescence despite androgens, making it imperative that these children are brought up as girls[1]). NB: if the stretched phallus is <25mm long at birth it is unlikely that it can ever be used for procreation, despite the best plastic surgery.

If there is uncertainty because the penis is so short, a paediatric endocrinologist may recommend 3 days' treatment with human chorionic gonadotrophin. If the baby is a boy the penis will grow (possibly even to normal length) after 48h.[1] Advise against registering the birth until a definite treatment plan is in place. Once registered, legal sex cannot be changed.

True hermaphroditism (10% are XY, 10% mosaic, and 80% XX). It is often best to raise these as girls. Two-thirds will menstruate.

The adrenogenital syndrome (Congenital adrenal hyperplasia—due to the excessive secretion of androgenic hormones because of deficiencies of 21-hydroxylase, 11-hydroxylase, or 3-β-hydroxysteroid dehydrogenase). Cortisol cannot be adequately produced, and the consequent rise in adrenocorticotrophic hormone leads to adrenal hyperplasia, and overproduction of cortisol precursors (which are androgenic). Incidence: 1:14000.

Clinical and biochemical features: Vomiting, dehydration, and ambiguous genitalia. Boys may show no obvious abnormality at birth, but will exhibit precocious puberty, or may have ambiguous genitalia (reduced androgens in 17-hydroxylase deficiency), or incomplete masculinization (hypospadias with cryptorchidism from 3β-hydroxysteroid dehydrogenase deficit). Hyponatraemia, (with a paradoxically high urine Na^+) and hyperkalaemia are common. ↑Plasma 17-hydroxyprogesterone in 90%; urinary 17-ketosteroids↑ (not in 17-hydroxylase deficit).

Emergency treatment: Babies may present with an adrenocortical crisis (circulatory collapse) in early life. Other presentations include hyponatraemic seizures in infancy (often misdiagnosed as a febrile convulsion). ►►Urgent treatment is required with 0.9% saline IVI (3–5g Na^+/day), glucose, and hydrocortisone 100mg/2–6h IV (all ages). Give fludrocortisone 0.1mg/day PO.

1 JO Ahlquist 1994 *BMJ* i 1041

Genetics, biosynthetic pathways, and the possibility of screening for congenital adrenal hypoplasia

The common cause of adrenal hyperplasia is one of ~10 gene defects (6p21.3; the gene is called CYP21) which causes deficiency of 21-hydroxylase (which mediates the penultimate step in cortisol biosynthesis). Corticotrophin-induced accumulation of 17OH-progesterone leads to ↑levels of testosterone (via hepatic conversion). Most affected infants are also salt losers, as 21-hydroxylase is needed for aldosterone biosynthesis, and in boys, this is usually the sole early manifestation (excess virilization may be early or delayed to adulthood).[1] Biochemical screening is rarely universal, but some centres use it in boys, aiming for diagnosis before life-threatening adrenal hypoplasia. (Girls are generally detected by finding virilization at neonatal examination providing the baby is not misdiagnosed as a boy[1]—prenatal diagnosis is possible, and treatable by giving the mother dexamethasone from early in pregnancy.) One difficulty is the diversity in time of onset and clinical presentation despite identical CYP21 mutations, making adrenal hypoplasia a continuum of disorders. Treatment is medical and surgical (clitoral reduction and vaginoplasty). Growth and fertility are also impaired.

1 I Hughes 1998 *Lancet* **352** 752

Congenital heart disease (CHD)

Incidence 8/1000 births. 2 key questions: *Is the defect compensated?* (unobtrusive); if not, *Is there cyanosis? Signs decompensation:* Poor feeding, dyspnoea, hepatomegaly, engorged neck veins, bradycardia. *Physiological categories:*[1] •Left to right shunt (ASD; VSD) •↓Systemic perfusion: weak pulse ± acidosis (hypoplastic L heart; aortic stenosis) •Pulmonary venous congestion (eg mitral stenosis) •Transposition streaming (of caval return→aorta) •↓Pulmonary blood flow (eg Fallot's) •Intracardiac mixing of 'blue' and 'red' blood (eg truncus arteriosus).

Acyanotic causes of uncompensated defects (The shunt is left to right.) Atrioseptal defects (ASD), VSDs, aortopulmonary window, patent ductus arteriosus (PDA). Later pulmonary hypertension may lead to a shunt reversal and subsequent cyanosis (Eisenmenger's syndrome, p 746).

Cyanotic causes (R to L shunt through VSD or ASD.) Fallot's tetralogy (p 746), transposition of the great arteries (TGA), other multiple defects; tricuspid or pulmonary stenosis/atresia associated with shunts.

Tests FBC, CXR, P_aO_2 (in air & 100% O_2), ECG, 3D echocardiogram, cardiac catheter.

VSD: (25% of cases) Symptoms: as above. Signs: harsh, loud, pansystolic 'blowing' murmur ± thrill; ± a diastolic apical inflow murmur. ECG: left (or combined) ventricular hypertrophy. CXR: pulmonary engorgement. Course: 20% close spontaneously by 9 months (*maladie de Roger*).
ASD: (7% of cases) Symptoms: above. Signs: widely split, fixed S_2 + midsystolic murmur (esp. at 2nd intercostal space at left sternal edge). CXR: cardiomegaly, globular heart (primum defects). ECG: RVH ± incomplete R bundle branch block.
Patent ductus: Presents with failure to thrive, pneumonias, heart failure, SBE. Signs: collapsing pulse, thrill, loud P_2, systolic murmur in pulmonary area. CXR: vascular markings↑, big aorta. ECG: LVH. Dexamethasone in preterm labour helps close PDAs. *Coarctation of the aorta:* Aortic constriction leads to difficulty in feeling the femoral pulses, ↑BP in the arms (may cause epistaxis), and reduced in the legs, absent foot pulses, ± systolic murmur at the left back, heart failure. CXR: rib notching. ECG: LVH.
Transposition of the great arteries (TGA): Cyanosis, CCF, ± a systolic murmur. CXR: egg-shaped ventricles. ECG: RVH. Balloon atrial septostomy allows oxygenated blood to reach the aorta via the right heart. Recorrection is possible.
Pulmonary stenosis: Pulmonary thrill with systolic murmur. See *OHCM* p 310.

Treatment •Treat heart failure in babies with nasogastric feeds, sitting upright, O_2, furosemide (=frusemide) eg 1mg/kg/24h IV slowly and digoxin 10μg/kg/24h PO. •Neonatal cardiologists may advise keeping ductus open in duct-dependent cyanotic conditions with prostaglandin E_1 (0.05–0.1μg/kg/min IV); intubate and ventilate before transfer to specialist unit. During transfer be alert to hypothermia, hypoglycaemia, hypocalcaemia, hypovolaemia. •Prevent endocarditis (p 194). Open-heart surgery using hypothermia and circulatory arrest is possible at any age, eg for: Fallot's tetralagy, VSD, TGA, total anomalous pulmonary venous drainage (in which pulmonary veins drain, eg into the portal system, causing severe CCF). Balloon valvuloplasty is reducing the need for open heart surgery in pulmonary stenosis (there is more of a problem with restenosis and residual incompetence with aortic valvuloplasty). It is also employed in aortic coarctation. Examples of palliative surgery: pulmonary artery banding to restrict blood flow; systemic to pulmonary shunts to enlarge an underdeveloped pulmonary arterial tree, before inserting a valve-bearing conduit.

Prenatal screening echocardiography[2] In the UK, this is feasible, provided there are 400 or so spare ultrasonographers.[3] Sensitivity: 88%; specificity and +ve predictive value: 100%. Intrauterine cardiac intervention is attractive to some.

1 S Howarth 1993 *Arch Dis Chi* **68** 707 2 I Stumpflen 1996 *Lancet* **348** 854 3 S Kleinert 1996 *Lancet* **348** 836

Murmurs and heart sounds in children

Benign flow murmurs are often heard in early systole at the left sternal edge. Lack of other features distinguishes them from malformations.

Questions to ask yourself while listening to the 2nd heart sound (S_2)

- Is it a double sound in inspiration, and single in expiration? (Normal)
- Is S_2 split all the time? (ASD—atrial septal defects)
- Is S_2 never split, ie single? Fallot's; pulmonary atresia; severe pulmonary stenosis; common arterial trunk; transposition of the great arteries (the anterior aorta masks sounds from the posterior pulmonary trunk.)
- Is the pulmonary component (2nd part) too loud? (Pulmonary stenosis)

NB: the 2nd heart sound is more useful diagnostically than the first.

Questions to ask yourself while listening to a murmur

Timing: •Ejection systolic crescendo–decrescendo (eg innocent murmur, semilunar valve or peripheral arterial stenosis).

- Pansystolic with no crescendo–decrescendo (VSD, mitral incompetence).
- Late systolic, no crescendo–decrescendo (mitral prolapse, *OHCM* p 306).
- Early diastolic decrescendo (aortic or pulmonary incompetence).
- Mid-diastolic crescendo–decrescendo (↑atrio-ventricular valve flow, eg VSD, ASD; or tricuspid or mitral valve stenosis). An opening snap (*OHCM* p 306) and presystolic accentuation suggest the latter.
- Continuous murmurs—usually crescendo–decrescendo (usually patent ductus, venous hum, or arterio-venous fistula).

Loudness: The 6 grades for systolic murmurs: ►Thrills mean pathology.
1 Just audible with a quiet child in a quiet room. 2 Quiet, but easily audible.
3 Loud, but no thrill. 4 Loud with thrill.
5 Audible even if the stethoscope only makes partial contact with skin.
6 Audible without a stethoscope.

Place:

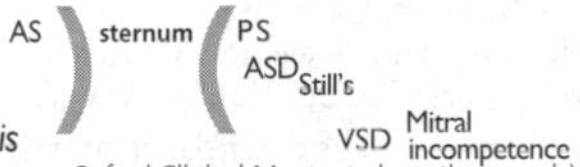

AS) sternum (PS
ASD Still's
VSD Mitral incompetence

AS=aortic stenosis; PS=pulmonary stenosis

(Use our *Oxford Clinical Mentor* to hear the sounds)

Accentuating/diminishing manoeuvres:

- Inspiration augments systemic venous return (the 'negative' pressure draws blood from the abdomen into the thorax), and therefore the murmurs of pulmonary stenosis and tricuspid regurgitation.
- Expiration augments pulmonary venous return and decreases systemic return, and therefore VSD, mitral incompetence, and aortic stenosis too. In (mild) pulmonary stenosis, the ejection click is augmented by expiration.
- Valsalva manoeuvre ↓ systemic venous return and benign flow murmurs, but ↑ murmurs from mitral incompetence and subaortic obstruction.
- Sitting or standing (compared with lying) ↓ innocent flow murmurs, but ↑ murmurs from subaortic obstruction or from a venous hum (a hum is best heard at the right base or below the left clavicle, or in the neck—it is abolished by gently pressing the ipsilateral jugular; patent ductus murmurs are similar, but do not change with posture).

Cardiac catheter findings

Pulmonary stenosis	RV pressure↑; pulmonary artery pressure↓
+ foramen ovale	as above with right atrial pressure↑ and P_aO_2↓
VSD	RV pressure↑; RV O_2 >R atrial O_2
ASD	right atrial pressure and oxygenation↑ compared to IVC
Patent ductus	RV pressure↑; pulmonary artery O_2 >RV O_2
Fallot's tetrad	see p 748; pulmonary artery pressure >RV; RV O_2 & P_aO_2↓

Still's murmur A common innocent murmur (*peak incidence:* 4–5yrs, eg during fevers or on routine examination). It is musical, low-pitched, vibratory and mid-systolic, the left sternal edge and the apex. It may radiate to the 2nd intercostal space. Differential diagnosis: VSD (but it is crescendo–decrescendo).

Cleft lip and palate

This is the most common facial malformation. It results from failure of fusion of maxillary and premaxillary processes (during week 5). The defect runs from the lip to the nostril. It may be bilateral, when there is often a cleft in the palate as well, with the premaxillary process displaced anteriorly. Palate clefts may be large or small (eg of the uvula alone). *Incidence:* 0.8–1.7/1000. *Causes:* Genes, drugs (benzodiazepines, antiepileptics, p 161), rubella. Other malformations are present in 50% (eg trisomy 18, 13–15, or Pierre Robin syndrome, when the mandible is too small, causing cyanotic attacks). *Prevention:* Possibly folic acid ± multivitamins (p94). *Treatment:* A long-term team approach is best (orthodontist, plastic surgeon, oral/maxillofacial surgeon, GP, paediatrician and speech therapist).[1] Feeding with special teats may be necessary before plastic surgery (usually, repair of the lip is at 3 months, and of the palate at 1yr; some surgeons do the lip eg at 1 week old). Repair of unilateral complete or incomplete lesions often gives good cosmetic results. Try to refer to expert centres. There is always some residual deformity with bilateral lesions. Complications: otitis media, aspiration pneumonia, post-operative palatal fistulae, speech defects (enlist a speech therapist's help). Avoid taking to SCBU (this can hinder bonding).

Other malformations in the head and neck

Eyes Anophthalmos: there are no eyes; rare; part of trisomy 13–15.
Ectopia lentis: presents as glaucoma with poor vision. The lens margin is visible; seen in arachnodactyly, Ehlers–Danlos (p 746), homocystinuria; incidence: <1/5000; autosomal-dominant (a-Dom) or recessive (a-R).
Cataract: rubella, Down's, others: recessive or sex-linked.
Coloboma: notched iris with a displaced pupil; incidence: 2/10,000; (a-R).
Microphthalmos: small eyes; 1/1000; due to rubella—or genetic (a-Dom).

Ears Accessory auricles: seen in front of the ear; incidence: 15/1000.
Deformed ears: Treacher–Collins' syndrome (p 758).
Low-set ears: associations—Down's syndrome; congenital heart disease.

Nose and throat Choanal atresia: this presents as postnatal cyanotic attacks. A nasal catheter does not pass into the pharynx because of malformation in the nose; incidence: <1/5000.
Congenital laryngeal stridor: this may be due to laryngeal webs, or laryngomalacia (the larynx is unable to stay open); incidence <1/5000.
Laryngeal atresia: this presents as the first breaths fail to expand the lungs. Immediate tracheostomy is needed. Branchial fistula: these open at the front of sternomastoid (a remnant of the 2nd or 3rd branchial pouch); incidence: <1/5000. Branchial and thyroglossal cysts: see *OHCM* p 148.

Skull and vertebrae Brachycephaly: short, broad skull from early closure (craniostenosis) of the coronal suture; incidence: <1/1000; a-Dom. Cleidocranial dysostosis: no clavicles, enabling the shoulders to meet. Slow skull ossification, no sinuses, high-arched palate; incidence <1/5000; a-Dom.
Craniofacial dysostosis: tower skull, beaked nose, exophthalmos.
Klippel–Feil syndrome (p 752): fused cervical vertebra (so the neck is short).

CNS Hydrocephalus: incidence 0.3–2/1000. Neonatal injury, infection, or genes (sex-linked) may cause aqueduct stenosis. Dandy–Walker syn. (p 744) Arnold–Chiari malformation (*OHCM* p 694).
Microcephaly: causes—genetic, intrauterine infection (eg rubella), hypoxia, irradiation. Incidence: 1/1000. Risk of recurrence: 1/50.

Spina bifida and **anencephaly** See p 228.

Fetal alcohol syndrome The severity depends on how much alcohol the mother has used in pregnancy. Features: microcephaly, short palpebral fissure, hypoplastic upper lip, absent filtrum, small eyes, IQ↓, cardiac malformations.

1 B Morgan 1998 *BMJ* i 1462

Some words about the head and neck

Acrocephaly: This term may be applied to tower headed conditions.

Arhinencephaly: Congenital absence of the rhinencephalon.

Arthrogryposis: This term implies contracture of a joint.

Brachycephaly: The head is too short.

Cephalocele: Tntracranial contents protrude. 'Kélé' means hernia in Greek.

Craniostenosis = craniosynostosis = premature closure of skull sutures.

Dolicephalic: The head is too long.

Dystopia canthorum: Intercanthal distance is increased, but not the interpupillary or (bony) interorbital distances.

Holoprosencephaly: Hypotelorism with cleft palate.

Lissencephalic: Bat-like brain with no convolutions (agyria).

Micrognathia: The mandible is too small.

Metopic suture: This is the same as the frontal suture.

Neurocranium: That part of the skull holding the brain.

Obelion: The point on the saggital suture crossed by a line joining the parietal foramina.

Oxycephalic = Turricephaly = acrocephaly = the top of the head is pointed.

Plagiocephaly: An asymmetrical, twisted head—eg associated with irregular closure of the cranial sutures.

Rachischisis: Congenital fissure of the spinal column.

Sinciput: The anterior, upper part of the head.

Viscerocranium: Facial skeleton.

Wormian bones: Supernumerary bones in the sutures of the skull.

Neural tube defects

Spina bifida:	Having an incomplete vertebral arch.
Spina bifida occulta:	The defect is covered by skin and fascia.
Meningocele:	Dura and arachnoid mater bulge through the defect.
Myelocele:	Segments of the cord are exposed with no covering.
Myelomeningocele:	The cord's central canal is exposed.
Anencephaly:	Absent skull vault and cerebral cortex.
Encephalocele:	Part of the brain protrudes through the skull.

Prevalence (% births) USA 0.1%; UK 0.4%; Wales 0.7%; Northern Ireland 0.9%; it increases with lower social class—and homozygosity for a point mutation (C677→T; prevalence ≈ 10%, interfering with folate metabolism).[1] Recurrence risks rise 10-fold if one pregnancy has been affected, 20-fold if 2, 40-fold if 3 pregnancies affected; and 30-fold if a parent is affected.

Neurological deficit is very variable, depending on the level of the lesion, and the degree to which the lower cord functions independently from the upper cord. The defect may progress after birth[1] (and after subsequent operations); subsequent hydrocephalus gradually worsens mental performance. A child who learns to walk during his second year may outgrow his ability to support himself during the next years (weight increases as the cube of surface area, power only as its square). Those with lumbosacral myelomeningoceles usually learn to walk with calipers by the age of 3, but few with higher lesions ever walk. An unstable condition exists when there is paralysis below L3, as unopposed hip flexors and adductors are likely to dislocate the hips. Only between 5% and 13% retain their ability to walk.

Postnatal surgery Firm guidelines on whom to treat often prove too simple to apply to the individual infant. The final outcome of early closure of the defect depends on the state of the kidneys after multiple UTIs, and the extent of delayed hydrocephalus (requiring ventriculoperitoneal CSF shunts). Early post-operative mortality may account for ~25% of deaths. Many operations may be needed for spinal deformity (often severe and very hard to treat).[2]

Intrauterine diagnosis A maternal serum α-fetoprotein >90u/mL at 18 weeks[2] detects ~80% of open spina bifidas, and 90% of anencephalics, but also 3% of normal singleton fetuses, twins, and some with exomphalos, congenital nephrosis, urethral valves, Turner's syndrome, trisomy 13, and oligohydramnios. Amniocentesis and skilled ultrasound ↑pick-up rates further.

Intrauterine surgery (*eg at 23 weeks' gestation*) This is very controversial.[3]

Hurdles for the developing child

- Urinary and faecal incontinence. Penile appliances, urinary diversions or intermittent self-catheterization (for girls) save laundry and bed sores.
- Social and sexual isolation, if a special school is needed.
- The mother who 'does it all' can prevent maturity developing.
- Immobility. Mobility allowances are small and of little help.

Prevention In mothers who have already had one affected baby, there is good evidence that folic acid (5mg/day is recommended by DoH) given from before conception (as the neural tube is formed by 28 days, before pregnancy may even be recognized) reduces the risk of recurrence of neural tube defects by 72%.[2] If no previous neural tube defects, 0.4mg of folic acid is now recommended in the months before conception and for 13 weeks after. See p 94. Many mothers do not take folate pre-conception, hence the call for folate-fortification of grain. This is adopted in the USA, but is not ideal, as pernicious anaemia may be masked.[1]

1 R Whitehead 1997 *Lancet* **350** 1642 2 DoH 1991 PL/CMO (91) 11 3 C Sobkowiak 1999 *Lancet* **353** 406

►►Resuscitation after delivery[APLS]

Most newborn babies are perfectly healthy, and the best plan is to return these babies to the mother without interference, so that breast feeding and bonding may start. Those who do not breathe need prompt action to save their lives. Remember mouth to mouth-and-nose breathing if there is no equipment. A paediatrician or nurse trained in advanced paediatric resuscitation should attend the following births: emergency Caesarean sections, breeches, multiple pregnancies, instrumental deliveries for fetal distress, intrapartum bleeding, prematurity, erythroblastosis, eclampsia.

Before birth Familiarize yourself with the equipment. Heat the resuscitation crib. Ask for a warm blanket. Wash your hands. Explain that you are here to welcome the baby. It helps if she has 100% O_2 if there is fetal distress.

At birth Determine the Virginia Apgar score (see below). ►If baby is in difficulty, do not delay for scoring, but proceed as follows:
•Set a clock in motion* •Cover the baby in the crib •Extract mucus from the oropharynx with suction. Use a laryngoscope to help with this if the baby may have inhaled meconium •Assess colour, heart rate, respiratory effort.

If baby is pink, pulse >100, and good respiratory effort give to mother. *Primary apnoea* = pulse <60 + cyanosis. Give O_2 by funnel and wait 1min. *Terminal apnoea* = pulse <60, pallor + floppiness. Do gentle suction; bag & mask ventilation or intubate. *Fresh stillbirth:* Asystolic terminal apnoea: start CPR.

►►Neonatal CPR Intubate and ventilate with 100% O_2 (ensure system has a reservoir bag, and a blow-off valve set to 30–40cmH_2O) at 30–40/min.

Start cardiac massage (120 compressions/min, using index and middle fingers 1 finger breadth below internipple line to depress the sternum ~1.5cm). Give 3 chest compressions for each ventilation. If the baby fails to improve give: •*Epinephrine (=adrenaline)* 10μg/kg IV or 20μg/kg via ET (repeat every 3–5min of arrest) •*Bicarbonate* 1mmol/kg IV (4.2%).

If little response think of: •Hypothermia—dry baby and keep under heat lamp •Pneumothorax, if ventilated •Hypoglycaemia—give dextrose 25%, 2mL/kg IV •Opiate toxicity—naloxone 10μg/kg IV if mother received opiate; repeated every 2–3min if needed. •Anaemia (heavy fetal blood loss?)—give 20mL/kg 4.5% albumen, then blood •Does the baby have lung disease or congenital cyanotic heart disease (p 224)? ►Transfer to SCBU for monitoring.

Endotracheal intubation is a key skill: use 3.5mm uncuffed, unshouldered tubes on term infants; 3.0 if 2.5–1.25kg (2.5 if smaller). Learn from experts. Always have larger and smaller sizes to hand. Practise on models saves lives.

Prognosis There has been no good recent research correlating Apgar scores with survival in otherwise uncomplicated births, but older studies indicate that if the Apgar score is 0 at birth, of the few survivors, most survive intact (>80%), and most of those who are neurologically abnormal after birth recover fully. If the Apgar is <4 at 1min 17% die (48% if of low birth weight). If the Apgar is <4 at 5min 44% die.

Apgar score	*Pulse*	*Respiratory effort*	*Muscle tone*	*Colour*	*On suction*
2	>100	strong cry	active movement	pink	coughs well
1	<100	slow, irregular	limb flexion	blue limbs	depressed
0	0	nil	absent	all blue	nil

* *Love set you going like a fat gold watch.*
The midwife slapped your footsoles, and your bald cry
Took its place among the elements...

Sylvia Plath, *Morning Song*

Examination of the neonate

The aim is to discover any abnormality or problem, and to see if the mother has any questions or difficulties with her baby. The following is a recommended routine before the baby leaves hospital—or during the first week of life for home deliveries.

Before the examination Find out the weight. Was the birth and pregnancy normal? Is mother Rhesus –ve? Find a quiet, warm, well-lit room. Enlist the mother's help. Explain your aims. Does she look angry or depressed? Listen if she talks. Examine systematically, eg from head to toes.

The head Circumference (30–38cm, p 294), shape (odd shapes from a difficult labour soon resolve), fontanelles (tense if crying or intracranial pressure↑; sunken, eg if dehydrated).
The eyes: Check for red reflex, corneal opacities and conjunctivitis?
The ears: Shape and position. Are they low set (ie below the eyes)? The tip of the nose, when pressed, is a useful indicator of jaundice in European children. Breathing out of the nose (shut the mouth) tests for choanal atresia.
The complexion: Cyanosed, pale, jaundiced or ruddy (polycythaemia)?
Mouth: Look inside. Insert a finger. Is palate intact? Is suck good?

Arms and hands Single palmar creases (normal or Down's). Note waiter's (porter's) tip sign of Erb's palsy (injury to C5 and 6 trunks). Clinodactyly.

The thorax Watch the respiratory movements. Note any grunting or intercostal recession (respiratory distress). Palpate the precordium and apex beat. Listen to the heart and lungs. Inspect the vertebral column for neural tube defects.

The abdomen Expect to feel the liver and spleen. Are there any other masses? Next inspect the umbilicus. Is it healthy? Surrounding flare suggests sepsis. Next, lift the skin to assess skin turgor. Inspect the genitalia and anus. Are the orifices patent? 93% of neonates pass urine within the first 24h. Is the urinary meatus misplaced (hypospadias), and are both testes descended? The neonatal clitoris often looks rather large. Bleeding PV may be a normal variant following maternal oestrogen withdrawal.

The lower limbs Test for congenital dislocation of the hip (p 632). Avoid repeated tests as it hurts—and may induce dislocation. Can you feel the femoral pulses (to exclude coarctation)? Note talipes (p 632). Are the toes: too many, too few, or too blue?

Buttocks/sacrum Are there 'mongolian spots'? These are blue and harmless. Tufts of hair ± dimples: is there spina bifida occulta? Any pilonidal sinus?

CNS Handling the baby. Now intuition can be most helpful in deciding whether the baby is ill or well. Is he jittery (hypoxia/ischaemia, encephalopathy, hypoglycaemia, infection, hypocalcaemia)? There should be some degree of control of the head. Do the limbs move normally, and is the tone floppy or spastic? Is the response absent on one side (hemiplegia)? The Moro reflex rarely adds important information (and is uncomfortable for the baby). It is performed by sitting the baby at 45°, supporting the head. On momentarily removing the support the arms will abduct, the hands open and then the arms adduct. Stroke the palm to elicit the grasp reflex. Use the ophthalmoscope (red reflex may be absent in retinoblastoma).

Is the baby post-mature, light-for-dates or premature (p 180)?

►Discuss any abnormality with the mother and father after liaising with a senior doctor.

Neonatal intensive care

Cost: >£600/day

Neonatal intensive care is a technological development of the basic creed of first aid—ABC; A for *a*irway, B for *b*reathing, and C for *c*irculation. Success depends on mastering this trinity, and designing the best *milieu intérieur* to encourage healing and growth without developing mental retardation or spasticity. As more physiological functions are taken over by machines, monitoring the state of the *milieu intérieur* becomes ever more vital. Monitor temperature, pulse, blood pressure (intra-arterial if critical), respirations (continuous read-out device), blood gases—transcutaneous oximetry (SpO_2, *OHCM* p 658) and CO_2 monitoring, or via intra-arterial electrode, U&E, bilirubin, FBC, daily weight, weekly head circumference.

The patient is usually a prematue baby. His mortal enemies are cold, hypoglycaemia (p 238), respiratory distress syndrome (p 240), infection (p 238), intraventricular haemorrhage, apnoea and necrotizing enterocolitis (p 244).

Cold With their small volume and relatively large surface area, this is a major problem for the premature and light-for-dates baby. The problem is circumvented by using incubators which allow temperature (as well as humidity and F_iO_2) to be controlled, and also afford some protection against infection. F_iO_2 is the partial pressure of O_2 in inspired air.

Neonatal apnoeic attacks *Causes:* Respiratory centre immaturity; milk aspiration; heart failure; infection; hypoxia; hypoglycaemia; $Ca^{2+}\downarrow$; seizures.

If stimulating the baby does not restore breathing, suck out the pharynx and use bag and mask ventilation. Avoid high concentrations of O_2 to prevent retinopathy of prematurity, which may follow repeated resuscitations.
Tests in apnoea: CXR; U&E; infection screen; glucose; Ca^{2+}; Mg^{2+}.
Prevention and treatment of apnoea: If aspiration is the problem, give small feeds every 2h, or continuously infused tube feeds. Monitor SpO_2 continuously; if hypoxia develops despite an ambient O_2 of 40%, CPAP or IPPV will be necessary. Aminophylline (0.15mg/kg/h IVI) may also be useful, but levels must be monitored. Reduce the dose for persistent tachycardia (>165/min). Abrupt withdrawal may cause further apnoea. If the apnoea is thought to represent seizures, phenobarbitone may be tried.

Retinopathy of prematurity (RoP)[1] Immature retinal vessels are sensitive to high P_aO_2, as occurs during repeated resuscitations. This may lead to retinal fibrosis, detachment and visual loss. Postnatal age of onset is *later* for the more immature baby. *Prevalence (lower limits):* Babies <1000g: 53%; ≤1250g: 43%; ≤1500g: 35%.
Classification: There are 5 types, depending on site involved, the degree of retinal detachment, and extent (measured as clock hours in each eye).
Treatment: Diode laser therapy[1] causes less myopia than cryotherapy.[2]
Screening: If <1500g or ≤31 weeks' gestation. If ≤25 weeks, screen ophthalmoscopically under 0.5% cyclopentolate pupil dilatation at 6 weeks old, and 2-weekly until 36 postmenstrual weeks. Often one examination is enough if 26–31 weeks' gestation. It is best done by an ophthalmologist.

Intraventricular haemorrhage (IVH) This occurs in >40% if birth weight <1500g. It may be subependymal, subarachnoid, or directly into a ventricle or brain tissue. Possible causes: hypoxia, hypercarbia, hypotension, bleeding disorder (p 244), and, rarely, birth trauma. Suspect IVH in any neonate who deteriorates rapidly in an unexplained way. Opisthotonos, cerebral irritability, shock, deteriorating feeding skills, a bulging fontanelle with a rapidly expanding head, an exaggerated (or absent) Moro reflex, fits and somnolence are telling signs, but a high proportion (~50%) may be 'silent'. *Tests:* Ultrasound and CT confirm the diagnosis. *Complications:* Mental retardation, cerebral palsy, post-haemorrhagic hydrocephalus. Many survive unscathed. It is uncertain whether late learning and behavioural disorders occur.
Treatment: Rest, head elevation, and control of fits (p 238).

1 B Fleck 1999 *Lancet* **353** 166 2 Cryotherapy for retinopathy group 1990 *Arch Ophth* **108** 1408

UK randomized trial of extracorporeal membrane oxygenation (ECMO) This important trial ($N = 185$ neonates of ≥35 weeks' gestation) showed that ECMO done after referral to one of the five UK ECMO centres reduced deaths from severe respiratory failure (oxygenation index ≥40). Typical diagnoses were pulmonary hypertension from meconium aspiration, diaphragmatic hernia, persistent fetal circulation, sepsis, and respiratory distress syndrome. The trial had to be stopped early because independent scrutineers found the results so strongly favoured ECMO over traditional measures: 30 out of 93 died in the ECMO group, compared with 54 out of 92 in the control group. The advantage was upheld irrespective of the primary diagnosis, or the type of referring centre. The number of infants suffering severe disability at follow-up at one year was one in each group.[1]

ECMO is a complex procedure providing life-support in specialized units during respiratory failure, which obviates the need for lung gas exchange.

Patients were excluded from the trial if there was severe bleeding, pre-existing CNS damage, substantial IVH, or exposure to high pressure ventilation for >10 days, or gestation was <35 weeks. NB: more premature babies *may* benefit, eg when problems with circuitry and systemic heparinization have been solved. The need for ECMO may be ~1 per 4000 live births.

1 UK collaborative trial of neonatal extracorporeal membrane oxygenation (ECMO) *Lancet* 1996 **348** 75

Ventilation of neonates

This is a practical skill which must be learned at the cot side. Nurses are often expert, and may be best placed to teach. Needs of apparently very similar babies will vary, so that what follows is only a rough guide to prepare your mind before receiving teaching. Continuous refinement in the light of transcutaneous and blood gas analysis is needed.

Pressure-limited, time-cycled continuous flow ventilation A continuous flow of gas that is heated and humidified is passed to the infant via an endotracheal tube. The nasotracheal route is preferred (fewer tube displacements), but insertion needs more experience. *Variables:* Air/O_2 mix; maximum inspiratory pressure (P_I); positive end-expiratory pressure (PEEP); inspiratory (T_I) and expiratory (T_E) times. The infant is able to make respiratory efforts between ventilator breaths (intermittent mandatory ventilation, IMV). Aim for a prolonged inspiratory time (1–1.5sec) and a T_I / T_E ratio of ≥1 for severe respiratory distress syndrome. If less severe, a T_I / T_E ratio of <1 may be tried (pneumothorax risk ↓).
Initial settings: Choose to give good chest excursion and air entry on auscultation and adequate transcutaneous O_2 readings. Typical settings might be T_I 1sec, 20–25 cycles/min, inspiratory pressure 14–16cmH_2O, and PEEP 5cmH_2O. Adjust in the light of blood gas analysis.

PEEP (Positive end-expiratory pressure) A loaded valve is fitted to the expiratory limb of the ventilator, so airways pressure stays ≥atmosphere. Levels >10cmH_2O are rarely used (venous return to the thorax ↓).

CPAP (Continuous positive airways pressure) Pressure is raised throughout the respiratory cycle, so assisting spontaneous inspiration. With skill, this method has few complications, and is useful as a first stage in ventilating a baby before it is known whether he will need IMV.

PTV (Patient-triggered ventilation) With traditional ventilation, the baby may fight the ventilator, trying to expire during inflations: hence the need for paralysis: but this makes the baby entirely dependent on the ventilator, fluid retention is common, and contractures may develop in limbs. One answer is PTV in which inspiratory and end-expiratory pressure is set by the operator, but the rate set by the baby.[1]

Muscle paralysis Pancuronium (0.02–0.03mg/kg IV; then 0.03–0.09mg/kg every 1.5–4h to maintain paralysis) prevents pneumothorax in infants 'fighting the ventilator' (eg needing an unexpectedly high P_I).

Pain relief Consider 5% dextrose IVI+morphine 100–200μg/kg over 30min, then 5–15μg/kg/h.[1,2] This is thought to be safe, and reduces catecholamine concentrations—a possible objective correlate of pain and stress.

Weaning from the ventilator Decrease the rate of IMV and lower the P_I by eg 2cm H_2O decrements. Try extubation when blood gases are adequate with a PEEP of ~2cmH_2O with spontaneous breathing.
Air leak: Air ruptures alveoli and tracks along vessels and bronchioles (pulmonary interstitial emphysema), and may extend intrapleurally (pneumothorax with lung collapse), or into the mediastinum or peritoneum. *Signs:* Tachypnoea, cyanosis, chest asymmetry. The lateral decubitus CXR is often diagnostic. Prompt 'blind' needle aspiration of a pneumothorax may be needed. Aspirate through the second intercostal space in the midclavicular line with a 25G 'butterfly' needle and a 50mL syringe on a 3-way tap. If the leak is continuous, use underwater seal drainage.

Retinopathy of prematurity p 232 Bronchopulmonary dysplasia p 235.

1 A Greenough 1992 *Arch Dis Chi* 67 69 2 *Drug Ther Bul* 1994 21

Bronchopulmonary dysplasia

This condition, also called *chronic lung disease of prematuritiy*, was first described in 1967, as a syndrome of chronic lung disease in premature babies who had had mechanical ventilation for respiratory distress syndrome. There is persistent hypoxaemia, and difficulty weaning from the ventilator.

Tests: CXR: hyperinflation, rounded, radiolucent areas, alternating with thinner strands of radiodensity.

Histology: Necrotizing bronchiolitis and alveolar fibrosis.

Mortality: About 40%.[1]

Early sequelae: Decreased cognition, cerebral palsy, feeding problems. O_2 desaturation during feeds is not uncommon.[2]

Late sequelae: By adolescence/early adulthood the main changes remaining are airways obstruction, airways hyper-reactivity, and hyperinflation.[1]

Pulmonary hypoplasia

Suspect this in all infants with persisting neonatal tachypnoea ± feeding difficulties, particularly if oligohydramnios has been noted in pregnancy (this is not a universal association, and, if swallowing is affected, there may be polyhydramnios—the Pena–Shokeir syndrome). Hypoplasia may be secondary to causes of oligohydramnios such as diaphragmatic hernia—or it may be a primary developmental abnormality. Diagnosis may be at postmortem, or, if facilities are available, by measuring functional residual capacity. CXR is likely to misleadingly reported as normal. The condition need not be fatal: postnatal catch-up growth has been well documented.[3]

1 W Northway 1992 *NEJM* **333** 1793 2 L Singer 1992 **90** 380 3 NR Aiton 1996 *BMJ* **i** 1149

Neonatal jaundice

To detect jaundice in non-Caucasian babies, press the nose.

Hyperbilirubinaemia (<200μmol/L) after the first day of life is common and may be 'physiological' (eg in binding free radicals). Mechanisms:
1 Hepatic immaturity in bilirubin uptake and conjugation.
2 Excessive removal and destruction of fetal red cells.
3 A low plasma albumin (so unconjugated bilirubin is left unbound).
4 Absence of gut flora impeding bile pigment elimination.
5 Poor fluid intake, or breast feeding (inhibiting factors—and is not a reason to stop breast feeding).

Jaundice within 24h of birth is always pathological. *Causes:*
- Rhesus haemolytic disease: +ve direct Coombs' test (DCT, p 242).
- ABO incompatibility: (mother O; baby A or B) DCT +ve or –ve. Send maternal blood for haemolysins (also for other rare blood group incompatibilities, eg anti-C, E, c, e, Kell, Duffy).
- Red cell anomalies: congenital spherocytosis (do blood film); glucose-6-phosphate dehydrogenase deficiency (do enzyme test).

Tests in all patients: FBC; film; blood groups; Coombs' test; urine for reducing agents; infection screen, p 238 (an important cause).

Prolonged jaundice (not fading after 7–10 days) Causes: Hypothyroidism (vital not to miss; do T_4 and TSH); *biliary atresia*—►Exclude this in *all* who continue to be jaundiced after 14 days by testing for conjugated and unconjugated bilirubin. *Galactosaemia:* urine tests for reducing agents (eg Clinitest®) are +ve, but specific tests for glycosuria are –ve. This test is insensitive. Red cell galactose-1-phosphate levels are diagnostic.

Kernicterus May occur if bilirubin is >360μmol/L (lower in prems).
Stage I: Sleepy; reduced suck; lethargic feeding.
Stage II: T°↑; restless; odd mouth movement; lid retraction (*setting sun*).
Stage III: Latent phase.
Stage IV: Subsequent cerebral palsy; deafness; IQ↓ (later).

Lesser levels of bilirubin (170–323μmol/L) are unlikely to give rise to permanent problems, and have little effect on later IQ unless the infant is preterm or light-for-dates (eg 0.009–0.018 IQ points/μmol/L).

Methods of reducing plasma bilirubin Phototherapy lamps may be used if the jaundice is mild. It is not a substitute for exchange transfusion. SE: cold; fluid loss (give 30mL/kg/day extra water). *Start phototherapy at the following plasma bilirubin levels:* Term baby at age 48h: 230μmol/L. (At 72h 250μmol/L; at 4 days 275μmol/L at 5 days 300μmol/L.) In prems or low-birth-weight babies reduce these thresholds by at least 25μmol/L. Stop phototherapy when levels fall (eg by >25μmol/L) below these thresholds. NB: this is a guide. Most units have their own protocol.

Exchange transfusion Uses warmed blood (37°C), crossmatched against maternal and infant serum, given via umbilical vein IVI. Aim to exchange 160mL/kg over ~2h (twice the blood volume). IV Ca^{2+} is not needed if citrate phosphate dextrose blood is used. Monitor ECG, U&E, Ca^{2+}, bilirubin and glucose. More exchanges may be needed if bilirubin goes on rising. *Stop the exchange transfusion* if the heart rate fluctuates by >20 beats/min. ►Ensure that the volumes exchanged always balance. If anaemic, consider a simple fresh blood transfusion (20mL/kg).
Plasma bilirubin levels at which exchange transfusion is indicated: Term baby at birth, 50μmol/L; at 12h, 125μmol/L; at 24h, 200μmol/L; at 36h, 250μmol/L; at 48h, 325μmol/L; at 72h, 350μmol/L; at 4 days, 375μmol/L; at 5 days, 400μmol/L. If the baby is premature or weighs <2.5 kg lower these thresholds (eg by 50μmol/L, after age 48h).

►►The ill neonate

Overwhelming infection Neonatal sepsis is common (1–10/1000 births), and it may quickly become overwhelming, when mortaility is 15–50%. Signs may be minimal, or as opposite.

Action: Clear the airway; intubate and ventilate if necessary. This will correct acidosis, so bicarbonate is rarely needed. Set up a colloid IVI (20mL/kg initially). Exclude hypoglycaemia; do blood gases.
Infection screen: •Blood-culture, virology, FBC, platelets, glucose.
•Lumbar puncture: CSF (p 258) for urgent Gram stain, cell count, culture, glucose estimation and virology. •Stool: for virology.
•Urine: microscopy, culture and virology. •ENT swabs: for culture.

Antibiotics: In early onset infection (<48h old) group B streptococci and *E coli* (as well as any other organism prevalent in your SCBU) are common pathogens. Dose example: benzylpenicillin 25mg/kg/12h + netilmicin 3mg/kg/12h both slowly IV. Monitor netilmicin levels, U&E and creatinine, adjusting the dose as indicated in the *Data sheet* if renal function is impaired. Cefotaxime is a good alternative (p 258). In late onset infection (>48h old) staphylococci are likely pathogens, so regimens include flucloxacillin (eg 125mg/6h IV over 3min) or a cefalosporin.

If the CSF suggests meningitis, see p 258. Note: a CSF WCC of up to $30/mm^3$ with 60% polymorphs may be normal in neonates.

Neonatal seizures (3–6/1000 births) *Causes:* Hypoxia; infection; hypoglycaemia; hypocalcaemia (<1.7mmol/L); plasma Mg^{2+} <4mmol/L; CNS damage (haemorrhage, hydrocephalus, CNS cysts, tuberous sclerosis).

Treatment: Turn on the side.
- Diazepam 0.1–0.3mg/kg IV slowly.
- Rule out (or treat) hypoglycaemia (5mL/kg 10% dextrose IV over 5min, then 100mL/kg/day IVI; then give hourly feeds reducing IVI rate as blood glucose estimations allow).
- Phenobarbitone 10mg/kg slow IV + 10mg/kg 1h later if needed. (Maintenance dose: reduce slowly from 2mg/kg/12h IV/PO. Monitor blood level. Aim for 30–45μg/mL >4h after a PO dose.)
- If seizures continue, give phenytoin 10–15mg/kg IVI in 0.9% saline (<1mg/kg/min). (Plasma level of 10–20μg/mL >1h post dose.)
- If fits continue, give pyridoxine 50mg IV.

Hypocalcaemia: Use low PO_4^{3-} milk + calcium gluconate 10%, 4.4mL/kg/day PO. IV dose: 0.2mL/kg diluted in 4.8mL/kg of 0.9% saline over 10min. Monitor ECG.

Hypomagnesaemia: Give magnesium chloride 10mg, 0.3mL/kg/6h PO.

Shock Causes include blood loss (placental haemorrhage, twin-to-twin transfusion; intraventricular haemorrhage; lung haemorrhage); capillary plasma leaks (sepsis, hypoxia, acidosis, necrotizing enterocolitis); fluid loss (D&V; ↑insensible loss, eg sweat; inappropriate diuresis); cardiogenic causes (hypoxia, hypoglycaemia, L to R shunts, valve disease, coarctation).

Signs: Pulse ↑; BP ↓; urine output ↓; coma.

Management: Ventilate as needed. Treat causes. Aim for a CVP of 5–8cmH_2O. Give colloid 10–20mL/kg IV over 30–60min, with dobutamine 5–15μg/kg/min as needed (which may be combined with dopamine 5–20μg/kg/min to produce the optimal effect). If the pH is <7.2, bicarbonate, eg 1–2mmol/kg IV as a 4.2% solution, may be indicated (once adequate ventilation is established).

Diagnosing neonatal sepsis

This is often difficult as signs may be nonspecific, and culture results take time—and time is most definitely *not* on your side. Signs include:

- Unusual crying • Sleepiness • Listlessness • Shock • Fits/apnoea
- Hypotonia • Vomiting • Rashes • T° ↑or ↓ • Bradycardia

Also: feeding difficulty, abdominal wall reddening (omphalitis), grunting, rib recession, use of respiratory muscles, tachypnoea and cyanosis.

Nonspecific and probably unreliable tests include C-reactive protein, FBC & film: looking at the ratio of immature to total neutrophils *may* help.

The furure: It is possible that looking for soluble immunological mediators may help: the ideal ones may be interleukin-1 receptor antagonist (IL-1ra), and interleukin-6 (IL-6). Specificity: 92 and 83%, respectively. Circulating intercellular adhesion molecule-1 (cICAM-1) is less reliable.

Blood and other cultures are definitive, but take ~72 hours.

1 MWeiss 1998 *Lancet* **352** 1271

Respiratory distress syndrome (RDS)

Insufficient surfactant is made so that the lungs are unable to stay expanded; re-inflation between breaths exhausts the baby, and respiratory failure follows. It is the major cause of death from prematurity.

Infants at risk: 100% if 24–28 weeks' gestation; 50% if 32 weeks. Also: maternal diabetes, male sex, second twin, Caesarean birth.

Prenatal prevention See p 102.

Signs Worsening tachypnoea (>60/min) in the hours after birth. Increased inspiratory effort, with grunting, flaring of the nasal alae, intercostal recession and cyanosis. CXR: diffuse granular patterns, with air bronchograms. Mild signs subside after ~36h.

Differential diagnosis *Transient tachypnoea of the newborn* is due to excess lung fluid. It usually resolves after 24h. *Meconium aspiration* (p 244); congenital pneumonia (group B streptococci); tracheo-oesophageal fistula (suspect if respiratory problems after feeds).

Treatment Learn this skill at the cot side. If gestation <~28 weeks, intubate at birth and, if >700g, give surfactant by ET tube, eg synthetic pumactant (100mg, repeat at 1h and 24h if needed: monitor P_aO_2 as needs may suddenly↓ or pork 'poractant' (Curosurf® 100–200mg/kg, ± second dose in 12h). Rock gently to promote spread in the bronchial tree.

- Wrap up warmly and take to SCBU incubator.
- Monitor blood gases (eg transcutaneously). Aim for a P_aO_2 of 7–12 kPa, enhancing the ambient O_2 with a perspex head box.
- If blood gases deteriorate intubate and ventilate (p 234), before the infant becomes exhausted. Start with CPAP, eg 5cmH_2O (p 234). A rising P_aCO_2 may indicate either that CPAP is too high, or that paralysis and further ventilation is needed (CPAP = continuous positive airways pressure).
- *Traditional ventilator settings:* Inspiratory pressure 20cmH_2O with 60% O_2; positive end-expiratory pressure 3–5cmH_2O; 20–25 breaths/min, with an inspiratory duration of 1sec. On connecting the endotracheal tube check chest movement is adequate and symmetrical. Listen for breath sounds. P_aO_2 is increased by ↑pressures (not too high). P_aCO_2 is decreased by lengthening the expiratory time, or ↑breath frequency by lessening inspiratory time. One trial indicates that *high-frequency oscillatory ventilation* is better (*N*=125 neonates ≤35weeks' gestation).[1] Get expert help.
- ►If any deterioration, consider: blocked tube, infection, faulty ventilator, pneumothorax.
- Fluids: avoid oral feeding. Give 10% dextrose IVI (p 246).

Signs of a poor prognosis Persistent pulmonary hypertension, large right to left shunt via the ductus.[2]

If, despite everything, hypoxia worsens, the baby is dying. Explain this to the mother, emphasizing that the baby will feel no pain. Encourage her to christen the baby. Seek senior advice and consider 115.5μg/kg/IM of papavaretum 7.7mg/mL (=0.15mL/kg of one 7.7mg ampoule diluted with 9mL water). Disconnect the tubes, so allowing the mother to hold the baby, and, in so doing, to aid her grief.[3]

1 DR Gerstmann 1996 *Pediatrics* **98** 1044 & E-BM **2** 83 2 FJ Walther 1992 *Paediatrics* **90** 899
3 Roy Col Paed & Child Health 1997 *Withholding or Withdrawing Life-saving Treatment in Children.*

3. Paediatrics

Rhesus haemolytic disease

Physiology When a RhD–ve mother delivers a RhD+ve baby a leak of fetal red cells into her circulation may stimulate her to produce anti-D IgG antibodies (isoimmunization). In later pregnancies this can cross the placenta, causing worsening rhesus haemolytic disease (*erythroblastosis fetalis*) with each successive Rh+ve pregnancy. first pregnancies may be affected due to leaks, eg: •Threatened miscarriage •APH, •Mild trauma •Amniocentesis •Chorionic villous sampling •External cephalic version.

An affected oedematous fetus (with stiff, oedematous lungs) is called a *hydrops fetalis*. Oedema occurs as the liver is devoted to producing new RBCs (so albumin ↓, leading to ↓oncotic pressure).

Clinical Rh disease ► *Test for D antibodies in all Rh–ve mothers, at booking, 28 and 34 weeks' gestation.* Anti-D titres <4u/mL (<1:16) are very unlikely to produce serious disease; it is wise to check maternal blood every 2 weeks. If >10u/mL, get the advice of a referral centre: fetal blood sampling ± intraperitoneal (or, with fetoscopy, intravascular via the cord) transfusion may be needed. Expect fetal Hb to be <7g/dL in 10% of those with titres of 10–100u/mL (75% if titres >100u/mL).

Do regular ultrasound and amniocentesis and if anti-D titre >4u/mL. Timing is vital. Do it 10 weeks before a Rh-related event in the last pregnancy (eg if last baby needed delivery at 36 weeks, expect to do amniocentesis at ~26 weeks). Fetuses tolerating high bilirubins may be saved risky transfusions (fatality 2–30%) if monitored by serial measurements of fetal Hb (by fetoscopy) and skilled daily ultrasound, to detect oedema, cardiomegaly, pericardial effusion, hepatosplenomegaly or ascites.

Anti-D is the most common antibody. Others: Rh C, D, E, c, e, Kell, Kidd, Duffy (all are IgG). Relatively low concentrations sometimes produce severe disease.

Signs

•Jaundice on day1 (or later)
•Heart failure (oedema, ascites)
•Progressive anaemia; bleeding
•Yellow vernix
•Hepatosplenomegaly
•CNS signs

Tests

Hb ↓ •Direct Coombs' +ve*
•Anti-Rh agglutinins present
•Mother Rh–ve, baby Rh+ve
•Anti-Rh titre ↑ in mother
•Reticulocytes ↑
•Bilirubin ↑
•Hypoglycaemia

Exchange transfusion *Indications and technique:* p 236.
If Hb <7g/dL, give the first volume of the exchange transfusion (80mL/kg) as packed cells, and subsequent exact exchanges according to response. ► Keep the baby warm.

Ultraviolet photodegradation of bilirubin (with phototherapy lamp) may be all that is needed for mild cases. Give extra water (30mL/kg/24h PO). Avoid heat loss. Protect the eyes.

Kernicterus See p 236.

Giving Rh–ve mothers anti-D Ig ► See p 109.

*The direct Coombs' test identifies red cells coated with antibody or complement and a positive result usually indicates an immune cause of haemolysis (OHCM p 584).

3. Paediatrics

Other neonatal problems

Necrotizing enterocolitis (NEC) This is death of bowel mucosa. Typically it occurs at the end of the first week of life in a prem infant on SCBU (it affects 1–2% of admissions to SCBU). If mild, a little blood and mucus may be passed per rectum. At worst, there is sudden abdominal distension, tenderness (± perforation), shock, DIC, and sloughing of the rectal mucosa. It may be sporadic or epidemic. *Treatment:* If mild, barrier nurse the baby; culture faeces; stop oral feeding; do plain erect and supine abdominal x-rays, to look for oedematous loops of bowel with intramural gas. If more severely affected, crossmatch blood; give metronidazole 7mg/kg/12h IV with penicillin and netilmicin (p 238). Do repeated radiology and girth measurement. Liaise early with a surgeon. Indications for laparotomy: progressive distension, perforation.

Meconium aspiration Only thick meconium is important (aspiration pneumonitis). Using a laryngoscope, the pharynx and trachea should be sucked out at birth. Intubate the trachea with the largest comfortable tube. 2–3 intubations with sucking withdrawals are repeated to clear as much meconium as possible. The obstetrician may try compressing the thorax as he passes the baby to the paediatrician, so minimizing inspiratory effort until the airway is clear (but this does not stop diaphragm effort). Ventilation with CPAP or IMV may be needed (p 234). Try a PEEP of 6cm H_2O and an inspiratory time of 0.5–0.75sec. Give penicillin + netilmicin (p 238).

Haemorrhagic disease of the newborn occurs from days 2–7 postpartum; it is due to lack of vitamin K (no enteric bacteria, or mother taking anticonvulsants). The baby is usually well, but develops unexplained bruising and bleeding. Prothrombin and partial thromboplastin times (PT and PTT) are prolonged; platelets normal. Prevention: vitamin K eg 2mg IM (oral route: see ref 1) ►*Formula milk already contains vitamin K.* *Treatment:* Give plasma (10mL/kg IV) and vit. K (eg 1mg IV) for active bleeding (monitor coagulation).

Disseminated intravascular coagulation (DIC) The baby is usually ill (and often infected), and may have petechiae, oozing from venepuncture sites and GI haemorrhage. Platelets ↓, fibrin degradation products ↑, INR and partial thromboplastin time ↑, schistocytes (fragmented RBCs).
Treatment: •Treat cause (eg infection, NEC); vitamin K 1mg IV.
•Platelet transfusion, to keep platelets $>30 \times 10^9$/L.
•Replace clotting factors with fresh plasma (eg 10mL/kg by IVI).
•If bleeding continues, consider an exchange transfusion.

Immune thrombocytopenia <10% of babies of women with autoimmune thrombocytopenia may develop thrombocytopenia after birth (p 142). *Alloimmune thrombocytopenia:* Affecting 1:2000 live births this is due fetomaternal incompatability of platelet antigens. It develops *in utero*. 40–60% of babies are first born (it recurs in 75–90% of subsequent pregnancies with same or increased severity). Of babies affected *in utero* 25% have a developmental abnormality; 10% an intracerebral haemorrhage *in utero*. Platelets continue to fall for 48h post-delivery. Severe thrombocytopenia is treated with compatible platelets or irradiated maternal platelets. IgG 1g/kg/24h IVI for 1–3 days may help. Cordocentesis from 24 weeks may be needed in subsequent pregnancies.[4] Diagnose by detecting maternal platelet alloantibody against fathers platelets (not detectable in 20%).

Minor neonatal problems

Milia: These tiny cream papules on the nose and sometimes on the palate (Ebstein's pearls) are sebaceous cysts. They disappear.

Erythema toxicum (neonatal urticaria): These are harmless red blotches, often with a central white vesicle which come and go in crops. They last ~24h (try ringing them), in contrast to septic spots which develop obvious pustules. If in doubt take a swab. Ask for a Wright's stain: neutrophils indicate sepsis; eosinophils suggest erythema toxicum.

Miliaria/heat rash: This itchy red rash fades rapidly when the baby is unwrapped.

Stork mark: These are areas of capillary dilatation on the eyelids, central forehead and back of the neck—where the baby is deemed to have been held in the stork's beak. They blanch on pressure and fade with time.

Harlequin colour change: One side of the face or body suddenly flushes for a few minutes. It is a shortlived vasomotor event.

Peeling skin: Common in postmature babies, it does not denote future skin problems. Olive oil prevents skin folds from cracking.

Petechial haemorrhages, facial cyanosis, subconjunctival haemorrhages: These temporary features generally reflect suffusion of the face during delivery (sometimes inaccurately referred to as 'traumatic asphyxia').

Swollen breasts: These occur in both sexes and occasionally lactate (witch 's milk). They are due to maternal hormones and gradually subside if left alone, but if infected require antibiotics.

The umbilicus: It dries and separates through a moist base at about day 7. Signs of infection: odour, pus, periumbilical red flare, malaise. Isolate the baby, take swabs and blood cultures, give antibiotics. Granuloma: exclude a patent urachus and cauterize with a silver nitrate stick

Sticky eye: (Common; usually from an unopened tear duct, p 482.) Swab to exclude *ophthalmia neonatorum* (p 100)/chlamydia (special swab).

Feeding anxieties: Healthy term babies require little milk for the first few days and early poor feeding is not an indication for investigation or bottle top-ups. The exceptions are babies of diabetic mothers, and light-for-dates babies, because of their risk of hypoglycaemia.

New babies may have difficulty co-ordinating feeding and breathing and briefly choke, gag or turn blue. Exclude disease, check feeding technique (too much? too fast?) and reassure.

Regurgitation is often due to overfilling a tiny stomach with milk and air. Check feeding technique; if bottle fed, is the teat too big for the mouth or the hole too small or the amount too great?

Winding during feeds may help but is not essential to health.

Red-stained nappy: This is usually due to urinary urates but may be blood from the cord or baby's vagina (oestrogen withdrawal bleed).

Sneezing: Neonates sneeze to clear amniotic fluid from the nose.

1 A new oral mixed micelle vit K formulation is becoming available: F Greer 1998 Arch Dis Chi **79** 300 & J Trip ibid page 295; see also G Draper 1994 BMJ **i** 867 & E Letsky 1996 *Br J Haematol* **95** 21

Enteral and parenteral feeding

Enteral feeding *Indications:* Any sick infant who is too ill or too young to feed normally (eg respiratory distress syndrome). It is best achieved by continuous infusion of expressed breast milk (from the baby's own mother) via a silastic nasojejunal tube (the least risk of aspiration). After entering the stomach, the tube enters the jejunum by peristalsis. Confirm its position by x-ray. Other milks: cow with added carbohydrate (eg Cow and Gate Plus®, New Ostermilk Two®); skimmed cow's milk with fats and minerals (eg SMA®); skimmed cow's milk with less whey (eg SMA Gold Cap®), in which the casein to whey ratio is similar to breast milk's. Volume to infuse (for neonates): ~150mL/kg/day. Breast milk is still probably the best food for premature infants—but add vitamin D 1000u/day and vitamin K 2–3μg/day—and extra phosphate if plasma phosphate is < 1.5mmol/L.

Indications for IV feeding •After surgery, trauma, or burns.
•When oral nutrition is poor; eg in ill, low-birth-weight babies.
•Necrotizing enterocolitis (when the gut must be 'rested').

Parenteral nutrition (PN) Day-by-day guide. ►All values are per kg/day.

			PROTEIN	CARBOHYDRATE		FAT	IONS		FLUID
Type of baby	Day of PN	Age days	Vamin®[1] (mL)	mL dextrose 5%	20%[2]	Intralipid 10% (mL)	mmol Na	K	PN vol (mL)/ total need[3]
Neonates	1	3	7	–	36	10	2.7	2.4	53/90
and	1	4&5	7	60	22	10	2.7	2.4	99/120
Low-birth-	1	≥6	7	120	6	10	2.7	2.4	143/150
weight	2	4&5	10	20	40	10	2.5	2.3	80/150
babies	2	≥6	10	80	25	10	2.5	2.3	125/150
	3	5	14	–	43	20	2.3	2.2	77/150
	3	≥6	14	60	28	20	2.3	2.2	108/150
	4	≥6	21	20	44	20	2.0	2.1	105/150
	5	>6	28	–	56	30	1.6	1.9	114/150
	M	>6	35	–	52–62	35	1.25	1.8	≥122/150
Infants	1		7	120	6	10	2.7	2.4	143/*
>1 month	2		14	80	23	10	2.3	2.2	127/*
& <10kg	3		21	20	44	20	2.0	2.1	105/*
	M		35	–	52	30	1.25	1.8	117/*
10–30kg	1&2		14	–	15	15	2.0	2.0	44/*
	M		28	–	21–26	20–30	1.5	1.5	69–84/*
>30kg	1&2		14	12	–	10	2.0	2.0	36/*
	M		21	–	4–30	20–25	1.5	1.5	45–76/*

Note: M = maintenance. *See p 250 for 24h fluid requirement.

1 Vamin® with 10% glucose. 2 If 10% dextrose is used, double the volume. Both dextrose solutions are needed. 3 This is the total volume of fluid required (60 and 75mL/kg for days 1 and 2). Ca^{2+} and other elements are given to infants as Ped-el® 4mL/kg/day if renal function good. **Vitamins** Solvito N®: add 0.5mL/kg/day (≤5mL/day) to Vamin® (protect from light). Add vitamins A, D, and K as Vitlipid N Infant®, 1mL/kg/day (≤4mL/day), to Intralipid®.
►These values are a guide only. *Individual needs vary greatly. Get an expert's advice.*
►Sterility is vital. Prepare using laminal flow units. Give into a central vein.

Regular checks *Daily:* Check weight; fluid balance; U&E; blood glucose; Ca^{2+}. Turbid plasma means too much Intralipid® has been given. Urine electrolytes and osmolality (every 48h from week 1). Test for glycosuria. Change IVI sets and filters. Culture: filters, Vamin® and Intralipid® samples. *Weekly:* Length and head circumference; skin fold thickness. LFTs; Mg^{2+}; PO_4^{3-}; alk phos; ammonia; lipids; FBC. Infection screen (p 238).

Complications Infection; acidosis; metabolic imbalances; hepatic dysfunction. If plasma PO_4^{3-}↓, consider giving PO_4^{3-} (0.25–0.5mmol/kg/day) as the potassium salt. Mix with dextrose, but not Vamin® or trace element mixtures.

Stopping IV nutrition Do in stages to prevent hypoglycaemia.

3. Paediatrics

►►The ill and feverish child

There are 2 distinct questions to ask: *How severe are the symptoms* and *How appropriate is the child's response to the illness?* The symptom may be severe (eg 'terrible diarrhoea all over the cot') without being biologically serious (if the baby is alert, drinking, wetting many nappies, and behaving as usual); but ANY apparently mild symptom should set your internal alarm bell ringing if:[1,2]

- < Half the usual amount of feed has been taken in the last day.
- There is breathing difficulty, or high-pitched continuous moans.
- There is a history of being pale, mottled, cyanosed, and hot.
- Dull expression; apathetic; uninterested in you; drowsy; dehydrated.
- Fewer than 4 wet nappies in the last 24h. • Blood in the diarrhoea.

For recognizing severe illness, and treating the moribund ►see p 175.

The above carry particular weight in the immunocompromized (eg neonates; post measles; AIDS; cystic fibrosis; leukaemia; chemotherapy for malignancy; absent spleen; B/T cell dysfunction).

Fever The most common 'emergency' presentation in paediatrics. In most, the cause is a viral infection, otitis media or pharyngitis/tonsillitis (p 556)—and the prognosis is good. Here, fever may have some *beneficial* effects (enhanced neutrophil migration and secretion of antibacterials, increased production and activity of interferon, increased T-cell proliferation).[1] The challenge is to identify those feverish children with serious bacterial infections who need prompt treatment.

Bacteraemia This occurs in ~4% of febrile children, sometimes without an obvious focus of infection; this is made more likely if the child is between 3 and 24 months of age with fevers of ≥40°C, and a WCC >15 × 10^9/L (but using these criteria alone, 50% of those with bacteraemia will be missed). An ESR >30mm/h and a raised C-reactive protein may also indicate bacterial infection. Examples of organisms: *Strep pneumoniae, H influenzae, N meningitidis.* If blind antibiotics are started (eg if there is shock), they must cover these organisms (p 258 and p 260). *Cefotaxime:* 50mg/kg/8–12h IV over 20min or *ceftriaxone* 20–45mg/kg once daily IM; use IVI route over 30min for top dose (50–80mg/kg/day; max 4g daily); 20–50mg/kg/day IVI over 1h if <7 days old).

Finding a focus of infection entails a good history and examination, CXR ± LP (if the child is ill, see above). If ill and no focus of infection is found, it may be wise to withold antibiotics, and to review the child yourself after 1h. Watching and waiting is not the easiest rôle, and depends critically on the presence of a skilled nurse whose opinions you trust. However, dividends may be great: eg if a rash or diarrhoea develops, you know you are observing the illness as it unfolds, and not an antibiotic side-effect.

Encephalitis (Rarer than septicaemia) This is characterized by consciousness↓, odd behaviour ± seizures. An infective cause is suggested by fever and meningism. Consider: herpes simplex (for aciclovir treatment, see p 256), mumps, rubella, influenza, measles, mycoplasma, rickettsia, toxoplasmosis (*OHCM* p 208). Note: non-infective causes (encephalopathy) include kernicterus (p 236), hepatic failure (eg Reye's syndrome), lead poisoning.

►Urinary infections often present as fever: get a 'clean catch' if you can, p 188.

►Consider malaria whenever the child has been to a malarious area (even for a 'stop-over'). Do not wait to see how the illness unfolds: do a thick blood film at once, and enlist expert help.

In prolonged fever, consider: endocarditis; Still's (p 758); malignancy.

1 MJ Kluger 1992 *Paediatrics* **90** 846   2 P Hewson 1990 *Arch Dis Chi* **65** 750

3. Paediatrics

Fluid regimens[APLS]

If tolerated, always use *oral* rehydration. Rehidrat® and Dioralyte® come in sachets, and contain glucose, Na^+ and K^+. Show mother how to make it up (water is the vital ingredient!). If breast feeding, continue.

Daily IV water, Na and K (mmol/kg/day) MAINTENANCE needs[1]

Age	*Weight*	*Water (mL/kg/day)*	*Na^+*	*K^+*
<0.5yr	<5kg	150	3	3
0.5–1yr	5–10kg	120	2.5	2.5
1–3yr	10–15kg	100	2.5	2.5
3–5yr	15–20kg	80	2	2
>5yr	>20kg	45–75	1.5–2	1.5–2

Use dextrose saline for these requirements (0.18% sodium chloride + 4% dextrose; few calories, but prevents ketosis). Pre-existing deficits and continuing loss must also be made good. Reliable input-output fluid balance charts are essential.

Calculating pre-existing deficit ≈ % dehydration × weight (kg) × 10—give eg as 0.45% saline over 24h (eg 750mL for a 10kg child who is 7.5% dehydrated). Add in K^+ (20mmol/500mL) once the child has passed urine.

Estimating dehydration *Mild dehydration:* •Decreased urine output.

5% dehydration: •Dry mucous membranes •Decreased urine output.

10% dehydration: The above + •Sunken fontanelle (but if crying, pressure↑) •Eyeball pressure ↓ (difficult to assess if young) •Pulse ↑ •Hoarse cry.

>10%: •↑ severity of the above, with: •Shock •Drowsiness •Hypotension. If a recent weight is known, this is useful in quantifying dehydration.

IV fluids for the first 24h in MILD dehydration If the oral route is impossible, give maintenance needs (above), and start oral fluids when possible.

IV fluids for the first 24h in 5–10% dehydration•Give maintenance water requirement (above) + the deficit. Keep the rate <25mL/kg/h.
- Measure and replace ongoing losses (eg from the bowel).
- Monitor U&E on admission, and at 2, 12 and 24h. Also do PCV.

►►IV fluid replacement in the first 24h in >10% dehydration
- If IV access fails, use the intraosseous route (p 309) and get help to retry IVI.
- 0.9% saline (or plasma, if desperate) at 25mL/kg/h IVI, while calculations are performed. Continuously monitor pulse, BP, ECG.
- Continue until BP rises, pulses are felt, and urine flows (catheterize).
- Then give the daily requirement and the fluid deficit as described above, making good continuing loss with 0.18% or 0.45% saline depending on type of dehydration.
- Measure plasma and urine creatinine and osmolality (p 280), and plasma bicarbonate. Metabolic acidosis usually corrects itself.

Guidelines for success: 1 Stay at the bedside; use clinical state + biochemistry to adapt IVI. 2 Be simple 3 Beware hidden loss (oedema, ascites, GI pools). 4 Measure U&E and urine electrolytes often.

Hypernatraemic dehydration: (ie greater water loss than salt, eg from wrongly made feeds). It causes intracellular dehydration (± fits, CNS thrombosis). Rehydrate slowly with 0.45% saline (replace deficit over 48h, lowering Na^+ by <12mmol/L/24h, and giving only 60% of maintenance volume) to avoid brain oedema (p 256). The chief danger is too rapid rehydration. Hyperglycaemia is common, but self-correcting.

1 APLS group 1993 *Advanced Paediatric Life Support* BMA

3. Paediatrics

►►Poisoning: general management

- Find the name and quantity of the poison ingested. The number of tablets dispensed is often recorded on the bottle. The dispenser may also have a record and be able to name the tablets; or try the BMA's *Drug Finder Index*.
- When was the poison ingested? Has he or she vomited since? If the child is *comatose*, enlist expert help. Proceed thus:
- Place in the *semi-prone recovery position*. Note the pupil size.
- Have *suction*, O_2, *a laryngoscope* and *endotracheal tube* to hand.
- Do ward test for *blood glucose*. Treat hypoglycaemia (p 262).
- If there is respiratory failure (do blood gases), summon expert help. Intubate and ventilate. Treat shock (with plasma). Note: the mean systolic BP in mmHg (± 1 sd) is 85 (± 15) at birth, 95 (± 15) at 1yr, 100 (± 10) at 4yrs and 110 (± 8) at 10yrs.
- Record the *level of consciousness*. Glasgow Coma Scale: p 680. Coma Scale if <4 yrs: p 257. Record the time.
- If narcotic poisoning is possible, give *naloxone* 10μg/kg IV, then 100μg/kg every few mins if no response (SC or IM all right, but slower action).
- Send blood and urine for a *drug screen*—and blood alcohol if indicated (give 10% dextrose IVI: the danger is hypoglycaemia).
- Do a gastric lavage (after intubating the trachea) if ingestion has been recent, or if salicylates suspected. Have the child held with his head lower than his trunk. The length of orogastric tube required is estimated by the length from the mouth to the ear lobe and thence to the xiphisternum. Pass the tube and keep the initial aspirate for analysis. Use gravity to drain 50mL of 1.4% sodium bicarbonate solution into the stomach. Aspirate after a few mins and repeat eg 10 times. Do not use lavage if petroleum products or corrosives have been ingested.
- Monitor TPR, BP, urine output and blood glucose frequently.

The alert child It is common to induce vomiting by ipecacuanha 10–15mL mixed with juice (200mL)—but this is of uncertain value. However, activated charcoal (p 254) does reduce absorption.

Some specific poisons For aspirin and paracetamol, see p 254.

- Atropine poisoning (eg from deadly nightshade) causes dilated pupils, dry skin and mouth, tachycardia, excitement. With Lomotil® (atropine and diphenoxylate) the pupils may be constricted.
- Iron poisoning is mild if <50mg/kg elemental iron is ingested (200mg ferrous sulfate tablet ≈ 60mg iron). After emesis, give 60mL milk. If >50mg/kg ingested, measure iron levels in clotted blood urgently. If >90μmol/L, give desferrioxamine 15mg/kg/h IVI up to a total of 80mg/kg/24h. Leave 5g in 50mL water in the stomach after gastric lavage. Beware hypotension.
- Tricyclic poisoning is often fatal with seizures, coma, cyanosis and arrhythmias if >10mg/kg (eg of amitriptyline) is taken.
- Paraffin or petrol (kerosine, gasoline): ►Avoid gastric lavage and emetics. Inhalation may cause lung collapse and consolidation. Do CXR. Lung complications may be delayed 12h.

►Contact a National Poisons Information Service.[1]

1 In UK, Belfast, tel. 01232 240503; Edinburgh, 0131 536 2300; Leeds, 0113 292 3547; London, 0171 635 9191

3. Paediatrics

Salicylate poisoning

Most children can tolerate ingesting 100mg/kg aspirin, and if there is no doubt that a smaller quantity has been ingested and the patient is well, he need not be admitted. Those who have ingested more than this may show deep respiratory movements, causing a respiratory alkalosis, but this is an early sign, before the dangerous metabolic acidosis sets in.

If the child is unconscious, the first step is to place him in the semi-prone recovery position and do a ward test for blood glucose so any hypoglycaemia can be corrected. Protect the airway with an endotracheal tube and perform a gastric lavage (p 252), even if 24h have elapsed since ingestion. Do an urgent plasma salicylate level with blood gases, U&E and bicarbonate. Blood samples taken within 6h of ingestion may be misleadingly low.

Serious poisoning is indicated by levels >2.5mmol/L—consider alkaline diuresis (under expert guidance in ITU, as there is significant morbidity) or activated charcoal, which is a much safer means of enhancing the elimination of salicylates. NB: charcoal tastes gritty—and patients may be vomiting after salicylate poisoning, so consider giving by wide-bore nasogastric tube, providing the airway is adequately protected by a cuffed endotracheal tube. A good regimen is 50g (or 1mg/kg body weight) of activated charcoal on admission, or after gastric lavage, then 25g/2–4h, until recovery or until plasma drug concentrations have fallen to safe levels. The dose of charcoal is more related to the quantity of poison ingested than to the size of the child, although the quantity of fluid with which it is mixed may need to be reduced. Charcoal is *not* contraindicated if the child is pregnant. Adding an emetic (ipecacuanha) to this regimen is of no benefit.[1]

An alternative is urinary alkalinization (in ITU, eg with small boluses of sodium bicarbonate 1.2% IV; do catheter urine pH every 15min—aim for ~8). If none of these measures is practicable, try haemodialysis or charcoal haemoperfusion, particularly if plasma salicylate is very high, eg >5.2mmol/L. Seek expert help.

Paracetamol poisoning

This is rare in infants as a 100mL bottle of paediatric paracetamol mixture typically contains only 2.4g of paracetamol. Serious hepatotoxicity is likely to occur if ≥150mg/kg is ingested. The initial features are nausea and pallor. Jaundice and an enlarged, tender liver occur after >48h. *Other features:* hypotension, arrhythmias, excitement, delirium, coma. *Management:* •Empty the stomach if within 2h of ingestion. •Give *N*-acetylcysteine if the plasma paracetamol level is above the line in the graph opposite. (Take sample ≥4h after ingestion.) The initial dose is 150mg/kg in up to 200mL (depending on the size of the child) of 5% dextrose infused over 30mins, followed by 50mg/kg IVI over the next 4h, and 100mg/kg IVI over the next 16h. This is very effective in preventing liver damage, but only if given within ~8h of ingestion.

Late presentations: Seek expert advice. Check often for hypoglycaemia.

1 G Bayly 1995 *Prescrib J* 35 12

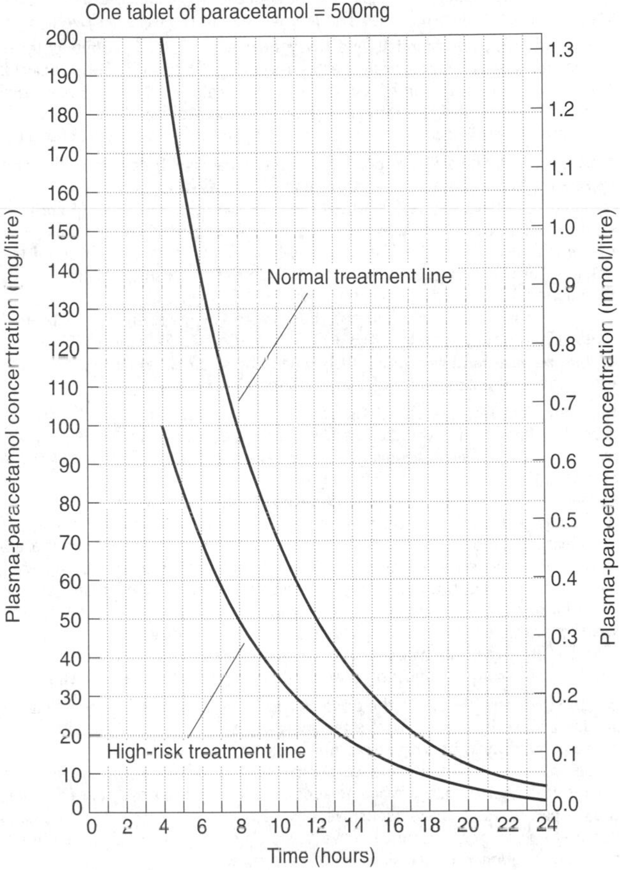

One tablet of paracetamol = 500mg

Plasma-paracetamol concentration (mg/litre)

200 190 180 170 160 150 140 130 120 110 100 90 80 70 60 50 40 30 20 10 0

Plasma-paracetamol concentration (mmol/litre)

1.3 1.2 1.1 1.0 0.9 0.8 0.7 0.6 0.5 0.4 0.3 0.2 0.1 0.0

Normal treatment line

High-risk treatment line

0 2 4 6 8 10 12 14 16 18 20 22 24

Time (hours)

Patients whose plasma-paracetamol concentrations are above the **normal treatment line** should be treated with acetylcysteine by intravenous infusion (or, provided the overdose has been taken **within 10–12 hours**, with methionine by mouth). Patients on enyzme-including drugs (e.g. carbamazepine, phenobarbitone, phenytoin, rifampicin, and alcohol) or who are malnourished (e.g. in anorexia, in alcoholism, or those who are HIV-positive) should be treated if their plasma-paracetamol concentrations are above the **high-risk treatment line**. We thank Dr Alun Hutchings for permission to reproduce this graph.

Graph for use in deciding who should receive *N*-acetylcysteine.
►1 tablet of paracetamol=500mg. 150mg=1mmol paracetamol.

►►Rising intracranial pressure[APLS]

Causes Meningoencephalitis; head injury; subdural or extra-dural haemorrhage (eg by shaking); hypoxia (eg near-drowning) may all cause sudden and life-threatening rises in ICP. The rise with brain tumours is slower.

Presentation Listless; irritable; drowsy; headache; diplopia; vomiting; tense fontanelle; ↓level of responsiveness—assess by Children's Coma Scale if <4yrs (see opposite), or by Glasgow Coma Scale if >4yrs (p 680); pupil changes (ipsilateral dilatation); rising BP and falling pulse (Cushing reflex); intermittent respiration. Later, ie chronic: papilloedema and hydrocephalus.

Management The aim is to prevent secondary damage. Help venous drainage by keeping head in the midline, elevated at ~20°. Give O_2. Fan/sponge (tepid water) if T° >40°C. Check for hypoglycaemia. Control any seizures (p 268).

- Intubate and hyperventilate: aim for P_aCO_2 of ~3.68kPa if *Coma Scale* is <8.
- Give mannitol 20% (check it is crystal-free), 7mL/kg IVI over 30min if the child is deteriorating—but discuss this with the neurosurgeon first.
- Dexamethasone 0.1mg/kg IV stat, then 0.05–0.1mg/kg/6h IV.
- Fluid restriction and diuresis, but avoid hypovolaemia (keep Na^+ 145–150mmol/L, osmolarity to 300–310, and CVP to 2–5cmH_2O).
- Measure pulse and BP continuously (check that cuff fits well).
- Remember the possibility of non-accidental injury.

Herpes simplex encephalitis This is the one form of encephalitis discussed in detail as it is treatable. ►*Think of the diagnosis in any febrile child with focal seizures or focal neurological signs associated with deteriorating consciousness.* Patients often present with subtle or non-specific signs. Nasolabial herpetic lesions are often absent. Neurological deficits may be mild or gross (eg hemiparesis). Focal or generalized seizures occur. Tests such as CT and CSF examination are often non-specific (unless polymerase chain reaction is available). MRI is better. EEG may show focal changes and periodic complexes. Herpes simplex antibodies are produced too late to guide management. Brain biopsy is diagnostic but seems rather drastic. It is therefore probably wise to start treatment with aciclovir as soon as the diagnosis is suspected. Give 5–10mg/kg/8h by IVI over 1h (250–500mg/m^2) eg for 2 weeks. Monitor U&E and urine output, adjusting dose in the light of these (see *Data sheet*).

Brain tumours ⅔ are in the posterior fossa. Key features in their diagnosis are a raised ICP with focal signs (below), ± false localizing signs (eg VI nerve palsy, due to its long intracranial course.

Medulloblastoma: This midline cerebellar tumour arises from the inferior vermis. It causes truncal ataxia and sudden falls. 75% are boys. It seeds along the CSF pathways. It is radiosensitive.

Brainstem astrocytoma: Cranial nerve palsies; pyramidal tract signs (eg hemiparesis); cerebellar ataxia; signs of ICP↑ are rare.

Midbrain and third ventricle tumours may be astrocytomas, pinealomas or colloid cysts (cause posture-dependent drowsiness). Signs: behaviour change (early); pyramidal tract and cerebellar signs; upward gaze defect.

Suprasellar gliomas: Visual field defects; optic atrophy; pituitary disorders (growth arrest, hypothyroidism, delayed puberty); diabetes insipidus (DI). Cranial DI is caused by ADH↓, so that there is polyuria and low urine osmolality (always <800mosmol/L) despite dehydration.

Cerebral hemispheres: Usually gliomas. Meningiomas are rare. Fits may be the presenting sign. Signs depend on the lobe involved (*OHCM* p 457).

Tests: EEG, skull x-ray, CT scans ± magnetic resonance imaging.

Treatment options: Excision, CSF shunting, radio- and chemotherapy.

Other space-occupying lesions Aneurysms; haematomas; granulomas; tuberculomas; cysts (cysticercosis); ►abscess—suspect whenever signs of ICP ↑, fever and a leukocytosis occur together; arrange urgent referral.

Other causes of headache Viruses; meningitis; sinusitis (frontal sinus not developed until >10yrs); hypertension (always measure BP); migraine (*OHCM* p 416; admit if hemiplegic). Signs requiring further assessment:
- Headaches of increasing frequency or severity.
- Age <6yrs.
- Headache unrelieved by paracetamol.
- Irritable; loss of interest/skills.
- Slowing of physical or cognitive development.
- Head circumference >97th centile, or greatly out of line.

Children's Coma Scale[1] (<4yrs)APLS

Best motor response This has 6 grades:

6 Carrying out request ('obeying command'): The child moves spontaneously, or to your request.

5 Localizing response to pain: Put gentle pressure on the patient's finger nail bed with a pencil then try supraorbital and sternal pressure: purposeful movements towards changing painful stimuli is a 'localizing' response.

4 Withdraws to pain: Pulls limb away from painful stimulus.

3 Flexor response to pain: Pressure on the nail bed causes abnormal flexion of limbs—decorticate posture.

2 Extensor posturing to pain: The stimulus causes limb extension (adduction, internal rotation of shoulder, pronation of forearm)—decerebrate posture.

1 No response to pain.

NB: record the best response of any limb.

Best verbal response This has 5 grades. If intubated *can the patient grimace?*

5 Orientated: The patient smiles, is orientated to sounds, fixes and follows objects.

	Crying	*Interacts*
4	Consolable	Inappropriate
3	Inconsistently consolable	Moaning
2	Inconsolable	Irritable
1	No response	No response

Score the highest out of either two columns.

Eye opening This has 4 grades.

4 Spontaneous eye opening.

3 Eye opening in response to speech: Any speech, or shout, not necessarily request to open eyes.

2 Eye opening to response to pain: Pain to limbs as above.

1 No eye opening.

An overall score is made by summing the score in the 3 areas assessed. Eg: no response to pain + no verbalization + no eye opening = 3.

►If >4 yrs, see *Glasgow Coma Scale*, p 680; scores may be hard to interpret.[1]

1 R Gemke 1998 *Lancet* **351** 926 & Advanced Life Support Group 1993 *Advanced Paediatric Life Support*, BMA

►►Meningitis[APLS]

Suspect this in any ill baby or child. The only signs may be unusual crying, poor feeding, or vomiting. Pay great attention to the fontanelle: in GI vomiting it becomes sunken; with meningitis it may be tense. ►*Get expert help from your senior and a microbiologist;* if confirmed, *notify your local consultant in Communicable Disease Control (CCDC).* If there is any hint of meningococcal disease, give penicillin at once (dose below). On lumbar puncture, if CSF is cloudy, start a broad-spectrum IV agent (eg ceftriaxone below) at once, while awaiting microscopy and further advice.

Meningeal signs: Stiff neck (unable to kiss knees), often absent if <18 months old; photophobia; Kernig's sign (resistance to extending knee, with hip flexed); Brudzinski's sign (hips flex on bending head forward); opisthotonos.

ICP↑: Irritable; drowsy; vomiting; fontanelle tense; pre-hernia, below.

Septic signs: Fever; arthritis; odd behaviour; rashes—*any*, do not *expect* petechiae with meningococcus; cyanosis; DIC; pulse↑; BP↓tachypnoea; WCC↑.

Other causes of meningism: Tonsillitis, pneumonia, subarachnoid bleed.

Lumbar puncture: Do this at once unless: focal signs; DIC; purpura (top priority is penicillin 50mg/kg max 2g for meningococcus); or if *brain herniation* is near (abnormal postures or breathing; coma scale <13, p 257; dilated pupils, doll's eye reflexes, BP↑, pulse↓, papilloedema). NB: preliminary CT is incapable of showing that LP would be safe.[1] *Technique:* There is no substitute for learning from an expert physician: the commonest error is aiming too low. What follows are simply some reminders. •Explain everything to the mother. •Ask an experienced nurse to help, by positioning the child fully flexed (knees to chin) on the side of a bed, with his back exactly at right angles with it. •Mark a point just above (cranial to) a line joining the spinous processes between the iliac crests. •Drape and sterilize the area; put on gloves. •Infiltrate 1mL of 1% lidocaine (=lignocaine). •Insert the LP needle aiming towards the umbilicus. •Catch 4 CSF drops in each of 3 bottles for an urgent Gram stain, culture, virology, and glucose (do blood glucose too). •Request frequent neurological observations. •Report to mother.

Tests: (after LP): FBC, U&E, culture blood, urine, nose swabs (and stool, for virology). C-reactive protein: is it >20mg/L? CSF lactate: is it >3mg/L? CXR. Fluid balance, TPR and BP hourly.

Treating pyogenic meningitis before the organism is known

- Protect airway and give high flow O_2 •Set up IVI: colloid in 10mL/kg boluses.
- If meningococcaemia likely use antibiotics as detailed on p 260.
- *Ceftriaxone* 80mg/kg/day IVI over 30min (50mg/kg if <7 days old) is standard. Alternative: *cefotaxime* 50mg/kg/8h (up to 200mg/kg/day in neonates) IV over 15min. Benzylpenicillin may also be used—50mg/kg/12h slowly IV for prems/neonates; 50mg/kg/8h for babies <1yr old. *Netilmicin* may be used in neonates (2mg/kg/8h slowly IV—monitor plasma levels, U&E and creatinine, ↓dose as needed; see *Data sheet*); with *ampicillin* in case of listeria. If >2 months, you can swap chloramphenicol 12mg/kg/6h IVI (half this if <2wks old; do levels) for the ceftriaxone (resistance is a problem; SE: marrow aplasia; high doses risk 'grey baby syndrome'—abdominal swelling, cyanosis, collapse). NB: in general, the intrathecal route is not required for antibiotic therapy.
- If pre-hernia signs, treat for ICP↑ (p 256), eg mannitol 0.5g/kg IVI.
- Once the organism is known and the right drug started, find its minimum inhibitory concentration (MIC) to the organism *in vitro*.

Complications Disseminated sepsis, subdural effusion, ataxia, paralysis, deafness, mental retardation, epilepsy, brain abscess.

CSF in meningitis	*Pyogenic:*	*Tubercular:*	*Aseptic:*
Appearance	often turbid	may be fibrin web	usually clear
Predominant cell	polymorphs eg $1000/mm^3$	mononuclear $10–350/mm^3$	mononuclear $50–1500/mm^3$
Glucose level	< ⅔ of blood	< ⅔ of blood	>⅔ of blood
Protein	1–5g/dL	1–5g/dL	<1.5g/dL

Preventing deaths from meningococcaemia

Because death is so swift, this can seem a hopeless task—as even when we doctors contract meningococcal disease, we simply think we have 'flu, and our families are surprised to find us dead in bed just hours after reporting sick. Nevertheless, good practice (and luck) *can* save lives, and the meningococcus is not always *that* fast.

- ►Do not expect meningeal signs always to be to the fore. Septicaemic features predominate in fatal illness.
- ►*Any* rash (or none) will do for the meningococcus. If you wait for purpura, you may be waiting until the disease is untreatable.
- ►For any acutely unwell child *leave your consulting room door ajar*. Explain that you or your deputy can be contacted *at any time* if:
  - –He seems to be worsening
  - –He seems to be unrousable
  - –A rash develops
  - –He starts crying in an odd way
- ►Beware fever+lethargy+vomiting, even if no headache or photophobia.
- ►Give parenteral penicillin *early*, before admission to hospital.

See OHCM p 710 for a discussion of heroic but non-standard ways that are being developed to aid management[1]—eg *extracorporeal membrane oxygenation*; use of *terminal fragment of human bactericidal/permeability-increasing protein* ($rBPI_{21}$) to ↓cytokines; *heparin with protein C concentrate* to reverse coagulopathy; *plasmapheresis* to remove cytokines, and correct acidosis—and *thrombolysis* (rTPA) to help limb re-perfusion.

1 *Lancet* 1997 **350** 1566

Meningitis: the organisms

The meningococcus, the pneumococcus, and, in the unvaccinated, *Haemophilus influenzae* are the great killers, but of these it is the meningococcus that is the swiftest and the most deadly. The interval between seeming wellbeing and coma may be counted in hours. If you suspect meningitis, give benzylpenicillin (opposite) before hospital admission.

Neisseria meningitidis Abrupt onset ± rash (purpuric or not, eg starting as pink macules over the legs). Septicaemia may occur without meningitis (Waterhouse–Friedrichsen, *OHCM* p 710), so that early LPs may be normal, and give false reassurance. Arthritis, conjunctivitis, myocarditis and DIC may coexist. *Typical age:* Any. Film: Gram –ve cocci in pairs (long axes parallel), often within polymorphs. Drug of choice: benzylpenicillin (G) 50mg/kg/4h IV. If penicillin-allergic, give cefotaxime (p 258) or chloramphenicol (below). Treat shock with colloid. *Prevention:* Rifampicin 10mg/kg/12h PO (if <1yr, 5mg/kg/12h) for 48h for close contacts, or ceftriaxone 125mg IM if under 12yrs (250mg IM stat if over 12yrs). Observe closely.

Haemophilus influenzae This is rare where immunization is the rule. Predisposing events: otitis (send swabs). Typical age: <4yrs. Gram stain: Gram –ve rods in pairs or chains. The lower the CSF glucose, the worse the infection. *Drugs:* ceftrixone (dose on p 258) or, where resistance is not a problem, chloramphenicol 12–25mg/kg/6h IVI (not in neonates) with ampicillin 30mg/kg/4h IV. Rifampicin (see below) may also be needed. If chloramphenicol is used, try to monitor peak chloramphenicol levels. Aim for 20–25µg/mL. Do not be surprised if you far exceed usual doses to achieve this. (Trough level: <15µg/mL.) As soon as you can, switch to PO (more effective). Dexamethasone (0.15mg/kg/6h IV for 4 days) has been reported by some to reduce post-meningitis deafness (eg from 15% to 3%).

Streptococcus pneumoniae Risk factors: upper respiratory infections, pneumonia, skull fracture, meningocele. *Typical age:* Any. Film: Gram +ve cocci in pairs. *Drug of choice:* Benzylpenicillin 25–50mg/kg/4h slow IV—or, if resistance likely (eg parts of Europe, USA), vancomycin (dose in children older than 1 month: 10mg/kg/6h IVI over 1h) with a third-generation cefalosporin (see ceftriaxone, dose on p 256) is advised. Monitor U&E.

Escherichia coli This is a cause of meningitis in the neonate (in whom the signs may consist of feeding difficulties, apnoea, fits and shock). Drug of choice: netilmicin 2mg/kg/8h slowly IV (p 238).

Group B haemolytic streptococci eg *via* mother's vagina (so swab mothers whose infants suddenly fall ill at ~24h-old). Infection may be delayed for a month. Drug of choice: benzylpenicillin 25–50mg/kg/8–12h slowly IV.

Perinatal listeriosis (*Listeria monocytogenes*) This presents soon after birth with meningitis and septicaemia (± pneumonia). Microabscesses form in many organs (granulomatosis infantiseptica). *Diagnosis:* Culture blood, placenta, amniotic fluid, CSF. Treatment: IV ampicillin with gentamicin. Further details and prevention: *OHCM* p 223.

TB can cause CNS infarcts, demyelination (hence cranial nerve lesions) and tuberculomas ± meningitis (long prodrome: lethargy, malaise, anorexia). Photophobia/neck stiffness are likely to be absent. The first few CSFs may be normal, or show visible fibrin webs, and widely fluctuating cell counts. *Treatment:* Seek expert help. *Dose example:* Isoniazid 10mg/kg/24h IV ?with vit. B_6 + rifampicin 10mg/kg/24h (≤600mg/day) for 1yr + (for 2 months) pyrazinamide 35mg/kg/ day + eg streptomycin 15mg/kg/day IM adjusted to give a peak plasma level <40µg/mL and a trough of <3µg/mL; an alternative is ethambutol 15mg/kg/day PO if old enough to report visual problems.

Other bacteria Leptospiral species (canicola); Brucella; Salmonella.

Causes of 'aseptic' meningitis Viruses (eg mumps, echo, herpes, polio), partially treated bacterial infections, cryptococcus (use ink stains).

Giving benzylpenicillin before hospital admission

- 300mg IM up to 1 year old
- 600mg if 1–10yrs
- 1.2g if >10yrs

Diabetes mellitus—some questions

What should the family know before the child leaves the ward?

- Insulin: the dose to use. Can the parent draw it up accurately, and can the child self-inject? Practise on oranges.
- Diet: What is it? Why is it important? Why must meals be regular? What does mother do if the child is hungry?
- Can blood sugar be monitored accurately? Watch her technique.
- What should she do if the blood sugar is not well controlled?
- Does she know what 'well controlled' means?
- What happens if he has too much insulin? What will happen as hypoglycaemia evolves? (Weakness, hunger, irritability, faintness, sweating, abdominal pain, vomiting, fits and coma). What action needs to be taken? Practise inducing hypoglycaemia (glucose <2mmol/L) on the ward, by omitting breakfast after morning insulin. Explain symptoms as they happen, and their amelioration with oral drinks (or Hypostop® oral jelly). If things get out of hand, for *hypoglycaemic coma*, give glucose 0.5 g/kg as a 25% IVI (or via rectal tube if no IV access, with glucagon 0.5–1mg IM or slowly IV). Then give 10% dextrose, 5mL/kg/h. *Expect a quick return to consciousness*. If not, recheck glucose; if low, give IV dexamethasone (p 256); if normal, ask yourself if there is a post-ictal state after a hypoglycaemic fit: don't give more glucose as this can promote cerebral oedema.
- What should happen if the child misses a meal, or is sick afterwards? What happens to insulin requirements during 'flu?
- Who does mother contact in emergency? Give written advice.
- Is the GP informed of discharge and follow-up arrangements?
- Encourage membership of a *Diabetic Association* (in UK, tel 0171 323 1531).

'What are the aims of routine follow-up in the diabetic clinic?'

- To achieve normoglycaemia through education and motivation.
- To prevent complications. So check growth and fundi (dilate the pupil). Blood: glucose, glycosylated Hb. Note: it is generally the case that retinopathy develops only after 10yrs of disease.
- If normoglycaemia is unachieved, choose the best compromise with the child's way of life and strict glucose control. Methods are available such as the Novopen® which allow great flexibility in the timing and dose of insulin. This device delivers a variable dose (2u/push) of insulin at the push of a plunger, and obviates the need for carrying syringes and drawing up insulin at inconvenient times (eg during a party).

Management of the new diabetic The management of ketoacidosis is described on p 263. If there is no ketosis IV fluids are seldom needed. A suitable initial dose is insulin 0.2u/kg SC followed by 0.35–0.5u/kg/12h SC, given 30min before breakfast and tea. ~70% of the dose should be as long-acting insulin. With help from the pancreas a 'honeymoon' period may follow in which insulin requirements fall to 0.1u/kg/day. *Diet:* 1500 kcal/m^2 or 1000kcal plus 100–200kcal for each year of age (depending on energy expenditure). Aim for 30% of this with each major meal, and 10% as a bedtime snack. Give 20% of the calories as protein, 50% as unrefined carbohydrate, and 30% as fat. Enlist the help of a paediatric dietitian.

Genes and environment Diabetes used to be a disease of the over-5s, but in the UK, incidence is rising in infancy from ~1:10,000 in 1985-90 to ~1.6/10,000 in 1990-1995. Islet cell antibodies are found in HLA-B8 (but not HLA-B15) individuals. If one child in a family has diabetes, risk to siblings is 5–10%. *Diagnostic criteria:* see OHCM p 474. * Mean duration of symptoms pre-diagnosis is 30 days. Feeding with cows' milk, and infant exposure to various enteroviruses, may be having an effect on incidence. We note with interest that twin studies show that, although at least 4 genes are thought to be important—and one (6q) partly determines islet sensitivity to damage, most of the susceptibility to diabetes is environmentally acquired, and patients with type I diabetes have antibodies to cows' milk albumin which react with β-cell (the insulin-producing cell) surface proteins. We also know that mumps, rubella and coxsackie viruses (± CMV) have potential to injure β-cell—but their exact rôle is unclear.

►►Diabetic ketoacidotic coma

Clinical features: Listlessness; vomiting; drowsiness; polyuria; polydipsia; weight loss. Examination: dehydration (p 250); deep, rapid respirations; ketotic ('fruity'/peardrop-smelling) breath; shock, coma.

Bedside tests: Urine: ketones +++; high ward test for blood glucose (may be falsely low if the patient is vasoconstricted).

The first 4h: airway (*recovery position*) breathing (O_2) circulation (*ECG monitor*).

- Weigh; FBC, U&E, glucose, Ca^{2+}, PO_4^{3-}, blood gas. Set up 0.9% saline IVI.
- Give 0.5mL/kg/min while doing calculations (+ plasma 10 mL/kg IV if BP↓↓).
- Calculate the fluid requirement. This is the maintenance fluid (eg 100mL/kg/day, p 250) + the water deficit. Assume that the patient is 10% dehydrated, so the water deficit is 100mL/kg.
- Give ⅓ of this volume over the first 4h as a 0.9% saline IVI.
- Determine plasma osmolality [2 (Na^+ + K^+)] + glucose + urea. If >340 mosmol/kg (hyperosmolar coma) give fluid as 0.45% saline.
- Insulin (eg Actrapid®) If >5yrs. 0.1u/kg stat IV, then 0.1u/kg/h IVI by pump in 0.9% saline. If no pump, give 0.25u/kg IM stat, then 0.1u/kg/h IM. Halve the dose to 0.05u/kg/h if glucose falls faster than 4mmol/h). If <5yrs old, give less insulin (eg 0.05u/kg/h IVI).
- When urine flows, start IV K^+, as guided by plasma K^+. If <5 mmol/L, give 6mmol/kg/day (keep concentration <30mmol/L). The danger is hypokalaemia. Aim for plasma K^+ of 4–5mmol/L.
- Even in severe acidosis bicarbonate's rôle is controversial (unfavourable shift in Hb–O_2-dissociation curve). If pH <7.0, consider bicarbonate 2.5mL/kg of 8.4% IVI over 2h. Check pH after 1h, and stop IVI if pH >7.15
- Repeat U&E, glucose. Do CXR, FBC, and do infection screen.
- Monitor TPR; continuous ECG; BP. Pass a nasogastric tube.
- Measure urine output and specific gravity (oliguria p 280).

Subsequent management: Measure glucose hourly. When <15mmol/L change IVI to dextrose saline (4.3% dextrose + 0.18% saline).

- Give next ⅓ of the 24h water requirement over the next 8h, and the last ⅓ over the subsequent 12h (oral fluids may then be possible, eg 15–30mL/h PO). NB: some regimens rehydrate more slowly (eg equal hourly rates over 36h) to avoid risking cerebral oedema (suspect if there is a set-back after 2–24h; mannitol is the only treatment which helps).
- Repeat U&E, PCV and blood gases (for acid–base balance) every 2–4h, until consciousness returns, and oral fluids are tolerated.

Pitfalls in diabetic ketoacidosis

- Infection: often patients are apyrexial. Perform an MSU, blood cultures and CXR. Start broad-spectrum antibiotics early if infection is suspected.
- Creatinine: some assays for creatinine cross-react with ketone bodies, so plasma creatinine may not reflect true renal function.
- Hyponatraemia may occur owing to the osmotic effect of glucose. If <120mmol/L, search for other causes, eg hypertriglyceridaemia. If >150mmol, treat with of 0.45% saline to start with, then 0.9% saline.
- Ketonuria does not equate with ketoacidosis. Normals may have ketonuria after 12h fasts. Not all ketones are due to diabetes, eg alcohol, if glucose normal. Test plasma with Ketostix® to demonstrate ketonaemia.
- Acidosis without glucose↑↑ may occur, but consider overdose (eg aspirin).
- Serum amylase is often ↑ (up to 10-fold) in the absence of pancreatitis.
- Cerebral oedema is a constant threat: prevent this by *slow* return to normal glucose and hydration. Monitor neurological status hourly.

Sleep problems and the parasomnias

Wakefulness A common problem is the child who wakes at 3am, ready to play, or wanting entry to the parent's bed. For those not appreciating these visitations from the pure of heart, the easiest thing is to refuse to play and buy ear plugs to lessen the impact of screaming—or to let the child into the bed. Or try extinguishing the behaviour by attending the child ever more distantly: cuddle in bed → cuddle on bed → sitting on child's bed → voice from doorway → distant voice. Try to avoid hypnotics (such as promethazine, chloral hydrate). If drugs are essential, consider triclofos sodium 25–30mg/kg.

Other causes of sleeplessness: Hunger/colic (infants); poor routines (preschool); worries (adolescence). Try behavioural therapy before hypnotics.

Day-time sleepiness: Causes: night sleep↓; depression; sleep apnoea (*OHCM* p 362); narcolepsy (*OHCM* p 698); and *encephalitis lethargicans* (there are sporadic cases affecting children, but nothing to match the pandemic of 1917–26)—suspect this condition whenever sleepiness occurs with extrapyramidal effects, oculogyric crises, myoclonus, inversion of diurnal rhythms, obsessional phenomena, and mood change. The cause is said to be viral (influenza, rarely measles), but Q fever and mycoplasma have also caused this syndrome, as has infiltration of the hypothalamus (eg by lymphoma). MRI: look for subcortical involvement.

Parasomnias Of all our non-insane automatisms, somnambulism is the most familiar and the most striking, literally, sometimes, as whole households may occasionally be endangered when the bloodiest dreams of junior somnambulists are enacted. The young are by far the most proficient sleepwalkers, but the old may emulate them when under stress, particularly if this is associated with excess alcohol or caffeine use, and lack of stage IV sleep (our deepest sleep). Any psychic event associated with sleep may be termed a parasomnia. Parasomnias comprise: •Arousal disorders (sleep walking, night terrors, and 'confusional arousal') •Sleep–wake transition disorders (rhythmic movement head-banging disorder) •REM sleep parasomnias (rapid eye movement sleep associated nightmares, sleep paralysis, hallucinations, and REM sleep behaviour disorders, involving motor enactment of dreams, sometimes with injury to self and others) •Miscellaneous disorders (sleep-talking; nocturnal enuresis; myoclonus nocturnus; and nocturnal bruxism, ie teeth grinding).

Suffering from night terrors is often a familial problem. The child awakens frightened, hallucinated and inaccessible—and is obviously alarmed.

It is common to observe movement in children during sleep: it is their *repetitive* nature which allows the diagnosis of rhythmic movement disorder. The movement may be body rocking, leg rolling, or head-banging (this 'jactatio capitis' may lead to subdurals, fractures, eye injuries, and erroneous accusations of physical abuse). If the jaw is involved, there may be tongue-biting, which may suggest nocturnal epilepsy. But do not try to be too obsessive in differentiating parasomnias from nocturnal epilepsy, for three reasons: the first is that our definition of epilepsy is tested to destruction by the parasomnias ('epilepsy is intermittent abnormal brain activity manifesting as simple or complex seizures'). The second reason is that those with clearly defined parasomnias are at risk of developing tonic–clonic nocturnal seizures later in life.[1] The third reason is that some parasomnias are signs of autosomal-dominant nocturnal frontal lobe epilepsy (ADNFLE). ADNFLE is associated with abnormalities in the gene encoding nicotinic acetylcholine receptor α_4-subunit (chromosome 20). In these individuals, correct diagnosis may be aided by EEG (rhythmic slow anterior activity) and video-polysomnography (shows sleep-related violent behaviour, sudden awakenings with dyskinetic or dystonic movements, and complex behaviours ± enuresis[2]).

Antiparasomniacs include bedtime clonazepam, amitriptyline, and carbamazepine.[3] If these do not work, self-hypnosis may help, or the simple expedient of waking the patient 30 minutes before the expected parasomnia.

1 R Silvestry 1995 *Neurophysiol Clin* **25** 19 2 A Oldani 1998 *Brain* **121** 205 3 M Bahro 1994 *Nervenarzt* 65 568

Sleep paralysis

When we sleep we trawl forbidden seas, arranging and being rearranged by the flotsam and jetsam of our waking lives. As our nets descend through the various stages of sleep, our Sovereign Reason or Will usually remains quietly on deck, but if by chance it descends with the nets then, like the tail wagging the dog, it adopts and propagates a life of its own, which may be full of danger. Because our vessel has been vacated, Marie-Celeste-style, we are judged, in Law, not to be responsible for our actions while asleep—be they theft, arson, or homicide. Without will or wind, our vessel, like Coleridge's *Mariner's*, is moved 'onward from beneath' by secret forces.* So here we have the model of Reason and Will residing, during sleep, either upstairs or downstairs: but in sleep paralysis, neither is the case—the tail cannot wag the dog, nor the dog wag his tail. Sleep paralysis may involve complete paralysis of all voluntary muscles, even the diaphragm. For anyone who has experienced it, it is frightening, unforgettable, and difficult to describe—perhaps like being aware during anaesthesia. Sleep paralysis was first described by Ishmael during a reverie on deck, sleeping between Queequeg, the cannibal whaler from the South Seas, and his harpoon, before Herman Melville embarks them on the *Pequod's* voyage to track down Moby Dick '. . . At last I must have fallen into a troubled nightmare of a doze; and slowly waking from it—half steeped in dreams—I opened my eyes, and the before sunlit room was now wrapped in outer darkness. Instantly I felt a shock running through all my frame; nothing was to be seen, and nothing was to be heard; but a supernatural hand seemed placed in mine. My arm hung over the counterpane... for what seemed like ages piled on ages, I lay there frozen with the most aweful fears ... thinking that if I could but stir it one single inch, the horrid spell would be broken... '

**Till noon we quietly sailed on,*
Yet never a breeze did breathe:
Slowly and smoothly went the ship,
Moved onward from beneath.
Under the keel nine fathom deep,
From the land of mist and snow,
The spirit slid: and it was he
That made the ship to go.

Samuel Taylor Coleridge Part v of *The Rhyme of the Ancient Mariner*

Epilepsy and febrile convulsions

EPILEPSY is a tendency to intermittent abnormal brain activity. It is classified according to whether signs are referable to one part of a hemisphere (partial epilepsy) or not (generalized). The 4 kinds of **generalized epilepsy:**

- *Tonic/clonic (grand mal):* Limbs stiffen (the tonic phase) and then jerk forcefully (clonic phase), with loss of consciousness.
- *Absences:* Brief (eg 10sec) pauses ('he stops in midsentence, and carries on where he left off'); eyes may roll up; he/she is *unaware of the attack.*
- *Infantile spasms:* Eg at 5 months. Jerks forwards with arms flexed, and hands extended ('Salaam attack'). Repeated every 2–3sec, up to 50 times. Here the EEG is characteristic. Treat with valproate or vigabatrin.
- *Myoclonic fits:* 1–7-year-olds; eg 'thrown' suddenly to the ground.

Partial epilepsy Signs are referable to part of one hemisphere.
Elementary phenomena: consciousness is not impaired.
Complex phenomena: (temporal lobe fits) consciousness ↓; automatisms (lip smacking, rubbing face, running); fits of pure pleasure.

Causes of seizures (Often none is found) Infection (eg meningitis); U&E↑, glucose↓, Ca^{2+}↓, Mg^{2+}↓; toxins, phenylketonuria, flickering lights (eg television) CNS disease—tuberous sclerosis, tumours (<2%), malformations. *Differential diagnosis:* Arrhythmias, migraine, narcolepsy, night terrors, faints (reflex anoxic seizures, p 267), tics, Munchausen's syndrome (*OHCM* p706).

Investigating epilepsy Always have an EEG done by an expert. Do CT only if there are infantile spasms, or unusual features, CNS signs, or the epilepsy is partial or intractible.[1] (MRI may be more sensitive, but is not so available and may require anaesthesia or sedation—but there is no radiation.)

A FEBRILE CONVULSION is diagnosed if the following occur together:

- A tonic/clonic, symmetrical generalized seizure with no focal features
- Occurring as the temperature rises rapidly in a febrile illness
- In a normally-developing child between 6 months and 5yrs of age
- With no signs of CNS infection or previous history of epilepsy
- When there are less than 3 seizures, each lasting <5min.

Differential diagnosis: Meningoencephalitis, brain lesions, trauma, hypoglycaemia, hypocalcaemia and hypomagnesaemia.
Lifetime prevalence: ~3% of children have at least one febrile convulsion.
Examination: A complete search to find any possible infection.
Tests: FBC, MSU, CXR, ENT swabs, LP (always if aged <1 year). Get help in deciding if an LP is needed. If it is not, review this decision in ~2h. If LP *is* indicated, be sure to exclude signs of ICP↑ (see p 258).
Management: Lie prone; diazepam (p 268);. Cool by tepid sponging when hot; 12mg/kg/4–6h of paracetamol syrup, 120mg/5mL. *Parental education:*

- Allay fear (eg a child is *not* dying during a fit).
- Febrile convulsions do not mean epilepsy, or, usually, risk of epilepsy.
- For the 30% who have recurrences (50% if first degree relative also affected), try teaching mother to use rectal diazepam, eg with one 5mg tube (Stesolid®) if 1–3yrs*, or one 10mg tube if older. This dose may also be used at home *during* seizures before calling for help.

Further prevention: Prophylactic anticonvulsants are almost never needed.[2]
Follow-up: Explain that fever with future pertussis and MMR vaccination should prompt oral paracetamol (p 214)—with rectal diazepam to hand.
Prognosis: If no focal signs, and the seizure lasts <30min, and is single only, 1% develop epilepsy. <1% have all these adverse signs: their risk of epilepsy is much higher (50%, eg if coupled with pre-existing CNS abnormality).

Treatment and prevention of epilepsy See p 268 and p 269.

1 R Appleton 1995 *Prescribers' J* 35 182 2 H Valman 1993 BMJ i 1743 *If <3yrs insert PR half way to the mark on the nozzle. ~2.5mL is expellable (don't worry about the bit left behind; this is allowed for in the dose formulation). NB: The regimen for CP ***diazepam Rectubes***® differs: their licence is for a 0.5mg/kg ***single*** dose–for adults and children >10kg (a typical weight for a 1yr-old), ***which should not be repeated for >12h*** (there are very few reports of respiratory problems at this dose: all survived).

Reflex anoxic seizures

Essence Paroxysmal, spontaneously-reversing brief (eg 15 second) asystole triggered by pain, fear, (eg at the time of venepuncture) or anxiety, or an overwhelming confrontation with reality, perhaps in the form of a bath which is unexpectedly hot or cold. During this time the child is deathly pale— ± hypotonia, rigidity, upward eye deviation, clonic movements, and urinary incontinence. The typical patient is aged 6 months to 2 years old (but may be much older).[1]

Prevalence It is hard to be exact, because misdiagnosis is so common, but one estimate is that 0.8% of preschool children are affected.[2]

Differential The most often confusing condition is epilepsy which is frequently misdiagnosed, because the trigger aspect to the history is ignored or unwitnessed. When in difficulty, refer to a specialist for vagal excitation tests, while under continuous EEG and ECG monitoring (ocular compression induces the oculo-cardiac reflex; do not do this test if there is glaucoma, or known arrhythmia, or if you lack experience: it is uncomfortable for the child). NB: tongue-biting is not described in reflex anoxic seizures.

Management Drug treatment is rarely, if ever, needed.[1] Atropine has been tried, to reduce sensitivity to vagal influences. Anticonvulsants are not indicated. Inserting a pacemaker is one option under review.

What to tell the parents Avoid the term 'seizure', as this is all that is likely to be remembered, *however* careful your explanation. *Pallid syncopal attack*, or *white breath-holding attacks* are useful synonyms. Emphasize the benign nature of the condition, and that the child usually grows out of it (but it may occur later in life, and in older family members).

1 R Appleton 1993 BMJ ii 215   2 C Lombroso 1967 *Paediatrics* 39 563–81

Epilepsy: management[APLS]

(Neonates: *see* p 238)

Stepwise treatment of status epilepticus Supportive therapy: •Secure airway; give O_2. Set a clock in motion. •Set up 5% dextrose IVI. •Measure BP, pulse, blood glucose, blood gases, Ca^{2+} (± Mg^{2+}). ►If hypoglycaemic, give glucose 0.5g/kg IV as a 25% solution, then 5–10mg/kg/min as 10% dextrose IVI.

Seizure control:[1] Proceed to the next step only if fits continue.

0min	Estimate the weight of the child: kg = 2 × [age in yrs + 4]. *Diazepam* 0.25–0.4mg/kg slow IV as Diazemuls® (less toxic to veins).*
5min	*Diazepam* repeated as above.
10min	*Paraldehyde* 0.15mg/kg PR in arachis oil, or IM. Rule of thumb: 1mL /yr; max 10mL PR (or 5mL if IM). Avoid contact with plastics/rubber.
20min	*Phenytoin* 18mg/kg IVI; max rate 1mg/kg/min. Monitor ECG.
50min	*Diazepam* 0.1–0.4mg/kg/h IVI. Get expert help. Transfer to ITU.
65min	Paralyse and ventilate: use *thiopentone* infusion.

►These times refer to elapsed time on the clock from the first drug, *not* gaps between each drug. Some authorities recommend starting ventilation earlier, and always be ready to do this to protect the airway.

Tests Pulse oximetry, cardiac monitor, glucose, blood gases, U&E, Ca^{2+}, magnesium, FBC, platelets, ECG. Consider anticonvulsant levels, toxicology screen, blood ammonia, lumbar puncture, culture blood and urine, EEG, CT, carbon monoxide level, lead level, amino acid levels.[2] Consider MRI + CT.

Once the crisis is over, start prophylaxis, eg with sodium valproate or carbamazepine, guided by regimen on p 269. Aim to use one drug only. Increase dose until fits stop, or toxic levels reached. *Out of the context of status, it is not known when to start prophylaxis.* After 2–3 fits is a rule of thumb.

Carbamazepine *SE:* Rash (± exfoliation); platelets↓, agranulocytosis, aplasia (all rare). It induces its own enzymes, so increasing doses may be needed.

Sodium valproate The sugar-free liquid is 200mg/5mL. *SE:* vomiting, appetite↑, drowsiness, thrombocytopenia (do FBC pre-op). Rare hepatotoxicity can be fatal (eg if co-existing unsuspected metabolic disorder). Routine monitoring of LFTs is needed, usually only in first 6 months of use.

Ethosuximide The syrup is 250mg/5mL. *SE:* D&V, rashes, erythema multiforme, lupus syndromes, agitation, headache. Indication: absence epilepsy.

Lamotrigine This is increasingly used in absences and intractable epilepsy as an add-on. **When given with valproate** the dose is 0.2mg/kg/24h PO for 2 weeks, then 0.5mg/kg daily for 2 weeks, then increasing by up to 0.5mg/kg every week. Usual maintenance dose: 1–5mg/kg/day (higher if combined with non-valproate anticonvulsants—eg 2.5–7mg/kg/12h PO).

Vigabatrin (May be first choice in infantile spasms and seizures in tuberose sclerosis.[1]) This GABA analogue blocks GABA transaminase (so GABA ↑ at GABA-ergic synapses, *OHCM* p 406). Consider adding it to regimens if partial seizures are uncontrolled. Vigabatrin starting dose: 40mg/kg/day PO (sachets and tabs are 500mg). Max: 100mg/kg/day. Blood levels do not help (but monitor concurrent phenytoin: it may fall by ~20%[3]). *SE:* Drowsiness, depression, psychosis, amnesia, diplopia and field defects (test every year).[1]

Phenytoin Rarely used as: **1** Dosage is difficult: a small increase may lead to big increases in plasma concentration. **2** Monitoring plasma levels is essential. Aim for 40–80μmol/L (10–20mg/L). **3** Toxic effects: nystagmus, diplopia, dysarthria, tremor and ataxia. **4** *SE:* Intellectual deterioration, depression, motivation↓, behavioural disorders, polyneuropathy, acne, coarse facial features, hirsutism, gum hypertrophy, blood dyscrasias, plasma Ca^{2+} and folate↓.

Education If fits are few, educate teachers on lifting bans on supervised swimming, and cycling etc. Showers are safer than baths. Emphasise importance of compliance (fits *may* ↓threshold for further fits: the concept of *kindling*).

*If IV access fails, try diazepam PR ~0.5mg/kg (not Diazemuls®, absorption is slow)—if using preloaded tubes (as Rectubes®) give 0.5mg/kg stat—eg ~one 10mg tube PR if ~6yrs old. 1 A Appleton *BMJ* 1998 **ii** 1322

Drug	Starting dose mg/kg/24h	Target dose for initial assessment of effect mg/kg/24h	Dose increment		Usually effective dose mg/kg/24h	Doses per day	Target trough drug level in plasma	
			Size mg/kg/24h	Interval in days			mg/L	µmol/L
Carbamazepine	5	12.5	2.5	7	10–25	2–3	4–10	17–42
Valproate	10	20	10.0	10	15–40	1–2	Not helpful	
Phenytoin	5	7	1.0	10	5–9	1–2	10–20	40–80
Phenobarbitone	4	6	2.0	10	4–9	1	15–40	60–180
Ethosuximide	10	15	5.0	5	15–40	1	40–99	280–700
Clonazepam	0.025	0.05	0.025	7	0.025–0.1	2–3	Not helpful	

When to use which drug
Tonic/clonic fits: first try sodium valproate or carbamazepine.
Absences: first choice, ethosuximide; second, sodium valproate.
Myoclonic or akinetic fits: sodium valproate or benzodiazepines.
Infantile spasms: prednisolone or nitrazepam (0.2–0.6mg/day PO).
Partial fits: first try carbamazepine; then sodium valproate.

Stopping anticonvulsants See *OHCM* p 451. The risk of seizure recurrence during the tapering down process is no greater if the tapering period is 6 weeks compared with 9 months.

1 Advanced Life Support Group *Advanced Paediatric Life Support* 1993 BMA 2 M Tunic 1992 *Paed Clin N America* (Oct, p1014) 3 *Drug Ther Bul* 1990 **28** 95

►►Asthma[APLS]

Asthma implies variable airways obstruction (peak flow varies by >20%, p 271), with wheeze, dyspnoea, or cough. *Prevalence:* >7% (>20% wheeze at some time); prevalence↑ if: ♂, birth weight↓, atopy, past bronchopulmonary dysplasia, passive or active smoking. *Differential:* Foreign body, pertussis, croup, epiglottitis, pneumonia, hyperventilation. *Signs of severe asthma:* (Patients may not be distressed). Too breathless to speak or feed; respirations ≥50 breaths/min; pulse ≥140; peak flow ≤50% predicted.
Life-threatening if: Peak flow <33% of predicted •Cyanosis •Silent chest •Fatigue or exhaustion •Agitation/reduced level of consciousness.

Treatment if >5yrs old: BTS guidelines[1,2] •Try to avoid provoking factors •Check inhaler technique •Address all fears •Have self-management plan •Check compliance •Prescribe peak flow meter •Start 1 step above that indicated by severity, gain rapid control (and the patient's confidence), then step down a rung •Double dose of inhaled steroid if control falters, or there is URTI •Rescue prednisolone may always be needed (≤40mg/day, halved if <4yrs old).
Step 1: Try occasional β-agonists. If needed more than daily, add step 2.
Step 2: Add inhaled steroid (eg fluticasone 50–200μg/12h or budesonide 100–400μg/12h) or cromoglicate, eg 20mg/8h as inhaled powder.
Step 3: Add inhaled salmeterol; or↑fluticasone (1000μg/12h+large vol. spacer).
Step 4: Add trial of: •Theophylline (eg Slo-Phyllin® <12mg/kg/24h PO) or: •Long-acting β-agonist tablet, or •Inhaled ipratropium/oxitropium.
Step 5: Add prednisolone tablets eg 5–10mg PO, as a once daily dose.
Dose examples: b-*agonists:* Sugar-free salbutamol is 2mg/5mL; eg 5mL/8h (0.1 mg/kg/8h if <2yrs). Inhalers are far more preferable: terbutaline 250μg per 4–6h (1 puff)—eg with spacer until 8yrs old. Salmeterol inhaled: eg 50μg per 12h; *Xanthines:* Theophylline, 5mg/kg/8h PO (syrup = 60mg/5mL). Try to monitor levels; bioavailability varies between brands. Capsules are 60, 125, or 250mg. Their enclosed granules may be spread on soft food.
NB: beware growth retardation from steroids (including, rarely, from inhalers: inhaled fluticasone has been found to be least problematic in this regard).[3]

Treatment of severe asthma ►A calm atmosphere is beneficial.[4] *Give these treatments if life-threatening signs are present (above) or the patient is not improving 15–30min after treatment has started.*

1 Sit the child up; high-flow 100% O_2
2 Salbutamol—5mg O_2-nebulized in 4mL 0.9% saline (2.5mg if <2yrs) ± 15μg/kg IV[4]
3 Prednisolone 1-2mg/kg PO (max 40mg) ± hydrocortisone 5mg/kg IV over 3min
4 Aminophylline 5mg/kg IV over 20min (omit if already on a xanthine); then IVI aminophylline (opposite). Do levels
5 Hydrocortisone 100mg IV/6h; add ipratropium 0.125–0.25mg to nebulizer
6 Oximetry + CXR if SpO_2 ≤92%
7 Treat any pneumonia
8 Chart peak flow before & after each nebulizer treatment; for normal values, see opposite
9 Repeat nebulizers as needed, eg at 30min, 1h, 2h 3h & 4h
10 Take to ITU if falling peak flow, exhaustion, confusion, feeble respirations, or coma

Before discharge ensure: •Good inhaler technique. •Has had discharge regimen for >24h. •Taking inhaled steroids *and* oral soluble prednisolone. •Written management plan. •Follow-up by GP in 1 week and in clinic in <4 weeks.[1]

Pitfalls[1] •Faulty inhaler technique. Watch the patient operate his device.
•Reluctance to diagnose until a serious attack occurs. Formerly, 50% of diagnoses were made after >15 visits to the GP. Things are now improving.
•Inadequate perception of, and planning for, the severe attack.
•Unnoticed, marked diurnal variation in airways obstruction. Always ask about nocturnal waking: it is a sign of dangerous asthma.
•Being satisfied with less than total symptom control.
•Forgetting to start prophylaxis—and not using oral prednisolone early.
•No direct access to hospital. •Failure to discourage smoking.

Peak flow* (litres/min) in normal boys and girls (5–18 years).

Height (cm)	*Mean*	*Third centile*	*Height (cm)*	*Mean*	*Third centile*
100	110		150	360	300
113	160	100	155	400	320
120	210	140	160	420	350
125	240	160	165	450	370
130	260	190	170	470	400
135	290	220	175	500	430
140	310	240	180	520	450
145	350	270	185	550	470
			190	570	500

Source: S Godfrey 1970 *Br J Dis Chest* 64 15 *To 2 significant figures

Guidelines for continuous IVI of aminophylline

(mg/kg/h)—after a loading dose† of 6–7.5mg/kg IV.

(Multiplying by 0.85 gives dose of theophylline)

	Aminophylline (mg/kg/h)
Neonates	0.15
Infants <6 months	0.47
6–9 months	1.0
Children 10–16 yrs	0.8

†Omit the loading dose if previous theophyllines have been taken. If the plasma theophylline concentration is known and is subtherapeutic, an additional loading dose may be given. Increasing the dose by 1mg/kg causes an increase in serum theophylline of ~2μg/mL).

Erythromycin *increases* the half-life of aminophylline, as do cimetidine, ciprofloxacin, propranolol, and contraceptive steroids. Drugs which *decrease* the half-life: phenytoin, carbamazepine, barbiturates, and rifampicin. Adjust the dose according to plasma concentrations.

►Aim for plasma level of 10–20μg/mL (55–110μmol/L). Serious toxicity (BP↓, arrhythmias, cardiac arrest) can occur at levels ≥25μg/mL.

1 BMJ 1997 **i** 315 & *Thorax* 1997 **52** sp. 1-24 ◄2► KJ Chau 1995 *Arch Paed Adol Med* **149** 201 3 O Walthers 1993 *Arch Dis Chi* **68** 673 & U MacFadyen 1995 *Prescrib J* **35** 174 4 GJ Browne 1997 *Lancet* **349** 301 & E-BM 1997 **2** 138

Abdominal pain

Acute abdominal pain Children often have difficulty in localizing pain, and other factors in the history may be more important. Pointers may be:

- Hard faeces suggest that constipation is the cause (p 206).
- In those of African origin, suspect sickle-cell disease (do sickling tests).
- Suspect TB (do a tuberculin test, p 208) if travel or other factors sugest TB risk.
- In children with pica (p 206), do a blood lead level.
- Abdominal migraine is suggested by periodic abdominal pain with vomiting especially if there is a positive family history.
- If any past UTIs, suspect GU disease (eg renal colic or hydronephrosis).

Common physical causes Gastro-enteritis, UTI, viral illnesses (eg tonsillitis associated with mesenteric adenitis) and appendicitis.

Some rarer causes Mumps pancreatitis; diabetes mellitus; volvulus; intussusception; Meckel's diverticulum; peptic ulcer; Crohn's/ulcerative colitis, Hirschsprung's disease; Henoch–Schönlein purpura and hydronephrosis. Consider menstruation or salpingitis in older girls.
►In boys always check for a torted testis.

Investigations ►Always microscope and culture the urine. Others: consider plain abdominal x-ray; ultrasound; FBC; ESR; IVU, barium studies.

Appendicitis (*OHCM* p 114) is rare if <5yrs, but perforation rates are high in this group (nearing 90%). Think: how can I tell this from other causes of abdominal pain? •Clues in the history: increasing pain in right lower quadrant, no previous episodes, anorexia, slight vomiting, absence of cough and polyuria. •Examination hint: fever and pulse↑ are likely; if the child appears well and can sit forward unsupported, and hop, appendicitis is unlikely. •Tests are unlikely to help when the clinical picture is uncertain.

Gastro-oesophageal reflux/oesophagitis Presents with regurgitation, distress after feeds, apnoea, pneumonia, failure to thrive and anaemia. *Tests:* Endoscopy and evaluation with an oesophageal pH probe is more reliable than barium studies. Ultrasound is not much help. *Treatment:* Reassurance; avoid over feeding (a common cause); lying on the front may help children, but avoid in infants, as this predisposes to cot death (such infants may be helped by lying on the left side). Drugs may be needed, eg an antacid + sodium/magnesium alginate, eg for term infants, Infant Gaviscon® dual dose sachets, 1 dose mixed with 15mL boiled (cooled) water. This paste is given by spoon after each breast feed. If bottle fed, give the dose dissolved in feeds. Children >4.5kg may have a whole dual dose sachet. Carobel® thickens the feeds. If this fails, some experts use cisapride (↑gastro-oesophageal sphincter tone by acting on post-ganglionic nerve endings) 0.2–0.3mg/kg/8h PO (SE: colic; diarrhoea, many drug interactions which ↑Q–T interval which is why the *BNF* rejects this unlicensed use).[1] Most resolve by 6–9 months.

Abdominal distension

Causes *Air:*	*Ascites:*	*Solid masses:*	*Cysts:*
Faecal impaction	Nephrosis	Neuroblastoma	Polycystic kidney
Air swallowing	Hypoproteinaemia	Wilms' tumour	Hepatic; dermoid
Malabsorption	Cirrhosis; CCF	Adrenal tumour	Pancreatic

Hepatomegaly Infections: many, eg infectious mononucleosis, CMV.
Malignancy: leukaemia, lymphoma, neuroblastoma (see below).
Metabolic: Gaucher's and Hurler's diseases, cystinosis; galactosaemia.
Others: sickle-cell disease, and other haemolytic anaemias, porphyria.

Splenomegaly All the above causes of hepatomegaly (not neuroblastoma).

Neuroblastoma This highly malignant tumour, derived from sympathetic neuroblasts, is thought to be an embryonal neoplasm, presenting with decreasing frequency from birth to 5yrs of age. *Prevalence:* 1:6000–

1:10,000. It is the most common solid tumour in the under-5s.[1] *The patient:* is likely to present with abdominal swelling. *Metastatic sites:* Lymph nodes, scalp, bone (causing pancytopenia and osteolytic lesions). In 92%, urinary excretion of catecholamines (vanillylmandelic and homovanillic acids) will be raised. *Treatment:* Refer to special centre. Excision (if possible) and chemotherapy (eg cyclophosphamide and doxorubicin). *Prevention:* Screening programmes (eg urinary catecholamine excretion) exist, but may only be detecting a small proportion of high-risk neuroblastomas.[1] *Prognosis:* This is adversely influenced by genetics (pseudodiploid karyotypes, chromosome 1p deletions, N-*myc* gene amplification), less mature catecholamine synthesis and excretion, and age. Those <1yr old do best, and if stage I and II disease, spontaneous remission may occur in 25%. If older, the disease is often disseminated by the time of presentation.

Recurrent abdominal pain At least 10% of children >5yrs suffer recurrent abdominal pains interfering with normal activities. The question is: is there organic disease? No cause will be found in most, if looked for, but this should neither encourage complacency (you may delay a diagnosis of *Crohn's*[2] (OHCM p 516) or *peptic ulcer*) or lead to an over-zealous diagnosis of underlying psychological problems (now thought to be less important—but do consider it: who is present when the pain starts; what, or who, makes the pain better?).[3] NB: long-term follow-up indicates a 4-fold ↑risk of psychological problems manifesting in adult life.[4]

Consider these causes: gastro-oesophageal reflux (above), small bowel dysmotility, gastritis, duodenitis, carbohydrate malabsorption (eg lactose, sorbitol), abdominal migraine. The rôle of these is unclear in children. *Who to investigate:* There are no hard rules. Be suspicious if the pain is unusual in terms of localization, character, frequency, or severity.

1 *Drug Ther Bul* 1997 **35** 77 & BNF 1998 **ii** page 30 2 I Booth 1991 *Arch Dis Chi* **66** 742 3 M Murphy 1993 *Arch Dis Chi* **69** 409 4 BMJ 1998 **i** 1196–200

Anaemia

The clinical problem You have the results of a full blood count, showing a low Hb (<11g/dL, p 292, the WHO criterion). How should you proceed?

1 Take a history (include travel and diet); examine the child.

2 If the MCV is <70fl suspect iron deficiency or thalassaemia. Features suggesting iron deficiency anaemia (IDA): poor diet, low socio-economic class, bleeding, stomatitis, koilonychia. Features suggesting thalassaemia: of Mediterranean or Thai extraction, short stature, muddy complexion, icteric sclerae, distended abdomen (from hepatosplenomegaly), bossed skull, prominent maxillae (from marrow hyperplasia).

3 If the MCV is >100fl suspect folate deficiency (eg taking phenytoin, malabsorption, p 185), or B_{12} deficiency (breast milk from a vegetarian mother, absent intrinsic factor, malabsorption, worms), or haemolysis.

4 If the MCV is 81–97fl (normocytic), suspect haemolysis, or marrow failure. This may be transient, after infections, or chronic (eg thyroid, kidney or liver failure). Marrow aplasia may follow toxins (eg chloramphenicol) or be inherited (Diamond-Blackfan and Fanconi anaemia, p 744 and 748).

5 Is the WCC or differential abnormal? Eosinophilia (>400 × 10^9/L) + anaemia = hookworms until proved otherwise, in the Tropics.

6 Next look at the ESR/CRP. This may indicate some chronic disease.

7 Look at the film. Do a reticulocyte count. Do thick films for malaria if indicated. Note RBC morphology (*OHCM*, p 572). A hypochromic microcytosis suggests IDA; target cells suggest liver disease or thalassaemia.

8 Further tests: transferrin for IDA; thick film for malaria; sickling tests + Hb electrophoresis for sickle-cell anaemia (do in blacks); B_{12}; red cell folate.

9 Prevention: no cows' milk if <1yr; if formula-fed, use iron-fortified; wean at 4–6 months. Adequate vitamin C intake; iron supplements if premature.

Iron deficiency anaemia This is the commonest nutritional deficiency (20% of the world's population). Despite fortification of breakfast cereals, this is common (12% of white children and 28% of Asian children admitted to hospital).[1] The chief behavioural effect is that iron deficient babies are less happy than others. Dietary causes are the most common—eg poverty, lack of education, or coeliac disease. In recurrent IDA, suspect bleeding (eg Meckel's diverticulum or oesophagitis). Treat with ferrous fumarate syrup (140mg/5mL), 2.5–5mL/12h PO (if <6yrs old; for prems: 0.6mg/kg/day), or Plesmet®/Sytron®. Warn of the dangers of overdosage. Aim for a rise in Hb of >1g/month (do reticulocyte count after 2 months). *Iron deficiency without anaemia:* ►Do not fall into the trap of thinking that if he's not anaemic he's not Fe deficient. CNS iron levels fall *before* RBC mass falls.[1] If in doubt, check ferritin. Treating a low ferritin may improve: •Memory •Lassitude •Developmental delay •Mood •Cognition •Concentration—not only in toddlers but in adolescent girls, facing the demands of puberty and menstruation.[2] NB: pica is a sign of iron deficiency.

Haemolysis Get expert help, and try to provide the expert with sufficient information to answer these 4 questions: •Any evidence of ↑ rate of RBC production, ie polychromasia, reticulocytosis, marrow hyperplasia?
- Is there decreased RBC survival? (Bilirubin ↑, haptoglobins ↓)
- Is there intravascular haemolysis? (Haemoglobinuria)
- Is there an inborn error of metabolism (eg G6PD deficiency), spherocytosis or is the defect acquired (usually with +ve Coombs' test)?

Sickle-cell disease ►*OHCM* p 588. *Pain relief:* Try warmth, hydration, and oral analgesia (ibuprofen 5mg/kg/6h PO, codeine phos 1mg/kg/4–8h PO up to 3mg/kg/day). If this fails, see on the ward and offer prompt morphine by IVI—eg 0.1mg/kg. Consider patient-controlled analgesia (PCA). Start PCA with morphine 1mg/kg in 50mL 5% dextrose, and try a rate of 1mL/h, allowing the patient to deliver extra boluses of 1mL when needed. Do respiration and sedation score every ¼h + pulse oximetry if chest/abdominal pain.[2]

1 A Emond 1995 *Arch Dis Chi* **74** 36–9 2 AB Bruner 1996 *Lancet* **348** 992

Purpura in children

If a child is ill with purpura he or she should be presumed to have meningococcaemia (and be given penicillin, p 258), leukaemia or disseminated intravascular coagulation (investigate initially with a visual blood film and WCC). If the child is well, and there is no history of trauma, the cause is likely to be Henoch–Schönlein purpura or idiopathic thrombocytopenic purpura, readily told apart by the normal platelet count in the former. (Aplastic anaemia is very rare.)

Idiopathic thrombocytopenic purpura *Presentation:* Acute bruising, purpura, and petechiae. Less commonly there is bleeding from gums, nose or rectum. If this is present to any large extent, or there is lymphadenopathy, hepatosplenomegaly, or pancytopenia, another diagnosis is likely. *Tests:* The peripheral blood film usually shows only simple thrombocytopenia. ITP may be a response to a virus, and it is worth looking for congenital CMV if the patient is <1yr old. Also look for Epstein–Barr virus and erythrovirus (formerly parvovirus B19). There may also be a lymphocytosis. It is not necessary to do a marrow biopsy, unless:

- Unusual features are present, eg possibly abnormal cells on a film.
- Platelet count is $<30 \times 10^9$/L or the count is not rising after ~2 weeks.
- Treatment is contemplated with steroids.

Platelet antibody tests are unhelpful. If there are features of SLE (may be associated) do DNA binding.

CT scans to exclude intracerebral haemorrhage may be needed if there is headache or CNS signs.

Natural history: The course may be gradual resolution over ~3 months, or the course may be more chronic (>6 months in 10–20%). The chronic form is compatible with normal longevity, and normal activities of daily living, provided contact sports are avoided.

Management: Consider admitting to hospital if:

- Unusual features, including excessive bleeding.
- Social circumstances.
- There are rowdy siblings at home who might engage in physical badinage (the risk of intracranial haemorrhage is <1%).

Splenectomy may benefit ⅔ of those with chronic ITP if >6yrs old, and have had ITP for >1yr. NB: Platelet transfusion is only indicated if very severe haemorrhage (and during splenectomy). Steroids and immunoglobulin are now not used (unfavourable risk/benefit ratio). Follow-up of 92 children with chronic ITP revealed only one death from bleeding, and this was associated with a major physical assault.[1,2]

Henoch–Schönlein purpura (HSP) This presents with purpura (ie purple spots/nodules which do not disappear on pressure—signifying intradermal bleeding) often over buttocks and extensor surfaces. There may be associated urticaria. The typical patient is a young boy. There may be a nephritis (with crescents, in ⅓ of patients—an IgA nephropathy—we could think of HSP as being a systemic version of Berger's syndrome, *OHCM* 694), joint involvement, abdominal pain (± intussusception), which may be severe enough to mimic an 'acute abdomen'. The fault lies in the vasculature; the platelets are normal. It often follows respiratory infection, and it usually follows a benign course over months. Complications (worse in adults): massive GI haemorrhage, ileus, haemoptysis (rare) and renal failure (rare).

1 O Eden 1992 *Arch Dis Chi* **67** 1056–8 2 MM Reid 1995 *Arch Dis Chi* **72** 125–8

Upper respiratory infections[1]

Stridor and epiglottitis ►►Acute stridor may be a terrifying experience for children and this fear may lead to hyperventilation, which makes symptoms worse. Causes: p 558. The leading causes to be distinguished are viral croup and epiglottitis (rare in the UK since vaccination): see table opposite. *Investigations:* A lateral neck x-ray may show an enlarged epiglottis (but do not insist on x-rays at the expense of upsetting the child).

Croup (Acute laryngotracheobronchitis) *Epidemics:* Autumn & spring. *Causes:* Parainfluenza virus (types 1, 2, 3), respiratory syncytial virus, measles (rare). Symptoms are caused by subglottic oedema, inflammation and exudate. *Management of croup:* Mostly at home. Anecdotal evidence suggests that a warm, humid environment is helpful, but mist tents have lost favour as they frighten children, and subsequent hyperventilation increases distress. Aim for minimal interference and careful observation by an experienced nurse. Watch for restlessness, rising pulse and respiration rate, increasing indrawing of the chest wall, fatigue and drowsiness. This will prompt intubation under general anaesthesia. If severe, admit to hospital, and buy time with nebulized epinephrine (=adrenaline) 1:1000. Nebulized budesonide also helps—loading dose: 2mg, then 1mg/12h eg as Pulmicort Respules®.[1,2] Oral dexamethasone 0.15mg/kg for each dose is equally effective, and cheaper.[2]

Management of suspected epiglottitis Accompany the child to hospital (complete airways obstruction may occur suddenly). ►*Avoid examining the throat.* This may precipitate obstruction. Once in hospital, summon the most experienced anaesthetist. Ask him to make the diagnosis by laryngoscopy. If the appearances are those of epiglottitis (a cherry-red, swollen epiglottis), electively intubate, *before* obstruction occurs. (A smaller diameter endotracheal tube than normal for that age may be needed—so don't precut all your tubes!) Then do blood cultures. The cause is usually *Haemophilus influenzae* type b, and strains resistant to ampicillin (and less so chloramphenicol) are prevalent, so the only safe initial treatment is a 3rd generation cefalosporin (eg cefotaxime 1–2g/8h IV adults, 25–50mg/kg/8h IV children). Hydrocortisone (1–2mg/kg/6h IV) is often given, but is not of proven value. Expect to extubate after about 24h (longer if the diagnosis turns out to be staphylococcal laryngotracheobronchitis, when flucloxacillin 50mg/kg/6h IV should also be given).

Diphtheria is caused by the toxin of *Corynebacterium diphtheriae*. It usually starts with tonsillitis ± a false membrane over the fauces. The toxin may cause polyneuritis, often starting with cranial nerves. Shock may occur from myocarditis, toxaemia, or conducting system involvement. Other signs: dysphagia; muffled voice; bronchopneumonia and airway obstruction preceded by a brassy cough (laryngotracheal diphtheria); nasal discharge with an excoriated upper lip (nasal diphtheria). If there is tachycardia out of proportion to fever, suspect a toxin-induced myocarditis. Monitor with frequent ECGs. Motor palatal paralysis also occurs.
Diagnosis is by swab culture of material below the pseudomembrane.
Treatment: Diphtheria antitoxin: 10,000–30,000U IM (any age) and erythromycin; give contacts 7 days' erythromycin syrup: <2yrs old 125mg/6h PO (500mg per 6h if >8yrs) *before swab results are known.* UK vaccination has been effective.
Prevention: Isolate until 3 –ve cultures separated by 48h. There is a resurgence of diphtheria in Moscow and St Petersburg. Those born before 1942 visiting Russia or the Ukraine who have *close local contacts* need a primary *low dose* course. Give a booster (0.5mL of Diftavax®; contains tetanus toxoid too) to diphtheria contacts whose primary immunization was >10yrs ago. Explain that it may not work. Schick tests are no longer available.

Sore throats See p 556. **Coryza** See OHCM p 206.

1 CW Godden 1997 *Arch Dis Chi* 76 155–7   2 A Thomson 1997 *Arch Dis Chi* 76 157–8

Viral croup	*versus*	*Epiglottitis (supraglottitis)*
Onset over a few days		Sudden onset
Stridor only when upset		Continuous stridor
Stridor sounds harsh		Stridor softer, snoring
Voice hoarse		Voice muffled/whispering
Barking cough		Cough not prominent
Likely to be apyrexial		Toxic and feverish (eg T° >39°C)
Can swallow oral secretions		Drooling of secretions

Note: the distinction may not be clear cut. If in doubt, admit to hospital.

Lower respiratory infections

Each year ~3 million infants die from acute respiratory infections (WHO). ►If severely ill, think of staphs, TB and HIV (pneumocystosis, *OHCM* p 334). In any chronic cough think of: •Pertussis •TB •Foreign body •Asthma •Smoking.

Acute bronchiolitis is the commonest lower respiratory tract infection in infants <1yr old. Coryza precedes cough, low fever, tachypnoea, wheeze, apnoea, intercostal recession, and cyanosis if severe. In winter, an epidemic of respiratory syncytial virus is the usual cause, and is identified by immunofluorescence of nasopharyngeal aspirates. Other causes: mycoplasma, parainfluenza, adenoviruses. Those <6 months old are most at risk. Signs that admission is needed are feeding difficulties, tachypnoea >50 breaths/min, and episodes of apnoea. *Tests:* CXR (eg hyperinflation); blood gases/oximetry; FBC. *Treatment:*[1] If severe, give 40% O_2; feed by nasogastric tube. 5% need ventilating (mortality ≈1%, rising to ~33% if symptomatic congenital heart disease). Nebulized ribavirin may help those at greatest risk (congenital heart disease; cystic fibrosis). Antibiotics and steroids are generally not indicated; the former may be used if secondary bacterial pneumonia is suspected.

Pneumonia[2] Signs: fever, malaise, feeding difficulties, tachypnoea and cyanosis. Older children may have typical lobar pnuemonia, with toxaemia and pleural pain. Auscultation: creps; bronchial breathing (easy to miss). CXR: consolidation. Cavitation suggests TB or a staphylococcal abscess. Take samples (blood; urine culture) before starting 'blind' antibiotics, eg penicillin G 25mg/kg/4h IV + erythromycin ethylsuccinate eg as Erythroped® syrup (250mg/5mL)—5mL/12h PO for babies ≤2yrs, 10mL/12h from 2–8yrs; if severely affected, give this dose 6-hourly. Alternative: ampicillin 25–50mg/kg/6h. High-flow O_2 may be needed. If compliance is a problem, once daily azithromycin may be the answer: 10mg/kg, ie 200mg (5mL) if 15–25kg, PO for 3 days. *Causes: Pneumococcus, Haemophilus, Staphylococcus, Mycoplasma* (hence the choice of erythromycin), TB, viruses.

Pulmonary tuberculosis ►Suspect; if from overseas, and their contacts, or HIV+ve. *Clinical features:* Anorexia, low fever, failure to thrive, malaise. Cough is common, but may be absent. *Diagnosis:* tuberculin tests (p 208); culture and Ziehl–Neelsen stain of sputa (× 3) and gastric aspirate. CXR: consolidation, cavities. Miliary spread (fine white dots on CXR) is rare but grave. *Treatment:* Seek expert help. 6-month supervised regimen: isoniazid 15mg/kg PO 3 times a week + rifampicin 15mg/kg/PO ac 3 times a week + pyrazinamide (first 2 months only) 50mg/kg PO 3 times a week. Monitor U&E and LFT before and during treatment. Stop rifampicin if the bilirubin rises (hepatitis). Isoniazid may cause neuropathy (give concurrent pyridoxine). ►Explain the need for prolonged treatment. Multiple drug resistance: *OHCM* p 199.

Whooping cough (*Bordetella pertussis*) is underdiagnosed. Bouts of coughing which end with vomiting which are worse at night, and after feeding suggest the diagnosis—particularly if associated with cyanosis. The whoop (not always present) is caused by forced inspiration against a closed glottis. Differentiation from pneumonia, asthma, bronchitis and bronchiolitis is aided by the (usual) absence of a fever >38.4 °C and wheeze. Peak age: 3yrs (a smaller peak at 30yrs, ie the reservoir in parents). In the UK, the illness is usually mild, with ~1% needing hospital admission (eg with a secondary pneumonia)—in one careful GP survey of 500 consecutive patients. *Diagnosis:* Culture is unsatisfactory (organisms often die on the way to the laboratory). Direct fluorescent antibody testing of nasopharyngeal aspirates is specific but insensitive. Absolute lymphocytosis is common (sometimes very high). *Incubation:* 10–14 days. *Complications:* Prolonged illness may occur (>3 months). Coughing bouts may cause petechiae (eg on the cheek), conjunctival haemorrhage or CNS damage. Deaths may occur (particularly in infants), as may late bronchiectasis. *Treatment/prevention:* Erythromycin, salbutamol and steroids are not very effective. Erythromycin is often used in those likely to expose infants to the disease (benefit is unproven). Admit if <6 months old (risk of apnoea). *Vaccine:* p 208.

1 K Rakshi 1994 *Arch Dis Chi* 71 463-9 2 SW Denny 1986 *J Paediatrics* **108** 635-96

The chesty infant

Many children with cough and wheeze do not fit into the categories opposite, and are too young for a diagnosis of asthma to be made with confidence. These infants often end up being treated with escalating bronchodilator therapy with frequent courses of antibiotics against uncultured organisms. While it is certainly true that asthma can begin in infancy, most of these chesty infants do not have asthma—but we tend to prescribe 'just in case'. As the natural history of symptoms is to vary from hour to hour, sometimes we *appear* to be successful. 'Happy wheezers' probably require no treatment, whereas those with chest symptoms starting very early in life need a sweat test to rule out cystic fibrosis. Between these two ends of the spectrum of 'chestiness' lie those who clearly need some help. These may benefit from relatively high-dose inhaled steroids, given regularly for 8 weeks or so.[1] Assess benefit by reference to reduction in sleep disturbance.

Aim to engage in a constructive dialogue with parents so that they understand that treatment is often unsuccessful, but that their child is unlikely to come to harm, while he or she is 'growing out of it'.

1 D Cochran 1998 BMJ i 1546

Renal failure and some renal diseases

Acute renal failure Essence: a rapidly rising K^+ and urea often with anuria (<100mL/day) or oliguria (<200mL/m²/day) and ↑BP.

Causes: GU obstruction, toxins (eg sulfonamides), glomerulonephritis (GN, *OHCM* p 380); haemoglobinuria; myoglobinuria; (*OHCM* p 394); ATN (opposite).

Plasma biochemistry: K^+↑, urea↑, PO_4^{3-}↑; Ca^{2+}↓, Na^+↓, Cl^-↓.

MSU: Are there red cell casts (=GN)? If no RBCs seen but Labstix +ve for RBCs, consider haemo/myoglobinuria (*OHCM* p 394).

Other tests: ECG, serum and urine osmolality, creatinine, acid–base state, PCV, platelets, clotting studies (DIC), C3, ASO titre, ANA (antinuclear antibody).

Radiology: ►Arrange prompt abdominal ultrasound. Are the ureters dilated (eg stones)? If so, urgent surgery may be required.

Treatment: •Treat shock and dehydration promptly (p 250).
- If the urine/plasma (U/P) osmolality ratio is >5 the kidneys concentrate well; the oliguria should respond to rehydration.
- If the U/P ratio is low, try for a diuresis: frusemide 1.5mg/kg IV slowly, maximum 20mg/day.
- If BP↑↑: nitroprusside (p 304).
- 24h fluid requirement: Avoid overhydration. Replace losses + insensible loss (12–15mL/kg). Aim for weight loss (0.5%/day).
- Give no K^+. Monitor ECG. Tall T-waves and QRS slurring prompt urgent lowering of K^+, with:
  1. Glucose (4g/kg) with soluble insulin (1u/4g of glucose) IVI over 2h.
  2. Resonium A® 0.5g/kg PO.
  3. Calcium gluconate (10%, 0.5mL/kg IV over 5min; monitor ECG: stop IVI if heart rate↓) to counteract electrophysiological effect of hyperkalaemia.
- High energy, protein limited diet to slow catabolism.
- Dialysis indications (a guide, only): K^+ >7mmol/L; urea >40mmol/L; HCO_3^- <13mmol/L; severe hypertension; overhydration.
- Monitor BP. •Improvement is ushered in with a diuretic phase.

Chronic renal failure

Causes: Congenital dysplastic kidneys, pyelonephritis, glomerulonephritis.

Clinical features: Weakness, tiredness, vomiting, headache, restlessness, twitches, hypertensive retinopathy, fits and coma.

Treatment: •Correct fluid and electrolyte imbalance.
- If diastolic BP >100mmHg consider propranolol (10–20mg/8–12h PO).
- Vitamin D (50 nanograms/kg of alfacalcidol each day PO) is helpful in reducing phosphate excretion, and promoting Ca^{2+} absorption, thereby preventing 'renal rickets'.
- Talk to with experts: haemodialysis, transplants, growth hormone treatment.

Haemolytic uraemic syndrome *Essence:* Microangiopathic haemolytic anaemia, thrombocytopenia, renal failure, and endothelial damage to glomerular capillaries. *Typical age:* 3 months to 3yrs. Epidemics may occur from *E coli* Verocytotoxin. Diarrhoea is usual but not *always* present.
Other causes: Shigella, HIV, SLE, drugs, tumour, scleroderma, BP↑.
Clinical features: Colitis→haemoglobinuria→oliguria ± CNS signs→encephalopathy→coma. LDH↑. WCC↑. Coombs' –ve. PCV↓. Fragmented RBCs.
Mortality: 5–30%. A few have many relapses—to form a condition rather like thrombotic thrombocytopenic purpura (TTP).
Treatment: Seek expert advice. Treat the renal failure (above). There is no evidence that fibrinolytic agents or anticoagulation help. Relapses in TTP may be preventable by steroids, splenectomy, or vincristine.

Causes of acute tubular necrosis (ATN)

- Crush injury
- Dehydration
- Septicaemia
- Burns
- Shock
- Malaria

Acute nephritis and nephrosis

Acute nephritis Essence: haematuria and oliguria (±hypertension and uraemia) produced by an immune mechanism in the kidney.

Causes: Often β-haemolytic streptococcus, which may cause a sore throat 2 weeks before an acute glomerulonephritis. Others:

- Henoch–Schönlein purpura
- Berger's disease (*OHCM* p 694)
- Infections: viruses; SBE; syphilis
- Toxins, heavy metals
- Malignancies
- Renal vein thrombosis

Uncomplicated presentation: Age peak: 7 years. Haematuria; oliguria; 50% have hypertension; periorbital oedema; fever; GI disturbance; loin pain.

Complications: **1** hypertensive encephalopathy (restless, drowsy, bad headaches, fits, visual disturbances, vomiting, coma). **2** Cardiac involvement: gallop rhythm, cardiac failure and enlargement, pulmonary oedema. **3** Uraemia: acidosis, twitching, stupor, coma.

Tests: •Urine microscopy (count red and white cells, hyaline, granular cellular casts; red cell casts mean glomerular bleeding). Phase-contrast detects abnormally shaped red cells, signifying glomerular bleeding. This change may not be present at first. 24h urine for protein and creatinine clearance. Check urine culture, and specific gravity (normal range: neonate 1.012; infants 1.002–1.006; child/adult 1.001–1.035).

- Blood: urea↑ in ⅔; ESR↑; acidosis. Complement (C3) often ↓ 2–8 weeks after onset (not in Henoch–Schönlein purpura). Find the cause: do ASO titre, antinuclear factor, syphilis serology, blood cultures, virology.
- Other tests: renal ultrasound, renal biopsy—check platelets, clotting and IVU (are there two kidneys?); parents' consent.

Treatment: Restrict protein when in oliguric phase. Give penicillin 10mg/kg/4h IV for the first few days, then PO for 3 months to prevent further streptococcal infection. Measure BP often. Treat severe hypertension (p 304). If encephalopathy, give nitroprusside 0.5–8μg/kg/min IVI (p 304).

Nephrotic syndrome (nephrosis) Essence: oedema, proteinuria (eg 4g/24h), hypoproteinaemia ± hypercholesterolaemia. In 90% the cause is unknown, but any of the causes of nephritis (above) may also cause nephrosis. Histology: usually minimal change. Symptoms: anorexia, GI disturbance, infections, irritability; then oedema (periorbital, genital), ascites, oliguria.

Urine: Frothy, albuminous; ± casts; Na^+↓ (secondary hyperaldosteronism).

Blood: Albumin↓ (so total Ca^{2+}↓); urea and creatinine usually normal.

Renal biopsy: Reserve this for older children with any of: haematuria, BP↑, urea↑, if protein loss is unselective (ie large molecular weights as well as small), and treatment 'failures'.

Complications: Pneumococcal peritonitis, so consider Pneumovax Ⅱ if >2yrs.

Treatment: Limit oedema with protein-controlled (3g/kg/24h), low Na^+ diet (<50mmol/24h). Consider frusemide (1–2mg/kg/24h slow IV or PO) and spironolactone (1.2mg/kg/12h PO). *For 'minimal change'* give prednisolone, eg up to 1mg/kg/24h PO (not if incubating chickenpox!) for 8–12 weeks, or for 1 week after remission-induction. Half the induction dose is then given, eg for 1 month, with subsequent tapering. 90% respond in 8 weeks. ~30% of responders have no relapse. 10–20% of these are cured after ≤4 courses of steroids. The rest may become dependent on steroids: if >0.5mg/kg/day of prednisolone is needed, growth may be slowed, especially at adolescence, and agents such as cyclophosphamide may be indicated (2–2.5mg/kg/day PO, SE: haemorrhagic cystitis, WCC↓, hair loss, infertility). Alternatives: chlorambucil 0.2mg/kg/day; ciclosporin (nephrotoxic, *OHCM* p 622).[1]

►Monitor BP. Meticulous control minimizes progression to renal failure.[1]

1 P Mason 1994 *BMJ* ii 1557

3. Paediatrics

Non-accidental injury (NAI)

NAI has, until recently, been an overtly endemic feature of our culture (eg floggings of 24 lashes of 'the cat' for 'misconduct' in 8-year-olds[1]). In some hospitals abused children arrive almost daily. Abuse may be physical, sexual, emotional, or by neglect. *Risk factors:* Birth weight <2500g; mother <30yrs; unwanted pregnancy; stress; social class IV and V *Suspect abuse if:*

- Disclosure by the child
- Inconsistent story
- Odd mode of injury*
- Late presentation, to an unknown doctor
- Odd constellation of signs
- The accompanying adult may not be a parent
- Parental financial problems
- Efforts to avoid full examination, eg after an immersion burn.
- Unexplained fracture; injury to buttocks, perineum or face. Ruptured tongue frenulum results from shaking; also look for vitreous/retinal bleeds, hyphaema (p 514), lens dislocation, bulging fontanelle, head circumference ↑ ± xanthochromia; ►if in doubt, do CT.[1] *Other telling signs:* Cigarette burns; linear whip marks (look for outline of a belt buckle, or the loop of a double electric flex); bruised *non-mobile* baby; signs of suffocation.

Imponderable questions Although non-medical, these need addressing because we are not simply technicians, and they influence what we do, how we react to child abuse, and how the rest of society perceives our rôle.

- Could *proving* of abuse be more destructive than the abuse itself?[2]
- Is it better for him to be loved and battered than neither?
- Is help from the extended family more desirable than the law?
- Is it possible that the parents will grow through crisis, as battering is brought to light, and help given?

Remember that the first aim is to prevent organ damage and murder. If this is a real danger ►*contact the duty social worker today*—eg for an emergency protection order. Offer help to the parents. Learn to listen, leaving blame and punishment to judges. Find out about local policies and referral routes. Remember that very often your duty is not to diagnose child abuse, but to recognize *possible* abuse, and then to get help.[3]

Sexual misuse This may be prevented by pre-school teaching about 'personal safety' and how to say 'No'. Once a child's claim is made, believe it (usually). Know your local guidelines. Follow them. Inform Social Services. If you do not, ask yourself with whom you are colluding. Forensic specimens (eg pubic hair, vaginal swabs) should be taken by an expert who knows how to be gentle, and to avoid a 'second rape'. Prepubertal venereal disease means abuse until proven otherwise. Does abuse cause psychological harm? It is impossible to be sure: although morbidity is increased, this may reflect antecedent events which themselves lead to the abuse (ie confounding variables, eg absent mother, stepfather, which themselves predict later morbidity).[4]

Repertoire of actions by the GP

- Liaise with health visitor or the National Society for the Prevention of Cruelty to Children (NSPCC), if in the UK; have the child put on a Social Services 'at risk' register.
- Admission to a place of safety (eg hospital or foster home).
- Continuing support for parents and protection for siblings.
- Prevention: encourage impulses to be shared, and not acted on.
- Attend a 'case conference' (eg with social worker, health visitor, paediatrician and police) to help decide what action to take. Note: it is not known if such conferences are the best way of making such decisions. Not all members will know the family.

*Look for injuries inconsistent with child's level of development. 1 H Carty 1995 BMJ **i** 344 2 K Hulme 1984 *Bone People*, Spiral 3 R Morton 1992 *Accidents & Emergencies in Children*, OUP 4 A Weiner 1991 BMJ **ii** 415

A possible sequence of events might be:[1]

Unexplained signs (or disclosure, or allegations), eg odd bruising

↓

'Testing of professional hypotheses'≈weighing it up in your own mind

↓

'Clarification by discussion with an experienced colleague' ≈ tell your boss

↓

'Reach a critical threshold of professional concern' ≈ you're both worried

↓

'Weigh the pros and cons of breaking confidentiality' ≈ try to do your best (Disclosing medical facts to social services without consent is 'illegal'.)

↓

'Sharing concerns with statutory agencies' ≈ phone Social Services/police

↓

'Act within a timeframe not detrimental to the child' ≈ aim to do it now

↓

'Contemporaneous records detailing all your sources' ≈ write it down now

↓

'Preliminary consultation with all concerned': don't promise to keep secrets

↓

'Strategic multidisciplinary discussion' ≈ is an abuse investigation needed?

↓

'If so, 'Instigation of child abuse investigation' ≈ plan a case conference

↓

'Must parents/child be present?' ≈ bend the ear of the conference chairman

↓

Tell parents and child (if appropriate) what your report to conference will be

↓

Case conference timed to let doctors fulfil their major rôle ≈ ?get a locum

↓

Register your dissent (if any) to the conference conclusions in its minutes

↓

Child is placed on a Register indicating that questions of abuse are unresolved

↓

'Establish networks for information exchange, discussion & advice' ≈ follow up by social services, or a national society protecting children from cruelty (NSPCC)

↓

Second (review) conference to weigh new evidence

↓

Death of a child

↓

Agencies must issue reports to the Area Child Protection Committee (in UK)

↓

Judge issues a life sentence ≈ male breadwinner removed from family for ~10yrs

↓

No ♂ rôle model for siblings ≈ perpetuation of a cycle of poverty and abuse

↓

Unexplained bruising in a member of the next generation

↓

*Man hands on misery to man**

---

1 DoH 1994 *Child Protection: Medical Responsibilities* and 1991 *Working Together Under the Children Act 1989*, HMSO ► NB: not all our efforts to protect children end thus. Successes are frequent.

Man hands on misery to man.
It deepens like a coastal shelf.
Get out as early as you can,
And don't have any kids yourself.

*Philip Larkin, *This Be The Verse*

(This might be thought a trifle pessimistic, particularly to readers of PD James's *Children of Men*, which records that, far from reducing misery, 100% childlessness produces universal panic.)

Sudden infant death syndrome (SIDS)

Definition 'Sudden death of an infant under 1 year of age, which is unexpected after a thorough case investigation, including a complete autopsy, examination of the death scene, and review of the clinical history.'[1]

SIDS is the leading 'cause' of death in infants aged over 1 week old.

Epidemiology Peak incidence: 1–4 months; higher incidence in lower socio-economic classes, passive smokers, males, premature babies and during winter; co-existing minor upper respiratory infection is common.

Theories These deaths were often attributed to direct mechanical suffocation, eg from a pillow, or from the family cat misplacing itself. It is now recognized that these deaths are just as common in families without cats, and in cots without pillows. There is no single cause which yet explains all cot deaths, but the following have been proposed:

Obstructive apnoea:	*Central apnoea:*	*Others:* Prolonged Q–T interval[2]
Inhalation of milk	Faulty CO_2 drive	Overheating/heat stroke
Airways oedema	Prematurity	Immature diaphragm
Pharyngeal collapse	Brainstem gliosis	Passive smoking; viruses

Preventing overheating and exposure to parental cigarette smoke are the main areas to concentrate on in prevention. The risk from passive smoking is dose-dependent, and often at least doubles risk. The face is an important platform for heat loss—and it is known that the incidence of SIDS is ~5–10-fold higher among infants usually sleeping prone (17-fold higher if sleeping in a room separated from parents):[3] ►so recommend sleeping supine (unless there is gastro-oesophageal reflux, Pierre Robin syndrome or scoliosis). Advise as follows:[4]

- Do not overheat the baby's bedroom. Aim for a temperature of 16–20°C.
- Do not use too much bedding, and avoid duvets if less than 1 year of age.
- If ill or feverish, consult a GP—do not increase the amount of bedding.
- Have feet come down to the cot's end to avoid migrations under blankets.
- While sleeping, avoid heaters, hot water bottles, electric blankets and hats unless ambient T° is very low. Do wrap up if going out in winter.
- Babies >1month do not need to be kept as warm as in hospital nurseries.

Autopsy is unrevealing; minor changes are common; petechial haemorrhages over pleura, pericardium or thymus, and vomit in the trachea may be agonal events. *Causes to exclude:* meningococcaemia; epiglottitis; heart defects; murder.[1]

How the GP can help the family on the first day

- A prompt visit to express sympathy emphasizing that no one is to blame.
- Explain about necessary postmortems and coroner's inquests. The parents may be called upon to identify the body.
- Bedding may be needed to help find the cause of death.
- Don't automatically suppress lactation (bromocriptine 2.5mg/12h PO for 1 week), as continued lactation may be an important way of grieving.
- Many parents will not want anxiolytics, but may want hypnotics.
- Admit a twin sibling to hospital (their risk is increased).

Subsequent help[4] Advise the parents of likely grief reactions (guilt, anger, loss of appetite, hearing the baby cry). Make sure that the coroner informs you of the necropsy result; take some trouble to explain these to the parents. Offer them a chance to talk to a consultant paediatrician. This can provide helpful reinforcement and encouragement to the parents and yourself. The parents may find an electronic apnoea alarm reassuring in caring for later infants. Ask if they would like to join a self-help group.[5]

1 *Lancet* Ed 1999 **353** 161 2 P Schwartz 1998 NEJM **338**; risk↑ if Q–T corrected for rate (QT^c) ≥440msec; NB: $QT^c = (Q\text{-}T)/(\sqrt{R\text{-}R})$ 3 P Pharoah 1996 *Lancet* **347** 2 4 DoH advice 1993 PL/COM (93) 4 5 Cot Death Helpline (24h) 0171 235 1721; 14 Halkin St, London SW1

Denver developmental screening test

Younger children may be examined while sitting on their mother's lap. Explain to her that the child is not expected to pass every test. Begin with a few very easy tests. Go slowly.

Test materials Ball of red wool, box of raisins, rattle with handle, small bottle, bell, tennis ball, 8 blocks (one inch cubes).

Administering the test •Draw a vertical line at the child's chronological age on the charts on p 290–1. If premature, subtract the months premature from the chronological age.

- The items to be administered are those through which the line passes. A parent may administer a test if the child wishes.
- Failure to pass an item passed by ≥90% of children may or may not be abnormal. Note how the child behaves during the test.

Test footnotes (See top corner of test boxes on p 290–1.)

1 When prone lifts head up, using forearm support (± hands).
2 No head lag as you pull by the hand from supine to sitting.
3 Child may use a wall or rail for help (but not a person).
4 Throws ball overhand 3 feet to within your reach.
5 Jumps over a distance (eg over an A4 piece of paper).
6 Walk forward, heel within one inch of toe.
7 Bounce a ball. He must catch it. Allow up to 3 trials.
8 Walk backwards, toe within 1 inch of heel.
9 Wave wool slowly before eyes: do eyes move 90° to midline?
10 Grasps rattle when it touches his finger tips.
11 Looks for ball of wool dropped out of sight over table's edge.
12 Child grasps raisin between thumb and index finger.
13 Overhand grasp of raisin between thumb and index finger.
14 'Copy this' (circle). Do not name or demonstrate.
15 'Which line is longer?'; turn upside down and repeat.
16 'Copy this' (cross). Pass crossing lines at any angle.
17 'Copy this' (square). You may demonstrate if he fails.
18 Two arms or two eyes or two legs only count as one part.
19 Name the pictures at the bottom of the chart.
20 'Give the block to Mum'. 'Put it on the table'. No gestures.
21 Answer ⅔ of: 'What do you do if you are cold/hungry/tired?'
22 Put this on/under/in front of/behind the chair. No gestures.
23 Answer ⅔: 'Fire is hot, ice is– '. 'Mum is a woman, Dad is a–'. 'A horse is big, a mouse is– '.
24 Define 6/8 of ball, lake, desk, house, banana, curtain, hedge, pavement. An verbal indication of understanding is passed.
25 Answer 3/3 of: 'What is a spoon/shoe/door made of?' (No others).
26 Smile, talk or wave, to elicit smile (3 tries). Do not touch.
27 While he plays with a toy, pull it away. Pass if he resists.
28 Child need not be able to tie shoes or button at the back.

►This test is poor at picking up articulatory or mild linguistic deficits—if this is suspected, liaise with speech experts. NB: an alternative version of this test (*Denver II*), contains more language items, new age scales, new categories of item interpretation and a behaviour rating scale.[1]

1 WK Frankenburg 1992 **89** *Paediatrics* 91

3. Paediatrics

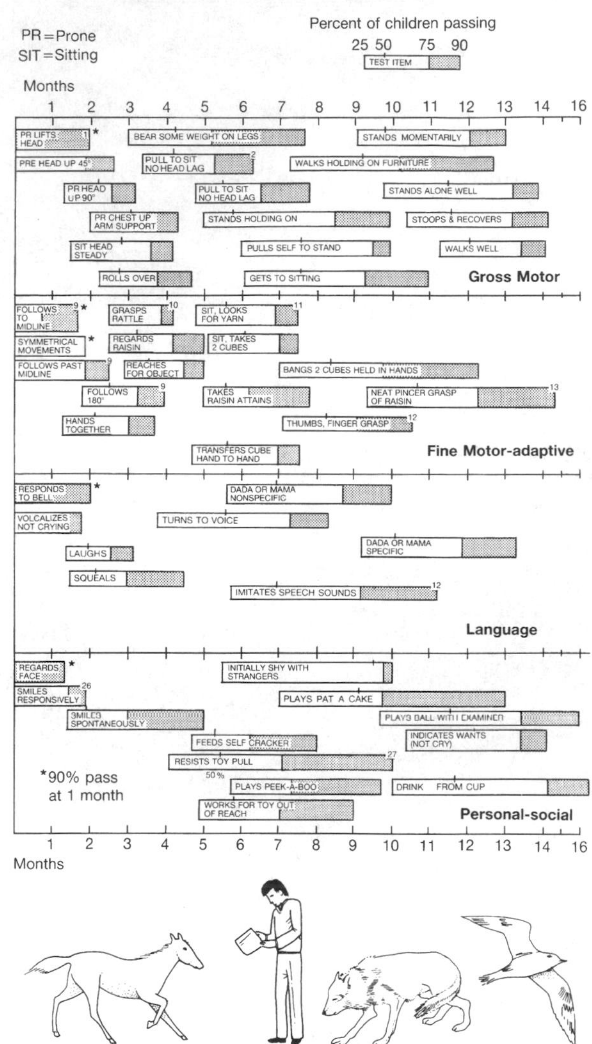

Denver developmental screening test. (After H Silver, C Kempe & H Bruyn 1977 *Handbook of Paediatrics*, Lange.)

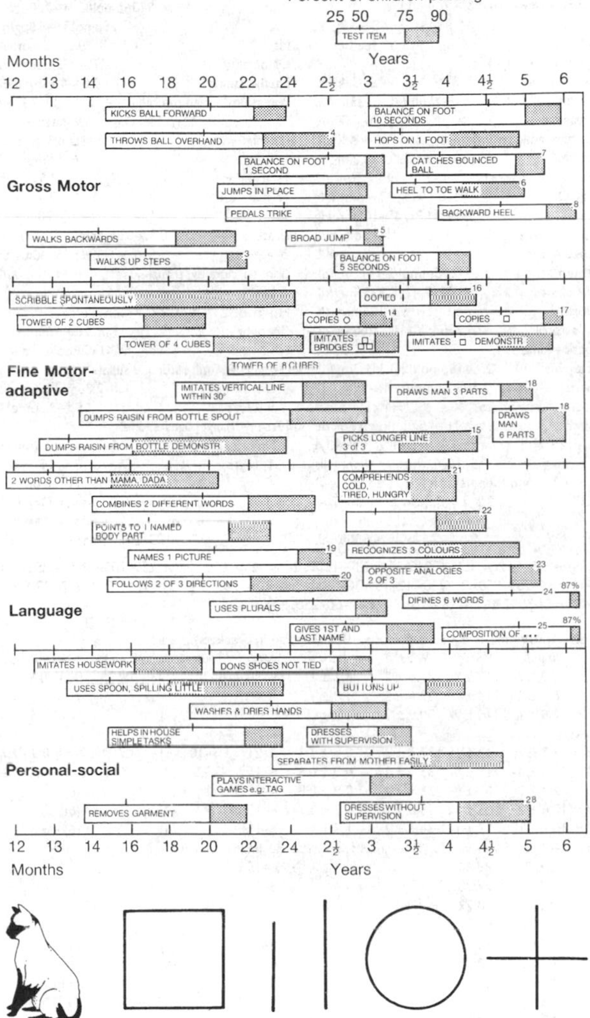

Percent of children passing
25 50 75 90
TEST ITEM
Months
Years
12 13 14 16 18 20 22 24 2½ 3 3½ 4 4½ 5 6
Gross Motor
KICKS BALL FORWARD
THROWS BALL OVERHAND
BALANCE ON FOOT 1 SECOND
JUMPS IN PLACE
PEDALS TRIKE
WALKS BACKWARDS
WALKS UP STEPS
BROAD JUMP
BALANCE ON FOOT 5 SECONDS
BALANCE ON FOOT 10 SECONDS
HOPS ON 1 FOOT
CATCHES BOUNCED BALL
HEEL TO TOE WALK
BACKWARD HEEL
Fine Motor-adaptive
SCRIBBLE SPONTANEOUSLY
TOWER OF 2 CUBES
TOWER OF 4 CUBES
TOWER OF 8 CUBES
IMITATES VERTICAL LINE WITHIN 30°
DUMPS RAISIN FROM BOTTLE SPOUT
DUMPS RAISIN FROM BOTTLE DEMONSTR
COPIES ○
IMITATES BRIDGES
PICKS LONGER LINE 3 of 3
COPIES □
IMITATES □ DEMONSTR
DRAWS MAN 3 PARTS
DRAWS MAN 6 PARTS
Language
2 WORDS OTHER THAN MAMA, DADA
COMBINES 2 DIFFERENT WORDS
POINTS TO 1 NAMED BODY PART
NAMES 1 PICTURE
FOLLOWS 2 OF 3 DIRECTIONS
USES PLURALS
GIVES 1ST AND LAST NAME
COMPREHENDS COLD, TIRED, HUNGRY
RECOGNIZES 3 COLOURS
OPPOSITE ANALOGIES 2 OF 3
DIFINES 6 WORDS
COMPOSITION OF . . .
87%
Personal-social
IMITATES HOUSEWORK
USES SPOON, SPILLING LITTLE
WASHES & DRIES HANDS
HELPS IN HOUSE SIMPLE TASKS
PLAYS INTERACTIVE GAMES e.g. TAG
REMOVES GARMENT
DONS SHOES NOT TIED
BUTTONS UP
DRESSES WITH SUPERVISION
SEPARATES FROM MOTHER EASILY
DRESSES WITHOUT SUPERVISION

Paediatric reference intervals

P = plasma; S = serum F = fasting

Biochemistry (1mmol = 1mEq/L)

Albumin^{P}	36–48g/dL
Alk phos^{P} (depends on age)	see below
α_1-antitrypsin^{P}	1.3–3.4g/dL
Ammonium^{P}	2–25µmL/L; 3–35µg/dL
Amylase^{P}	70–300u/L
Aspartate aminotransferase^{P}	<40u/L
Bilirubin^{P}	2–16µmol/L;0.1–0.8mg/dL
Blood gases, arterial	pH 7.36–7.42
P_aCO_2	4.3–6.1 kPa; 32–46mmHg
P_aO_2	11.3–14.0 kPa; 85–105mmHg
Bicarbonate	21–25mmol/L
Base excess	–2 to +2mmol/L
Calcium^{P}	2.25–2.75mmol/L;9–11mg/dL
Neonates:	1.72–2.47; 6.9–9.9mg/dL
Chloride^{P}	98–105mmol/L
Cholesterol^{P,F}	≤5.7mmol/L;100–200mg/dL
Creatine kinase^{P}	< 80u/L
Creatinine^{P}	25–115µmol/L; 0.3–1.3mg/dL
Glucose (lower in newborn. Fluoride tube)	2.5–5.3mmol/L; 45–95mg/dL
IgA^{S}	0.8–4.5g/L (low at birth, rising to adult levels slowly)
IgG^{S}	5–18g/L (high at birth, falls and then rises slowly to adult level)
IgM^{S}	0.2–2.0g/L (low at birth, rises to adult level by one year)
IgE^{S}	< 500u/mL
Iron^{S}	9–36µmol/L; 50–200µg/dL
Lead^{EDTA}	<1.75µmol/L; <36µg/dL
Mg^{2+} ^{P}	0.6–1.0mmol/L
Osmolality^{P}	275–295mosmol/L
Phenylalanine^{P}	0.04–0.21mmol/L
Potassium^{P} mean mmol/L:	Day 1: 6.4 Day 2: 6; Day 3: 5.9 (later 4–5.5)
Protein^{P}	63–81g/L; 6.3–8.1g/dL
Sodium^{P}	136–145mmol/L
Transferrin^{S}	2.5–4.5g/L
Triglyceride^{F,S}	0.34–1.92mmol/L (≡30–170mg/dL)
Urate^{P}	0.12–0.36mmol/L; 2–6mg/dL
Urea^{P}	2.5–6.6mmol/L; 15–40mg/dL
Gamma-glutamyl transferase^{P}	<20u/L

Hormones—a guide. ►Consult lab

Cortisol^{P}	9am 200–700nmol/L midnight <140nmol/L (mean)
Dehydroepiandrosterone sulfate^{P}:	
Day 5–11	0.8–2.8µmol/L (range)
5–11yrs	0.1–3.6µmol/L
17α-Hydroxyprogesterone^{P}:	
Days 5–11	1.6–7.5nmol/L (range)
4–15yrs	0.4–4.2nmol/L
T_4 ^{P}	60–135nmol/L(not neonates)
TSH ^{P}	<5mu/L (higher on Day 1–4)

B=boy; ^{EDTA}=edetic acid; ^{F}=fasting G=girl; ^{P}=plasma; ^{S}=serum.

Alk phos u/L: 0–½yr 150–600; ½–2yr 250–1000; 2–5yr 250–850; 6–7yr 250–1000; 8–9yr 250–750; 10–11yr G=259–950, B ≤730; 12–13yr G=200–750, B ≤ 785; 14–15yr G=170–460, B=170–970; 16–18yr G=75–270, B=125–720; >18yr G=60–250, B=50–200.

Haematology mean ± ~1 s.d. Range × 10^9/L (median in brackets)

Day	*Hb g/dL*	*MCV fl*	*MCHC%*	*Retic%*	*WCC*	*Neutrophils*	*Eosins*	*Lymphs*	*Monos*
1	19.0 ± 2	119 ± 9	31.6 ± 2	3.2 ± 1	9–30	6–26 (11)	.02–.8	2–11	0.4–3.1
4	18.6 ± 2	114 ± 7	32.6 ± 2	1.8 ± 1	9–40				
5	17.6 ± 1	114 ± 9	30.9 ± 2	1.2 ± .2					
Weeks									
1–2	17.3 ± 2	112 ± 19	32.1 ± 3	0.5 ± .03	5–21	1.5–10 (5)	.07–.1	2–17	0.3–-2.7
2–3	15.6 ± 3	111 ± 8	33.9 ± 2	0.8 ± 0.6	6–15	1–9.5 (4)	.7–.1	2–17	0.2–2.4
4–5	12.7 ± 2	101 ± 8	34.9 ± 2	0.9 ± 0.8	6–15	(1)		(6)	
6–7	12.0 ± 2	105 ± 12	33.8 ± 2	1.2 ± 0.7	6–15	(4)		(6)	
8–9	10.7 ± 1	93 ± 12	34.1 ± 2	1.8 ± 1	6–15	(4)		(6)	
Months—all the following Hb values are Medians/Lower limit of normal									
3	11.5/9	88/80			6–15	(3)		(6)	
6	11.5/9	77/70			6–15	(3)		(6)	
12	11.5/9	78/72			6–15	(3)		(5)	
Years									
2	11.5/9	78/74			6–15	(3)		(5)	
4	12.2/10	80/75			6–15	(4)		(4)	
6	13/10.4	82/75			5–15	(4.2)		(3.8)	
12	13.8/11	83/76			4–13	(4.9)		(3.1)	
14B	14.2/12	84/77			4–13	(5)		(3)	
14G	14/11.5								
16B	14.8/12	85/78	30–36	0.8–2	4–13	2–7.5 (5)	.04–.4	1.3–3.5	.2–.8
16G	14/11.5								
18B	15/13								

Note *Basophil range:* 0–0.1 × 10^9/L; B_{12}^{S}, ³ 150ng/L.
Red cell folate ^{EDTA} 100–640ng/mL. **B = boys; G = girls.**

Platelet counts do not vary with age; range: 150–400 × 10^9/L.

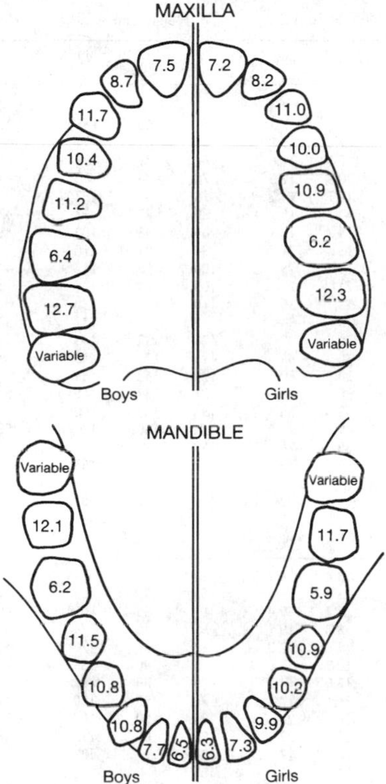

Mean times of eruption (in years) of the permanent teeth.

Deciduous teeth	Months		Months
Lower central incisors	5–9	First molars	10–16
Upper central incisors	8–12	Canines	16–20
Upper lateral incisors	10–12	Second molars	20–30
Lower lateral incisors	12–15		

A 1-year-old has ~6 teeth; 1½yrs ~12 teeth; 2yrs ~16 teeth; 2¼yrs ~20.

Centile tables

Age	Weight (kg)			Height (cm)			Skull circumference (cm)		
Centile—Boys	3	50	97	3	50	97	3	50	97
Birth term	2.5	3.5	4.4	–	50	–	30	35	38
3 months	4.4	5.7	7.2	55	60	65	38	41	43
6 months	6.2	7.8	9.8	62	66	71	41	44	46
9 months	7.6	9.3	11.6	66	71	76	43	46	47
12 months	8.4	10.3	12.8	70	75	80	44	47	49
18 months	9.4	11.7	14.2	75	81	87	46	49	51
2 years	10.2	12.7	15.7	80	87	93	47	50	52
3 years	11.6	14.7	17.8	86	95	102	48	50	53
4 years	13	15	21	94	101	110			
5 years	14	19	23	100	108	117	49	51	54
6 years	16	21	27	105	114	124			
7 years	17	23	30	110	120	130			
8 years	19	25	34	115	126	137	50	52	55
9 years	21	28	39	120	132	143			
10 years	23	30	44	125	137	148			
11 years	25	34	50	129	142	154			
12 years	27	38	58	133	147	160	51	54	56
13 years	30	43	64	138	153	168			
14 years	33	49	71	144	160	176	53	56	58
15 years	39	55	76	152	167	182			
16 years	46	60	79	158	172	185			
17 years	49	62	80	162	174	187			
18 years	50	64	82	162	175	187			

Centile tables—Girls

Age	Weight 3	Weight 50	Weight 97	Height 3	Height 50	Height 97	Skull 3	Skull 50	Skull 97
Birth term	2.5	3.4	4.4	–	50	–	30	35	39
3 months	4.2	5.2	7.0	55	58	62	37	40	43
6 months	5.9	7.3	9.4	61	65	69	40	43	45
9 months	7.0	8.7	10.9	65	70	74	42	44	47
12 months	7.6	9.6	12.0	69	74	78	43	46	48
18 months	8.8	10.9	13.6	75	80	85	45	47	50
2 years	9.6	12.0	14.9	79	85	91	46	48	51
3 years	11.2	14.1	17.4	86	93	100	47	49	52
4 years	13	16	20	92	100	109			
5 years	15	18	23	98	107	116	48	50	53
6 years	16	20	27	104	114	123			
7 years	18	23	30	109	120	130			
8 years	19	25	35	114	125	136	50	52	54
9 years	21	28	40	120	130	142			
10 years	23	31	48	125	136	148			
11 years	25	35	56	130	143	155			
12 years	28	40	64	135	149	164	51	53	56
13 years	32	46	70	142	156	168			
14 years	37	51	73	148	160	172	52	54	57
15 years	42	54	74	150	162	173			
16 years	45	56	75	115	162	174			
18 years	46	57	75	–	–	–			

Measure height exactly: •Feet together •Straight legs; loose arms •Buttocks, shoulders and heels touching wall •Hair firmly compressed •Ear canal level with infraorbital margin •Take reading in expiration.

More up-to-date charts are being designed to take into account new growth data, and to amalgamate American, WHO, and European centile divisions.[1]

1 The 1990 nine centile UK charts are available from Harlow Publishing, Maxwell St, South Shields, NE33 4PU Tel. 0191 427 0195. See TJ Cole 1994 BMJ **i** 641 & DMB Hall 1995 BMJ **ii** 583. NB: the 1995 Castlemead (Buckler) charts have not met with approval from paediatric growth experts because the upper centile on the weight chart is too low, classifying too many children as obese—but these charts have the (unproven) advantage of being based on serial measurements, not cross-sectional data.

Centile growth charts[1]

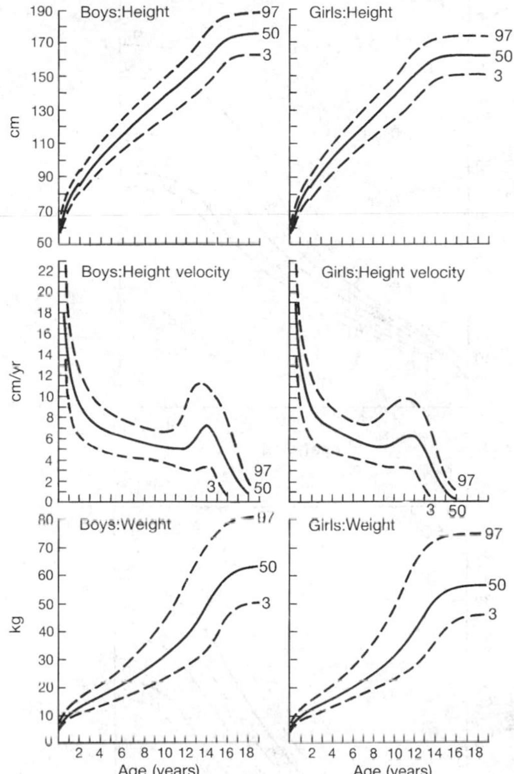

►It is worthwhile to plot all children on growth charts. See p 185 for ethnic growth charts.

Note: the figures at the end of each of the curves refer to centiles. If a child is 'growing along the third centile' this means that only 3% of children from a healthy population have a growth rate as low or lower than such a child. Not all human populations are the same, so that while such a child might be said to be abnormally small if he was a well-fed Caucasian, this need by no means be the case if he is of Chinese or Bangladeshi extraction. Serial growth measurements tend to correlate well with each other when plotted on simple charts—ie children tend to stay within a given centile. However, measurements on velocity charts do not correlate with each other and this makes it easier to give firm guidelines on when to say that a child is abnormal, based on a single reading. Immediate action needs to be taken if a child is below the third centile on the velocity chart—even on one reading.[2] Another action point is being below the 0.4 centile for height (only 1 in 250 will be below this line).

1 After J Tanner, *Arch Dis Childh* **41** 613–35   2 C Brook 1986 BMJ **ii** 1186

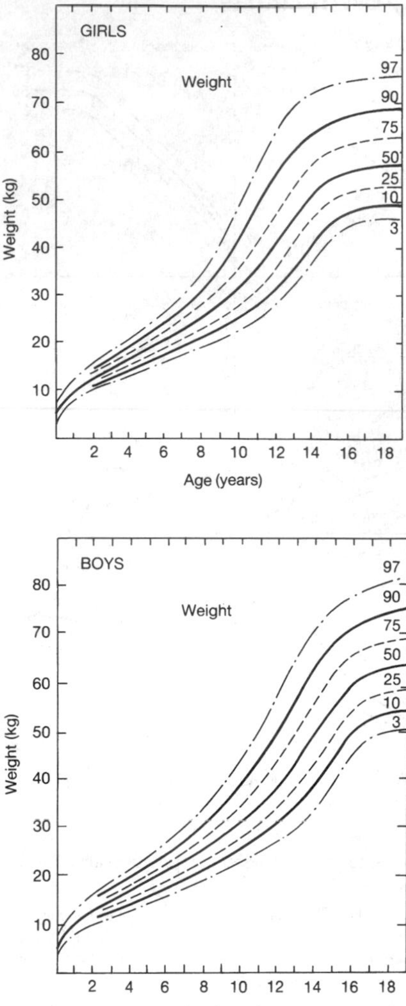

Cross-sectional standards for weight and height attained at each age (English girls and boys). The central line represents the mean, or 50th centile. The two dashed lines above and below it represents the 75th and 25th centiles respectively; ie 25% of the sample fell below the lower line and 25% above the upper line. Other centile lines are also provided. (From D Sinclair *Human Growth after Birth*, OUP, modified from JM Tanner.)

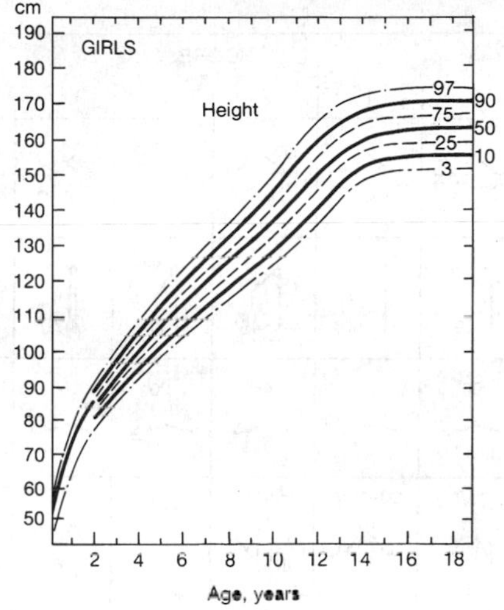
cm
GIRLS
Height
97
90
75
50
25
10
3
190
180
170
160
150
140
130
120
110
100
90
80
70
60
50
2
4
6
8
10
12
14
16
18
Age, years

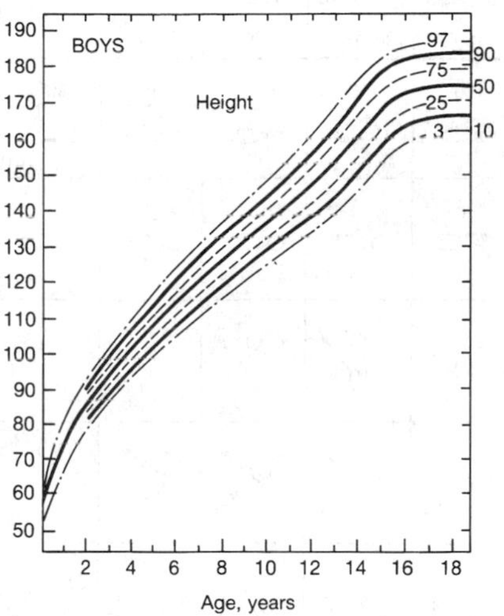
BOYS
Height
97
90
75
50
25
3
10
190
180
170
160
150
140
130
120
110
100
90
80
70
60
50
2
4
6
8
10
12
14
16
18
Age, years

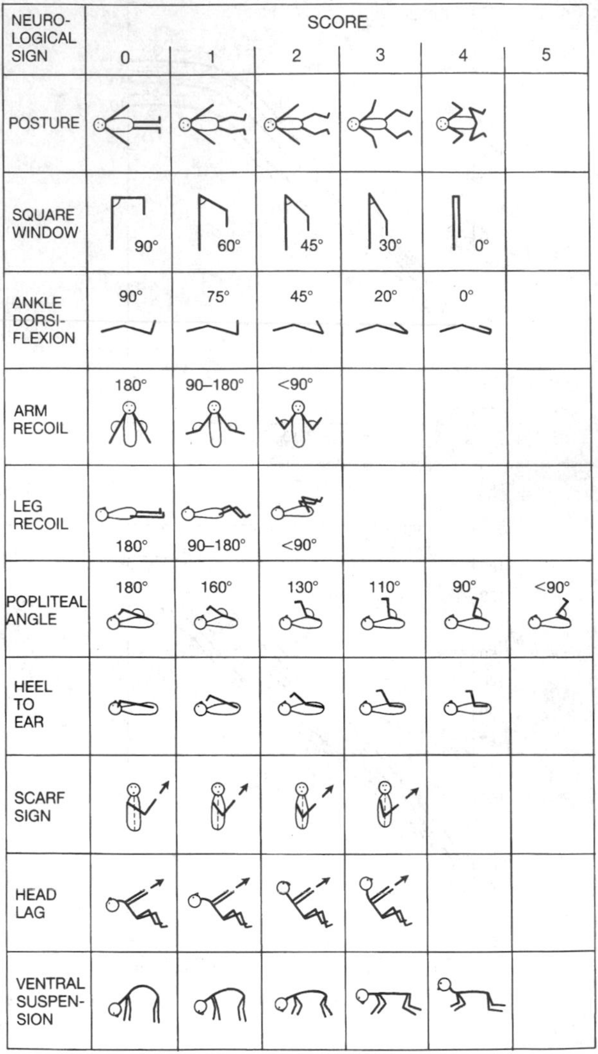

NEURO-LOGICAL SIGN	SCORE 0	1	2	3	4	5
POSTURE						
SQUARE WINDOW	90°	60°	45°	30°	0°	
ANKLE DORSI-FLEXION	90°	75°	45°	20°	0°	
ARM RECOIL	180°	90–180°	<90°			
LEG RECOIL	180°	90–180°	<90°			
POPLITEAL ANGLE	180°	160°	130°	110°	90°	<90°
HEEL TO EAR						
SCARF SIGN						
HEAD LAG						
VENTRAL SUSPEN-SION						

Assessment of gestational age: Dubowitz system. Neurological criteria. (By kind permission of the *Journal of Paediatrics*.)

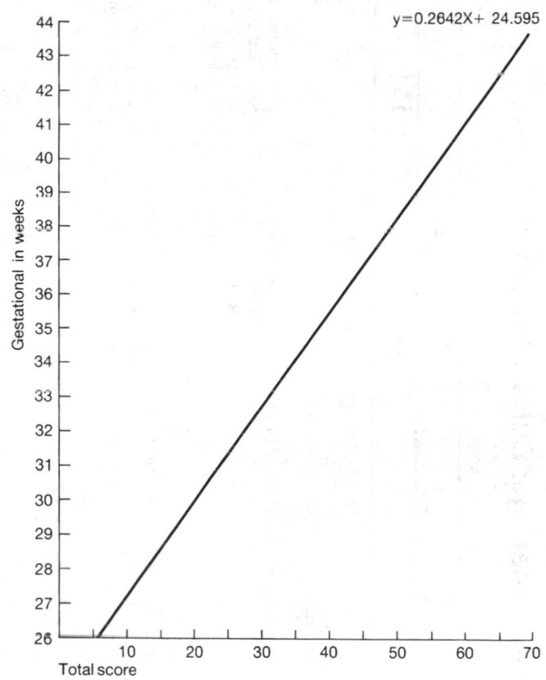

Assessment of gestational age: Dubowitz system. Graph for reading gestational age from total score. (By kind permission of the *Journal of Paediatrics*.)

Assessment of gestational age: Dubowitz system

Physical (external) criteria

	Score				
External sign	**0**	**1**	**2**	**3**	**4**
Oedema	Obvious oedema hands and feet: pitting over tibia	No obvious oedema hands and feet: pitting over tibia	No oedema		
Skin texture	Very thin, gelatinous	Thin and smooth	Smooth: medium thickness Rash or supericial peeling	Slight thickening Superficial cracking and peeling, especially hands and feet	Thick and parchment-like: superficial or deep cracking
Skin colour (infant not crying)	Dark red	Uniformly pink	Pale pink: variable over body	Pale Only pink over ears, lips, palms, or soles	

Skin opacity (trunk)	Numerous veins and venules clearly seen, especially over abdomen	Veins and tributaries seen	A few large vessels clearly seen over abdomen	A few large vessels seen indistinctly over abdomen	No blood vessels seen
Lanugo (over back)	No lanugo	Abundant long and thick over whole back	Hair thinning especially over lower back	Small amount of lanugo and bald areas	At least half of back devoid of lanugo
Plantar creases	No skin creases	Faint red marks over anterior half of sole	Definite red marks over more than anterior half: indentations over less than anterior third	Indentations over more than anterior third	Definite deep indentations over more than anterior third
Nipple formation	Nipple barely visible: no areola	Nipple well defined: areola smooth and flat diameter <0.75 cm	Areola stippled, edge not raised: diameter <0.75 cm	Areola stippled, edge raised diameter >0.75 cm	
Breast size	No breast tissue palpable	Breast tissue on one or both sides <0.5 cm diameter	Breast tissue both sides: one or both 0.5—1.0 cm	Breast tissue both sides: one or both >1 cm	

Assessment of gestational age: Dubowitz system

Physical (external) criteria

	Score				
External sign	**0**	**1**	**2**	**3**	**4**
Ear form	Pinna flat and shapeless, little or no incurving of edge	Incurving of part of edge of pinna	Partial incurving whole of upper pinna	Well-defined incurving whole of upper pinna	
Ear firmness	Pinna soft, easily folded, no recoil	Pinna, soft, easily folded, slow recoil places, ready recoil	Cartilage to edge of pinna, but soft in recoil	Pinna firm, cartilage to edge, instant	
Genitalia •Male	Neither testis in scrotum	At least one testis high in scrotum	At least one testis right down		
•Female (with hips half abducted)	Labia majora widely separated, labia minora protruding	Labia majora almost cover labia minora	Labia majora completely cover labia minora		

Nomogram for calculating the body surface area of children

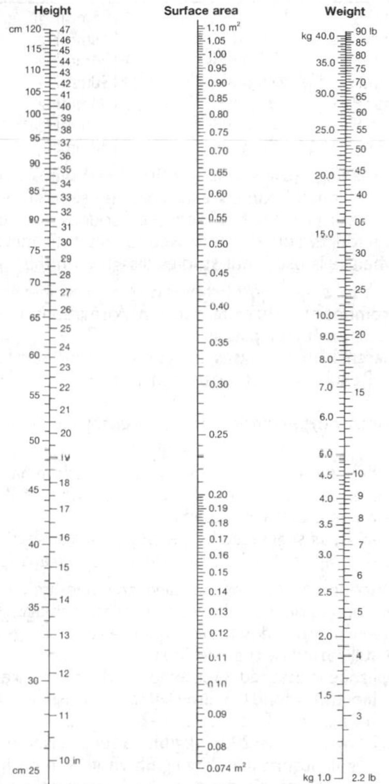

►►IM epinephrine (adrenaline) in anaphylaxis

Age	mL of 1:10,000*	Age	mL of 1:1000
3–5 months	0.5mL	2yrs**	0.2mL
6–11 months	0.75mL	3–4yrs**	0.3mL
12 months	1.0mL	5yrs**	0.4mL
		6–12yrs**	0.5mL; adult 0.5–1mL

Doses may need repeating every 15min, until improvement occurs. Also: •O_2 (± IPPV) •Hydrocortisone (4mg/kg IV) •Chlorpheniramine (0.2mg/kg) •Colloid (20mL/kg IVI). NB: Weight (kg) ≈ 2(Age in yrs + 4). OK if 1–10yrs.

*Eg as Min-I-Jet Adrenaline® (10mL 1:10,000 epinephrine).

**For underweight children, halve the dose, or, if weight known, give 10µg/kg (=0.01mL/kg of 1:1000). Epinephrine dose by endotracheal tube: 100µg/kg. If bronchospasm is a feature, give salbutamol 2mg nebulized too. After the emergency, take blood at 1–5h for mast cell tryptase; refer to an allergist. Self-use of pre-loaded pen injections may be needed (eg EpiPen®; strength is 0.3mL of 1:2000, or 0.3mL of 1:1000). See P Ewan 1998 *BMJ* i 1442

Blood pressure in childhood[1,2]

Age	Significant hypertension[1]		Severe hypertension[1]	
(Years)	Systolic	Diastolic	Systolic	Diastolic
At birth	≥96mmHg*		≥106mmHg*	
<2	≥112mmHg	≥74mmHg[k4]	≥118mmHg	≥82mmHg[k4]
3–5	≥116mmHg	≥76mmHg[k4]	≥124mmHg	≥84mmHg[k4]
6–9	≥122mmHg	≥78mmHg[k4]	≥130mmHg	≥86mmHg[k4]
10–12	≥126mmHg	≥82mmHg[k4]	≥134mmHg	≥90mmHg[k4]
13–15	≥136mmHg	≥86mmHg[k5]	≥144mmHg	≥92mmHg[k5]
16–18	≥142mmHg	≥92mmHg[k5]	≥150mmHg	≥98mmHg[k5]

Note Take ≥3 readings (using a snugly fitted cuff whose bladder width is >75% of upper arm length) some weeks apart (in general) before hypertension is diagnosed. Because the fifth Korotkoff sound (K5) is often not heard in childhood, the fourth sound (K4) is used for diastolic measurement, until adolescence, when K5 is used (but studies disagree on this[1,2]).

Commoner causes of hypertension *Newborn infants:* Renal artery stenosis (or thrombosis), congenital renal malformations, coarctation of the aorta, bronchopulmonary dysplasia.
Infants: Renal parenchymal diseases, aorta coarctation, renal artery stenosis.
6–10 years old: Renal artery stenosis, renal parenchymal diseases, primary hypertension.
Adolescence: Primary hypertension, renal parenchymal diseases.

Clinical assessment *Ask about:* Family history (phaeochromocytoma, *OHCM* p 554 & 788); GU symptoms. Examine for abdominal masses, bruits, endocrine diseases, coarctation and Turner's syndrome (p 758). **Tests:**
Urine: MSU, creatinine clearance, catecholamines.
Blood: FBC, U&E, lipids, as suggested by the physical examination.
Others: Echocardiography; renal ultrasound, isotope scans (p 188) ± IVU.

Treatment Discourage smoking; manage any obesity. *Drugs:* Indications: severe hypertension (as defined above); end organ damage. The following is a suggested sequence: move down the sequence (using drugs in combination, as neeed) if BP still raised, if the previous drug is being taken in a suitable dose, and compliance is assured. Get expert help: doses are provisional.
1 *Diuretics:* Eg chlort(h)alidone 0.5–2mg/kg/day PO; frusemide 0.56mg/kg/12h.
2 *b-adrenergic antagonists:* Eg atenolol 1–2mg/kg/day PO (unlicensed use).
3 *Vasodilators:* Eg hydralazine 200μg/kg/6h PO (unlicensed use).
4 *ACE inhibitors:* Eg captopril 0.5–2mg/kg/8h PO if >6 months old; neonates may need < one-tenth of this dose. CI: renal artery stenosis; possibility of becoming pregnant. ►See *OHCM* p 299. Check U&E 1–2 weeks after starting.

Hypertensive emergencies (Eg in glomerulonephritis, haemolytic uraemic syndrome, or head injury.) Get expert help. Use sodium nitroprusside 0.5–1μg/kg IV then 1–8μg/kg/min IVI by pump to allow precise control of IVI rate. Cover IVI with foil to prevent photodeactivation. Monitor BP continuously, ↑dose slowly to the required level. CI: severe hepatic impairment. Withdraw over >10–30min to prevent rebound hypertension. In prolonged use (>1 day), monitor blood and plasma cyanide levels (keep to <38μmol/L and <3μmol/L respectively). Note: labetalol is an easier to use alternative, starting dose recommended:[2] 0.1–1mg/kg/dose IV, then up to 2mg/kg/h IV.

*Doppler is needed–it is often only possible to record systolic pressure. Reference intervals need adjusting if the child is taller or shorter than expected for age (tables are available[2]); compared with a 50th height-centile child the reference interval is 1-4mmHg lower for a child on the 5th height-centile (1–4mmHg *higher* if on 95th height-centile)[2].

1,2 Task force on blood pressure control in children. Report of the second task force on blood pressure control in children. *Paediatrics* 1987 **79** 1-25 & *ibid*: 1996 *Paediatrics* **98** 649–58

Milks for preterm babies

If weight gain is not satisfactory on human milk, a formula milk is needed—provided the failure of breast feeding cannot be attributed to to poor technique (p 176). See p 177 for how to express breast milk.

Water This is the most important nutrient. Water comprises 50–70% of weight gain (eg of 15g/day) in preterm babies.
Insensible water loss (IWL) falls with increasing body weight, gestational age and postnatal age; it increases with ↑T° (ambient and body) and low humidity. In a single-walled, thermoneutral incubator with a humidity of 50–80% IWL≈30–60mL/kg/day. This may double in infants on phototherapy under a radiant heater.
Faecal water loss ≈ 5–10mL/kg/day (except during diarrhoea).
Urine loss: if ~90mL/kg/day, there is no excessive renal stress.

An intake of 180mL/kg/day (range 150–200mL) of human or formula milk meets the water needs of very low birth weight infants (VLBW; <1500g) under normal circumstances. In infants with heart failure water restriction is necessary (eg 130mL/kg/day).

Energy 130kcal/kg/day (range 110–165) meets the needs of the LBW infant in normal circumstances, and can be provided by formulas with similar energy density to human milk (65–70kcal/dL) in a volume of 180–200mL/kg/day. If a higher energy density is required keep it <85kcal/dL. The problem with energy densities above this is fat lacto-bezoars and U&E imbalance.

Protein Aim for between 2.25g/100kcal (2.9g/kg/day when fed at 130kcal/kg) and 3.1g/100kcal (4g/kg/day). Lysine should be as high as possible. Precise guidelines on taurine and whey:casein ratios cannot be given. At present LBW formulas are whey-predominant. Signs of protein deficiency: a low plasma urea and prealbumin.

Fat Aim for 4.7–9g/kg (fat density 3.6–7.0g/100kcal). Longer chain unsaturated fatty acids (>C12) are better absorbed than saturated fatty acids. Aim to have ≥4.5% of total calories as the essential fatty acid linoleic acid (500mg/100kcal). No recommendations can be made about cholesterol, carnitine or choline.

Carbohydrates Aim for 7–14g/100kcal (<11g/100dL), with lactose contributing 3.2–12g/100kcal (<11g/100dL). Lactose is not essential; substitutes are glucose (but high osmolality may cause diarrhoea) or sucrose (± starch hydrolysates, eg corn syrup oils).

Vitamins A reasonable daily supplement is Vitamin A: 300μg (1μg = 3.33U). Vitamin D: 20μg (1μg colecalciferol=40U vitamin D_3). Vitamin E: 5mg. Vitamin K: 3μg. Vitamin B_1: 50μg. Vitamin B_2: 200μg. Vitamin B_6: 100μg. Vitamin C: 20mg. Folic acid: 60μg. Niacin, biotin and pantothenic acid need not be added. Giving the above supplement would not be toxic, even if the milk being given contained the maximum permitted limit of vitamins. When the baby has reached 2kg the vitamin intake should be reconsidered.

Elements Na^+: 6.5–15mmol/L. K^+: 15–25.5mmol/L. Ca^{2+} 1.75-3.5mmol/100kcal. PO_4^{3-}: 1.6–2.9mmol/100kcal. Ca^{2+}:PO_4^{3-} ratio: 1.4-2.0:1. Magnesium: 0.25-0.5mmol/100kcal. Iron: if breast fed, give 2-2.5mg Fe/kg/day (the recommended total intake). Formula-fed infants may need a supplement to achieve this. Iodine: 10–45μg/100kcal. Manganese: 2.1μmol/100kcal. ►1cal=4.18 joules.

This is our world of broken. . .

Tonight you hold a weakening baby in your arms, uncertain as to whether to give him milk or oxygen. Then you realize that the breast is dry, and the oxygen is exhausted. Welcome to our world of broken. . . broken promises, broken equipment, the broke hospital breaking the backs of its staff and the hearts of these parents as their son slips through your fingers. The broken chromosome, the broken Hippocratic Oath and now your broken sleep all conspire against you.

It is too glib to say that somehow all these broken pieces will be fitted together into some new pattern—by the arrival of money, or hope, or ideas. There will always be pieces missing and the pattern never makes sense for long. But all around you, feel the ghosts of past physicians, the thousands in your predicament, who have walked your way. Link arms with theirs for a moment—a bond unbreakable as invisible, and saying to you "Don't quit: not yet. . ." It is the hardest thing to pick yourself up from a series of defeats—but know this for sure: our job *is* worth doing.

Now back to that infant in your arms, and remember that, sigh as you may, you have always got some oxygen left in your own lungs to share: your respiratory reserve is the tail-end of your vital capacity—and as for the milk: well. . . no one is expecting you to work miracles: but you can always try (p 177).

Talking with parents about their child's mortal illness

Impending death is always a hard subject to approach—especially, it might be thought, when the death concerned is that of a child. Although death in childhood is now a rare event at least in Britain, there will be few mothers who have not thought of the death of their child—probably from the moment of its first stirrings within her. This is important to appreciate as the mother's and father's preparedness for a child's death is a key factor in determining the pacing of interviews in which mortal diagnoses are imparted. Pacing is important because it acknowledges that the acceptance of a mortal diagnosis is not an event, but an unfolding process of the mind. This process may be marked by uncontrollable outbursts, weeping, anger and reproach. These reactions need saluting as they arise, and the interviewer should resist impulses to suppress or turn away from these negative emotions. There is also an additional temptation when faced in medicine by a difficult and uncertain task: it is to lessen one's insecurity by surrounding oneself with professional talismans: the white coat, medical terminology, scientific objectivity, brief and evasive prognostications and an attitude of lofty condescension. Divesting yourself of these things takes practice. We are all at times frightened of appearing naked before our patients—with nothing to offer and with nothing to shield ourselves against impertinent realities.

A criticism of the above is that it consists of unsubstantiated platitudes. However, the tentacles of clinical science are now embracing even this most difficult and sensitive area. Carefully structured, tested interviews yield the following guidelines:[1]

- Ask both parents to be present (plus a nurse whom they trust).
- Take steps to avoid being interrupted. Allow sufficient time.
- Call the family by name.
- Do not avoid looking at the family (mutual gaze promotes trust).
- Name the illness concerned. Write it down.
- Give the address and telephone number of a patient's group where further support can be obtained. Find this by telephoning a central directory of groups (the UK the number is: 0171 240 0671).
- Outline the support available throughout the illness.
- Elicit what the parents now know. Clarify or repeat as needed.
- Answer any questions. Acknowledge that it is difficult to absorb all the information so arrange early follow-up.
- Explain that you will be telling the child's GP straight away that you have had a full discussion with him or her. (Parents are likely to seek his advice: make sure he is fully and promptly informed.)

What about the children themselves? Studies have indicated that children's insight into their impending death may be greater than adults'. So do not assume that a child under your care cannot understand. But expect this understanding to be expressed in different ways. We know that children learn to behave as society expects them to behave. Thus a dying child will play with toys while parents are around, but then engage in frank discussion when alone with peers. The child may have learned that speaking about death makes his parents cry—so he or she will avoid the topic.

Hope Hope in the face of stark evidence represents our minds at work reframing reality and putting events in their place—but hope itself is a burden. Total despair is manageable because it is dead: but when hope keeps our despair alive, it serves to sharpen the claw moving towards our face. It is easy to admire the uncrushable, intoxicating hope parents bring to us: it is much harder to protect them from the vulnerability which accompanies hope.

1 H Woolley 1989 *BMJ* i 1623

Intraosseus transfusion[1]

Immediate vascular access is required in paediatric practice in the following circumstances: cardiopulmonary arrest, severe burns, prolonged status epilepticus, hypovolaemic and septic shock. In many cases rapid intravenous access is not easily obtained, and intraosseous infusion is a relatively safe, easy and effective means of obtaining vascular access, and is recommended for life-threatening emergencies in young children in whom other methods of access have failed.

Contra-indications: Osteoporosis, osteogenesis imperfecta, and infection or fracture at the site of insertion.

Preparation: Set trolley: Dressing pack, Betadine®, needles, 10mL syringe, lidocaine (=lignocaine) 1% (5mL), scalpel, intraosseous needle, paediatric infusion set, 10mL 0.9% saline, adhesive tape.

Choosing the site of insertion: The proximal tibia is the best site. Other sites are the distal tibia, or distal femur. Choose a point in the midline on the flat anteromedial surface of the tibia, two finger-breadths below the tibial tuberosity. The patient's leg should be restrained, with a small support placed behind the knee.

Procedure:

- Sterilize the skin with antiseptic, infiltrate with lidocaine (=lignocaine) as necessary. (Puncturing the skin with the scalpel is not usually necessary.)
- Insert the intraosseous needle at an angle of 60–90 degrees away from the growth plate, and advance with a boring or screwing motion into the marrow cavity. Correct location of the needle is signified by a decrease in resistance on entering the marrow cavity.
- Stabilize the needle in the cortex, and verify the position by aspirating marrow, or by the easy flushing of 5–10mL of 0.9% saline, without any infiltration of surrounding tissue. The needle should stand upright without support, but should be secured with tape.
- Flushing with heparin-treated saline may prevent clotting.
- Connect to IV infusion—but better flow rates are often achieved by syringing in boluses of fluid (standard bolus is 20mL/kg of crystalloid or colloid).

Complications: These are infrequent, but there may be extravasation of fluid, or cellulitis, fractures, osteomyelitis, pain, and fat or bone microemboli. These are more common with prolonged use—so intraosseous infusion should be discontinued as soon as conventional IV access is attained.

NB: Intraosseous delivery may also be used in adults.[2]

1 DH Fisher 1990 NEJM **322** 1579–81 2 G Bratteb 1993 BMJ **ii** 627

1998 European paediatric basic life-support algorithm

This algorithm assumes that only one rescuer is present, and no equipment.

Remove yourself and the infant from danger

↓

Check responsiveness *(shake & shout)*

↓

Open the airway *(remove obstructions; head tilt; chin lift)*

↓

Check breathing *(look, listen, feel; if breathing, place in recovery position)*

↓

Give 2 breaths *(have up to 5 goes at giving 2 rescue breaths sufficient to raise the chest)*

↓

Assess for signs of life (10sec only) *(signs of circulation, eg pulse; now phone for help at once)*

↙ ↘

Circulation present: Continue rescue breathing

No circulation: compress chest & give breaths *(100 compressions/min 5 strokes to 1 ventilation; check circulation every minute)*

Compress sternum to ⅓ of the chest's depth; use the heel of one hand. If >8yrs, the adult 2-handed method may be needed. For an infant, 2 fingers are sufficient, positioned in the middle of a line joining the nipples. Perform resuscitation for ~1 min before going for help.

How to give the rescue breaths to a child Ensure head tilt and chin lift. Pinch the soft part of his nose. Open his mouth a little, but maintain chin up. Take a breath, and place your lips around his mouth (good seal). Blow steadily into his mouth over 1–1.5sec. Does his chest rise? Take your mouth away, and watch for the chest to fall. Take another breath, and repeat this sequence up to 5 times. ***With an infant*** Do as above, but cover the nasal apertures and the mouth with your lips. If the chest does not move, respiratory obstruction may exist ►►move on to **'Removing foreign body' sequence** for obstructed airway—ie:

- Remove any obvious obstructions. Recheck that there is adequate head tilt and chin lift, but do not overextend the neck.
- Do up to 5 back blows between the scapulae to dislodge hidden obstructions (hold prone, positioning the head lower than chest).
- If this fails, do 5 chest thrusts: turn to supine; over 12sec, give 5 sternal thrusts (same position as for compressions, but be sharper and more vigorous). Remove any foreign bodies which have become visible.
- Tilt head and lift chin to reopen the airway, and assess breathing.
- If not breathing; do 5 more rescue breaths: does the chest move now?
- If not, for a child, give 5 abdominal thrusts (directed towards diaphragm); use the upright position if the child is conscious; supine if not.
- Repeat these sequences until breathing is established, alternating chest and abdominal thrusts. *Do not give abdominal thrusts to infants.*

When breathing place in the recovery position—as near to the true lateral position as possible, with mouth dependent to aid draining of secretions. The position must be stable (eg use pillows placed behind back). The degree of movement is determined by risk of spinal injury.

Cardiac arrest: *1998 paediatric advanced life-support*[1]

Each step assumes the previous one has been unsuccessful

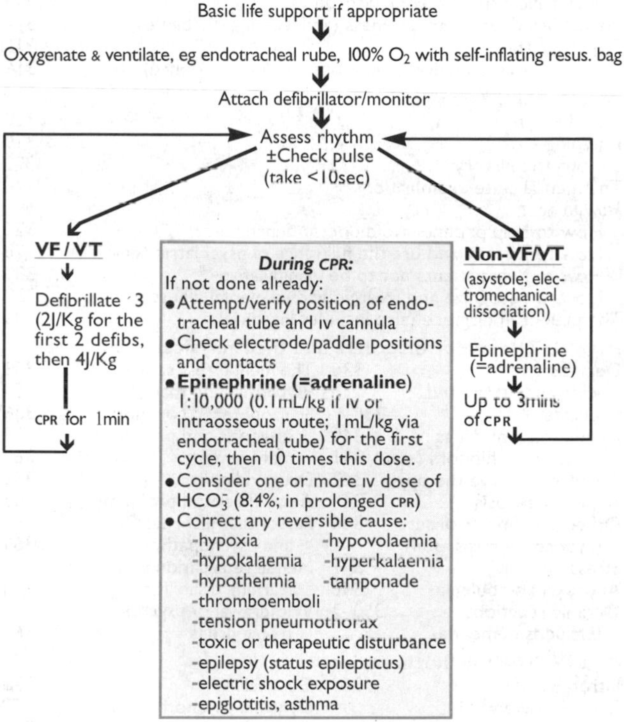

Basic life support if appropriate

↓

Oxygenate & ventilate, eg endotracheal rube, 100% O_2 with self-inflating resus. bag

↓

Attach defibrillator/monitor

↓

Assess rhythm
±Check pulse
(take <10sec)

VF / VT

↓

Defibrillate ×3 (2J/Kg for the first 2 defibs, then 4J/Kg

CPR for 1min

↓ (back to Assess rhythm)

Non-VF/VT

(asystole; electromechanical dissociation)

↓

Epinephrine (=adrenaline)

↓

Up to 3mins of CPR

↓ (back to Assess rhythm)

During CPR:

If not done already:

- Attempt/verify position of endotracheal tube and IV cannula
- Check electrode/paddle positions and contacts
- **Epinephrine (=adrenaline)** 1:10,000 (0.1mL/kg if IV or intraosseous route; 1mL/kg via endotracheal tube) for the first cycle, then 10 times this dose.
- Consider one or more IV dose of HCO_3^- (8.4%; in prolonged CPR)
- Correct any reversible cause:
  - -hypoxia
  - -hypovolaemia
  - -hypokalaemia
  - -hyperkalaemia
  - -hypothermia
  - -tamponade
  - -thromboemboli
  - -tension pneumothorax
  - -toxic or therapeutic disturbance
  - -epilepsy (status epilepticus)
  - -electric shock exposure
  - -epiglottitis, asthma

Treat acidosis with good ventilation. Sodium bicarbonate may worsen intracellular acidosis and precipitate arrhythmias, so use it only in severe acidosis after prolonged resuscitation (eg 1mmol/kg, by slow IV bolus).

1 Algorithm of the *European Resuscitation Council Guidelines* (*Resuscitation* 1998 **37** 97–110)

4. Psychiatry

Relevant pages in other chapters Puerperal psychosis p 148; consultation analysis p 422–4; social and ethnic matters p 462 & 436; prescribing and compliance p 460; behavioural questions in childhood p 206.

*This chapter should be read in conjunction with the American Psychiatric Association's *Diagnostic and Statistical Manual of Mental Disorders* (DSM-IV), 1994, ISBN 0-89042-062-9

Major adult psychiatric diagnoses defined in *International Classification of Diseases*

Affective (mood) disorders:		Organic reactions	
Depressive disorders	336	Acute	350–2
Mania	354	Chronic (dementia)	350–2
The neuroses		Schizophrenia	356–60
Anxiety neurosis	344	Paranoia & other psychoses	354
Obsessional neurosis		Mental retardation	364
Phobias	346	(ie developmental disabilities)	
Depersonalization	346	Personality disorders	364
Hysteria	334	Alcoholism	362
Sexual disorders	380	Drug problems and addiction	362

Problems with classificatory systems No system can be equally successful in guiding treatment and in illustrating basic biological distinctions. For example, depression spans the neurosis/psychosis division, and mania has both affective (mood) and psychotic components.

- There is no such thing as a correct classificatory system—only more or less useful ones. It is instructive to bear in mind that in ancient times (as reported by Borges) one approved classification of animals had as its first 6 categories: 1 Those animals that belong to the Emperor. 2 Embalmed ones. 3 Those that are trained. 4 Suckling pigs. 5 Mermaids. 6 Fabulous ones. We do not know how many mermaids and other fabulous beings are included in the above classificatory system.
- Not all the diagnostic categories have the same value. If a patient with some features of schizophrenia (eg hallucinations) is subsequently found to have an organic psychosis (eg caused by a brain tumour) the schizophrenic element is usually subsumed under the more powerful diagnostic category of organic illness. This is an example of the 'hierarchy of diagnosis', in which organic illness 'trumps' schizophrenia and affective disorders, which in turn 'trumps' neurosis, but does preclude multiple diagnoses, eg schizophrenia with depression and substance abuse disorder.
- Each patient is unique—and is none is simply a member of a class, and it is a fundamental error to appear to abandon our patients, once he or she has been categorized. Because of its tragic essence, it is possible for mental illness to be a humanizing experience for those affected (patient, family, and friends)—as well as being an intensely destructive one, and there is much to be said for the idea that we should embrace our patients, rather than analyse them. Nevertheless, as ever, the holistic must, on occasion, give ground to reductionist analysis, for diagnosis is the single best tool we have to help our patients.

Introduction to psychiatry

Doctors have never been particularly important because nothing that happens to our bodies ever really matters. In historical terms, the importance of what happens to our bodies rarely outlives the times in which we live. Even the exceptions to this doctrine prove a different rule—for example, we recall forever the human images burnt on to stone at their moment of immolation in Nagasaki and Hiroshima. Surely what happened to these bodies was important, and transcended the times in which they lived? True. But it is all the more true that it was not the way they lived, but the way they died that was important, and it is not the body nor its image on stone which is important, but the image left on our mind. And so it is with psychiatrists, psychologists, and psychiatric nurses who play such a large rôle in determining whether we live and die in hope or despair, who mitigate our madness and give meaning, purpose and dignity to the mental sufferings of so many of us. So when we think of these men and women going about their work, we think of them burnishing humanizing images not on stone, but on the mind itself. How they do it is the subject of this chapter.

Mental health and mental illness

The essence of mental health Ideally, healthy humans have:

- An ability to love and be loved. Without this cardinal asset, human beings, more than all other mammals, fail to thrive.
- The power to embrace change and uncertainty without fear—and to face fear rationally and in a spirit of practical optimism.
- A gift for risk-taking free from endless worst-case-scenario-gazing.
- Stores of spontaneous *joie de vivre*, and a wide range of emotional responses (including negative emotions, such as anger; these may be important for motivation, as well as being a natural antidote to pain).
- Efficient contact with reality: not too little; not too much. (As T S Eliot said, humankind cannot bear very much reality.)
- A rich fantasy world enabling hope and creativity to flourish.
- A degree of self-knowledge to encourage the humane exercising of the skill of repairing the self and others following harm.
- The strength to say "I am wrong", and to learn from experience.
- An adequate feeling of security and status within society.
- The ability to satisfy the requirements of the group, combined with a freedom to choose whether to exercise this ability.
- Freedom of self-expression in whatever way he or she wants.
- The ability to risk enchantment and to feel a sense of awe.
- The ability to gratify his own and others' bodily desires.
- A sense of humour to compensate if the above are unavailable.

Happiness need not be an ingredient of mental health; indeed the merely happy may be supremely vulnerable. All that is needed is for their happiness to be removed. The above are important as they are what a person needs should this misfortune befall him. The above may also be seen as a sort of blueprint for our species' survival.

The essence of mental illness Whenever a person's abnormal thoughts, feelings or sensory impressions cause him objective or subjective harm which is more than transitory, a mental illness may be said to be present. Very often the harm is to society, but this should not be part of the definition of mental illness, as to include it would open the door to saying that, for example, all rapists or all those opposing society's aims are mentally ill. If a person is manic, and is not complaining of anything, this only becomes a mental illness (on the above definition) if it causes him harm as judged by his peers (in the widest sense of the term). One feature of mental illness is that one cannot always rely on patients' judgment, and one has to bring in the judgment of others, eg family, GP or psychiatrist. If there is disparity of judgment, there is much to be said for adopting the principle of 'one person one vote', provided it can be shown that the voters are acting solely in the interests of the person concerned. The psychiatrist has no special voting rights here—otherwise the concepts of mental health and illness become dangerously medicalized. Just because the psychiatrist or GP is not allowed more than one vote, this does not stop them from transilluminating the debate by virtue of their special knowledge.

For convenience, English law saves others from the bother of specifying who has a mental illness by authorizing doctors to act for them. This is a healthy state of affairs only in so far as doctors remember that they have only a small duty to society, but a larger duty to their patient (not, we grant, an overriding duty in all instances—eg when murder is in prospect).

Learning disabilities (mental impairment/retardation) This is a condition of arrested or incomplete development of mind which is especially characterized by subnormality of intelligence.

Dignity on the ward

Apart from showing our mentally ill patients sympathy, nothing is more to be desired than that we should give them dignity—not the dignity which they deserve (who among us would merit an ounce of dignity on this measure?) but the dignity which confirms to our patients that, mad, bad or rambling, they are, root and branch, body and mind, just as human as their doctors—perhaps more so, because they are suffering.

So much, someone might say, for the platitudes, but what might giving dignity actually entail?

- We should ask our patients how they would like to be addressed. "Miss Hudson" may be preferred to "Agatha, dear". Dignity is about giving choice, and then respecting stated preferences.
- We should wear name badges so patients can label us just as easily as we can label them.
- Allow patients to wear their own clothes—and clothe them decently if they have none.
- Offer the right to choose whether to take part in medical research.
- Do not presume that patients will want to be seen by students.
- Offer personal space—both to stow their belongings, and to walk in, in private, whether alone, or with visitors.
- Make every effort to explain and agree treatment plans with your patient. Explain the options, and describe some of the side-effects of drugs you may recommend.
- Explain what to do if a crisis develops. It's a great help to know that you will be seen in 4 hours, rather than be left to moulder all week-end.

These 8 points are the basis of the UK *patient's charter* in mental health.

Our patients' other needs: Maslow's hierarchy[1]

Maslow states that a healthy personality (ie fully functioning and self-actualizing) entails the meeting of a hierarchy of needs:

1 Biological needs (eg oxygen, food, water, warmth).
2 Safety needs (no present threats to safety).
3 Love, affection, and 'belongingness' needs.
4 Esteem needs (self-respect, and need for respect from others: see above).
5 Self-actualization needs (the need to *be* and *do* that which we feel born to do: his or her calling. If these needs are not met, restlessness and tenseness result. To meet this need we should teach ourselves and others:
   - To be aware of the inner self and to understand our inner nature.
   - To transcend cultural conditioning.
   - To feel joy and the worth of living.
   - To transcend the trifling and to grapple with life's serious problems.
   - To refresh consciousness by appreciating beauty and all good things.

1 http://www.connect.net/georgen/maslow.htm

Odd ideas

It is important to decide whether a patient has delusions, hallucinations or a major thought disorder, because if these are present the diagnosis must be: schizophrenia; affective disorder; an organic disorder; or a paranoid state—and it is *not* a neurosis or a personality disorder.

Patients may be reluctant to reveal odd ideas. Ask gently: "Have you ever had any thoughts which now seem odd; perhaps that there is a conspiracy against you, or that you are controlled by outside voices or the radio?"

Hallucinations are a sensory experience (auditory, visual, gustatory or tactile) in the absence of a stimulus. The often-encountered pre- or post-sleep (hypnagogic/hypnopompic) hallucinations are not indicative of pathology. A pseudo-hallucination is one in which the patient knows that the stimulus is in his mind (such as a voice heard within himself, rather than over the left shoulder). They are more common, and need not indicate any mental illness, although they may be an important sign—for example, that a genuine hallucination is being internalized before being disbanded altogether (ie the person hears a voice but no longer believes it represents an autonomous agent). Visual and tactile hallucinations (without auditory hallucinations) suggest an organic disorder, while auditory hallucinations suggest psychosis.

NB: 2–4% of the general population experience auditory hallucinations, but only ~30% of these have a mental illness.[1]

Delusions These are beliefs which are held unshakably, irrespective of any counter-argument, and which are unexpected, given the patient's cultural background. The belief is usually (but not always) false. If the belief arrives in the mind fully formed, and with no antecedent events or experiences which account for it, it is said to be *primary*, and is strongly suggestive of schizophrenia. Such delusions form around a 'delusional perception', as illustrated by the patient who, on seeing the traffic lights go green (the delusional perception) knew that he had been sent to rid his home town of materialism. Careful history-taking will usually reveal that the delusion is secondary—for example, a person who is depressed may come to think of himself as being literally worthless.

Ideas of reference The patient cannot help feeling that other people are taking notice of the very thing he feels ashamed of. What distinguishes this from a delusion is that he knows the thoughts come from within himself, and are excessive. It is important to distinguish delusions and hallucinations from obsessional thoughts. With any odd idea, get a clear description so that you can decide whether the person hears the thought as a voice (hallucination); whether they believe that the voice is being put into their head—thought insertion (a delusion), or whether they know that the thought really comes from themselves, although it is intrusive (obsessional). An obsessional thought is a sign of neurosis, not psychosis.

Major thought disorder This is recognized from the person's speech. He jumps from one idea to another in a bizarre way (see mania—flight of ideas, p 354—and schizophrenia, p 358).

Note On establishing that an hallucination or a delusion is present, ask yourself: **1** What other evidence there is of psychopathology. Hearing the voice of a recently died spouse is a common hallucination, which does not indicate mental illness. **2** Could the odd ideas be adaptive—and the patient be better off ill? The answer is usually 'No', but not always: a woman once believed she saw aeroplanes flying over her house, and that this information was taken from her head by the British Ministry of Defence. She 'knew' she was playing a key rôle in the defence of Britain. When she was cured of these delusions she committed suicide.

1 M Romme 1994 *BMJ* ii 670

Some causes of odd ideas

A typical problem is trying to diagnose a young man presenting with hallucinations and or delusions. The question often is: *Are these odd ideas due to schizophrenia, drug abuse, or physical illness?*

- Most auditory hallucinations not associated with falling asleep or waking up are caused by schizophrenia or depression.
- In ~90% of those with non-auditory hallucinations, the cause is substance abuse, drug withdrawal, or physical disease.[1]
- Evidence that substance abuse is to blame includes:
  - *The history:* Ask the patient, the family, and friends about abuse. Be precise about timing. If ≥4 weeks elapse between abuse and starting of odd ideas, substance abuse is an unlikely cause.[1]
  - *Severity of symptoms:* If symptoms are severe, and the quantity of drug ingested is trivial, the drug is unlikely to be causative.
  - *Drug-seeking behaviour:* Be on the look-out for this.
  - *Physical examination:* This may reveal signs of drug abuse (eg injection marks ± cellulitis), chronic alcohol abuse (eg spider naevi, liver palms, atrophic testes), or a physical medical illness (eg brain tumour).
  - *Blood or urine tests* may disclose the substance abused or give a hint of abuse (MCV↑ and gamma GT↑ in alcohol abuse).
  - *Imaging:* Consider CNS imaging if the patient is elderly with nothing to suggest substance abuse, or there are CNS signs.
- NB: middle-age is not a typical time for schizophrenia to present: alcohol abuse or a primary CNS condition is more likely.
- Diagnosing a *substance-induced psychotic disorder* implies that the patient responds to the hallucinations or delusions as if they were real. If the patient recognizes the ideas for what they are, then consider diagnosing *substance intoxication, substance withdrawal* or, if there is past but no current exposure to hallucinogens, the diagnosis may be 'flashbacks'—ie *hallucinogen persisting perception disorder.* This condition presents episodically up to 5 years after exposure to an hallucinogen, with flashback hallucinations, any visual hallucinations or phenomenon such as: geometric visual hallucinations, seeing flashes of colour, or intensified colours, seeing dots, spots or flashes, seeing trailing images or after-images, seeing complementary coloured images of objects gone from view, seeing halos, seeing things too small (micropsia), or seeing things too big (macropsia). These phenomena may be self-induced or triggered by darkness, stress or fatigue.[1]

1 American Psychiatric Association 1994 *Diagnostic and Statistical Manual of Mental Disorders* (DSM-IV) page 313, ISBN 0-89042-062-9

Introduction: psychiatric skills

On beginning psychiatry you are likely to feel unskilled. A 'medical' problem will come as a relief—you know what to do. Do not be discouraged: you already have plenty of skills (which you will take for granted). The aim of this chapter is to build on these. No one can live in the world very long without observing mood swings in both himself or his fellows, and without devising ways to minimize what is uncomfortable, and maximize what is desirable. Anyone who has ever sat an important exam knows what anxiety is like, and anyone who has ever passed one knows how to master anxiety, at least to some extent. We have all of us survived periods of being 'down', and it is interesting to ask how we have done this. The first element is time. Simply waiting for time to go by is an important psychotherapeutic principle. Much of what passes as successful treatment in psychiatry is little more than protecting the patient, while time goes by, and his (and his family's) natural processes of recovery and regeneration bring about improvement. Of course, there are instances when to wait for time to go by could lead to fatal consequences. But this does not prevent the principle from being a useful one.

Another skill with which we are all more or less adept is *listening*. One of the central tenets of psychiatry is that it helps our patients just to be listened to. Just as we all are helped by talking and sharing our problems, so this may in itself be of immense help to our patients, especially if they have been isolated, and feel alone—which is a very common experience.

Just as spontaneous regeneration and improvement are common occurrences in psychiatry, so is relapse. Looking through the admissions register of any acute psychiatric ward is likely to show that the same people keep on being readmitted. In one sense this is a failure of the processes of psychiatry, but in another sense each (carefully planned) discharge is a success, and a complex infrastructure often exists for maintaining the patient in the community. These include group support meetings, group therapy sessions, social trips out of the hospital. We all of us have skills in the simple aspects of daily living, and in re-teaching these skills to our patients we may enable them to to take the first steps in rebuilding their lives after a serious mental illness.

So *time*, *listening* and the *skills of daily living* are our chief tools, and with these simple devices much can be done to rebuild the bridges between the patient and his outside world. These skills are simple compared with some of the highly elaborate skills such as psychoanalysis and hypnosis for which psychiatry is famous. The point of bringing them to the fore is so that the newcomer to psychiatry need not feel that there is a great weight of theoretical work to get through before he starts doing psychiatry. On the contrary, you can engage in the central process of psychiatry from your first day on the wards—using the knowledge and experience gained as a foundation on which to build the constructs required for the more specific and effective forms of psychotherapy.

4. Psychiatry

Listening

►Don't just do something—*Listen!* (Aphorism from Dr Anthony Storr)

Once we had the good fortune to work on an acute psychiatric ward with a surgeon, who, before he accustomed himself to the ways of psychiatry would pace aimlessly up and down the ward after he had clerked in his patients, wondering when the main action would start, impatient to get his teeth into the business of curing people. What he was expecting, no doubt, was some sort of equivalent to an operating list, and not knowing where to find one he was at a loss, until he gradually realized that taking a history from a psychiatric patient is not a 'pre-op assessment', but the start of the operation itself. Even quite advanced textbooks of psychiatry appear to have missed the insight of this surgeon, describing psychotherapy as something which should only happen after 'a full psychiatric history' and after assessing what aspects of his problems are to be dealt with in treatment. Of course, there is no such thing as a full psychiatric history. In describing the salient psychological events of a single day even the best authors (eg James Joyce in *Ulysses*) require substantial volumes.

In taking the history and agreeing with the patient what tasks should be attempted, treatment has already started—and indeed for some patients this process is all that is required.

Taking a history sounds like an active process, and suggests a list of questions, and the format of our page on this process (p 322) would seem to perpetuate this error. It is not a question of taking anything. It is more a question of receiving the history, and of allowing it to unfold. If you only ask questions, you will get only answers as replies.

As the history unfolds, sit back and listen. Avoid interruptions for the first 3min. Be prepared for periods of silence. If prompts are needed try '. . . and then how did you feel?' or just '. . . and then. . .'; or repeat the last words the patient spoke. Do not be overanxious if the patient appears not to be covering major areas in the history. Lead on to these later, by taking more control as the interview unfolds. At first you will have to ask the relevant questions (p 322) in a rather bald way (if the information is not forthcoming during the initial unstructured minutes), but it is important to go through this stage as a prelude to gaining information by less intrusive methods. Always keep in mind the chief aims of making a diagnosis, defining problems, and establishing a therapeutic relationship.

What is the point of all this listening? Listening enables patients to start to *trust* us. Depressed patients often believe they will never get better. To believe that they *can* get better, patients need to trust us, and this trust is often the start of the therapeutic process. In general, the more we listen, the more we will be trusted. Our patients' trust in us can be one of our chief motivations, at best inspiring us to pursue their benefit with all vigour. A story bears this out. One summer's day, in 334 BC, Alexander the Great fell ill with fever. He saw his doctor, who gave him a medicine. Later he received a letter saying his doctor was poisoning him as part of a plot (it was an age of frequent, and frequently fatal intrigue). Alexander went to his doctor and drank the medicine—then gave him the letter. His confidence was rewarded by a speedy recovery. We think it is unreasonable to expect *quite* this much trust from our patients, and one wonders what can have led Alexander to such undying trust in his doctor. We strongly suspect that such a doctor, above all else, must have been a good listener.

Note that listening, as with any interaction with patients, may have side-effects. It is certainly possible for listening to open up a can of worms (p 347), and then the difficulty is in deciding whether to dissect out each worm in turn, or hurriedly to try to put the lid back on.

Lifeworlds, and how how to keep them intact

Even if we all listen the same way, what we will hear will depend on our own expectations, anxieties and past experience. Take this dialogue:[1]

Doctor: "How long have you been drinking that heavily?"
Patient: "Since I've been married"
Doctor: [impatiently] "How long is that?"
Patient: [giggling] "Four years".

Perhaps the doctor is worrying about the length of time her liver has been exposed to excessive alcohol, or perhaps he just wants his notes to look complete. He needs facts in historical 'linear' time, but the patient chooses to answer in terms of event-time, or personal time. This is Mishler's great distinction between the the 'voice of medicine' and the 'voice of the lifeworld'.[2] The doctor above has forced his patient to submit to his own world. Sometimes this may seem unavoidable: the chief thing is to recognise when this is happening, and to be pre-emptive by biting your tongue. What would this patient have gone on to say if her doctor had not time-raped her? What did those giggles signify? We will never know, but they might have explained her coming death.

1 G Elwyn 1999 BMJ i 186 2 E Mishler 1984 *The Discourse of Medicine: Dialectics of Medical Interviews*, Norwood, NJ, Ablex

Eliciting the history

Introduce yourself, and explain how long the interview will take. Describe its purpose. Find out how the patient came to be referred, and what his expectations are (eg about treatment). If the patient denies having any problems or is reluctant to start talking about himself, do not hurry him. Try asking 'How are you?' or 'What has been happening to you?' or 'What are the most important things?' Another approach for hospital patients is to indicate why the GP referred the patient and then ask what the patient thinks about this. Sit back and listen, without interrupting, noting exact examples of what he is saying. Take more control after ~3 minutes, to cover the following topics.

Presenting symptoms Agree a problem list with the patient early on, and be sure that this is comprehensive, eg by asking 'If we were able to deal with all these, would things then be all right?' Then take each problem in turn and find out about onset, duration, effects on life and family; events coinciding with onset; solutions tried; reasons why they failed. The next step is to enquire about mood and beliefs during the last weeks (this is different from the mental state examination, p 324, which refers to the mental state at the time of interview). Specifically check for: **suicidal thoughts, plans or actions**—the more specific these are, the greater the danger. Discussing suicide does not increase the danger. Questions to consider: 'Have you ever felt so low that you have considered harming yourself?' 'Have you ever actually harmed yourself?' 'What stopped you harming yourself any more than this?' 'Have you made any detailed suicide plans?' 'Have you bought tablets for that purpose?'

Depression—ie low mood, anhedonia, self-denigration ('I am worthless'; 'Oh that I had not been born!'), guilt ('It's all my fault'), lack of interest in hobbies and friends plus biological markers of depression (early morning waking, decreased appetite and sexual activity, weight loss); **mania** (p 354); symptoms of **psychosis** (persecutory beliefs, delusions, hallucinations, p 316); **drug** and **alcohol ingestion**; **obsessional thoughts**; **anxiety**; **eating disorders** (eg in young women—often not volunteered, and important). Note **compulsive behaviour** (eg excessive hand-washing).

Present circumstances Housing, finance, work, marriage, friends.

Family history Physical and mental health, job and personality of members. Who is closest to whom? Any stillbirths, abortions?

Birth, growth and development How has he spent his life? Ask about school, play (alone? with friends?) hobbies, further education, religion, job, sex, marriage. Has he always been shy and lonely, or does he make friends easily? Has he been in trouble with the law? What stress has he had and how has he coped with it? (Noting early neurotic traits—nail-biting, thumb-sucking, food fads, stammering—is rarely helpful.)

Premorbid personality Before all this happened, how were you? Happy-go-lucky, tense, often depressed? Impulsive, selfish, shy, fussy, irritable, rigid, insecure? ►Talk to whomever accompanies him (eg wife), to shed light on premorbid personality (as well as on current problems).

Next examine the mental state (p 324 & 353). You may now make a diagnosis. Ensure that the areas above have been covered in the light of this diagnosis so that the questions **'Why did he get ill in this way at this time?'** and **'What are the consequences of the illness?'** are answered. Making a diagnosis entails a balancing of symptoms—eg is depression or anxiety more of a problem; and how much is explicable given the patient's background and personality (perhaps enough to obviate the need for making *any* diagnosis)?

4. Psychiatry

The mental state examination

This assesses the state of mind at the time the interview is being conducted. Make records under the following headings.

- *Observable behaviour:* Eg excessive slowness, signs of anxiety.
- *Mode of speech:* Include the rate of speech, eg gabbling (pressure of speech) or slow and retarded. Note its content.
- *Mood:* Note thoughts about harming self or others. Gauge your own responses to the patient. The laughter and grandiose ideas of manic patients are contagious, as to a lesser extent is the expression of thoughts from a depressed person.
- *Beliefs:* Eg about himself, his own body, about other people and the future. Note abnormal beliefs (delusions), eg that thoughts are overheard and ideas (eg persecutory, grandiose). See p 316.
- *Unusual experiences or hallucinations:* Note modality, eg visual.
- *Orientation:* in time, place and person. What is the date? What time of day is it? Where are you? What is your name?
- *Short-term memory:* Give a name and address, and test recall after 5 minutes. Make sure that he has got the address clear in his head before waiting for the 5 minutes to elapse.
- *Long-term memory:* Current affairs recall. Who is the Monarch? (This tests many other CNS functions, not just memory.)
- *Concentration:* Months of the year backwards; see p 353.
- Note the patient's *insight* and the degree of your *rapport*.

Non-verbal behaviour *Why are we annoyed when we blush, yet love it when our friends do so?* Part of the answer to this question is that non-verbal communication is less well controlled than verbal behaviour. This is why its study can yield valuable insights into our patients' minds, particularly when analysis of their spoken words has been unrevealing. For example, if a patient who consistently denies being depressed sits hugging himself in an attitude of self-pity, remaining in a glum silence for long periods of the interview, and when he does speak, uses a monotonous slow whisper unadorned by the slightest flicker of a gesticulation or eye contact—we are likely to believe what we see and not what our patient would seem to be telling us.

Items of non-verbal behaviour:

- Gaze and mutual gaze
- Facial expression
- Smiling, blushing
- Body attitude (eg 'defensive')
- Dress: *'the apparal oft proclaims the man'*
- Hair style
- Make-up
- Body ornament (eg ear-rings, tattoos)

Signs of auditory hallucinations:

- Inexplicable laughter
- Silent and distracted while listening to 'voices' (but could be an 'absence' seizure, p 266)
- Random, meaningless gestures

Anxious behaviour:

- Fidgeting, trembling
- Nail-biting
- Shuffling feet
- Squirming in the chair
- Sits on edge of chair

Signs of a depressed mood:

- Hunched, self-hugging posture
- Little eye contact
- Downcast eyes; tears
- Slowness of: thought; speech; movement

What is a mental state?

A true description of a mental state entails valid knowledge about a person's current emotions plus his or her reactions to those emotions. These reactions are themselves emotional (eg being annoyed or dumbfounded at finding oneself in love again)—as well as giving rise to beliefs and attitudes, and, as our way of validating knowledge about emotions is to find out what effect these emotions have on us the involved observer, the situation is necessarily complex, paradoxical, subjective, error-prone, contradictory—and fascinating. This combination nicely sums up what it is to be human, and explains why describing and communicating mental states is the central puzzle that confronts not just psychiatrists and their patients, but also all true artists. All the great poets and songwriters can summon up and make sense of diverse mental states (herein lies their genius)—but none can control them or their infinite progeny (what happens next). This might be said to be the proper province of psychiatry. If doctors could control mental states at will, then it is not necessarily the case that the job of psychiatry is done (there remains the problem of the will)—but at least the job would be half done (and, no doubt, there would be some unfortunate side-effects). Drugs, psychotherapy and behavioural methods are the chief tools available for this task, and they all, crucially, impinge on mental state. You cannot tell if these modalities are helping if you cannot access your patient's mental state, which is why the page opposite is *so* important. But if you think you can access mental states *just* by applying the formulaic regimen opposite, you will often fail, because any trip into the mind of another is not just a voyage without maps, it is ultimately a creative and metaphysical enterprise.

On this view, knowledge of mental states is a difficult and doubtful—but often this is not so: take for example the mental state of a baby being put to the breast after separation from his or her mother, or of an audience giving a standing ovation, or screaming fans waving to their idol, and we know without doubt that the these mental states comprise unalloyed satisfaction, pleasure, and adulation. Note that so often it is non-verbal behaviour which allows valid judgment about mental states: don't rely on words—those capricious tokens of disguise and deception.

Helping patients avoid doctor-dependency

A patient may become over-dependent on his or her doctor in many spheres of medicine. This is a particular danger in psychiatry because of the intimate and intense rather one-sided or asymmetrical relationship which may be built up between the patient and his psychiatrist—who is likely to come to know far more about the patient's innermost hopes and fears than many of his close friends. This encourages the patient to transfer to the therapist thoughts and attitudes that would more naturally be directed to a parent-figure. This process (known as transference) powerfully stimulates doctor-dependency, sometimes with serious consequences.

Signs of non-therapeutic dependency Repeated telephonings for advice, the inability to initiate any plan without help from the therapist, and the patient's disallowing of attempts by the therapist to terminate treatment (eg by threatening relapse).

Assessing whether dependency is a problem Clearly, in the examples above the patient's dependency on his doctor is non-therapeutic. At other times, for example early on in treatment, doctor-dependency may be quite helpful. In these circumstances the danger is that the doctor will be flattered by his patient's dependency on him. Most therapists either want to be loved by their patients or want to dominate them (or both), and it is important to know, in each session with each patient, just where you lie within the space marked out by these axes. Ask yourself 'Why do I look forward to seeing this patient?' 'Why do I dread seeing Mr X?' 'Why do I mind if this patient likes me?'

►When you feel good after seeing a patient always ask yourself why (it is so often because he is becoming dependent on you).

Avoiding dependency Planning and agreeing specific, limited goals with the patient is one way of limiting dependency. If the patient agrees from the outset that it is not your job to provide him with a new job, wife, or family the patient is more likely to have realistic expectations about therapy.

Planning discharge from the beginning of therapy is another important step in limiting doctor-dependency. Discharge is easy to arrange from the hospital outpatient department, but for the general practitioner the concept of discharge is diluted by the fact of his contractual obligation to the patient— who is perfectly within his rights to turn up the day after being 'discharged' and demand that therapy be started all over again. He must have more subtle methods at his disposal to encourage the patient to discharge himself. For example, he can learn to appear completely ineffective, so that the dependency cycle (patient presents problem → doctor presents solution → patient sabotages solution → doctor presents new solution) is never started. Another approach is to bore your patient by endlessly going over the same ground, so that the patient seizes control and walks out as if to say 'I've had enough of this!'

The foregoing makes patients out to be perpetual seekers after succour and emotional support—and so it can seem at times; but a great mystery of clinical medicine is that, spontaneously and miraculously, these patients *can* change, and start leading mature and independent lives. So do not be downcast when you are looking after these poor people: there is much to be said for simply offering a sympathetic ear, staying with your patient through thick and thin, and waiting for time to go by, and for the wind to change. Of course, the wind may change back again, but, if it does, you will not be back at square one, for you will be able to inject the proceedings with the most powerful psychotherapeutic agent of all: namely hope.

How to identify and use the full range of psychiatric services

Any good psychiatric service will have much more to it than out-patient clinics and hospital wards. The latter are very important, but it is not true to say that the most significant psychiatric interventions go on in this location. Alternatives to the cycle of outpatient/inpatient doctor-led treatments include:

- Responsive community psychiatric teams
- On-call community psychiatric nurses (CPNs)
- Crisis intervention teams
- Drop-in services during weekends and unsocial hours
- Telephone helplines
- Self-help groups
- Mental illness hostels
- Occupation centres (voluntary or statutory)
- Sheltered work
- Supervised living quarters so patients are not alone
- Self-running group homes

These components of any comprehensive service are not only important in keeping patients out of hospital (a prime aim of those who are purchasing care—as well as of patients and doctors); they are also important in gradually normalizing the patient's relationship with his environment.

How to help patients not to be manipulative

Fireships on the lagoon We have all been manipulated by our patients, and it is wrong to encourage in ourselves such stiffness of character and inflexibility of mind that all attempts by our patients to manipulate us inevitably fail. Nevertheless, a patient's manipulative behaviour is often counter-productive, and reinforces maladaptive behaviour. A small minority of patients are *very* manipulative, and take a disproportionate toll on your resources, and those of their family, friends and colleagues. We are all familiar with these patients who Ford Madox Ford describes as being like fireships on a crowded lagoon, causing conflagration in their wake.[1] After destroying their family and their home we watch these people cruise down the ward or into our surgeries with some trepidation. Can we stop them losing control, and causing melt-down of our own and our staff's equanimity? The first thing to appreciate is that, unlike an unmanned ship, these people *can* be communicated with, and you *can* help them without resorting to hosing them down with cold water.

Setting limits One way of avoiding becoming caught up in this web of maladaptive behaviour is to set limits, as soon as this behaviour starts.[2] In a small minority of patients, the therapist may recognize that their needs for time, attention, sedation and protection are, for all practical purposes, insatiable. Whatever the therapist gives, such patients come back for more and more, and yet in spite of all this 'input' they do not appear to get any better. The next step is to realize that if inappropriate demands are not met the patient will not become sicker (although there may be vociferous complaints). This realization paves the way for setting limits on patients' behaviour, specifying exactly what is and is not acceptable.

Take for example the patient who demands sedation, threatening to 'lose control' if it is not given immediately, stating that he cannot bear living another day without sedation, and that the therapist will be responsible for any damage which ensues. If it is decided that drugs do not have a part to play in treatment, and that the long-term aim is for the patient to learn to be responsible for himself, then it can be simply stated to the patient that medication will not be given, and that he is free to engage in destructive acts, and that if he does so this is his responsibility.

The therapist explains that in demanding instant sedation he usurps her professional rôle, which is to decide these matters according to her own expert judgment, and that such usurpation will not be tolerated. If there is serious risk of real harm, admission to hospital may be indicated, where further limits may be set. If necessary, he is told that if he insists on 'going crazy' he will be put in a seclusion room, to protect others.

Another method is to abdicate the power you have to bring about the end the patient or his family desires. So if, for example, the father of a patient who has been labelled 'psychotic' is very keen for repeated admissions for his son, while at the same time hotly resenting the suggestion that the family is in some way exacerbating the condition, an experienced therapist might make progress along these rather dangerous lines: 'It is clear that your wife cannot cope with your son when he is hearing his voices. Although we know that they are quite harmless, they are obviously more upsetting to her than to your son. So just ring the ward when you cannot cope, and send him in—or your wife. It doesn't matter who comes in'. Such strategies (which may be very effective) clearly need careful planning and agreement from all concerned in caring for the family.

1 Ford Madox Ford 1915 *The Good Soldier*, Penguin 2 G Murphy 1960 *Am J Psychotherapy* **14** 30–47

How to help patients be less lonely

*Being unwanted is the worst disease that any human being can experience.**

Loneliness is not a condition you will find in many psychiatric classifications—yet it is the root of much psychopathology. Some people, of course, *like* to avoid their fellows. For them, intrusion into their private world may cause despair; but, for most of us, these intrusions are welcome, and necessary for health. Loneliness seriously affects 1 in 10 older people, and can contribute to alcoholism, depression, and suicide. Suspect that loneliness is important whenever you find your hand being gripped for comfort after one would have thought that a social encounter was over—also whenever there is a verbal outpouring and a 'defeated demeanour'.[1]

Do not assume that loneliness means social isolation. Someone who has brief visits 3 times a day, from, say, a nurse, a care assistant, and a 'meals on wheels lady' is not socially isolated, but may be very lonely. But if he or she gets on well with just one of these visitors, this can be enough to banish loneliness. So this is the first lesson: *be nice to people, and take trouble to find out their hopes and fears*. But more is possible: in general, it is depressing waiting for the doorbell to ring, so tailor your suggestions in the light of your patient's mobility. This needs initiative on your patient's part: but do not think you must treat your patient's depression *before* you tackle a lonely life-style: tackling this may be the route out of depression. Areas to think about include:

- What facilities already exist? Is there a local pub, day centre, or lunch club available? "God, I wouldn't be seen dead in one of those places!" we so often hear. But take time to point out that it does not matter initially whether they get anything out of a social interaction. After all, they may meet someone of like mind, so enabling these artificial crutches to be thrown away.
- Is the person religious? If so there will often be activities and outings to plan and talk about, and reminisce over—even if they are not actually enjoyed at the time.
- Housing: if the person is already planning a move, ask for their views about small local communities, rather than anonymous high-rise flats. Will they be near family, and other people who speak their own language (metaphorically and literally)?
- Adult education classes are a good (but often expensive) way to meet like-minded people—and with the acquisition of new skills, confidence improves and social interaction becomes more pleasurable.
- Involvement with community action groups may be a source of friends (and a source of frustration and disappointment—but do not expect your interventions to be without side-effects: the thing is to plan for them).
- Details of local community activities can be found in the UK at the local *Council for Voluntary Services*. Other organizations advertise at local libraries.
- Befriending schemes can be very helpful to those who are housebound.
- Technology forums such as the Internet may provide relief from boredom and loneliness—and for some this will offer the best chance of meeting with a kindred spirit, unlimited by the constraints of time and space.
- Befriending others, and offering telephone support, may be a way forward whether or not one is housebound. Some local authorities will give help to get telephones.

*A saying of Mother Teresa's **1** A Forbes 1996 *BMJ* **ii** 352. **Useful UK addresses:**
University of the Third Age, 26 Harrison St, London WC1 tel. 0171 837 8838
Names of leaders of local religious groups: Contact, 15 Henrietta St, London WC2E 8QH, tel. 0171 240 0630
Age Concern: 1268 London Road, London SW16 4EJ, tel. 0181 679 8000
Cruse: Bereavement line: 0181 332 7227
Saga Holidays: Bouverie House, Middelburg Square, Folkstone, Kent CT20 1AZ

How to recognize and treat your own mental illnesses

Doctors have a higher than average incidence of suicide and alcoholism, and we must all be prepared to face (and try to prevent) these and other health risks of our professional and private lives. Our skill at looking after ourselves has never been as good as our skill at looking after others, but when the healer himself is wounded, is it clear that his ability to help others will be correspondingly reduced? Our own illnesses are invaluable in allowing us to understand our patients, what makes people go to the doctor (or avoid going to the doctor), and the barriers we may erect to resist his advice. But the idea of an ailing physician remains a paradox to the average mind, so that we may ask: ►Can true spiritual mastery over a power ever be won by someone who is counted among her slaves?[1] If the time comes when our mental state seriously reduces our ability to work, we must be able to recognize this and take appropriate action. The following may indicate that this point is approaching:

- Drinking alcohol before ward rounds or surgeries.
- The minimizing of every contact with patients, so that the doctor does the bare minimum which will suffice.
- Inability to concentrate on the matter in hand. Your thoughts are entirely taken up with the workload ahead.
- Irritability (defined as disagreeing with >1 nurse/24h).
- Inability to take time off without feeling guilty.
- Feelings of excessive shame or anger when reviewing past débâcles. To avoid mistakes it would be necessary for us all to give up medicine.
- Emotional exhaustion (defined as knowing that you should be feeling pleased or cross with yourself or others, but on summoning up the affairs of your heart, you draw a blank).
- Prospective studies suggest that introversion, masochism, and isolation are important risk factors for doctors' impairment.

The first step in countering these unfavourable states of mind is to recognize that one is present. The next step is to confide in someone you trust. Give your mind time to rejuvenate itself.

If these steps fail, try prescribing the symptom. For example, if you are plagued by recurring thoughts about how inadequately you treated a patient, set time aside to deliberately ruminate on the affair, avoiding distractions. This is the first step in gaining control. You initiate the thought, rather than the thought initiating itself. The next step is to interpose some neutral topic, once the 'bad' series of thoughts is under way. After repeated practice, the mind will automatically flow into the neutral channel, once the bad thoughts begin, and the cycle of shame and rumination will be broken.

If no progress is made, the time has come to consult an expert, such as your general practitioner. Our own confidential self-help group for addiction and other problems is the British Doctors' and Dentists' Group and may be contacted via the Medical Council on Alcoholism (UK tel. 0171 487 4445). If you are the expert that another doctor has approached, do not be deceived by this honour into thinking that you must treat your new patient in any special way. Special treatment leads to special mistakes, and it is far better for doctor-patients to tread well-worn paths of referral, investigation and treatment than to try illusory short cuts.

1 Thomas Mann 1924 *The Magic Mountain*, page 132–3, Penguin

Patients in disgrace: the fat-folder syndrome

One of the rôles of the psychiatrist is to act as the terminus for patients who have been shunted from hospital department to hospital department. These patients offer their doctor an 'organ recital' of incapacitating physical symptoms for which no physical cause can be found (somatization). She knows that 'there must be something wrong'. In the end, the patient is sent in disgrace to the psychiatrist because the doctor declares that there is 'nothing wrong' and that the patient is 'just a hypochondriac'. The psychiatrist then has to do much work undoing the cycle of symptom-offering and investigation, by acknowledging that there *is* something wrong. The aim is then to reframe symptom-offering into problems which need to be solved. This may start with an acceptance by the doctor that the patient is distressed and looking for helpful responses from her carers which are yet to be defined. After establishing rapport, the psychiatrist will agree a contract with the patient—that he will provide regular consultations for listening to how the patient feels and will try to help, on condition that she acknowledges that past investigations have not helped, and that she agrees not to consult other doctors until a specified number of sessions have elapsed. In addition, cognitive therapy (p 370) which examines the way that conscious thoughts and beliefs perpetuate disability, *can* lead to meaningful symptom reduction.[1]

Hysteria

This is a mental disorder in which there are signs or symptoms of disease (in the absence of pathology) which are produced *unconsciously* (so hysteria is different to malingering or lying, and does not, contrary to lay use, mean histrionic). Examples: paralysis, blindness, amnesia—eg in a patient who was homosexually raped: he had no conscious memory for the event, but felt an irresistible urge to write insulting letters about the person who had raped him. In deciding if phenomena are hysterical, ask:

- Has a physical cause been carefully discounted?
- Is the patient young? Beware making the first diagnosis if >40yrs old.
- Have the symptoms been provoked by stress? Ask the family.
- Is there secondary gain?—ie is it worthwhile perpetuating symptoms? Many physical illnesses have gain for the patient, so this sign is only useful if it is absent (so ruling out hysteria).
- Do the symptoms 'make sense' (eg aphonia in a news-reader)?
- Indifference to what should constitute a major handicap (*la belle indifférence*) is of marginal diagnostic use.

Most hysterical conversion reactions subside spontaneously, but if they do not it is important to refer early to a psychiatrist, before the hysterical phenomenon becomes habitual. Epidemic hysteria may occur, in which whole communities become involved, starting with the more suggestible members. In an hysterical fugue the patient disappears for a few days, making pointless journeys about which he has no recollection.

Prognosis in hysteria Follow-up over ~6yrs shows that ~5% of those referred to a neurological hospital who had hysteria diagnosed turned out to have organic illness.[2] However, these patients may not be typical of those diagnosed with hysteria (ultimate diagnoses included dystrophia myotonica and spinocerebellar degeneration).

Treatment of hysteria Exploring the stresses in the patient's life may help, as on p 388–96. In general, be ready to recognize the psychological components of physical illness, and get expert psychiatric help, while leaving the door open for reappraisal if new features develop.

[1] A Speckens 1996 *EBM* 1 80 2 H Crimlisk 1998 *BMJ* i 582

4. Psychiatry

Depression

The spectrum of depression Each year 40% of the population have quite severe feelings of depressed mood, unhappiness, and disappointment. Of these, ~20% will experience a clinical depression, in which low mood is accompanied by sleep difficulty, change in appetite, hopelessness, pessimism, or thoughts of suicide. *Diagnosis* of major depression:

- Loss of interest or pleasure—*anhedonia* in daily life with dysphoric mood (ie 'down in the dumps') plus ≥4 of the following (the first 5 are 'biological' symptoms)—present nearly every day for at least 2 weeks:
- *Poor appetite* with *weight loss* (or, rarely, increased appetite).
- *Early waking*—with *diurnal mood variation* (worse in mornings).
- *Psychomotor retardation* (ie a paucity of spontaneous movement, or sluggish thought processes), or *psychomotor agitation*.
- Decrease in *sexual drive* and other appetites.
- Evidence of (or complaints of) reduced *ability to concentrate*.
- Ideas of *worthlessness*, inappropriate *guilt* or *self-reproach*.
- Recurrent *thoughts of death* and *suicide*, or *suicide attempts*.

Why is major depression so often missed? •Lack of knowledge. •Preoccupation with physical disease. •Stigma of psychiatric labels. •A tendency to underrate severity. •It is not so easy to spot depression if it coexists with other illness (so often the case).[1]

Classification Classify as: •*Mild; moderate; severe.* •*With/without biological features.* •*With/without delusions or hallucinations.* •*With/without manic episodes* (ie bipolar not unipolar). These replace the old reactive/endogenous labels. *Differential diagnosis (DSM-IV):* Bipolar disorder (manic depression, or, if less severe, 'cyclothymic disorder'); substance-induced mood disorder; schizophrenia, dementia; mood disorder due to a general medical condition.

Why people get depressed: some ideas •Genetics: identical twins reared apart show 60% more concordance for depression than dizygotic twins.

- Biochemistry: there are excess 5-hydroxytryptamine ($5HT_2$) receptors in the frontal cortex of brains taken from suicide victims. See *OHCM* p 406.
- Endocrinology: cortisol suppression (dexamethasone suppression test, *OHCM* p 550) is abnormal in ~30%. Melatonin is also implicated (p 404).
- Stressful events (eg new births, job loss, divorce, illness): present in 40%.
- Freudian reasons: depression mirrors bereavement—but the loss is of a valued 'object', not a person. There is ambivalence in an important relationship, with hostility turned inwards. Another idea which some animal work supports is learned helplessness: if punishment is not contingent on actions of the person, but is perceived as random, the response is the helplessness which is, some believe, the hallmark of depression.
- Vulnerability factors: physical illness, pain, and lack of intimate relationships may allow depression to arise and be perpetuated.

Management There is no clear distinction between the low moods we all get and illness needing vigorous treatment, but the lower the mood and the more marked the slowness, the more vigorous the treatment needs to be.

- Presence of biological features or stressful life events suggests a good response to *antidepressants* (p 340)—particularly if symptoms are severe. Not everyone will want drugs. Discuss all options openly. Alternative therapies such as St John's Wort *do* work, and may be acceptable.
- Delusions or hallucinations prompt a physical treatment, ie *ECT* (p 342) or *drugs* (antidepressants ± antipsychotic drugs, p 360).
- The depressive phase of bipolar illness is treated as above, but note:
  1 Be cautious with the physical treatments: they may induce mania.
  2 Lithium prophylaxis may be needed (p 354).
- *Psychological treatment* (eg cognitive therapy, p 388–96) is part of the treatment of *all* depression; it may be all that is needed in milder depressions.
- *Reasons to admit:* Social circumstances; high suicide drive; isolation.

Who is likely to benefit from antidepressant drugs? (p 340)

Those who have had low mood or loss of desire for pleasure (anhedonia) most of the day for at least the last 2 weeks who show 4 or more of the following 7 markers of severe depression:

- **S**uicide plans in existence, or ideas of self-harm.
- **U**nexplained or unbidden feelings of guilt or worthlessness.
- **I**nability to function—eg psychomotor retardation or agitation.
- **C**oncentration impaired.
- **I**mpaired appetite.
- **D**ecreased sleep (especially early morning waking).
- **E**nergy low, or unaccountable fatigue.

►Enquire about these phenomena *whenever* depression is possible. NB: treatment may still be needed if the above criteria are not met: listen to their story—drugs may be needed later. Patients will often not accept that they could be depressed because "there is nothing to *make* me depressed". It helps to suggest that they could still be depressed, and that treatment could be very helpful. Give them time to go away and think about it, perhaps discussing it with someone they know. They usually return and are successfully treated. This may not be over-medicalizing a patient's symptoms: there is evidence that such patients are simply inexperienced in understanding their depression: when they *next* become depressed, their views much more nearly match those of their doctor.[1]

1 See J Ogden 1999 *Br J Gen Pr* **49** 123 & the Kendrick injunction 1996 BMJ **ii** 829

Suicide and attempted suicide

As we all know, Nature has implanted in us a dominant will to live; what the average mind may be quite unprepared for is the person who with equal but opposite energy pursues his own destruction, urgently discarding all that is partial and provisional, to achieve his end.* He differs from many self-poisoners—who are a very common problem. In girls aged 15–19 the incidence is >1%/yr in some areas. Most self-poisoning does not end in death—but in some places suicide accounts for half of adolescent deaths, and is a growing problem in the elderly.[1,2] 'Overdoses' account for 4.7% of all general hospital admissions in those aged 12–20yrs.

Understanding suicide behaviour Suicide behaviour may be a way of:

- Keeping honour and autonomy, and avoiding shame (the noble Roman in us will prefer to die by his own hand than be forced to walk on his knees).
- Avoiding something ghastly, eg pain, or another bout of depression.
- Controlling change in families, eg when a member is about to leave.
- Communicating important messages in a not-to-be ignored way.
- Gaining power in family transactions, by escalating conflict.

Causes of suicide behaviour Depression is a leading cause. A common antecedent is an argument with a boyfriend. Emotional immaturity, inability to cope with stress, weakening of religious ties, unemployment, and availability of guns and drugs (psychotropics are the most popular poison) are also important, as is 'copy-cat' behaviour: when a celebrity tries suicide, others will follow. Children who are bullied or placed under intolerable stress to succeed may opt for suicide, eg in Japan—where completed suicide is the cause of death of >600 children/yr. Common reasons are falling behind with homework—and if this reflects your own state after trudging through too many *OHCS* pages, shut this book, and have a good holiday. Australia has the highest suicide rates in 15–24yr-olds: 16/100,000.

There are 6 stages in trying to help the survivors:[1]

- Assessment. • Agreement of a contract offering help (p 339).
- Discussion with the family as to how problems might be tackled.
- Problem-solving by facilitating the patient's understanding of her predicament, and by pointing out how she has coped with problems in the past. The aim is to engender a greater ability to cope in the future as well as helping immediate personal and social problems.
- Prevention: open-access, walk-in clinics or 24h phone service.
- Follow-up—either with family or with the patient alone.

Assessment Think of a target with 3 concentric rings. *The inner ring* is the circumstances of the attempt: what happened that day; were things normal to start with? When did the feelings and events leading up to the act start? Get descriptions of these in detail. Was there any last act (eg a suicide note)? What happened after the event? Was this what did he/she expected? *The middle ring* is the background to the attempt: how things have been over the preceding months. Might the attempt have been made at any time over the last months? What relationships were important over this time? *The outer ring* is the family and personal history (p 322).

After the above, come to the *bulls-eye*—the intentions lying behind the attempt, and the present feelings and intentions. Does the attempt represent a wish to die (a grave, not-to-be-ignored sign); a wish to send a message to somebody; or a wish to change intolerable circumstances? Ask: 'If you were to leave hospital today, how would you cope?' Examine the mental state (p 324) to find out if there is any mental illness. *Summary:* • Any plan? What? When? Where? • Are the means available? • Ever tried before? How seriously? • Preparations (making a will, giving things away).[3]

Before arranging hospital admission, ask what this is *for*. Is it only to make you feel happier?—or to gain something that cannot be gained outside hospital. Ask: *Why will discharge be safer in a few weeks rather than now?*

1 D Aldridge 1992 BJGP **42** 482 2 N Retterstol 1993 *Suicide*, CUP 3 R Vinning 1995 BMJ **i** 126

How to cope with threats of suicide

Suicide behaviour is powerful. *Boyfriend:* 'After last night, I think we should separate—we'd better just be good friends. . .' *Girlfriend* thinks: 'You are not going to treat me like that', but says: 'So we are not getting married after all?' 'Well not for a little while, maybe.' 'So you don't love me . . . I knew you loved Amanda more than me.' Exit to bathroom, where she swallows handfuls of her mother's tranquillizers. Next day in hospital the boyfriend says 'I'm so sorry—I didn't know you loved me that much.' He thinks: 'No one has ever thought that much of me. . . Fancy wanting to kill herself because I wouldn't marry her! I feel guilty; I should not have led her to this. . .' Whereupon he proposes marriage. This disastrous ending may be complicated by threats of suicide from jilted Amanda.

The psychiatrist may become enmeshed in these webs of suicide threats, and may wrongly assume that because someone threatens suicide, they should be admitted to hospital (compulsorily if necessary) so that they can be kept under constant surveillance, and suicide prevented. This reasoning has 3 faults. The first is the idea that it is possible to prevent suicide by admission. There is no such thing as constant surveillance. Second, hospital admission may achieve nothing if it simply removes the patient from the circumstances which he must learn to cope with. Third, reason is that it is necessary to distinguish between suicide gestures, which have the object of influencing others' behaviour, and a genuine wish to die.

Before death, many suicides see a GP, and it is wise to be alert to undercurrents of suicide which only somtimes surface during consultations. Ask *unambiguously* about suicide plans (p 322). On deciding that a threat is more manipulative than genuine, very experienced therapists may influence the person's use of suicide behaviour by forcing him to face the reality of his suicide talk, eg by asking: 'When will you kill yourself?' 'How will you do it?' 'Who will discover the corpse?' 'What sort of funeral do you want? Cremation, burial, with or without flowers?' 'Who will come?'

The standard pointers to risk of death from a suicide attempt are being male, older, unemployed, with prolonged psychiatric or painful illness, ± drug abuse. Recent attempts to validate this list have failed. It is better to think dynamically of risks and protective factors (such as family support), with suicide occurring after key events which accumulate risk.[1]

►*All suicide threats must be taken seriously*—but the emphasis will differ depending into which group the patient falls. In both groups it may be helpful to form a *contract* with the patient, eg:

- The therapist will listen and help if the patient agrees to be frank, and to tell the therapist of any suicide thoughts or plans.
- Agreement about which problems are to be tackled is made explicit.
- The type of change to aim for is agreed.
- Specification of who else will be involved in treatment (eg other members of the family, friends, the patient's GP).
- An agreement about the timing and place of sessions.
- An agreement about the patient's responsibility to work effectively with the therapist, and to carry out any 'homework'.

*If in doubt about the energy with which we may pursue our own destruction, let us call to mind a notable Japanese pilot who, during World War II, persistently volunteered to be a Kamikasi pilot to run a suicide mission against US ships, in the defence of Okinawa. The authorities just as persistently refused his request–he had a wife and 3 daughters. He kept on reapplying, determinedly. Not wanting to risk her husband's failure again, and not not wanting to stand in Destiny's way, his wife killed their 3 daughters, and then herself, so removing the obstacle to her husband's mission–and on May 28, 1945, he finally took to the air, and achieved his end.

1 L Appleby 1996 BMJ ii 884

Tricyclic and related antidepressant drugs

These improve mood and ↑synaptic availability of norepinephrine or 5HT. The 3 kinds: tricyclic and related drugs; MAOI (below); SSRIs (p 341).

Explain to sceptical patients that drugs *do* work; also discuss side-effects.

In agitated patients, offer a sedative antidepressant, eg:

Amitriptyline (≥50mg/8–24h PO. Starting dose example: 50mg at night).
Dothiepin (50mg/8–24h PO. Start with 50–75mg at night).
Doxepin (75mg/8–12h PO. Start with 10–50mg at night).
Trimipramine (25–50mg/8h PO. Start with 50mg 2h before bedtime).

Less sedative antidepressants include the following:

Clomipramine (50mg/8–24h PO. Start with 10mg/24h). This drug is particularly helpful if there are phobic or obsessional features.
Imipramine (10–25mg/8–24h PO, up to eight 25mg tablets/day).
Lofepramine (70mg/12h PO. Start with 70mg/24h; few anticholinergic SE).
Nortriptyline (25mg/6–24h PO. Start with 10mg/12h).
Protriptyline (5–10mg PO morning, noon and at 4pm—to avoid insomnia, up to six 10mg tablets/day). This is a stimulant.

Build up dose over ~10 days (eg to amitriptyline 150mg/24h PO); maintain this if side-effects allow for ≥1 month, before deciding if ineffective. After 2––5 months it may be appropriate to reduce the dose (eg amitriptyline 75–100mg at night). ►In the elderly use the smaller doses indicated above.

Unwanted tricyclic effects Convulsions (dose-related), arrhythmias, and heart block occur (particularly with amitriptyline, which is contraindicated in the weeks after a myocardial infarct; it is particularly dangerous in overdose—so prescribe in small volumes; review suicidal drive often).

Anticholinergic effects (dry mouth, blurred vision, constipation, urinary retention, drowsiness, and sweating) may occur with any tricyclic or related drug, particularly nortriptyline, amitriptyline, and imipramine. Explain these to the patient. Indicate that these effects will diminish with time. Until they do, advise against driving and operating machinery.

Hepatitis and agranulocytosis also occur, particularly with mianserin, eg up to 3 months after treatment is started (do monthly FBCs during this period).

Interactions The Pill may reduce the effect of tricyclics. Side-effects may be worse if phenothiazines are used concurrently. The effect of some hypotensives (eg clonidine but not β-blockers) may be reduced.

Lack of response[1] •Is the diagnosis correct? •Are there other diagnoses (eg cancer or CNS disease)? •Is he taking the tablets?—at full dose for >1 month? Do not expect a response before this. Consider an SSRI (p 341), ECT (p 336)—or or a monoamine oxidase inhibitor (MAOI)—but *not with* a tricyclic (tricyclics must not be given within 21 days of MAOIs). Try phenelzine 15–30mg/8h PO. The danger is hypertensive crises caused by certain foods and drugs, eg cheese, yeast (Marmite®), pickled herring, narcotics, common cold remedies, levodopa, tricyclics. This may occur up to 2 weeks after stopping MAOIs. Patients must carry a card declaring use of MAOIs, and foods to be avoided. But do not be put off their use: the incidence of crises is only ~17/98,000 patient years.[2] Benefits may be great, eg if there is oversensitivity to rejection by friends, some lightening of mood related to circumstances, hostility, overeating, oversleeping, marked fatigue, panic, irritability, or hypochondriasis.[2] Moclobemide (150–300mg/12h PO pc) is a new reversible MAO-A inhibitor said to have few of the problems of older MAOIs; CI: confusion, phaeochromocytoma); hypertension has sometimes occurred.[3]

Antidepressants in adolescent depression Careful meta-analyses of 12 papers indicate that tricyclics are no more effective than placebos in this group, but SSRIs (p 341) may be effective.

1 M Hornig-Rohan 1994 *Psychiatric Ann* **24** 220 2 C Bass 1989 BMJ **ii** 345 3 *Drug Ther Bul* 1994 **32** 6

Selective serotonin reuptake inhibitors (SSRIs)

Mode of action* 5HT (serotonin) re-uptake inhibition (*OHCM* p 406). NB: Serotoninergic system dysfunction is a feature of drug-free depressed people (CSF and brain 5HT metabolite levels↓; ↑CNS density of binding sites). There is evidence that the *STin2.9* allele of the serotonin transporter gene confers susceptibility to unipolar depression in >10% of patients.

Effects of SSRIs SSRIs are effective antidepressants (response rate ≈ that of tricyclics: 60–70%). Compared with old tricyclics, eg amitriptyline...

- SSRIs are less toxic in overdose—so more suitable if ↑suicide risk; but new tricyclic-related drugs (eg lofepramine) are much safer than amitriptyline.
- SSRIs are less sedating.
- SSRIs are just as prone to patients stopping medication owing to side-effects.
- SSRI are ~30 times the price: if all patients needing an antidepressant used SSRIs, the excess cost in the UK would be >£350 million (enough to purchase 22 million hours of services from psychiatric nurses).[1]

Side-effects (all SSRIs) Nausea (20%), dry mouth (10%) blurred vision (10%), seizures, and anorgasmia. 300–400 people die each year from poisoning with tricyclic related compounds. If patients need to drive there is some evidence that this is safer with paroxetine than with tricyclics.

Despite >60 trials of SSRIs and their detailed meta-analyses, no clear advantages have been shown, with apparent equality in drop-out rates, suggesting that from patients' view points they are little different. One problem is that transferring treatment drop-out rates from a trial environment to routine consulting room or ward life is problematic as in trials there is much pressure and organization to ensure that the patient 'carries on taking the tablets'—for the short duration of a trial.[2] Although there is also evidence (at least for fluoxetine) that if the lower doses now recommended are used (20mg/day) drop-outs are less than with low-dose régimes of tricyclics,[2] the effect is small, and the data are suspect because of the anomaly of finding that if the dose of fluoxetine is increased, the drop-out rate also falls. Another problem is that in many studies standardized interviews were not used (it is hard to assess trials where inclusion depends on impressions—although this is exactly how depression is diagnosed in the real world!).

Treatment régimes ►Monitor closely: suicide risk is greater early on.

Sertraline: 50mg/24h PO, ↑ if needed by 50mg steps every few weeks to a maximum of 200mg/day; within 8 weeks reduce to a maintenance dose of 50–100mg/day PO. SE: dyspepsia, sweating, AST↑ (if so, discontinue). It is the SSRI least likely to cause agitation or sedation.

Fluoxetine: 20mg/24h PO. SE: anxiety, insomnia, drowsy, confusion, fever, weight↓, Na^+↓, platelets↓, prolactin↑, vaginal bleeding when drug stopped. If rash or lung fibrosis, discontinue. $t_{1/2}$ ≈ 3 days. CI: last ⅓ of pregnancy.[3] NB: fluoxetine is the best-researched drug for depression in children and adolescents (20mg/day), so in this group, the above caveats do not apply.[4]

Fluvoxamine maleate: 100mg/12–24h PO (max 300mg/day). SE: agitation, headache, tremor, fits, pulse↓, AST↑ (discontinue). CI: epilepsy.

Paroxetine: 20mg each morning (↑in 10mg steps to 50mg—40mg if old). SE: dystonia, Na^+↓. Anorgasmia rare. Withdrawal signs: sweats, tremor.

Caution Epilepsy, pregnancy/lactation, ECT. Toxic interactions: MAOI, sumatriptan, Li^+, theophylline (fluvoxamine), haloperidol (fluoxetine), β-blockers (fluvoxamine), warfarin. Anticonvulsant antagonism. Withdrawal dystonia (p 366).

*NB: newer SSRIs (eg nefazodone) also block serotonin receptors; experience with them is limited—as with blockers of central presynaptic α_2-adrenoceptors (noradrenaline↑ + 5-HT↑)—eg mirtazapine—*Drug Ther Bul* 1999 **37** 1 (SE: dry mouth in 25%, sedation, appetite↑, weight↑, WCC↓)

1 J Edwards *BMJ* 1998 **i** 1180 2 *BMJ* 1993 **ii** 1124-6 3 *NEJM* 1997 **335** 1010 4 E Emlie *E-BM* 1998 **3** 105

Electroconvulsive therapy

Indications *Depression* if: •Not responding to antidepressants, or •Psychotic features are present, or •Needing to be controlled fast (eg patient refusing to drink, high suicide risk, or postpartum): electroconvulsive therapy (ECT) is the fastest acting physical treatment. Emergency ECT is possible, but should rarely be necessary.

Schizoaffective depression: (depression with signs of schizophrenia).

Mania: If not responding to drug treatment.

Contraindications Recent subdural/subarachnoid haemorrhage. Cautions: recent stroke, myocardial infarct, arrhythmias. SE: anterograde amnesia; anaesthesia complications. **Consent** (p 400). Try to involve relatives, but they cannot consent for another adult. **Typical course length** 6 sessions (2/week).

Technique •Check the patient's identity. •Must be nil by mouth for >8h.

- Ensure a detailed medical history and physical examination has been done, and any illnesses investigated and treated as far as possible. High anaesthetic risk?—See p 762; seizure threshold ↑ if on concurrent benzodiazepines, anticonvulsants, or methohexital (=methohexitone) >1.2mg/kg; also ↑risk of heart complications if on tricyclics. Liaise between psychiatric and anaesthetic staff. Do benefits outweigh risks?
- Give calm reassurance away from the site where ECT is going on. (It may be distressing to watch ECT actually happening.)
- Are the consent forms in order (p 400)? In the rare instances in the UK where ECT is given without consent, a second opinion from the Mental Health Commission must state that the treatment is necessary (p 400).
- Ensure that fully equipped resuscitation trolleys are present including a functioning defibrillator and suction apparatus, and pulse oximeter.
- Ensure that the anaesthetist (senior and ECT trained) knows about allergies or drugs interfering with anaesthesia. For countering ECT-induced vagal stimulation, he/she is most likely to use atropine or methscopolamine before using an ultra-short-acting anaesthetic agent (eg methohexital) with muscle relaxation (eg with suxamethonium) to minimize the seizure.
- The ECT machine: checked recently? Reserve machine to hand? What charge/energy is to be given? Which waveform will be used (bidirectional or modified sinusoidal, or unidirectional)? Study manufacturer's information.
- Establish if unilateral (side of non-dominant hemisphere) or bilateral positioning of electrodes is to be used. Unilateral causes less anterograde amnesia. If dominance is uncertain (if left-handed) use bilateral positioning.
- In unilateral ECT, position one electrode (A) 4cm above the midpoint between the auditory meatus and the lateral angle of the eye, and the other (B) 10cm away from A, above the ear—see diagram opposite.
- In bilateral ECT (used eg if rapid response vital, if unilateral ECT has failed, or if previously successful—but there may be troublesome cognitive side-effects): place electrodes over the same spot (A) on opposite sides of head.
- Put electrode jelly on the chosen sites (not enough to allow shorting).
- When the anaesthetist gives the word, give the shock. Be prepared to restrain the patient if paralysis is incomplete. While the current passes, the muscles will contract. This will cease as the current ceases. After ~10sec, further clonic spasms occur, lasting about 1min. The only sign may be lid fluttering. Clonus is probably needed for ECT to be fully effective.
- Put the patient in the coma position. Do BP and pulse, etc until conscious. Ask the anaesthetist to consider IV midazolam for those (few) who become very agitated during the recovery process.

Note: ECT may be frightening for patients and relatives—partly because it has had a bad press; so explain, step-by-step, what will happen; and patients should not witness other patients having ECT. The author (JML) also finds it helpful to tell patients that he would opt for ECT, if the right indications pertained, on a psychiatrist's recommendation, because it can be so effective—indeed life-saving. ECT is not recommended for children.[1]

What is the correct 'dose' of ECT?

There is no universal answer to this question. Be sure that you have adequate training on this issue by the consultant in charge of the session. Dose is better measured in millicoulombs (mC) than milliamps. It depends on *seizure threshold*, which varies 40-fold among patients. A moderately 'suprathreshold' dose (50–200% above seizure threshold) usually gives seizures of adequate duration, while aiming to minimize cognitive side-effects.[1] Doses need changing depending on response, and dose of methohexital in the anaesthetic: also, seizure threshold rises by ~80% as courses progress. NB: a 'good' seizure is one which is of adequate duration (~15 seconds during early sessions; duration is less important later), with both a tonic and a clonic phase. Some ECT machines allow monitoring of the EEG which is useful as anaesthesia renders seizure analysis difficult. If the seizure lasts >2mins, tell the anaesthetist, who will provide a bolus of diazepam, or more of the general anaesthetic agent.

1 Royal College of Psychiatrists ECT *Handbook* 1995 & T Baker 1995 *Lancet* **345** 65

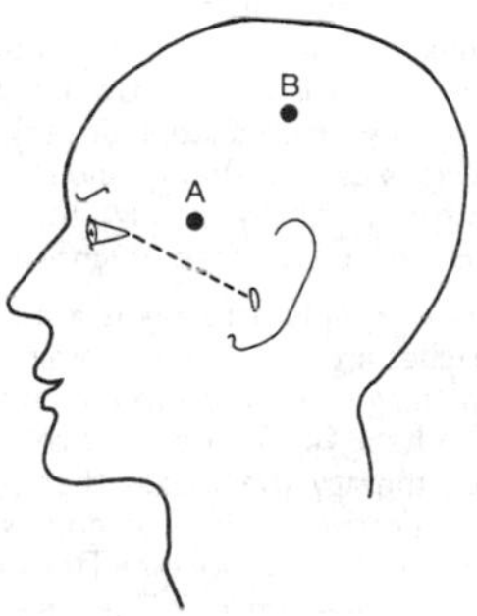

Electrode positions (see text)

Anxiety neurosis

Neurosis is the major psychological condition of our age—affecting at least one person in seven. It produces enormous suffering, and staggering losses to economies, in the UK estimated to reach £5.6 billion/yr (⅓ the cost of the NHS).[1] Neurosis refers to maladaptive psychological symptoms not due to organic causes or psychosis, and usually precipitated by stress. Apart from free-floating anxiety and depression, such symptoms are: fatigue (27%), insomnia (25%), irritability (22%), worry (20%), obsessions, compulsions, and somatization (p 744).[2] These are judged to be more intense than normal—ie out of proportion to the stress that precipitates them. Symptoms are not just part of a patient's normal personality, but they may be an exaggeration of personality: a generally anxious person may become even more so—ie develop an anxiety neurosis—as a result of job loss. The *type* of neurosis is defined by the chief symptom (eg anxiety, obsessional, depressive). Before diagnosing neurosis, consider carefully if there is underlying depression which needs treating with antidepressants.

Symptoms of anxiety:[3] Tension, agitation; feelings of impending doom, trembling; a sense of collapse; insomnia; poor concentration; 'goose flesh'; 'butterflies in the stomach'; hyperventilation (so tinnitus, tetany, tingling, chest pains); headaches; sweating; palpitations; poor appetite; nausea; 'lump in the throat'; unrelated to swallowing (globus hystericus); difficulty in getting to sleep; excessive concern about self and bodily functions; repetitive thoughts and activities (p 346). *Children's symptoms:* Thumb-sucking; nail-biting; bed-wetting; food-fads; stammering.

Types •Generalized anxiety disorder •Panic disorder •Simple phobia •Post-traumatic stress disorder •Agoraphobia •Social phobia •Obsessive-compulsive disorder

Possible causes •Stress (eg work—or lack of it, noise, a hostile home).
- Life events (p 336, eg gaining a spouse; losing a job or moving house).
- Intrapsychic theories (eg anxiety is excess psychic energy and is a manifestation of repressed hostility or conflicting drives). Neurotic behaviour is seen as a way of reducing excessive energy, and is more likely to occur if the person has failed to pass normally through the oral, anal, and genital stages of development. Evidence for these psychoanalytic ideas is scant.

Treatment *Symptom control:* Simple listening is a potent way of reducing anxiety. Explain that headaches are not due to a brain tumour, and that palpitations are harmless. Anything you can do to enrich the patient's relationship with others is likely to help. *Graded exposure* to the anxiety-provoking stimulus is a well-validated therapy (behaviour therapy, p 370).[4] *Anxiolytics* may be indicated to enable effective work to be done with the patient. *Dose example:* diazepam 5mg/8h PO for <6 weeks. The problems of benzodiazepine treatment (see p 366), severely limit their usefulness.

Progressive relaxation training: The patient is taught to tense and relax groups of muscles in an orderly way—eg starting with the toes and working up the body. By concentrating on this, anxiety and muscle tone are reduced. Deep breathing exercises bring about similar changes. The patient must practise often before benefit occurs. Commercial cassette tapes are available for repeated use, to help the learning process.[5]

Hypnosis: This is a powerful mechanism for reducing anxiety. Initially the therapist induces progressively deeper trances using such techniques as guided fantasy and concentration on various bodily sensations, such as breathing. Later, some patients will be able to induce their own trances.

1 J Holmes 1994 BMJ **ii** 1070 2 Off Pop Cens 1996 *B J Psych* **271** 70–1 3 M Lader 1994 BMJ **ii** 321 4 I Marks 1994 BMJ **ii** 1071 5 Adelph One, High St, Bottisham, Cambridge, UK (tel. 01223 811679)

Some remarks on the nature of anxiety

Anxiety is the engine in us, and also our steering-wheel, weaving us in and out of the fast or slow lanes of our lives. Some of us deliberately seek out anxiety as a way of feeling alive (think of the tightrope walker, or the falconer who places the meat for his bird between his own eyes). The lives of others are dominated by the imperative of minimizing anxiety, to the extent that some people never leave home, either physically or metaphorically. Anxiety implies heightened awareness, which is why it is one of the dominant colours in the artist's metaphysical palette. The artist makes us anxious so that we see familiar objects differently. Anxiety, up to a point, makes us sit up, and take note; beyond a certain level (different in all of us, and different at different times) anxiety is counter-productive: we become preoccupied with the feeling itself, which chokes our ability to act (*angere*, Latin for to choke, gives us both angina, and anxiety—*OED 1e* vol i 378.) So anxiety is no more a disease or a symptom than the circulation of the blood is a disease or symptom: rather it is one aspect of our human condition: it's part of the way we work. Just as our circulation can fail, so our ways of interacting with anxiety can fail. The most arresting manifestation of this phenomenon is panic (Pan is the god of groundless fear)—ie becoming petrified on being caught in the heart-stopping glare of events beyond our control. The strategies we adopt to recover our equilibrium are revealing: song, humour, camaraderie, and faith in God, gin, or our own genius. When these remedies fail, we turn to the psychiatrist and the strategies of cognitive therapy, hypnosis, and ritual relaxation. When these remedies fail in their turn (not always the case!), we are left on our own: this aloneness is another aspect of the human condition, and out of it grows our creativity and originality, born from the painful union of anxiety, fear and hope.

Other neurotic disorders

Anxiety neurosis has 4 subgroups: •Panic disorder (episodes of extreme anxiety and impending calamity) •Generalized anxiety disorder •Mixed anxiety and depressive disorder •Depressive disorder.

Phobic disorders These involve symptoms of anxiety occurring in specific situations only, and leading to their avoidance. These are labelled according to specific circumstance: agoraphobia (*agora,* Greek for market place) is fear of crowds, travel, or situations away from home; social phobias (where he might be minutely observed, eg small dinner parties); simple phobias, eg to dentists, intercourse, Friday the 13th (triskaidecophobia), spiders (arachnophobia), beetles (paint them red, and put black spots on and they become charming ladybirds). There may also be free-floating 'fear of fear', or fear of disgracing oneself by uncontrollable screaming.☎

It is important to find out exactly what the phobic stimulus is. It may be very specific, eg travelling by car, not bicycle. Why are some situations avoided? If because the patient is deluded that he is being followed or persecuted, paranoia rather than phobia is suggested. Panic attacks are lessened by paroxetine (p 341) ± cognitive therapy (p 370).[1]

Obsessive-compulsive disorder Compulsions are senseless, repeated rituals. Obsessions are stereotyped, purposeless words or phrases that come into the mind. They are perceived by the patient as nonsensical (unlike delusional beliefs), and, although out of character, as originating from themselves (unlike hallucinations or thought insertion). They are often resisted by the patient, but if longstanding, the patient may have given up resisting them. An example of non-verbal compulsive behaviour is the rambler who can never do a long walk because every few paces he wonders if he has really locked the car, and has to return repeatedly to ensure that this has, in fact, been done. Cleaning (eg handwashing), counting, and dressing rituals are other examples. *Pathophysiology:* Positron emission tomography (*OHCM* p 794) reveals increased blood flow to the orbitofrontal cortex, and reduced blood flow to the caudate nucleus. Successful treatment is reflected by some normalization of metabolism in these areas.[2] *Treatment:* Behaviour (or cognitive) therapy (p 370). Clomipramine (start with 25mg/day PO) and SSRIs (eg fluoxetine, start with 20mg per day PO) really can help (even if patients are not depressed):[3] see p 340.

Depersonalization This means an unpleasant state of disturbed perception in which objects (eg parts of the body) are experienced as being changed ('as if made of cotton wool'), becoming unreal, remote, or automatized. There is insight into its subjective nature, and it is not a feature of psychosis. Depersonalization may be primary, or part of another neurosis.

Hysteria *Clinical details:* p 334. *Case history in a depressed man:* p 388–96.

Treatment: Behaviour therapy (p 370) is often suitable, provided the patient really wants to change. Antidepressants (p 340) may also help, if combined with behavioural therapy.

☎See also the Internet link http://www.sci.rehabm.uab.edu/

[1] S Oehrberg 1996 *E-BM* **i** 81 **2** R Ramsay 1995 *BMJ* **ii** 167 **3** M Piccinelli 1995 *Br J Psych* 1995 **166** 424
4 D Wilkinson 1991 *BMJ* **ii** 191 **5** L Dillner 1992 *BMJ* **i** 1073 **6** C Krasucki 1995 *Lancet* **345** 1240
7 M Friedman 1994 *Psych Clin N America* **17** 256–77 **8** K Armstrong 1995 *Soc Work* **40** 83
9 CM Chemtob 1997 *Am J Psychiatry* **154** 415–17 **10** W Busuttil 1995 *Br J Psy* **167** 495

Stress, post-traumatic stress disorder, and 'razing out the written troubles of the brain and other rooted sorrows'

Signs of stress: insomnia, sleep-walking and other parasomnias (p 264), intrusive thoughts, dyspepsia, chest pain, fainting, palpitations, transitory hypertension, hyperventilation (± pins-and-needles), abdominal distension, nausea, irritability, over- or under-eating, depression, poor concentration, poor decision-making, and pre-occupation with trivia.

There are many biological consequences of stress, eg depression; increased weight, BP, and alcohol intake; peptic ulcers; irritable bowel syndrome; delayed wound healing (interleukin-1β mRNA↓); and migraine.

Relieving stress Smoking, alcohol and chattering are the most popular methods. If drugs must be given, and there is no asthma, heart failure or heart block, propranolol (eg 10mg/8h PO) may ↓autonomic symptoms, but side-effects are common. Some people try safer alternatives, eg exercise, singing, progressive relaxation (p 344), or counselling (p 376).

Post-traumatic stress disorder After great psychological trauma (near-death, shell-shock, rape, crimes of passion, etc) there may be: •Anxiety •Depression •Obsessive recall •Compulsive guilt at one's own survival* •Alcohol abuse •Irritability •Bed wetting •School/work refusal. Symptoms may be swift, or take *years* to come to light.[4,5] *Treatment* may focus on psychotherapeutic reliving of the emotional trauma, with skilled interpretation by the therapist, but success is elusive, and Macbeth's 'sweet oblivious antidote to cleanse the stuffed bosom of theat perilous stuff which weighs upon the heart' has yet to be found. After wars the 'talking cures' of psychotherapy may cause more harm than good: here the best advice may be to try to forget or ignore the past:[5] Macbeth's doctor replied (*Act V*) that such a patient 'must minister to himself', when he had been unreasonably but royally requested to 'pluck from the memory a rooted sorrow' and 'raze out the written troubles of the brain'—and perhaps tragic literature *can* offer more than medicine here. *Critical incident stress debriefing* is a more prosaic approach, using principles of proximity, immediacy, expectancy, and simplicity—eg by colleagues[6] or in the format of group discussions of the most troubling aspects of the trauma in question, with ventilation of feelings, normalization of emotional responses, and education into psychological insights.[7-9] In one study, 85% showed improvement with this.[10] *Prognosis:* Predicting when a given trauma will cause acute, delayed, or chronic post-traumatic stress disorder, or whether it will be a stimulus to growth and have salutary effects on overall functioning (sometimes the case[8-10]) is impossible. Presence of co-morbid disorders (eg depression) may be important, as well as age at exposure, and social networks. *Prevention:* This may involve promoting closely knit teamwork, techniques of stress inoculation (by exposure), and desensitization by experience with real casualty management (eg when preparing for war).

The many men so beautiful!
And they all dead did lie:
An a thousand thousand slimy things
Lived on; and so did I.

ST Coleridge, *see* R Holmes, *Selected Poems,* Harper Collins, 311

Anorexia and bulimia nervosa[1]

Anorexia epidemiology: Incidence: 4–16/10⁶/yr. ♀:♂≈20:1. Prevalence: 1–2% of schoolgirls (prevalence is higher in upper socio-economic classes). It is the third most common chronic illness in teenage girls. There is evidence that anorexia is a manifestation of attitudes such as 'I hate my body' engendered by western media stereotypes of long-legged gawky beauties—but note that negative body images are very common, but eating disorders are rare.

Definition of anorexia: There are 4 diagnostic criteria:

1 The person chooses not to eat, leading to potentially dangerous weight loss interfering with normal functioning, eg BMI <17 (p 473), or, more strictly, a weight less than 85% of weight expected, taking into account height, sex, and population the patient belongs to—see p 185 & 473).
2 Intense fear of becoming obese, even when underweight.
3 Disturbance of weight perception (ie feeling fat when thin).
4 Amenorrhoea: ≥3 consecutive cycles absent (when not on the Pill).

Symptoms: These usually start at ~16–17yrs (12 in boys) and may be precipitated by dieting. She attaches excessive importance to weight reduction (an over-valued idea), and she may become deluded that she is repulsively fat when she is, in fact, very malnourished. Excessive exercise, and induced vomiting may occur; there may be abuse of laxatives, diuretics and appetite suppressants. The patient sees her self-worth as being embodied in her shape and weight. Many patients may also have episodes of binge eating, followed by remorse, vomiting, and concealment. Depression and suicide attempts commonly coexist.

Physical complications of weight reduction: Sensitivity to cold, constipation, amenorrhoea, faints, weakness, fatigue, BP↓, K^+↓, glucose↓.

Causes: Single factor theories are not favoured. 10% of ♀ siblings may be affected, but this is more likely to show the importance of family behaviour in maintaining symptoms than any direct genetic effect (but concordant pairs of monozygotic twins are described). Rarely, hypothalamic tumours turn up in people originally diagnosed as having anorexia (amenorrhoea *before* weight loss is suspicious). Some workers see the relentless pursuit of thinness as a struggle for control and to gain an identity. Dietary problems in early life, parental preoccupation with food, and family relationships that leave the person without a sense of identity may also be important. There is little foundation for the view that the chief problem is psychosexual immaturity.

Treatment: What is the urgency? If extreme weakness, fainting, K^+↓ or glucose ↓, then prompt admission to hospital, possibly under the Mental Health Act, may be needed for feeding (IV if needed). In other circumstances work on building up a trusting relationship with the patient. Work on several fronts simultaneously: •Gaining of weight (agreed targets; aim for weight gain of 1.5kg/week, and a final body mass index of 20–25—special foods are not required).[2] •Treat the medical complications of starvation •Helping with relationships (eg family therapy) •Cognitive–behavioural therapy (p 370).[3] On admission privileges are removed, and restored as weight rises. *Prognosis:* 2% of anorectic patients die (by starvation), and 16% remain seriously underweight after 4–8yrs. Cardiac complications are the commonest cause of death (K^+↓ and prolonged Q–T interval predispose to arrhythmia).

Bulimia

Bulimia is common, affecting ~10% of young women. Diagnostic criteria: •Recurrent episodes of binge eating •During binging a lack of feeling of control •Regular use of mechanisms to overcome the fattening effects of binges (eg vomit-induction, laxatives, excessive exercise) •Persistent overconcern with body weight •Body weight higher than required for the diagnosis of anorexia (anorexia trumps the diagnosis of bulimia).

Physical complications: Stomach rupture, haematemesis and metabolic complications following excessive (eg self-induced) vomiting. There may be painless enlargement of the salivary glands, tetany and seizures. Russell's sign: calluses form on the back of the hand, following its repeated abrasion against incisors during inducement of vomiting.[1]

Management: Consider behavioural or cognitive techniques (p 368–82). For example, the patient may agree to limit eating to one room in the house, and to eat only at mealtimes. She may agree not to have food in the house, and when shopping, she may agree to buy only those items on a shopping list which she has made when satisfied after a meal. It may help to shop with a friend, and with only sufficient money to buy the items on the list. *Drugs:* These are rarely used, but a small randomized trial shows that fluoxetine (p 341) aids weight reduction, and reduces craving for carbohydrates[4]—but effects are short-term and a big problem is relapse on stopping medication.

1 *Drug Ther Bul* 1992 13 2 P Beaumont1993 *Lancet* 341 1635 ◄3► CG Fairburn 1995 *Arc Gen Psy* 52 304 4 J Edwards 1992 BMJ i 1644

Organic reactions

Acute organic reactions (Acute confusion, delirium) The central feature is impaired consciousness with onset over hours/days. It is difficult to describe; take any opportunity to be shown it. You have the sense when trying to communicate that he is not really with you. He is likely to be disoriented in time (doesn't know day or year) and, with greater impairment, in place. Sometimes he is very quiet/drowsy; sometimes agitated, and you are called when he is disrupting the ward. On other occasions the patient appears deluded (for example accusing staff of plotting against him/her) or to be hallucinating. If there is no past psychiatric history, and in the setting of a general hospital (ie the patient is physically ill or has had recent surgery), mental illness is rare but acute confusional state is common. A confusional state is particularly likely if the symptoms are worse at the end of the day.

Differential diagnosis: If agitated, consider anxiety (usually readily distinguished on history-taking). If onset uncertain consider dementia.

Causes: Infection; infarction; drugs (benzodiazepines, opiates, anticonvulsants, digoxin, L-dopa); U&E imbalance; hypoglycaemia; hypoxia; epilepsy; alcohol withdrawal; trauma. For a full list, see p 351.

Investigations: U&E, FBC, blood gases, blood glucose, appropriate cultures, LFT, ECG, CXR. Consider skull x-ray, LP and CT scan.

Management: ►Find the cause. Examine the patient with above causes in mind; do necessary tests. Start relevant treatment—eg O_2.

1 If agitated and disruptive, sedation may be needed before examination and tests are possible. Use neuroleptics (eg haloperidol 5–10mg IM/PO; or, chlorpromazine 50–100mg IM/PO). Wait 20mins to judge effect + further dose as needed. NB: in alcohol withdrawal use diazepam (*OHCM* p 682).

3 Nurse ideally in *moderately lit* quiet room with same staff in attendance (to minimize confusion). Repeated reassurance and orientation. In practice a compromise between a quiet room and a place where staff can keep under close surveillance has to be made.

Chronic organic reactions (dementia) *Prevalence:* ~6% of those >65yrs.

Cardinal features: Worsening memory and global intellectual deterioration without impairment of consciousness. Get a good history from friends/relatives. Exclude depression (may need a drug trial).

- Behaviour: restless; no initiative; repetitive, purposeless activity; sexual disinhibition; social gaffes; shoplifting; rigid routines.
- Speech: syntax errors; aphasia; mutism.
- Thinking: slow, muddled; delusions. Poor memory. No insight.
- Perception: illusions, hallucinations (often visual).
- Mood: irritability, depression (early); emotional blunting with sudden mood changes and emotional incontinence (later).

Identifying treatable causes: •Haematology: FBC, B_{12}, red cell folate (macrocytosis suggests alcoholism, or B_{12} or folate deficiency. ESR (malignancy).

- Biochemistry: U&E, LFT, GGT, Ca^{2+} (renal/hepatic failure, alcoholism, malignancy, endocrine causes leading to $Ca^{2+}\downarrow$). T_4 (hypothyroidism).
- Serology: for *syphilis* (*OHCM* p 218). After counselling carers, *test for HIV* if at risk.
- Radiology: CXR (evidence of malignancy). CT scan (hydrocephalus, tumours, subdural haematoma, CNS cysticercosis, *OHCM* p 248).

Management: If treatable causes have been excluded, explain this to the relatives, who may feel unable to look after the immobile, incontinent, aggressive patient. A walking frame, an indwelling catheter, thioridazine (eg 25mg/6h PO), day care, holiday admission, and an attendance allowance can transform this picture. If not, long-stay institutional care may be needed. Consider arranging power of attorney.

Causes of organic reactions:

	Acute organic reactions:	Chronic organic reactions:
Degenerative		*Alzheimer's Lewy*body dementia[1] (eosinophilic intracytoplasmic neuronal inclusion bodies) Creutzfeldt–Jakob, Pick's or Huntington's diseases
Other CNS	Cerebral tumour or abscess, subdural haematoma, epilepsy, acute post-trauma psychosis	Brain tumour, subdural haematoma, multiple sclerosis, Parkinson's, normal pressure hydrocephalus
**Infective*	Many, eg meningoencephalitis, septicaemia, cerebral malaria, trypanosomiasis	Late syphilis, chronic or subacute encephalitis, CNS cysticercosis, cryptococcosis, HIV
Vascular	Stroke (or TIA), hypertensive encephalopathy, SLE	Thromboembolic multi-infarct (arteriosclerotic) dementia, hypertension, anaemia
Metabolic	*U&E imbalance, *hypoxia, *liver and kidney failure, non-metastatic cancer, porphyria, *alcohol withdrawal	Liver and kidney failure non-metastatic or metastatic cancer
Endocrine	Hyperthyroid or Addisonian crisis, diabetic pre-coma, hypoglycaemia, hypo/hyperparathyroidism	T4↓, Addison's, hypoglycaemia hypopituitarism, hypo-/hyperparathyroidism
Toxic	*Alcohol, many drugs (check *Data sheet Compendium*), lead, arsenic, mercury	*'Alcoholic dementia', barbiturate or bromide abuse, too much manganese or carbon disulfide
Deficiency	Thiamine↓ B_{12}↓ folate↓ nicotinic acid↓	Thiamine↓; B_{12}↓; folate↓ nicotinic acid↓ (pellagra)

* = leading causes

Help for relatives of demented patients

- Alzheimer's disease is usually progressive, with mental functioning getting steadily worse; some problems (eg aggression) *may* improve over time. Both the rate of change and the length of life vary greatly. **Should you try to explain to your relative what the diagnosis is?** There is no easy answer. There is no evidence that knowing causes depression (but he may be depressed if he realizes his memory is fading). The advantage of frank talking is that he can participate in his care (so the vexed issue of stopping driving may be easier to handle). Also, during the early stages, he can give consent to future treatments. Most (71%) people *would* want to be informed if they got Alzheimer's.
- Take every opportunity to talk about your predicament with other people in the same position. This is often just as useful as talking to doctors. The Alzheimer's Disease Society exists to put you in touch: UK *tel*: 0171 306 0606.
- Accept offers of help, eg with care-giver training programmes, and of daycare for your relative (you certainly deserve, and need, a break from time to time).
- Lock up any rooms in the house which you do not use. Your relative will not notice this restriction—and this may make your life much easier.
- Lock drawers which contain important papers or easily-spoiled items to prevent him storing inappropriate things in them, such as compost, or worse.
- Remove locks from the lavatory—so he/she cannot get locked in.
- Normal sexual relationships will stop. Spouses should try not to fall into the trap of asking 'What's the matter with me?' NB: medroxyprogesterone acetate 100–200mg/2 weeks IM may help if hypersexuality becomes a problem.
- Prepare yourself psychologically for the day when he/she no longer recognizes you. This can be a great blow, unless you prepare for it.
- In the UK, apply to Social Services for *Attendance Allowance* + *council tax rebate*.

1 Lewy-body dementia is characterized by Lewy bodies in brainstem and neocortex, and a fluctuating but persisting cognitive impairment, parkinsonism, and hallucinations. It is a common form of dementia.

Alzheimer's dementia (AD)

This is the major neuropsychiatric disorder of our times, dominating not just psychogeriatric wards, but the lives of many thousand sons, daughters and spouses who have given up work, friends, and all their accustomed ways of life to support relatives through the last long years. The struggle of caring for loved ones through terminal illness always puts us on our mettle: never more so than when that loved one's personality disintegrates, and the person who is loved is gone long before their eventual death.

Suspect Alzheimer's disease in adults with any enduring, acquired deficit of memory and cognition—eg as revealed in the mental test score and other neuropsychometric tests (p 353). Onset may be from 40yrs (or earlier, eg in Down's syndrome)—so the notions of 'senile' and 'pre-senile' dementia are blurred (and irrelevant).

Genetics This is complex (defective genes on chromosomes 1, 14, 19, 21; the apoE4 variant is a major risk-factor, also bringing forward age of onset).

Diagnosis is often haphazrd, as the exact form of dementia used not to influence outcome, provided routine blood tests are normal. This view is hard to justify now that *specific* treatments are available for Alzheimer's. Specialist assessment with neuroimaging for all would be ideal (this would help rule out frontal lobe dementia and Lewy-body dementia, and Pick's disease).

Histology (rarely used) •Deposition of β-amyloid protein in cortex (a few patients have mutations in the amyloid precursor protein).
- Neurofibrillary tangles and an increased number of senile plaques.
- A deficit of neurotransmitter acetylcholine from damage to an ascending forebrain projection (nucleus basalis of Meynert connecting with cortex).

Presentation In stage I of AD there is failing memory and spatial disorientation. In stage II (which follows after some years) personality disintegrates (eg with increased aggression and focal parietal signs, eg dysphasia, apraxia, agnosia and acalculia). Parkinsonism may occur. She may use her mouth to examine objects (hyperorality). In stage III she is apathetic (or ceaselessly active—akathisia), wasted, bedridden and incontinent, ± fits and spasticity.

Mean survival 7 years from onset.

Management *Theoretical issues:* Potential strategies—the MRC menu:
- Preventing the breakdown of acetylcholine, eg donepezil, below.
- Augmenting nerve growth factor (NGF), which is taken up at nerve endings, and promotes nerve cell repair.
- Stimulating nicotinic receptors which may protect nerve cells.
- Inhibition of the enzymes that snip out β-amyloid peptide from APP, (amyloid precursor protein), so preventing fibrils and plaques.
- Anti-inflammatories to prevent activation of microglial cells to secrete neurotoxins (eg glutamate, cytokines) which stimulate formation of APP.
- Regulation of calcium entry (mediates the damage of neurotoxins).
- Preventing oxidative damage by free radicals; ± a rôle for vitamins & HRT.

Practical issues: ►See *Help for relatives of the demented*, p351. Exclude treatable dementias (B_{12}, folate, syphilis serology, T_4, ?HIV).

Treat concurrent illnesses (they contribute significantly to confusion). In most people the dementia remains and will progress. Involve relatives and relevant agencies. Alzheimer's Disease Society (0171 306 0606, in UK).

Liaise with an expert about increasing CNS acetylcholine by inhibiting the enzyme for its breakdown (donepezil; rivastigmine). Antioxidants such as extract of ginkgo biloba have been endorsed by randomized trials.[1] These agents may delay need for institutional care, but not necessarily its duration.[2]

Prevention Keeping alert, and engaged with current and family affairs and enjoying education seems sensible. HRT appears to offer some protection.[3]

1 P Le Bars 1998 *E-BM* **2** 80 2 C Kelly 1997 *BMJ* **i** 693 3 M Tang 1996 *Lancet* **348** 429

Mental test score

This is a quantifiable, standardized way of measuring someone's mental functioning. It is most useful for serial measurements. Maximum score 34; normal ≥29; a change of ≥5 is meaningful. See also the *Mini-Mental State Examination*, OHCM, p 77.

Knows his name	score 0 or 1
Knows his age	score 0 or 1
Time, to nearest hour	score 0 or 1
Time of day	score 0 or 1
Teach name and address: test recall after 5min:	
Mr John Brown	score 0, 1 or 2
42 West Street	score 0, 1 or 2
Gateshead	score 0, 1 or 2
Day of the week	score 0 or 1
Date of month	score 0 or 1
Current year	score 0 or 1
Place: eg hospital	score 0 or 1
name of hospital	score 0 or 1
name of ward	score 0 or 1
name of town	score 0 or 1
Recognizes 2 people	score 0, 1 or 2
Birthday	0 or 1
Town of birth	0 or 1
School	0 or 1
Former occupation	0 or 1
Name wife, sibling or next of kin	0 or 1
Monarch's name	0 or 1
Prime minister's or head of state's name	0 or 1
Give years of:	
World War I	0 or 1
World War II	0 or 1
Months of year backwards	0, 1 or 2
Count 1–20	0, 1 or 2
Count 20–1	0, 1 or 2

Other *possibly* significant questions Increasingly, do you find that:
- You forget what you are saying or reading in mid-sentence?
- When you enter a room full of people whose names you well know, the only name that *actually* comes into your mind is Alzheimer?
- You have to rely on lists whereas previously this was not necessary?
- Thought is slow or imprecise, harmonizing poorly with motor control?
- Mental agility is lacking, with powers of concentration declining?
- Are there difficulties executing fast movements of eyes or limbs, or difficulties in walking?—eg with spastic ataxic gait or quadriparesis of *HIV-1-associated cognitive/motor complex*—or psychomotor retardation, ± release reflexes such as a snout response, or hyperactive deep tendon reflexes).[1]

1 RW Price 1996 *Lancet* **348** 445

Psychosis (including mania)

►Beware labelling people: and remember that even during the best of times, there is only a thin veil separating us from insanity. In its most florid form, psychosis is the archetype of the layman's 'madness', and it signifies a state of mind in which contact with reality is lost and all the landmarks of our normal mental processes have been suspended and turned awry, with an abandoning of constraints imposed by reason and morality. However, the *usual* picture is much less obvious: the patient may be sitting alone, quietly attending to his or her voices.

Key features suggesting psychosis are: hallucinations, delusions, and thought disorder—defined on p 316 & 358. If one of these features is present, the diagnosis is limited to 4 entities: schizophrenia (p 358), a disorder of affect (ie mania or depression, p 336), a paranoid state, or an organic, ie physical, disease. So the term psychosis is not in itself a diagnosis, but is a useful term to employ, while the underlying diagnosis is being formulated.

Mania and hypomania We normally adapt our pace to the obstacles we encounter—but in mania we march round in circles, like a tornado picking up internal speed as we go, with the potential to destroy everything beneath the conquering tread of an unfettered will, while exhibiting these signs:

•Euphoria	•Hyperactivity	•Hallucinations	•Over-assertiveness
•Appetite↑	•Pressure of speech	•Disinhibition	•Grandiose delusions
•Insight↓	•Sexual desire↑	•Spending sprees	•Self-important ideas

Less severe states are termed *hypomania*. If depression alternates with manic features, the term *manic depressive psychosis* is used—particularly if there is a history of this in the close family. Cyclical mood swings without the more florid features (listed above) are termed *cyclothymia*.

Treatment and prophylaxis: Sedation may be required, eg chlorpromazine 25–150mg/4–8h PO, droperidol 5–15mg/4h IV, or a benzodiazepine. Zuclopenthixol acetate, 50–100mg IM into a buttock is an alternative (perhaps), if you you know that the patient can tolerate neuroleptics; it lasts 2–3 days. If compliance is good, and U&E, ECG, and T_4 normal, give lithium carbonate 125mg–1g/12h PO as follows. (Note: intracellular levels take time to build up.)

- Adjust the dose to achieve a plasma level of ~0.7–1.0mmol/L Li^+, measured on the 4th–7th day of treatment, 12h (± ½h) after the preceding dose.
- Check Li^+ levels weekly until the dose has been constant for 4 weeks; then monthly for 6 months, and then every 3 months, if stable. Do more often if on diuretic, low salt diet or pregnant (avoid Li^+ if possible).
- If levels are progressively rising, suspect progressive nephrotoxicity.
- Do plasma creatinine and TSH every 6 months; Li^+ affects thyroid and kidney (hypothyroidism; nephrogenic diabetes insipidus).
- Avoid changing proprietary brands, as Li^+ bioavailability varies.
- Make sure you know how to contact the patient by phone if Li^+ levels are high (>1.4mmol/L prompts urgent contact with patient to adjust dose).
- Toxic effects: blurred vision, D&V, K^+↓, drowsiness, ataxia, coarse tremor, dysarthria, hyperextension, seizures, psychosis, coma, and shock.

Refractory mania: consider carbamazepine (*OHCM* p 450), valproate, ECT.
NB: not everyone will need Li^+ prophylaxis after one episode of mania. Numbers needed to treat to prevent one relapse ≈3.

Organic psychoses These follow some physical stimulus: narcotics; amphetamines; cocaine; lysergic acid; alcohol; glue or solvent abuse; CNS trauma or tumour; epilepsy; puerperal psychosis (see p 148, the stimulus is birth); associated stress, life events, and tiredness are also important.

Paranoid states This implies paranoid symptoms (delusions or hallucinations) which concern a patient's relationships with others, and in whom using one of the other 4 categories of psychosis (above) is unjustified. A common form is a persecutory delusion ('there is a conspiracy against me'). Morbid jealousy (the Othello syndrome—p 754) is a rarer example.

4. Psychiatry

Schizophrenia: *history & current concepts*

Schizophrenia is a common mental disorder which typically presents in adulthood with delusions (p 316), hallucinations, and disordered thought (positive symptoms). There is also a more chronic picture with withdrawal, apathy, emotional blunting and slowness of thought (negative symptoms). *Incidence:* ~0.15/1000/yr. *Prevalence:* ~3/1000. It is a disorder with major implications, for the patient, his or her family, and it forms the basis for much of the chronic workload of psychiatrists and psychiatric nurses.

Past models Schizophrenia has been viewed as *a behavioural disorder*—ie a pattern of well-learned avoidance responses. The behaviour *is* the illness. *As a family disorder:* Schizophrenia is seen as a way of facing intolerable family stresses. Here a 'schizophrenogenic' mother gives conflicting messages (the 'double bind') to her daughter who is having difficulty with her exams: 'Your exams are very trying, and I do so understand why you have locked yourself in your room. I'll do anything I can to help. You must realize you are putting me and your father under a lot of stress: if this leads us to separate, it will be your fault.' Most mothers are very supportive of their schizophrenic offspring, and it is important not to suggest to her by your attitude that you are looking for a schizophrenogenic mother, or else you stand to lose the trust of the person best placed to help your patient in very many ways.

Newer models of schizophrenia Schizophrenia is now often thought of as a *physical/chemical disorder:* For example, images showing CNS function (positron emission tomography and single photon emission tomography) show subtle changes affecting the hippocampus and temporal lobe (where glutamate receptor subtypes are reported to be missing) in schizophrenia. The cerebral ventricles are also enlarged. Concepts derived from cognitive neuroanatomy are increasing being employed to throw light on the nature of schizophrenia. We now evidence that:

- Schizophrenic patients with poverty of speech show low blood flow in the dorsolateral prefrontal cortex (DLPFC) on the left.[1]
- During auditory hallucinations muscle activity resembling phonation can sometimes be detected in the tongue. Pre-vocal speech can be made audible by microphones, and the speech may correspond with what the hallucinations are telling the patient to do.
- We are all prone to paralysis of the will, contrary to the views of the boldest soldiers in their pre-psychotic phases, such as Othello, for whom 'to . . . be in doubt is [at] once to be resolved'. When psychosis arrives, and paralysis of the will becomes chronic, we can expect to find disconnections in the pathways of willed action. Imaging the brain during tasks involving choice (as opposed to the same manual task but pre-specified) shows that these pathways connect the anterior cingulate cortex, the basal ganglia, the dorsolateral prefrontal cortex, and the supplementary motor area.
- In schizophrenic patients there is an abnormal lack of connectivity between DLPFC and the superior temporal cortex.

One conclusion from this and other evidence is that we should regard schizophrenia as a white-matter neurodevelopmental encephalopathy affecting the interconnections of the associative centres of the brain (ie there is no distinct focal lesion). The initial event may be intrauterine stresses such as poor nutrition or infection. Frith has postulated that these events lead to a *defect in self-monitoring* such that the patient does not appreciate that he or she has willed inner speech, and these pre-vocal words therefore take on the characteristics of hallucinations.[2] Negative features arise from failure of the will due to events (or lack of events) in the dopaminergic pathways of willed action described above).

1 PF Liddle 1992 *Br J Psychiatry* **160** 179–86 2 C Frith 1995 *Lancet* **346** 615

Testing neurodevelopmental models of schizophrenia[1]

To the casual observer, a young man's first schizophrenic episode seems like a bolt from the blue: unheralded, and cataclysmic. But we now know that there are subtle but significant differences in early behaviour of those going on to get schizophrenia, eg there is excess solitary play ($p<0.05$; $N=5362$) and walking is delayed by a few months ($p<0.005$).[2]

Twin studies In monozygotic twins discordant for schizophrenia, it is always the twin with the smaller temporal lobes and larger ventricles who has the schizophrenia.[1]

One abiding difficulty with studying the behaviour and CNS characteristics of those with chronic schizophrenia is that it is impossible to tell for sure whether the events observed or the structural differences measured are the cause or the the effect of the schizophrenia. Suffering family breakdown or living in an institution, or taking neuroleptic medication are themselves highly significant events.

Studies of first-episode patients Some of these confounding events can be obviated by imaging the brains of those undergoing their first-ever schizophrenic event. Such studies show reduced brain volumes (↓by 3%), along with more specific deficits in medial temporal lobe structures such as the amygdala (known to be important in the recognition and expression of emotion) and hippocampus (needed for memory function). Emotion and memory are affected in schizophrenia, and the volume of these areas is reduced, typically by ~10%).[1,3] The thalamus is is also abnormal, and may be the source of hallucinatory events.[3]

No-episode-yet 'patients' If neurodevelopmental models of schizophrenia are correct, then it is predicted that individuals who have not yet had their first episode will nevertheless have structural brain anomalies. We now have evidence that this is the case.[3] The most important known risk factor is family history (risk↑ by 40-fold if a first-degree relative is affected, but no strongly linked genes have been found). On MRI, these people (aged 16–25) have anomalies similar to first-episode patients.

So, in this sense, schizophrenia is becoming a little more predictable, and, in time, this may pave the way for early detection and novel treatments.

1 P Harrison 1999 *Lancet* **353** 3 2 P Jones 1994 *Lancet* **344** 1398 3 S Lawrie 1999 *Lancet* **353** 30 (here, thalamic volumes were smaller in the high-risk group than in those with schizophrenia)

Schizophrenia: *diagnosis and prognosis*

First rank symptoms[1] Reliable, specific markers, seen in ~70% of patients.

- Thought insertion: 'Someone is putting thoughts into my head.'
- Thought broadcasting: 'People hear my thoughts as they occur.'
- Thought withdrawal: 'Thoughts are being taken out of my head.' (Thoughts may also stop in midflow, resuming on a different tack.)
- Passivity feelings: 'Someone is controlling my thoughts and movements; I'm their robot.'
- Hearing 'voices commenting on my actions' or referring to the patient in the third person (or the repeating of thoughts—*écho des pensées*).
- Primary delusions, in addition to the thought-delusions above.
- Somatic hallucinations, ie the experience of being the passive and reluctant recipient of bodily sensations imposed by some external agency—eg the experience of being sexually penetrated.

Other hallucinations/delusions occur in depression, mania, and organic reaction, so fleeting or fragmentary delusions and hallucinations, and negative symptoms (flattening of affect, poverty of speech, illogical thought, avolition, anhedonia) are less helpful, as are symptoms which it is hard to agree on—eg emotional detachment; coldness; lack of empathy—'as if a pane of glass separates me from others'; incongruity of affect—eg laughing at bad news; and *knight's move thoughts* which change direction, and fly off at tangents, often having a logic, albeit a strange one: 'his ideas seemed to move on a deeper level, like roots spreading below a layer of compost . . . a code uncracked which waits for a clue or an inspiration.'[2]

The presence of one first rank symptom is very suggestive of schizophrenia, but presentation may not be florid with delusions and hallucinations—also suspect the diagnosis in those who have become withdrawn, with negative symptoms (see above).

If psychotic features with *no* first rank symptoms, look meticulously for depression or mania. Ask yourself: is the content of the delusion or hallucination suggestive of either depression or mania (guilty or grandiose)?

Drugs (eg amphetamines) can cause schizophrenia-like symptoms. Taking a good history, and understanding the underworld vocabulary of drug abusers (OHCM p 184–5) will usually point you in the right direction.

The most frequent symptoms:	
Lack of insight	97%
Auditory hallucinations	74%
Ideas of reference (p 316)	70%
Suspiciousness	66%
Flatness of affect	66%
Voices speaking to patient	65%
Delusions of persecution	62%
Thought-delusions	~50%

The most frequent behaviour:	
Social withdrawal	74%
Underactivity	56%
Lack of conversation	54%
Few leisure interests	50%
Slowness	48%
Overactivity	41%
Neglect of appearance	30%
Odd postures or movements	25%

Better prognosis if: Sudden onset; no negative symptoms; supportive home. Also: premorbid psychosocial evolution, high scores on measures of expressed emotion, female sex, and negative family history (data from WHO's *disability assessment schedule*[3]). Overall, 10% only ever have one episode. With treatment, only ~7% of patients stay in hospital for >2yrs after first admission. 28% go at least 2 years without needing further hospital admission. The lifetime risk of schizophrenia in the general population is ~1%.

The family Get expert help. Create agreed care plans, specifying all options. Is housing adequate? Monitor family stress levels (plan what to do if levels rise). Family education about schizophrenia, and problem-solving skills reduces relapses, hospitalizations, and improves drug compliance.[4]

1 K Schneider 1959 *Clinical Psychopathology*, Grune & Stratton & N Andreasen 1995 *Lancet* **346** 477
2 Graham Greene 1957 & 1995 *Under the Garden*, Penguin ISBN 0-146-00057-9 p45. *See also* American Psychiatric Association 1994 *Diagnostic & Statistical Manual of Mental Ddisorders* DSM-IV, Washington DC, American Psychiatric Press 3 P Huguelet 1995 *Encephale* **21** 93 ◄4► J Mari 1996 E-BM **i** 121

4. Psychiatry

Schizophrenia: *management*

Aims These are to treat the patient and the illness as well as possible—and to provide support and advice to the relatives. *Is hospital admission needed?* Yes, if the patient is a danger to himself or others, or hospital is the only place where you can be sure the patient will get the treatment he needs. Treat acute symptoms with neuroleptics, eg chlorpromazine 25mg/8h PO, up to 1g/day (500mg if elderly); child: 0.5mg/kg/4–6h PO, if >6yrs $\frac{1}{3}$–$\frac{1}{2}$ adult dose, max 75mg daily. These usually reduce hallucinations and delusions within 3 weeks (but may not make the patient *feel* better—side-effects include tardive dyskinesia, apathy, drowsiness, depression, dry mouth, hypotension, arrhythmias, weight gain, impotence and extrapyramidal effects, photosensive rashes, and jaundice). By 3 months they reach full effect. Longer-term management includes helping the patient engage in as normal a life as possible, in a planned way. Aim to reduce relapse risk by continuing neuroleptics, and trying to ensure a stress-free environment. Relatives need help to be neither critical nor overprotective. Cognitive therapy (p 370) reduces psychotic symptoms. Sessions are devoted to systematically reviewing the start of symptoms. Patients are questioned in detail to reveal faulty reasoning, and then encouraged to monitor psychotic symptoms, and develop coping strategies, eg: •Changing the focus of attention •Relaxation techniques •Modifying exacerbating behaviours. The use of these have been confirmed in trials,[1] and note how their effects may be more humanizing than the ready resort to the 'liquid cosh' (below).

Psychotic violent patients (150 people have been killed in the UK in 1991–7.)

- Recognize early warning signs: tachypnoea, clenched fists, shouting, chanting, restlessness, repetitive movements, pacing, gesticulations. Your own intuition may be helpful here. At the first hint of violence, get help. If alone, make sure you are nearer the door than the patient.
- Do not be alone with the patient; summon the police if needed.
- Try calming and talking with the patient. Do not touch him. Use your body language to reassure (sitting back, open palms, attentive).
- Get his consent. If he does not consent to treatment, emergency treatment can still be given to save life, or serious worsening of the patient's condition—on the verbal authority of any doctor.
- Use minimum force to achieve his welfare (but may entail 6 strong men).
- If one of the following IM drugs is needed, monitor BP every 4h.
- Later, liaise with colleagues about long-term care. Will the outside world be at risk if community care is used? If so (or if the person is at danger from suicide or self-neglect) the UK government requires entry of the patient into a *supervision register*, with a key worker (eg a community psychiatric nurse) trained in risk-management and assessment, who can coordinate multidisciplinary review meetings to monitor progress. These requirements may be counter-productive,[2] if no extra funds are available and the key worker's chief aim is to keep people out of hospital.

Usual adult ORAL doses	Max licensed IM dose; halve in elderly
Group 1 phenothiazines:[Sed]	
• Chlorpromazine 25–100mg/8h	50mg IM
Group 2 phenothiazines:[Ach]	
• Thioridazine 25–100mg/6h	No injection available
Group 3 phenothiazines:[Ex]	
• Trifluoperazine 5–10mg/12h	No injection available
The butyrophones:[Ex]	
• Droperidol 5–20mg/4–8h	5–10mg/4h IM/IV (child: 0.5–1mg/day)
• Haloperidol 0.5–5mg/12–8h (rarely adults need 120mg/day and adolescents 30–60mg/day) *Initial child's dose:* 25–50µg/kg/day.	2–30mg IM, then 5mg/1h, max total: 60mg ►Move to PO route as soon as you can

Sed=sedative; Ach=anticholinergic SEs eg vision$\downarrow$, BP$\downarrow$
Ex=extrapyramidal effects: restless ± parkinsonism which may be helped by orphenadrine 50mg/8h PO

NB: doses are difficult, some patients require more than the licensed dose; if so, liaise with a colleague, and follow this advice from the Royal College of Psychiatrists: •Be cautious in those over 70yrs •Do an ECG; beware a long Q-T interval •Increase doses slowly (less than once weekly), and stop increased dose if no benefit after 3 months •Review often •Consider alternatives, eg clozapine (below).

•Akathisia (restlessness) and parkinsonism (use orphenadrine 50 mg/8h PO or benzhexol 1-4mg/6h PO—only if needed). •Dystonic reactions (eg torticollis, opisthotonus, often occurring in the first weeks of treatment, and responding to biperiden 2.5-5mg IM or IV slowly, up to 4 times daily.

•Tardive dyskinesia (chewing, grimaces, choreoathetosis) may be irreversible; but try tetrabenazine 12.5-50mg/6-24h PO (eg after waiting to see what happens for ~6 months after stopping the drug). Neuroleptic poisoning: *OHCM* p 749.

Other side-effects: BP↓, ejaculation delay, depression, fits, jaundice, corneal opacities, rash, WCC↓, and the rare (but fatal) neuroleptic malignant syndrome (hyperthermia, rigidity, dystonia, consciousness disturbance).

Maintenance treatment with drugs Up to two-thirds will relapse if antipsychotic medication is discontinued within the first 5 years of treatment.[2] As there is no way of predicting who needs prophylaxis, and because a psychotic relapse is likely to be devastating, the best plan is to offer prophylaxis to everyone, in the lowest effective dose, and by depot injections if concordance/compliance is a problem. Low-dose fluphenazine decanoate (5mg IM every 2 weeks) is probably as effective as 25mg/2 weeks IM, and some claim it causes less anxiety and depression.[3] On either dosage, ~40% of patients will show evidence of a mild relapse over the first year. At the first sign of relapse, increase the dose to control symptoms. Continuous treatment with oral chlorpromazine[2] may also be effective. Aim to keep doses <100mg/day.

Treatment failures: The 30% who do not respond to standard neuroleptics may benefit greatly from clozapine. SE: agranulocytosis in 0.5% (fatal in ~10% so special precautions are needed*; fits (in 14% if dose ≥600mg/day PO); myocarditis; sedation—but *not* tardive dyskinesia: its antagonism of striatal D_2 receptors is weak compared with S_2 and S_{1C} antagonism (*OHCM* p 407).[4,5] Risperidone (blocks D_2, $5HT_2$, α_1 and α_2 adrenoceptors) is a novel agent which may improve both positive and negative symptoms. 'Limbic selective antipsychotic agents' are under development—eg sertindole, which is a potent antagonist of $5HT_2$ receptors, D_2 receptors, and adrenergic α_1 receptors, while having little effect on GABA, benzodiazepine, glutamate, muscarinic or histamine (H_1) receptors. It inhibits the number of spontaneously active neurones in the mesolimbic ventral tegmental area, without affecting substantia nigra dopamine neurones (in animals—and in one human controlled trial—it was better than haloperidol in controlling negative symptoms in schizophrenia: they were equal in positive symptoms). Other new agents include olanzapine and quetiapine.

*Try to prevent WCC↓ and agranulocytosis by: • Only starting clozapine in hospital. • Explain that any symptoms of infection must be reported immediately. • Taper off conventional neuroleptic • Monitor WCC and differential every week for first 18 weeks, then every fortnight if OK. • If all is well for 1yr, monitor monthly; and for 4 weeks after stopping. • Avoid co-therapy with WCC-lowering drugs. • If WCC <3 x 10^9/L (or neutrophils <1.5) at any time, stop clozapine permanently • Other SE: drowsiness, anxiety, agitation, constipation, ileus, dysphagia, hypersalivation, priapism, hyperglycaemia, U&E & CK & LFTs↑, myocarditis, pancreatitis.

1 R Ramsay 1995 *BMJ* ii 167 2 I Marks 1994 *Br J Psy* 165 179 3 http://www.cochrane.co.uk (1997)
4 S Hirsch 1986 *BMJ* ii 515 5 S Hirsch 1993 *BMJ* i 1427 6 S Dursun 1993 *BMJ* ii 200

Drug problems and addiction (▶ See OHCM p 184)

Definitions *Tolerance:* A drug's early effects are later achievable only by using higher doses. *Withdrawal syndrome:* The physical effects experienced when a tolerance-inducing drug is withdrawn. *Dependence:* Only continued doses prevent physical or psychological withdrawal (compulsive activity to achieve this is called *drug addiction*). The drugs involved are the opiate derivatives, amphetamines, cocaine (p 550), lysergic acid, hydrocarbons ('glue sniffing'), barbiturates and, to a lesser extent, cannabis. Addiction may be psychological (restlessness and craving when the drug is withdrawn) or physical, such as the 'cold turkey' which occurs in narcotic withdrawal—dilated pupils, D&V, tachycardia, sweating, cramps, and piloerection.

This may be ameliorated by giving methadone, eg 20–70mg/12h PO, reducing by 20% every 2 days, ideally as part of a regimen in which a contract is made with the patient (p 339). Special clinics are available for this, or, with equally good results, treatment may be conducted in primary care, provided the GP has an interest and ongoing commitment.[1] In the UK, 40% of prescriptions for methadone are given by GPs. However most GPs are unwilling to become too closely involved for fear of attracting too many addicts, who might end up abusing them, and their staff, with the added risk of their methadone ending up on the black market.

A non-addictive alternative is lofexidine (a α_2-noradrenergic agonist related to clonidine): dose example: 0.2mg/24h PO, increased by 0.2–0.4mg increments/day (max 2.4mg/day); a 5-day régime may be better than standard 10-day ones.[2] SE: drowsiness, BP and pulse↓, dry mouth, rebound hypertension on withdrawal.

Narcotic abusers must, by UK law, be notified to the Home Office. Barbiturate withdrawal may cause seizures and death, and withdrawal should be as an inpatient, giving one-third of the previous daily dose as phenobarbitone. Lower the dose over 14 days.

When to suspect drug addiction •Convictions for crime, to buy drugs.
- Any odd behaviour, eg with visual hallucinations, elation or mania.
- Unexplained nasal discharge (cocaine sniffing ▶ See p 550).
- The results of injections: marked veins; abscesses; hepatitis; AIDS.
- Repeated requests for pain killers—with only opiates being acceptable.

Counselling parents about how they can counsel their children
- If possible, father and mother should agree a plan together, along with someone who knows the child (eg teacher or GP).
- Accept the child; and try not to seem authoritarian or bossy.
- Find out what the child's attitudes are to drugs. He may think that hard drugs are no more harmful than alcohol and tobacco.
- Bring the subject up with the younger siblings so that they know how to say no to offers of drugs.
- Confidential phone advice is always available (in the UK dial 100 and ask for Freefone Drug Problems).

The dangers of HIV infection (*OHCM* p 212) if drugs are injected has altered the approach to long-term management. It is important to try to maintain a relationship between the health team and the addict, and to educate the patient about avoiding high-risk behaviour. There is controversy over the extent to which addicts should be supplied with clean needles and controlled doses of addictive drugs. See *OHCM* p 184–5.

1 M Gossop 1999 *BJGP* **49** 31 2 J Bearn 1998 *Drug Alcohol Dependence* **50** 227–32

Alcohol-related problems

Repeated drinking harms a person's work or social life. Addiction implies:[1]

Difficulty or failure of abstinence	Often aware of compulsion to drink
Narrowing of drinking repertoire	Priority is to maintain alcohol intake
Increased tolerance to alcohol	Sweats, nausea, or tremor on withdrawal

Questions •Can you control your drinking? •Have you thought you should cut down? •Do friends comment on your drinking, or ask you to cut down? •Has alcohol led you to neglect family or work? •What time do you start drinking? Do you drink before this? •Go through an average day's drinking. •Have you been in trouble with the law (violent crime)?

Alcohol and organ damage •Liver: (normal in 50% of alcoholics). Fatty liver: acute, reversible; hepatitis—80% progress to cirrhosis (hepatic failure in 10%); cirrhosis: 5yr survival 48% if alcohol intake continues (if it stops, 77%). •CNS: poor memory/cognition→ may respond to multiple high-potency vitamins IM; cortical/cerebellar atrophy; retrobulbar neuropathy; fits; falls; accidents; neuropathy; Korsakoff's/Wernicke's encephalopathy (*OHCM* p 712). •Gut: D&V; peptic ulcer; erosions; varices; pancreatitis. •Marrow: Hb↓; haemolysis; MCV↑. •Heart: arrhythmias; cardiomyopathy.

Alcohol and drug metabolism Regular heavy drinking *induces* hepatic enzymes, but binging *inhibits* enzymes. So the answer is not to indulge in both and hope for the best, but to be alert with agents such as phenytoin, warfarin and tolbutamide. Chronic heavy drinkers are especially likely to convert paracetamol into hepatotoxic (*N*-acetyl-*p*-benzoquinoneimine).[2]

Alcohol contraindications Driving (planes, trains, vehicles); hepatitis; cirrhosis; peptic ulcer; drugs (antihistamines); carcinoid; pregnancy—the fetal alcohol syndrome (IQ↓, short palpebral fissure, absent filtrum, small eyes).

Withdrawal signs (Delirium tremens) Pulse↑; BP↓; tremor; fits; visual or tactile hallucinations, eg of animals crawling all over one. *Treatment:* •Admit; monitor vital signs (beware BP↓). •For the first 3 days give diazepam generously—eg 10mg/6h PO or PR if vomiting—or IVI during fits). Chlordiazepoxide is an alternative. Clormethiazole is best avoided as dependence is quickly engendered, and respiratory depression occurs unpredictably. Avoid phenothiazines (liver damage). After the first days, reduce diazepam (eg 10mg/8h PO from day 4–6, then 5mg/12h PO for 2 more days).

Treatment Key determinants of success are the patient's commitment and willingness to comply with treatment—so it is worth taking time to explore issues of concordance between your own ideas and those of your patient.

Treat any co-existing depression (p 336–8). Refer to a specialist service. Group psychotherapy in self-help organizations such as *Alcoholics Anonymous* may help, ± agents which produce an unpleasant reaction if alcohol is taken (eg disulfiram 800mg stat then ↓ to 100–200mg/24h PO over 5 days Reducing the pleasure that alcohol brings (and craving when it is withdrawn) with *naltrexone* 25–50mg/24h PO (an opioid receptor antagonist used in opiate addictions) can halve relapse rates.[3] SE: vomiting, drowsiness, dizziness, cramps, joint and muscle pain. CI: hepatitis; liver failure. *Cost:* ~£3.20/day. Liaise with experts on its best use. *Acamprosate* (*OHCM* p406) can treble abstinence rates. CI: pregnancy, severe liver failure, creatinine >120μmol/L; SE: D&V, libido fluctuation; dose example: 666mg/8h PO if >60kg & <65yrs old.

Non-pharmacological, physician-based brief interventions for problem drinkers: (Education, counselling, goal-setting + monitoring of γGT in those who have social or physical problems from alcohol, but who do not exhibit full dependency.) 4 out 8 randomized studies have shown that γGT falls in the intervention group, but none has shown convincing improvement in alcohol-related morbidity. More costly, specialized interventions fare no better.

Prevention See p 454.

1 RE Meyer 1996 *Lancet* **347** 162 2 *Drug Ther Bul* 1996 **34** 36 3 JP Volpicelli 1995 *Lancet* **346** 456

Personality disorders and psychopathy

Personality comprises lasting characteristics which make us the sort of people we are: easygoing or anxious; placid or histrionic; ambitious or stay-at-home; fearless or timid; self-satisfied or doubting; optimistic or pessimistic. (Personality *can* change and develop, and it may even change quickly, eg after religious conversion in which a timid man is remoulded into a fearless activist.) Personality is a spectrum lying between these opposites. Statistical analysis reveals that all these distinctions may in fact overlap, and are describable in terms of a few orthogonal dimensions (eg neuroticism/psychoticism; introvert/extrovert). Those with abnormal personalities may then be defined as occupying the extremes of the spectrum. Abnormal personality only matters if it is maladaptive, causing suffering either to its possessor or his associates. In general, psychological symptoms which are part of a personality disorder are harder to treat than those arising from other causes.

Psychopathy refers to a persistent personality disorder characterized by antisocial behaviour, inability to make loving relationships, and lack of guilt. Typically, the patient is impulsive, and regards his closest associates without affection. He does not know how to like or love them. Rather than leading to shame and guilt, his irresponsible actions are more likely to lead to prison. Reason is intact (but is used wholly for selfish ends). Note that psychopathy has forensic overtones. If a criminal act is seen as being part of a psychopathy then the Courts have the option of specifying psychiatric treatment (in a secure hospital if necessary) rather than just prison, so raising difficult questions about psychopathy and responsibility.
Causes: Brain damage, social factors, parental psychiatric illness or laxity have been suggested, but none is pre-eminent.
Treatment is problematic as patients are seldom in a frame of mind which is likely to promote change. Peer group pressure (as may occur in group therapy, p 372) may be a motivating force. It is rarely wise to use drugs, but there is evidence that SSRIs (p 341) may be beneficial in aggressive personality disorders.

Other personalities *Obsessional personality:* The rigid, obstinate bigot who is preoccupied with unimportant (or vital) details.
Histrionic personality: The self-centred, sexually provocative (but frigid) person who enjoys (but does not feel) angry scenes.
Schizoid personality: The cold, aloof, introspective misanthrope.

Mental retardation (mental handicap) and learning disabilities

Those with IQs of 50–70 account for 80% of people with learning disabilities. There is useful development of language, and learning difficulty only emerges as schooling gets under way. Most can lead an independent life. If the IQ is 35–49, then most can talk and find their way about. In severe learning disability (IQ 20–34) limited social activity is possible. If less than this, very simple speech may be achieved. Special schooling and medical services are needed, as are adequate care and counselling for the families involved. Further information is available from MENCAP.[1] For the causes of retardation see p 204.

1 123 Golden Lane, London EC1Y 0RT, UK, tel. 0171 454 0454

Managing psychopathy: beyond medicine and the law

Psychiatrists are sometimes unfairly criticized for abandoning psychopaths—as if they were too much trouble. This easy criticism does not take into account civil liberties: the patient must either want treatment, or they must have a *treatable* mental illness before they can be detained against their will (or admission must be likely to prevent deterioration). Preventive detention is problematic as the rule 'innocent until proven guilty of a crime' is central to the requirements of justice.[1]

Renewable sentences: It is against this background that the suggestion has arisen that those with a history of psychopathic violence should receive care outside current penal and health set-ups. Such people, it is argued by the National Association for the Care and Resettlement of Offenders (NACRO), could be detained at the end of their sentences if they are still thought to be a risk to others. For this to take place, courts would need to have new powers, and there is also a need for new specialist services. However, this is no guarantee against injustice occurring: for example, a man without psychopathy who poisoned his wife might be free to marry again after 10–15 years in prison, but a man with psychopathy who had held a hostage without harming them might never be free to try to rebuild his life.

1 J Warden 1998 BMJ ii 1270

Withdrawal of psychotropic drugs

Withdrawing benzodiazepines ►*The withdrawal syndrome may well be worse than the condition for which the drug was originally prescribed.* So try to avoid their use, eg relaxation techniques for anxiety, or, for insomnia, a dull book, sexual intercourse and avoiding night-time coffee may facilitate sleep. If not, limit hypnotics to alternate nights.

One-third of those taking benzodiazepines for 6 months experience withdrawal symptoms if treatment is stopped, and some will do so after only a few weeks of treatment. Symptoms appear sooner with rapidly eliminated benzodiazepines (eg lorazepam compared to diazepam or chlordiazepoxide). It is not possible to predict which patients will become dependent, but having a 'passive dependent' or neurotic personality appear to be partially predictive. Symptoms often start with acute anxiety or psychotic symptoms 1–2 weeks after withdrawal, followed by many months of gradually decreasing symptoms, such as insomnia, hyperactivity, panic attacks, agoraphobia and depression. Irritability, rage, feelings of unreality and depersonalization are common, but hallucinations less so. Multiple sclerosis is sometimes misdiagnosed as these patients may report diplopia, paraesthesiae, fasciculation and ataxia. Gut symptoms include D&V, abdominal pain and dysphagia. There may also be palpitations, flushing and hyperventilation symptoms. The problem is not so much how to stop benzodiazepine treatment, but how to avoid being manipulated into prescribing them unnecessarily. This issue is addressed on p 330.

Method of withdrawal: •Augment the patient's will to give up by elaborating the disadvantages of continuous prescribing. •Withdrawal is harder for short-acting benzodiazepines—so change to diazepam. •Agree a contract with the patient—that you will prescribe a weekly supply, but will not add to this if the patient uses up his supply early. •Withdraw slowly (eg by ~2mg/week of diazepam). Warn the patient to expect withdrawal symptoms, and not to be alarmed.

Withdrawing monoamine oxidase inhibitors (MAOI) Abrupt withdrawal of phenelzine leads to panic, shaking, sweats and nausea in ~¼ of patients. Tranylcypromine has amphetamine-like properties and may be addictive.

Withdrawing tricyclic drugs 4 withdrawal syndromes (all rare):
- Cholinergic activation: abdominal cramps, D&V, dehydration.
- Insomnia, followed by excessively vivid dreaming on falling asleep.
- Extrapyramidal symptoms, eg restlessness and akathisia.
- Psychiatric symptoms: anxiety, psychosis, delirium or mania.

Keep up treatment for ≥6 months post-recovery. Rate of withdrawal: 25mg/5 days (amitriptyline). NB: there are no reports of these withdrawal symptoms from non-tricyclic antidepressants (eg mianserin, trazodone).

Because of withdrawal symptoms it is tempting to stop treatment at the earliest opportunity—but this is a mistake. The severely depressed continue antidepressants for ~6 months after recovery. For amitriptyline, the maintenance dose during this phase of treatment is ~75mg/24h PO. Further slow reductions should be made before stopping the drug.

Phenothiazines Withdrawal symptoms have not been reliably reported.

SSRIs Paroxetine is associated more than other SSRIs with a specific extrapyramidal withdrawal syndrome (eg orofacial dystonias)—and a specific warning has been received from the Committee on Safety of Medicines.

4. Psychiatry

Introduction to the psychotherapies

'As usual, it was dialogue that combed out my muddle . . .'[1]

Medicine has three great branches: *prevention*, *curing by technical means*, and *healing*—and psychotherapy is the embodiment of healing: a holistic approach in which human dialogue and the relationship between doctor and patient is used in a systematic way not only to relieve stress and suffering, but to augment self-esteem and a sense of life's meaning, by producing changes in cognition, feelings, and behaviour.[2] It stands in stark contrast to the most visibly successful but increasingly questioned technical, machine-based sphere of medicine, and we accord it great prominence, in the hope that the explicit descriptions here, and their reverberations throughout our books will produce corresponding reverberations in our minds as we set about our daily work in *any* branch of medicine, to remind us that we are not machines delivering care according to automated formulae, but humans dealing with other humans. So, taken in this way, psychotherapy is the *essence* of psychiatry—and the essence of all psychotherapy is communication. The first step in communication is to open a channel. The vital rôle that listening plays here has already been emphasized (p 320).

It is not possible to teach the skills required for psychotherapy in a book, any more than it is possible to teach the art of painting in oils from a book. So what follows hereafter (p 370–96) is a highly selective tour round the gallery of psychotherapy, in an attempt to show the range of skills needed, and to whet the reader's appetite. It is not envisaged that the reader will try out the more complicated techniques without appropriate supervision.

The psychotherapies may be classified first in terms of *who is involved* in the treatment sessions: an individual, a couple, a family, or a whole group; and secondly they may be classified by their *content and methods* used: analytic, interpersonal, cognitive, behavioural. All psychotherapies are aimed at changing aspects of the patient.

Behavioural therapies (more details: p 370) aim to change behaviour, eg if avoiding crowded shops (agoraphobia) is the issue, a behavioural approach focuses on the avoidance-behaviour. Such approaches will define behavioural tasks which the patient is expected to carry out between sessions.

Cognitive therapy (p 370 & p 388–96) focuses on thoughts and assumptions, promulgating the idea that we respond to cognitive representations of events, not to raw events alone. If this is so, cognitive change may be required to produce emotional and behavioural change. So in the above example of agoraphobia, the therapist would encourage articulation of thoughts associated with entering crowds. The patient might report that she becomes anxious that she might be about to faint—fearing that everyone will think her a fool. These thoughts would be looked at using a Socratic approach: 'Have you in fact ever fainted? How likely would you be to faint? If someone fainted in front of you in a shop, what would you think? *Are* they foolish?'

Longer-term psychoanalytical therapies (p 378) are concerned with the origin and meaning of symptoms. They are based on the view that symptoms arise from earlier experiences and unresolved issues, particularly from childhood. The therapist adopts a non-dominant stance, encouraging the patient to talk without inhibitions. The therapist encourages change by suggesting interpretations for the content of the patient's talk.

Which psychotherapy is most successful? This is tackled on p 386.

1 A Miller 1990 *Timebends*, Octopus, London (page 83) 2 J Holmes 1994 BMJ ii 1070

Definitions of psychotherapy

There are important differences in how people use the term psychotherapy. The first recorded definition states that

> ***Psychotherapy includes every description of therapeutics that cures by means of the intervention of the psychical functions of the sufferer.*** (F van Eeden 1892 *Med Mag* **i** 233).

This definition is worth bearing in mind because, uniquely, it focuses on the content of the intervention made by the patient, not on the specifics of the therapist's intervention. The most general modern definition, and the one employed in this section, is summarized thus:

> ***Psychotherapy denotes treatment of mental disorders and behavioural disturbances using such psychological techniques as support, suggestion, persuasion, re-education, reassurance, and insight in order to alter maladaptive patterns of coping, and to encourage personality growth.*** (Dorland's *Medical Dictionary*)

Some commentators feel that it is important to draw a distinction between counselling and psychotherapy—but using the above definition (or indeed *any* definition that recognizes the great heterogeneity of psychotherapy) no valid distinction can be made, unless it is between the various *types* of psychotherapy. The main issue to bear in mind is that psychotherapy can be categorized as more or less specific, and more or less involved in, and driven by, theory.

So is 'just being nice to patients' in the normal course of one's medical activities an example of psychotherapy at work? The answer is 'no'—not because being nice is therapeutically neutral, but because one's attention is not focused on planning change through the systematic use of interpersonal techniques.

The issue of training is very important, and here are some questions that might usefully be addressed to anyone offering psychotherapy:

1 Is there proof of efficacy? Ask for evidence of long-term results.
2 What qualifications does the therapist hold? Is he or she supervised?
3 Is the recommended regimen tailored to the patient's unique needs?
4 How will progress be monitored?
6 Is confidentiality assured?
5 Is there support and follow-up after the formal programme ends?

Behavioural and cognitive therapies

Behavioural therapy is designed to treat symptoms such as phobias, obsessions, eating and sexual disorders, as well as more general anxiety and mild depression. In those with obsessive-compulsive disorders, rituals (eg hand-washing) respond better than ruminations. The therapy is not suitable *on its own* for those with schizophrenia, dementia or severe depression.

The first step is to analyse the behaviour that the patient wants to change in great detail. If the patient has agoraphobia (say), find out what somatic and psychological symptoms he has, such as palpitations, and fear of fainting ('fear of fear'), and then relate these to exact points in the behaviour—eg on merely planning to go out, or on entering a particular shop. Next ask the patient to make a hierarchy of such situations, starting with the least threatening. Treatment starts with graded exposure to the least threatening situation (systematic desensitization) combined with teaching a method of anxiety reduction. This might be systematic relaxation, in which groups of muscles are stressed and relaxed in an orderly sequence. For example, while sitting in a chair, the toes are pressed firmly into the ground, and then the knees are pressed firmly together, and then the hands on the knees, and then the fingers of one hand into the opposite palm, each finger in turn. Each pressing lasts for about 30sec and is followed by a period of relaxation, and it is this which counteracts the feelings of anxiety as systematic desensitization through the hierarchy gets under way.

Concordance/compliance (p 390) needs fostering by providing written information about reasons for practising the new behaviours, and by explaining that major benefits of treatment only come after hard work. It is wise to enlist the help of the spouse to give encouragement at each achievement.

Rituals such as hand-washing which is provoked by a particular stimulus (eg going to the toilet) are treated by repeated exposure to the stimulus while encouraging avoiding the ritual. The therapist illustrates what the patient has to do ('modelling'). Patients may be taught to interrupt obsessional thoughts, eg by doing a particular activity each time they start.

Cognitive therapy We respond to cognitive representations of events, not raw data.[1] The fundamental idea is that mood and thoughts can form a vicious cycle. Using the example of depression: low mood leads to gloomy thoughts and memories (eg dwelling on exams you did badly at, rather than those in which you performed well). These gloomy thoughts make you feel more depressed (mood) and this lowering of mood makes your thoughts even more gloomy. Cognitive therapy tackles this vicious circle by tackling the thoughts. Take for example the thought: 'I'm a failure, and all my friends are avoiding me'. In cognitive therapy the process is to: •Clarify exactly what the thought is (do not let it be just a vague negative belief) •Look for evidence for and against the proposition in the thought •Look for other perspectives •Come to a conclusion.

The therapist encourages the patient to find other explanations by challenging him, eg by examining what 'I'm a failure' really means. 'What are the important areas in your life?' 'What do you count as success or failure?' The patient may cite lack of promotion as evidence of failure—countered by the therapist pointing out that failing to achieve some goal is different from being a global failure. There are many kinds of biased thinking which cognitive therapy helps patients to recognize: eg 'black and white thinking', overgeneralizing (as in the case of treating one failure as a symbol of everything).
Uses of cognitive therapy are many, eg in: •Depression •Neurosis •Chronic fatigue syndrome •Psychosis (eg in challenging or counteracting delusions).

1 M Reinecke 1996 *Cognitive Therapy with Children and Adolescents*, Guilford Press, ISBN 1-57230-022-1

4. Psychiatry

Group psychotherapy

The rationale underlying group psychotherapy is that the group provides an interactive microcosm in which the patient can be confronted by the effect his behaviour has on others, and be protected during his first attempts to change. This implies that group psychotherapy (as with all forms of psychotherapy) is only practical for those who want to change. It has also been found that the most suitable patients are: 1 Those who enter into the group voluntarily, and not as a result of pressure from relatives or therapists; 2 Those who have a high expectation from the group, and do not view it as inferior to individual therapy; 3 Those who have adequate verbal and conceptual skills. Patients who are unlikely to benefit include those with severe depression, acute schizophrenia, or extreme schizoid personality (the aloof, cold, hypersensitive introvert); hypochondriacs; narcissistic (very self-centred) or paranoid (suspicious and pessimistic about the rôle of others) patients; and sociopathic types (they have low thresholds for frustration and little sense of responsibility)—but sociopathy is notoriously difficult to treat by *any* means, and group therapy may be the least bad option, as other members of the group may provide the only valid mirror that can be held up to these people, and other people *may* provide the impetus for change.

Clearly the selection procedure needs to be carried out by an experienced psychotherapist. He will aim for a group of, say, 6–8 members balanced for sex, and avoiding mixing the extremes of age. He will decide if the group is to be 'closed', or whether it will accept new patients during its life. He will usually take on a co-therapist of the opposite sex, and he will prepare the patients in detail before the group starts. The life of the group (eg 18 months) will develop through a number of phases ('*forming*'→'*norming*'→'*storming*'). First there is a settling-in period when members seem to be on their best behaviour, seeking to be loved by the therapist, and looking to him for directive counselling (which he rarely provides). Next is the stage of conflict, as the patient strives to find his place in the group other than through dependency on the leader. Frustration, anger and other negative feelings are helpful in allowing the patient to test the group's trustworthiness. It is worth learning that expressing negative feelings need not lead to rejection—and this is a vital prelude to the next stage of intimacy, in which the group starts working together.

Various models of group therapy are used, and typically the therapist will need to steer the group away from outside crises and searches for antecedent causes towards the here and now—eg by asking 'Who do you feel closest to in the group?' or 'Who in the group is most like you?' 'Who would you say is as passive (or aggressive) as you are?' But the therapist must avoid sacrificing spontaneity. He learns to use what the group gives him, eg 'You seem very angry that John stormed out just now'. He avoids asking unanswerable questions, especially those beginning with 'Why?'. His task is to encourage interaction between members and to facilitate learning and observation by members. Special methods used to augment this process include written summaries of group activities, video and psychodrama.

4. Psychiatry

Crisis intervention

Occupying the interval between the spilling of our lives and their congealing into history, crisis intervention recognizes that moments of maximum change are times of greatest therapeutic opportunity.[1] The heroic policeman who intervenes between the blade and the self's autotarget is, by this action, in the prime position, if he only knew it, to cut through to the heart of the matter, by entering into *dialogue* (and this takes courage too, for there are no rules of engagement, and your only tools are those your patient gives you). During the rescue you may concentrate on these questions:

- What events have led to the person's difficulties? Concentrate on his thoughts and actions in the last few days.
- What is his mental state at the moment (p 324)? It is vital to know about depression, suicidal ideas and psychosis.
- When his mental state allows, get to grips with methods he has used in the past to combat stress and resolve crises.
- Who are the significant people in the persons's life?
- What help can the person rely on from family and friends?
- What solutions has the person (or his or her family, school, or employer) tried in the present crisis? How have they failed?

Subsequent therapeutic strategies

- If the person has been very severely affected by the crisis, it will be appropriate to offer, and sometimes insist upon, his abandoning of his normal obligations and responsibilities. Temporarily relieving the patient of his responsibilities is necessary to allow concentrated contact ('intensive care') with a therapeutic environment—eg a hospital or crisis unit.
- Ensure by taking practical steps that the patient's commitments are adequately looked after (eg arrange transport of children to foster parents).
- Decide on the best way of lowering arousal (time spent talking is often preferable to administering anxiolytics, which may only serve to delay the natural process of adaptation). If the patient is shocked, stunned or mute, take time to establish the normal channels of communication.
- As soon as the person is receptive, promote a sense of hope about the outcome of the crisis. If there is no hope (a mother, consumed by grief, after losing all her children in a fire), then this too must be addressed.
- The next step is to encourage creative thinking about ways whereby the patient might solve the problems. Start by helping him think through the consequences of all options open to him. Then help compartmentalize his proposed solutions into small, easily executed items of behaviour.

As the immediate crisis passes, and the patient has reasonable psychological functioning, it will be necessary to put him back in charge of his own life. A period of counselling is likely to be appropriate. This is described on p 376. Making a contract about therapy is important in encouraging the patient to transfer from the 'sick rôle' to a self-dependent, adult rôle.

Crisis intervention often focuses on loss of face, loss of identity, or loss of faith—in oneself, in one's religion, one's goals or one's roots. 'Perhaps there is an advantage in being born. . . without roots, for one accepts more easily what comes. The rootless have experienced. . . the temptation of sharing the security of a religious creed or a political faith, and for some reason we have turned the temptation down. We [the counsellors] are the faithless; we admire the dedicated, the Doctor Magiots and the Mr Smiths for their courage and their integrity, for their fidelity to a cause, but through timidity, or through lack of sufficient zest, we find ourselves the only ones truly committed—committed to the whole world of evil and of good, to the wise and to the foolish, to the indifferent and to the mistaken. We have chosen nothing except to go on living, 'rolled round on Earth's diurnal course, With rocks and stones and trees'.'[2]

1 Sylvia Plath 1963 *A Birthday Present* in *Ariel*, Penguin, page 50
2 Graham Greene *The Comedians* Penguin, 279 & William Wordsworth *Lucy* (see OHCM p 568)

4. Psychiatry

Supportive psychotherapy

There are many people who need continuous psychotherapy, as they find daily activities pose unending stress. The smallest decisions are insurmountable problems, and the patient, lacking even a glimmer of insight, seeks support at every turn. What can we offer here?

- Reassurance—eg that his problems are not unique; he is not mad.
- Clarifying problems; instituting practical help (eg practising for a job interview); explanation (eg about claiming benefits).
- Teaching how to recognize that stress is building up, and how to take the first small steps to reduce anxiety (p 344).
- Positive feedback when he moves away from passive dependency.
- Encouragement in taking even the smallest step towards clearly defined goals—which should be set within his limitations.
- Help to change the patient's social world (job changes, protection from a hostile family, reducing social isolation).
- Counselling for relatives and friends. (Get permission first!)

Counselling

Good novelists (and counsellors) are somehow large enough to embody the world—so their characters (clients) are not just recreated in their own image. *Nothing* human is alien to them. Such exercise of the imagination is what enables virgins to counsel prostitutes—which they *can*, if they are submerged in and are fully aware of human affairs outside themselves.

In its basic (non-directive) form this involves focusing on helping the person clarify what it is they want to do, and what would be needed to achieve it. It does not entail advice, which would run counter to the process of empowering the patient. Fundamental counselling skills consist in listening, understanding and reflecting—see p378 (± summarizing, the use of silences, interpretation—p 378—and confrontation). Other points:

- History-taking: note how previous stress has been coped with.
- Production of an agreed full inventory of problems.
- Redefining problems in terms of attainable goals.
- Use of therapeutic contracts to negotiate small behaviour changes.
- Aim for adult relationships between patient, family, and therapist, so that duties are agreed, eg about frequency and duration of therapy, and what will be expected of the patient by way of 'homework', eg learning anxiety-reducing techniques, and carrying out 'rewards' such as cooking an extra-nice meal with the family if the patient achieves an anxiety-provoking task such as shopping.
- Allowing the expression of negative feelings such as anger—not acted out in reality, but talked about in a cathartic way.
- Reassurance. This is not so simple as it sounds. The therapist must not only give overt reassurance, but also by his demeanour he must reassure the patient that *whatever* he reveals (eg incest or baby battering), he will not be condemned, but accepted. Note: this is one advantage of computer-based psychiatric history taking—the computer is not shocked when the patient tells of drinking two bottles of gin a day: it simply goes on to ask: 'What about whisky?'

Questioning non-directive counselling: Is being non-directive a way of evading responsibility? Is it dishonest to hide our attitudes? What do we lose by being dispassionate? Compassion, perhaps? Note that not all counselling is analytic/expressive and non-directive. 'Problem-solving' models of counselling (see opposite) are sometimes directive—and may be most appropriate when the therapist already knows the client well.

Counselling in primary care

~30% of UK general practices employ a counsellor. This huge growth reflects the fact that people love to be listened to, and that GPs themselves may not have the time or inclination to satisfy this need in all cases. It is hard to prove the effectiveness of counselling, especially as skills and training vary markedly. But this does not mean it is ineffective.

However, one careful randomized study[1] (*N*=136) found that brief psychotherapy-type non-directive counselling offered no additional objective benefit to routine GP care for people with emotional distress—but, importantly, satisfaction was higher. It is pointed out that maybe too few counselling sessions were offered, or that the GPs were already effective counsellors, or that more focused counselling would have been more effective.[2] There are 3 facets to counselling in general practice:

1. In some patients, problem-solving strategies are used, with the counsellor using a non directive approach.
2. In coping strategies, the therapist helps the patient to make the most of the position they are in (eg afflicted by a chronic disease).
3. In cognitive therapy, we concentrate on elucidating negative thinking processes, and helps the patient learn how to intervene in negative cycles of thinking.

1 K Friedli 1997 *Lancet* **350** 1662 2 A Tylee 1997 *Lancet* **350** 1643

Psychodynamic psychotherapy

Psychotherapy can be classified into three main types.[1] 'Type A': where therapy is part of a general package of mental health interventions, eg someone with depression might be prescribed antidepressants, be attending a Day Hospital, and receive individual psychotherapy. 'Type B': an eclectic form of therapy tailored to the needs of the patient, often delivered by psychologists, eg a depressed patient offered some counselling sessions with a cognitive slant, followed by marital therapy. 'Type C': formal model-based therapy. The types of analytic therapy described below would be good examples.

Not all patients benefit from brief, symptom-focused cognitive-behavioural treatments. Psychodynamic psychotherapy is suitable for patients who have deeply ingrained maladaptive patterns of emotion and behaviour—ie personality disorders. Here past experience, especially of intimate relationships with parents, influence the present in ways of which the patient may be unaware. This basic idea derives from Freud and his famous followers such as Bowlby, Klein, and Winnicott.[2]

Key concepts of psychodynamic psychotherapy include:

1) *Psychological defences:* Just as the immune system protects our physical integrity, so psychological vulnerability is shielded by psychological defences. As with the immune system, overactive defences can lead to trouble. Primitive defences like repression (turning a blind eye to unpleasant experience) or splitting (dividing the world into black and white) can be maladaptive. We need to be able to think about and process experience if we are to learn from it. Thus a person who has been sexually abused as a child may as an adult enter abusive relationships without realizing the connection.

2) *Transference and counter-transference:* The past patterns (transfers) our present reactions to people. If we have trusted our parents, we will be likely to trust our doctors, teachers, and friends. The intense psychotherapeutic relationship brings these assumptions to the fore where they can be examined, understood, and learned from. The doctor in turn has unconscious reactions to her patients based on the past, ie counter-transference. For example, if her mother was an alcoholic she may be oversolicitous, or rejecting, with alcoholic patients. The doctor's reactions are also a key to the patient's feelings: if a patient makes us feel rejected (as alcoholics often do), perhaps that person himself was rejected as a child and has turned to the bottle in compensation.

How does psychodynamic psychotherapy work? The therapist provides a secure *frame*—a regular time and place and her own consistency and acceptingness. The patient *narrates* stories about himself and his life—usually about three per session. The therapist *listens* carefully, both to the stories and to her reactions to them. She then makes *linking hypotheses*, or *interpretations* which offer *meaning* to to the patient. Previously inexplicable behaviour begins to make sense. At the same time the patient forms a close relationship with the therapist based on *empathy*, *genuineness*, and *non-possessive warmth* (shown experimentally to be key therapeutic factors)—and, where necessary *challenge*. These may be novel experiences for the patient which can be *internalized*. The patient can *work through* his difficulties in the comparative safety of the therapeutic relationship, especially his reactions to *ending*, which will bring up previously unprocessed losses.

Psychodynamic psychotherapy can be (a) time-limited (brief dynamic psychotherapy) which is suitable for patients with circumscribed problems, eg unmourned grief, or (b) open ended, which in the UK NHS is usually about two years, but in private practice may be longer, and is suitable for patients with severe personality disorders.

Acknowledgement: We thank Dr Jeremy Holmes for supplying this page. 1 NHSE 1996 *Psychotherapy Services in England*, London, HMSO 2 A Bateman & J Holmes, *Introduction to Psychoanalysis*, Routledge

Does this type of psychotherapy have any real value?

This is a frequently asked question: to approach an answer let us focus first on psychodynamic psychotherapy, and then on what counts as value.

'The liberating and therapeutic value of analysis would seem to arise not simply from revelation and instruction on the part of the analyst, but from the creation by the patient of a new view of his personality and his own free assent to this view'.[1]

In an NHS-world where value equates with such things as 'number of new hips inserted per day' it is handy to reflect on what Wittgenstein said about sense and value in his *Tractatus:*

'The sense of the world must lie outside the world. In the world everything is as it is and happens as it does happen. In it there is no value. If there is a value which is of value, it must lie outside all happening and being-so. For all happening and being-so is accidental'.

So new hips have no value on their own. Value lies outside the world of things—and one route out of this world is psychodynamic psychotherapy. All 'getting better' involves a journey which can be modelled and mapped. There are many diferent types of map but none depicts such broad horizons as the psychotherapies here described.

1 Iris Murdoch 1950 (see *Existentialists and Mystics,* Chatto, 1997, p105)

Sex therapy for couples

This is one example of therapy with couples: often the problem is not specifically sexual, and sexual difficulties are likely to recede once other aspects of the relationship improve. This page is relevant when specific sexual dysfuntions remain.

Start with a full (joint) description of the problem. This may be premature (or delayed) ejaculation, female frigidity (anorgasmia), impotence or dyspareunia (eg from spasm—vaginismus—or other physical causes). How did the problem start (eg after childbirth)? Was there ever a time when sex occurred as desired? Is the problem part of some wider problem? What does your partner expect from you? Are you self-conscious or anxious during sex?

Sexual history Early experiences; present practices; orientation to either or both sexes. Has there been difficulty with other partners? When did you meet? What attracted you to each other?

Drugs Alcohol, hypotensives (impotence); tricyclics (delayed ejaculation); β-blockers, finasteride, contraceptive steroids and phenothiazines (loss of libido). Note: other causes of impotence include diabetes mellitus, cord pathology, hyperprolactinaemia.

Principles of behavioural therapy for sexual difficulties comprise:

1 Defining the task which the couple wishes to accomplish.
2 Reducing the task to a number of small, attainable steps.
3 Asking the couple to practise each small step in turn.
4 At the next session, discussing difficulties encountered.
5 Ameliorating maladaptive attitudes.
6 Setting the next task.

How do these principles work, eg when the problem is premature ejaculation and vaginismus? (Both are related to performance anxiety.) One sequence (to agree with the couple) might be:

1 A ban on attempted sexual intercourse (to remove fear of performance failure). Education and 'permission' giving (ie to talk about and engage in 'safe' sexual fantasies) is vital.
2 Touching without genital contact, 'for your own pleasure', initially, with any non-genital part of the body, to explore the range of what is pleasurable, and then to concentrate on whatever erogenous zones are discovered ('sensate focus').
3 Touching as above 'for your own and your partner's pleasure'.
4 'Homework' using a vaginal dilator and lubricating jelly.
5 Touching with genital contact, first in turn, later together. Problems in taking the initiative may surface at this stage. If premature ejaculation is the problem, the partner stimulates the penis, and as orgasm approaches the man signals to his partner—who inhibits the reflex by squeezing his penis at the level of the frenulum.
6 Concentrate on playing down the distinction between foreplay and intercourse, so that anxiety at penetration is reduced.
7 Vaginal containment in the female superior position so that she can stop or withdraw whenever she wants. She concentrates on the sensation of the vagina being filled.
8 Periods of pelvic thrusting, eg with a 'stop/start' technique.

Sexual universals

There is a great deal more to helping people with sexual difficulties than is outlined opposite—which is just one approach to one common problem. A good place to start in furthering understanding of these issues is the BMJ's *ABC of Sexual Health*.[1]

In any therapy the following universals need to be addressed:

- Never assume that your patient is too old or too ill for sexual issues to be relevant. Assume that everyone has a sex life, albeit sometimes in fantasy only.
- Psychological approaches are always important, whatever physical props are offered.
- Psychological events have physical sequelae, and physical events have psychological sequelae.
- All pleasure, including all erotic pleasure, is either purely sensory or arises from associations of ideas: this offers many points of intersection for negative operators, such as distraction, spectatoring, guilt, anxiety, fear of failure, pain, and inappropriate stimulation.

1 M Ramage 1998 *BMJ* **ii** 1509

Family therapy[1]

This is typically a problem-orientated, goal-directed psychotherapy which stresses the importance of social interactions, so treatment aims to includes family members. Therapy is based on the assumption that people have the resources and potential for growth and the resolution of life's difficulties. When someone's attempted solutions to these difficulties are consistently failing, the therapist's task is to step in and unblock the person's repeated application of these failed solutions, by prescribing new behaviours based on shared insights occurring during the process of family interaction.

The *mechanisms* of family interaction need careful study, and with four or more people in the room it is hard for the therapist to keep track of all verbal and non-verbal behaviours, so he has a team, which has various roles:

1) Observation and direction of the interaction via a one-way mirror, and an earphone for communicating instructions to the therapist: *verbal* (eg *ask the husband* 'What do you do when your wife cries?') or *non-verbal* (eg *Now turn to look at his wife*). The interaction is videotaped (with consent), and before the end of the session the therapist retires behind the screen to formulate insights gained, share the team's hypothesis for the mechanism of the psychopathology, and to check this by reviewing salient points on the videotape. A 'prescription' is formulated and the therapist relays this to the family. This prescription is usually a simple item of behaviour, and it may be negotiated between the members of the family. It is based on the answers family members give to the following sorts of questions, which allow problems to be defined in concrete terms and define the sequences and circularities of family behaviour:
   - What does he do (or say) that makes you say he is depressed?
   - When he said that, what did you reply?
   - What do you do when he behaves like that? Does it help?
   - What does your mother do when your father shouts at you?
   - Does this happen more indoors, or away from home?
   - How long does it last? How do you try to get over it?
   - How is this a problem to you? (Depressed? So what!)
   - What have other people suggested? What does your mother say?
   - Who is the first to see the depression? Your mother or father?
   - How do you see the relationship between your sister and mother? How does your mother see it? And your sister?
   - If I asked her if she's feeling better, what would she say?
   - Of the four of you, who can cheer her up the most?
   - What do you want therapy to do? When do you want to change?
   - What is the smallest step towards this goal?
   - Who wants this change most—you, your husband or your son?
2) The therapist and team co-worker may join the family and interview them with the co-worker, discussing points for clarification with the therapist *in front of the family*. The co-worker wears an earphone for communications from the other members of the team. The session is interrupted after half-an-hour, and the other members of the team join the therapist and co-worker for a discussion of what they have observed (*Reflecting*). The family then makes observations on the observations of the team, and finally an agreement between the family and the team is reached about any work the family may do before the next session.[2]
3) The whole team join the family (usually at the family's request) and the session can work in either of the above forms eg appropriate modifications.
4) Co-therapists join the family, either in clinic or at home, working on communication skills based interventions, eg in those with schizophrenia.[3]

Change usually occurs fairly quickly, eg needing 6–12 sessions, or as few as one.

1 Based on HG Procter's Southwood House approach (Bridgwater, Somerset, UK); M Palazzoli 1980 *Family Proc* **19** 3-12 and M Palazzoli 1978 *Paradox and Counter-paradox*, Jason Aronson 2 M White 1995 in *Re-authoring Lives*, Dulwich Centre 3 Mari Streiner 1996 *E-BM* **1** 121

Play therapy[1,2]

The people who have most experience in psychotherapy with children are parents. They hold the key cards for influencing a child's behaviour. These comprise love, mutually understood channels of communication, systems of valid rewards, and a shared knowledge of right and wrong. It is the families without these which are most likely to need the help of professionals. The following guidelines are offered[1] to help these children:

- Take time early on to make friends with the child. Don't rush.
- Accept the child on his own terms—exactly as he is.
- Avoid questioning, praising or blaming. Be totally permissive.
- Don't say 'Don't', and only restrain if about to harm himself.
- Show the child that he is free to express any feeling openly.
- The responsibility to make choices is the child's alone.
- Follow where the child leads: avoid directing the conversation.
- Use whatever he gives you. Reflect his feelings back to him.
- Encourage the child to move from acting-out his feelings in the real world, to expressing them in words and play.
- Prepare the parents for change in the child.

In play therapy the child and the therapist play together with toys which give the child an opportunity to verbalize his innermost fantasies. As Virginia Axline explained to one of her 5-year-olds,[2] play therapy is 'a time when you can be the way you want to be. A time you can use any way you want to use it. A time when you can be you.'

Verbatim example of play therapy in action with 6-year-old Dibs[2]
He walked around the playroom. Then he picked up a doll. 'Well, here is sister. I'll get her to eat some nice rice pudding, only I'll poison her, and she'll go away. . . forever and ever.' 'You want to get rid of the sister?' the therapist remarks. 'Sometimes she screams and scratches, and hurts me and I'm afraid of her. . . She's five now . . . She'll go to the same school as I go to next year.' 'And how do you feel about that?' 'Well, I don't care. . . she doesn't bother me like she used to.' He went over to the easel and picked up a jar of paint, adding further colours and stirring it well. 'This is poison for the sister. She'll think it is cereal and she'll eat it and then that will be the end of her.' 'So that is poison for the sister and after she eats it, then that will be the end of her?' Dibs nodded 'I won't give it to her yet a while, I'll wait and think it over.'

Before play therapy Dibs had been sullen, mute and unco-operative for years on end. No one had ever been able to engage him in normal family or school activities—an impossible child—until play therapy, by allowing him to express negative feelings, unlocked those reserves of resilience, creativity and zest for life which lie dormant in the heart of every child.

NB: play therapy is not the sum total of child psychotherapy: the above is given simply to illustrate the various issues involved. Also, play is a prominent part of therapies which are not play therapy. For example, play can prepare children for procedures such as micturating cystograms and MRI examinations.[3] Play is also used for promoting self-care in diabetes.[4]

1 V Axline 1969 *Play Therapy*, Ballantine
2 V Axline 1966 *Dibs: in Search of Self: Personality Development in Play Therapy*, Gollancz
3 D Pressdee 1997 *Clin Radiol* **52** 945–47
4 M Bannister 1996 *Prof Nurse* **12** 109–12

Art or art therapy?

Art can do more than soothe and placate the tortured, the tired, or the timid. It goes further even than healing (p 465), by approaching humanity by way of self-knowledge—a route which may entail wounding in equal measure to repair. Researchers have shown, seemingly idiotically, that reading poetry relieves stress. This is rather like finding out that if plants are put out in the rain they get wet—whereas the real conclusion is that rain makes them *grow*. It is this propensity to generate growth and development which is the essence of art, and, as we have observed elsewhere, growth and development are the essence of childhood. This implies that there is some relation between art and our pre-verbal, pre-logical life. We all once knew how to paint and draw: a well of knowledge that has, for most of us, been pierced by the reductionist logic of our mature years, so that this ability, like life itself, has leaked away, without our really knowing how or why or where. So we look into the well and it's empty.[1] The answer is to dig deeper, not to try to move the well to a better site—for as the ancient proverb states: *you can move a city, but you cannot move a well.*

Are these fascinating or futile observations of any use to our patients? To answer this question we might do best to look to two extremes: those individuals with a logico-verbal deficit (eg those with some forms of schizophrenia), and those with logico-verbal excess (eg overworked students). In the first category, art therapy has a much talked of relevance. Vittorino Andreoli has pointed out that artistic expression is a form of non-verbal communication that, once decoded, is most relevant to therapy and communication with the therapist. 'In pathologies where there is pronounced logic-verbal deficit, such as schizophrenia, this form of non-verbal communication becomes essential.'[2]

As for the rôle of art in those with logico-verbal excess, suffice it to recall the words of the greatest logico-verbal exponent of all time, Marcel Proust, who tells us, in *La Prisonnière* that '. . . Music, very different in this respect from Albertine's society, helped me to descend into myself, to make there a fresh discovery. . . As the spectrum makes visible to us the composition of light, so the harmony of a Wagner, the colour of an Elstir* enable us to know that essential quality of another person's sensations into which love for another person does not allow us to penetrate. . .'[3] But we have to move on in our researches from *La Prisonnière* to *Temps Retrouvé* to find the purpose of life and perhaps of art itself, which is to reveal the mystery of objects, people, and ideas through the exploration of unconscious memory: '. . . Certain people, whose minds are prone to mystery, like to believe that objects retain something of the eyes which have looked at them, that old buildings and pictures appear to us not as they originally were but beneath a perceptible veil woven for them over the centuries by the love and contemplation of millions of admirers. This fantasy, if you transpose it into the domain of what is for each of us the sole reality, the domain of his own sensibility, becomes the truth.'[4]

1 WH Auden (1937)—*As I walked out one morning:*

In headaches and in worry	*It was late, late in the evening*
Vaguely life leaks away,	*The lovers they were gone;*
And Time will have his fancy	*The clocks had ceased their chiming,*
To-morrow or to-day . . .	*And the deep river ran on.*

From *Tell me the Truth About Love* Faber & Faber ISBN 0-571-17444-2 2 P Pina 1996 *Lancet* **348** 603 3 Marcel Proust 1923 *The Captive* (p210) vol 7 of *Remembrance of Things Past–A la Recherche du Temps Perdu* tr. CK Scott Moncrieff (1931; vol 9, Chatto) 4 *Time Regained* (1927; vol 8 in French, vol 12 in the illustrated English translation (p248) by Andreas Mayor; vol 3 in the third translation) *Elstir is an imaginary impressionist painter.

Comparing the psychotherapies

▸Is it true that 'Everyone has won and all must have prizes'?[1]

One reason why it is hard to demonstrate that one form of psychotherapy is better than another is the high proportion of patients (~80%) who benefit from almost any intervention. A small (but perhaps useful) difference between 2 treatments is likely to be swamped by the large proportion of patients who will benefit from either technique.

The methodological problems of comparing different studies of varying validity have now been addressed in a systematic way (using techniques which themselves are not beyond criticism) and yield the following 'conclusions' from research which has met most of the ideal design criteria[1]: randomness; independent assessment; therapy being given by comparable, experienced therapists working for equal amounts of time on their respective patients; well-matched groups; and adequate sample size.

	Which is better?[1]		
	First item	Second item	Tie
Psychotherapy *vs* minimal or no treatment	9	0	5
Psychotherapy *vs* group psychotherapy	2	2	9
Time limited *vs* time unlimited psychotherapy	2	1	5
Non-directive *vs* other psychotherapies	0	1	4
Behaviour therapy *vs* analytic psychotherapy	6	0	13
Drugs *vs* psychotherapy	7	0	1
Drugs *vs* psychotherapy and drugs	0	6	5
Medical régime alone (eg for asthma) *vs* psychotherapy plus medical régime	1	9	1

The chief finding is the large number of ties, except when psychotherapy is compared with minimal treatment (it is better) and when it is combined with drugs, which confer a more-or-less consistent increased benefit.

The diagnoses in the above studies were mixed (ie depressed, neurotic or schizophrenic, with rather over-inclusive USA criteria), and so the question arises as to whether patients with different diagnoses respond differently to psychotherapy. The few consistent findings are that behaviour therapy is especially suited for treating circumscribed phobias, obsessive compulsive, sexual, and habit disorders, and that cognitive therapy is good for depression and may be more effective than antidepressants in preventing relapse.[2] It may also be more helpful than behaviour therapy in bulimia.[3] Family intervention is known to be particularly helpful in preventing relapse in emotional families with a schizophrenic member.

It is very hard to quantify improvement with psychodynamic therapy (psychoanalysis and its descendants)—but there *are* convincing trials of its use in helping with chronic disease, eg irritable bowel syndrome[4]—but in other cases, therapy may last for years, and often it is not clear what the exact goal of therapy is, or who should have it. So purchasers of health care (p 435) are reluctant to fund this type of care[5]—but this should not blind purchasers to the very real and large benefits randomized trials have 'proved' in the well-focused, usually brief psychotherapies above.[6]

It is said that the most suitable patients for psychotherapy are the YAVIS people (young, attractive, verbal, intelligent and successful). Research bears this out to some extent. Low socio-economic status, reclusiveness, and having a repressive morality are all known to be negatively correlated with improvement from traditional psychotherapies.

1 The dodo's verdict for the race in *The Adventures of Alice in Wonderland*: see L Luborsky 1975 *Arch Gen Psych* **32** 995 2 T Fahy 1993 BMJ **ii** 576 3 C Fairburn 1993 *Arch Gen Psy* **50** 419 4 E Guthrie 1993 *Br J Psych* **163** 315 5 G Andrews 1993 *Br J Psychiatry* **162** 447–51 6 J Holmes 1994 BMJ **ii** 1070

4. Psychiatry

Excerpts from the diary of a psychotherapist 1: treatment goals*

Formulation My patient, Mr X Smith, is a previously well 68-year-old farmer with one son. His wife died a year ago after a long illness in which her left leg was amputated. He is very sad, feeling low and depressed whatever the external environment is like. He feels guilty about the care he was able to offer his wife in her last illness. He feels a burden to his son, and has restricted all his contacts with the outside world because he feels that people dislike him. He is somewhat suicidal, and this is why he was referred to me by his general practitioner (who had started him on an appropriate dose of amitriptyline). He fulfils the DSM-IV criteria for major depression (p 336).

'Thank you for telling me in so much detail about your thoughts and feelings, Mr Smith. In this, the first of our 12 sessions, I would like to start by encouraging you to talk about your wife, although this may be painful at times.' My first goal is to help the patient overcome the guilt surrounding his wife's death. I wouldn't be surprised if he *wanted* her to die, if the illness was long and painful; it may take a few sessions before he feels ready to tell me about this. 'What did you feel like when you took your wife to the ward for the last time, knowing that she wouldn't be coming home again? . . . Was there anything else you could have done for her, in the circumstances?'

My second goal is to help Mr Smith reinstate himself in his social world, and I can start this process right now by getting him to go over his previous contacts with friends and family before his wife's illness, and ways he could go about reawakening these contacts. Mr Smith said he could not get in touch with his previous best friend—it had been so long since they had been together, because of his wife's illness, and it would seem rude now to have neglected him so long. 'Did he know that your wife was ill?' 'Yes.' 'Well, I wonder if he might understand if you explained to him. Might it be worth a try?'

My third goal is to reassure him and to instil a sense of hope. 'One of the reasons why it's hard to get going after such a deep loss as yours is because its hard to face up to the loss and allow yourself to feel all the painful feelings that go with such a loss. Here today you have started to let yourself feel these things. This is good. It will get easier as time goes by, and I'm sure that together we will be able to get over this depression. Yes, it is depression you are in the throes of now—but it doesn't go on for ever. You *will* get better.'

*This example is adapted from G Klerman *et al* 1984 *Interpersonal Psychotherapy of Depression*, Basic Books, New York. Our psychotherapist belongs to the school of interpersonal psychotherapy (IPP)—chosen because it offers an internally consistent approach, and its methods have been vindicated in fairly well-controlled 'outcome' research in which IPP has been assessed alone and in conjunction with amitriptyline, and minimal, 'placebo', psychotherapy.

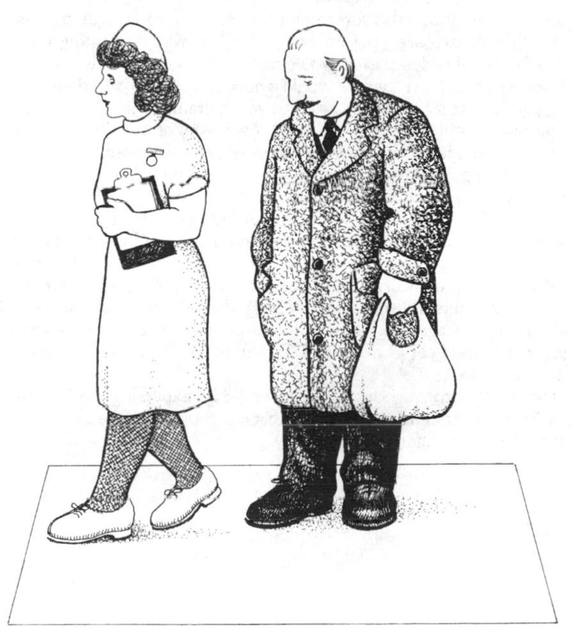

Excerpts from the diary of a psychotherapist 2: other people

Mr Smith seemed reluctant to talk about his wife, so we spent the first half of the session talking about his son and how he was coping with the loss of his mother, and finding out whether he had been able to talk to his son about his loss. We surveyed previous important relationships that he had had in years gone by, with both family and friends. In the second half of the interview I addressed his reluctance to talk about his wife, and he admitted that he found it very painful to do so. He admitted that somewhere deep down he was pleased that it wasn't him that had died, and that such feelings made him feel bad and guilty. He then began to bring forward disturbing material about his wife's last months—how she became demented, did not recognize him, and became abusive.

I let him talk about this for some time, but not so long as to miss the opportunity to explore how he was getting on with recreating his social life. He felt that his depression would make him an unattractive companion in his local pub and that people would ignore him. I confronted him on this, saying gently that if he had not tried to go to the pub, how could he know that people would treat him like that? We talked about the possibility of doing some voluntary work for his favourite charity at weekends.

He said he had developed a troublesome limp in his left leg, and that his doctor had been doing x-rays to find out the cause.

I checked for concorance (compliance) between Mr Smith and his GP's views on what dose of amitriptyline he should take, by looking at the number of tablets in his bottle (which I had asked him to bring with him), and we talked about the desirability of taking his medicines in full dosage if side-effects allowed (his dry mouth and slightly blurred vision had not been too troublesome, we agreed). He was not surprised that the tablets were not having much effect yet as his GP had warned him that they take a few weeks to start to work.

I stressed that throughout therapy I would be expecting frank discussion about his thoughts and feelings, and that he should feel free to bring forward topics which affected him greatly.

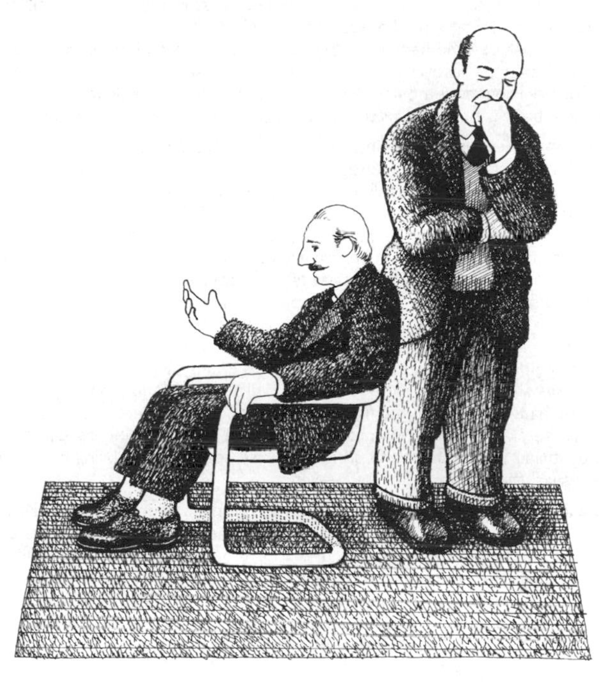

Excerpts from the diary of a psychotherapist 3–5: change begins

Session 3 Mr Smith reported that he had started to lead a more active life. He had joined a club and visited the pub once, where he had had a short conversation with an old acquaintance. He told of how much his wife, with her restricted personality, had confined his life over decades, and how now, being free from the constraints she placed on him, he was feeling guilty. This guilt was enhanced whenever he did something of which his wife would have disapproved, for example, driving his car at night.

I encouraged him to talk about his everyday lifestyle, and he described how he still behaved as if his wife was still alive, carefully leaving room for her on 'her' side of the double bed, and moving about the house as if to expect her in the next room. He admitted that he heard his wife's voice calling him from time to time, and he needed reassurance that this hallucination was not a sign that he was 'going mad'.

He told of how he had come to the realization that he, not she, could choose either to restrict himself, or to allow himself to do as he pleased. He was frightened by the new degree of freedom his wife's death had given him, and he was uncertain as to how he was going to use this new freedom.

Session 4 He came in limping, explaining that his doctor had had all the test results back, and he had been to a neurologist—and that no cause could be found for the weakness. He described how the limp had been inhibiting his plans for socializing, but as he spoke he smiled, and seemed quite unconcerned by it. *La belle indifférence* of an hysterical reaction?—I wondered to myself, remembering his description of his late wife's leg amputation. Perhaps he was not ready to socialize yet, and this limp was useful to him as it allowed him to get out of his commitment to himself to re-establish his links with old friends. He is a bit old for an hysterical reaction (but only if this is his first). We went on to cover the same ground as earlier, going over his wife's death, and his reactions to it. I slipped in a few questions about his war experience as a radio operator, and he told me of how he had had to leave the front because he lost his voice.

This session seemed to meander over the same ground as earlier. I thought that maybe there was something else he wanted to bring up, but if there was, there was no sign of it—yet.

Session 5 He started off by saying that he was much improved, and that he was concerned that he might be wasting my time. He went on to describe how he had begun to learn new rules to live by. I suggested that sessions need not just be concerned with his symptoms alone—especially as these were now improving. We could also concentrate on his experience of learning to live according to a new lifestyle. He was pleased at this suggestion, and went on to talk of plans for creating his new life.

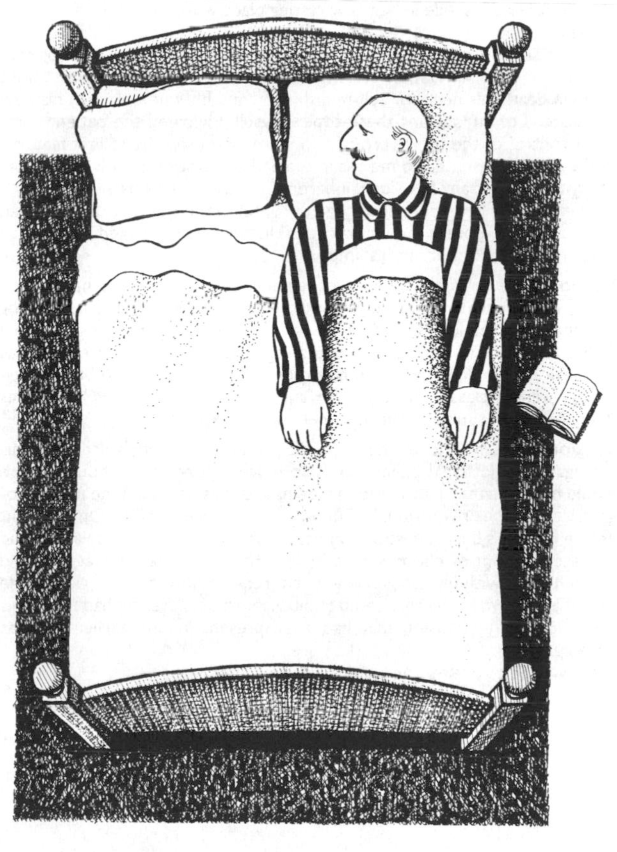

Excerpts from the diary of a psychotherapist 6–8: revelations

Session 6 Mr Smith described persisting, frenzied feelings, as if he had to get everything done before something dreadful happened. He had been doing more and more socializing, and was preparing to go on holiday for a weekend with a friend, while his son looked after the farm. This would be his first holiday without his wife. What was the meaning of these frenzied feelings? He related it to a fear of his own death, as a punishment, just when his new life was starting to look promising. He talked about his feelings about not having provided his wife's grave with a tombstone—as if he could not leave his wife in her new resting place while he went off enjoying himself.

In this session I encouraged him to talk at length about his new plans. I was also on the look out for setbacks due to unrealistic assumptions about his own death, his need for self-punishment, and his wife's place in his new life. Instead of introducing these topics myself, I allowed the patient complete control of the topics brought forward, and used the salient features as they were presented to me. As in the earlier sessions, I took the opportunity to counter any false logic inherent in these cognitions.

Our rapport had been steadily growing, but none the less there was an atmosphere of anxiety in our dialogue. He never fully relaxed, except for when he was talking about his limp.

Session 7 He arrived in a much more confident mood, having had several chats with a recently widowed lady who was still very depressed. In talking to her he realized just how much he had improved. This insight gave him a feeling as of rebirth, and he was redoubling his efforts to socialize (so far as his weak leg would allow), as if to make up for lost time. He had started taking evening classes in navigation and these were going well. He was interested in the subject, and was meeting new people.

Session 8 We went over the same old ground of his wife's death and his feelings about it. We'd been over it so much before that I thought there would be no further information to be had. But as he talked, he made progressively deeper revelations about why he was feeling guilty. On the night before his wife's final admission to hospital she had become unbalanced and had accused him of having secret lovers. He lost his temper at this, and found himself with his hands round her throat, wanting to strangle her. He only stopped when she spluttered and became blue. After he had made this revelation all the tension that had been present in our earlier sessions evaporated.

He was able to leave this session without limping.

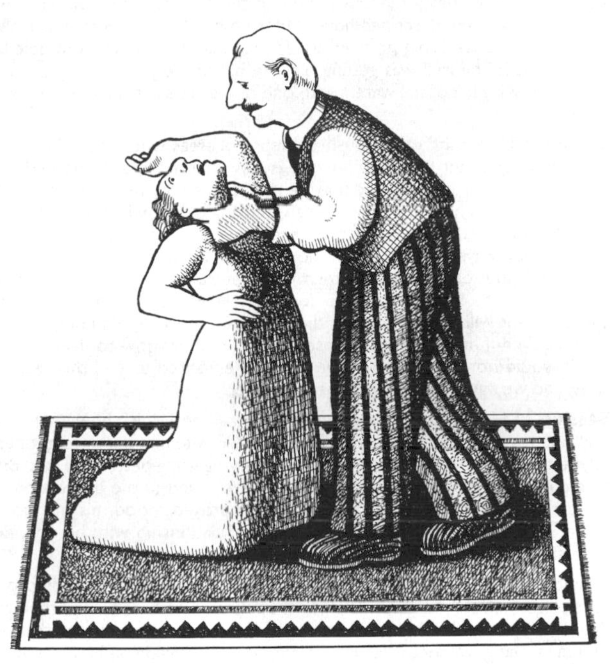

Excerpts from the diary of a psychotherapist 9–12: termination

Session 9 I decided to make the timing of the end of therapy explicit: 'There are only three more sessions to go after to day, and I thought this would be a good opportunity to discuss how much progress you think you have made.' The advantage of making termination explicit early is that it provides a definite goal, and that if Mr Smith is going to relapse because he is unready to accept the end of termination, this has a chance of occurring when there are still one or two more sessions to go. He appeared to accept that therapy should end after another three sessions. I explored his reactions to this carefully, giving him an opportunity—if he felt like it—to say how he felt let down or abandoned by myself.

He went on to give details of his navigation classes. He has been doing well—sometimes being the first person in the class to come up with the correct answer. He described how at first he had been reluctant to make friends in the class: 'They all seem so *old!*' He said that he was now able to accept that he himself was getting old. He has active plans to try out his navigation skills in coastal waters with one of the class members who owns a small boat.

Session 10 Mr Smith ran through a number of areas where he believes he has made significant progress: how he is now able to live his life without making 'space' for his wife, and how he is able to enjoy things without feeling guilty, and sometimes without even thinking of his wife at all, for brief periods (not a yardstick of success that I am necessarily happy with, but one cannot always explain that it is not so much the topics of our thoughts that matter, but our reaction to them). He seems to be fairly pleased with the new life he has constructed for himself. He is confident that his improvement will continue, but, rather disappointingly, he did not go on to say that even if he did have a relapse, he would know how to deal with it, and it would not be the end of the world. He wanted to end this session early, and we agreed to this proposal together.

Session 11 He discussed his attitude to therapy, describing how at first he was anxious and suspicious, and then how later, when he began to get better, he thought he should be feeling guilty about getting better too fast. But he did not feel guilty—he just felt pleased. We talked of the depression as of something in the past, dwelling on his improved mood, his increased sense of comfort with himself, his improved relationship with his son, his widening range of activities and his new friends.

Session 12 No new material was brought forward—perhaps a good prognostic sign indicating that it really was the appropriate time to end therapy. We reviewed Mr Smith 's progress again, and made arrangements that he should see his own doctor for maintaining and then tailing off his drug therapy. He thanked me, and we parted.

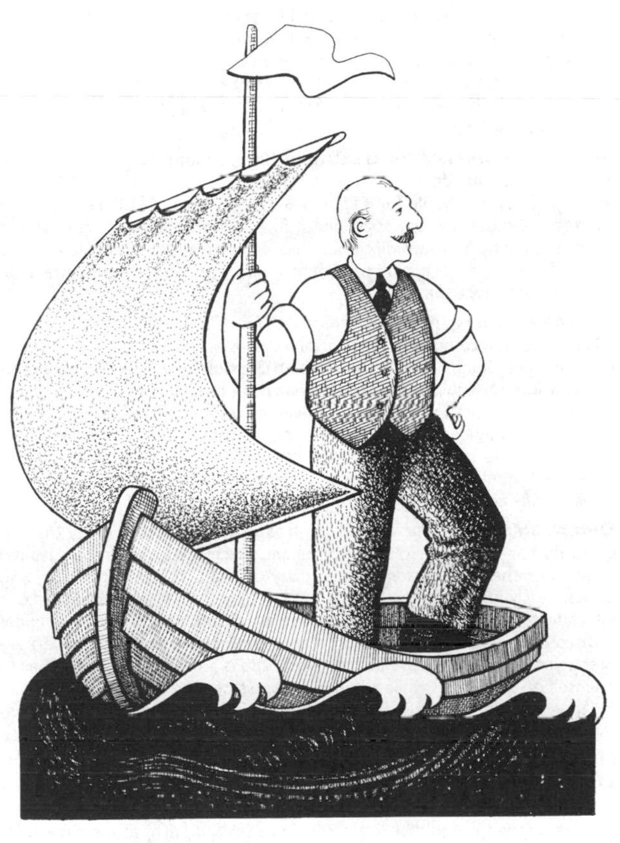

Compulsory hospitalization

►The patient must have a mental disorder, ie mental illness (p 314), mental impairment (p 314) or psychopathy (p 364), and need detention for treatment of it, or to protect himself or others, before compulsion may be used (if voluntary means have failed).

Admission for assessment (Mental Health Act* 1983, section 2)
- The period of assessment (and treatment) lapses after 28 days.
- Patient's appeals must be sent within 14 days to the mental health tribunal (composed of a doctor, lay person and lawyer).
- An approved social worker (or the nearest relative) makes the application on the recommendation of 2 doctors (not from the same hospital), one of whom is 'approved' under the Act (in practice a psychiatric consultant or senior registrar).

Section 3: admission for treatment (for ≤6 months)
- The exact mental disorder must be stated.
- Detention is renewable for a further 6 months (annually thereafter).
- 2 doctors must sign the appropriate forms and know why treatment in the community is contraindicated. They must have seen the patient within 24h. They must state that treatment is likely to benefit the patient, or prevent deterioration.

Section 4: emergency treatment (for for ≤72h)
- The admission to hospital must be an urgent necessity.
- May be used if admission under section 2 would cause undesirable delay (admission must follow the recommendation rapidly).
- An approved social worker or the nearest relative makes the application after recommendation from one doctor (eg the GP).
- The GP should keep a supply of the relevant forms, as the social worker may be unobtainable (eg with another emergency).
- It is usually converted to a section 2 on arrival in hospital.

Detention of a patient already in hospital: section 5(2) (≤72h)
- The doctor in charge (or, if a consultant psychiatrist, his or her deputy) applies to the hospital administrator, day or night, so it is often helpful to obtain early joint care for these patients with a consultant psychiatrist.
- A patient in an A&E department is not in a ward, so cannot be detained under this section. Common law is all that is available, to provide temporary restraint 'on a lunatic who has run amok and is a manifest danger either to himself or to others'[1] while awaiting an assessment by a psychiatrist.[2]
- Plan where the patient is to go before the 72h has elapsed, eg by liaising with psychiatrists for admission under section 2.

Nurses' holding powers: section 5(4) (for ≤6h)
- Any authorized psychiatric nurse may use force to detain a voluntary 'mental' patient who is taking his own discharge against medical advice, if such a discharge would be likely to involve serious harm to the patient (eg suicide) or others.
- During the 6h the nurse must find the necessary personnel to sign a section 5 application or allow the patient's discharge.

Renewal of compulsory detention in hospital: section 20(4)
- The patient continues to suffer from a mental disorder and would benefit from continued hospital treatment.
- Further admission is needed for the health or safety of the patient—which cannot be achieved except by forced detention.

Section 136 (for ≥72h) allows police to arrest a person 'in a place to which the public have access' and is who believed to be suffering from a mental disorder. The patient must be conveyed to a 'place of safety' (usually a designated A&E department) for assessment by a doctor (usually a psychiatrist) and an approved social worker. The patient must be discharged after assessment or detained under sections 2 or 3.

Section 135 This empowers an approved social worker who believes that someone is being ill-treated or is neglecting himself to apply to a magistrate to search for and admit such patients.

*This Act operates in England and Wales; arrangements in Scotland are slightly different.
1 Lord Justice Keith, 1988 *The Times* May 28 2 R Jones 1991 *Mental Health Act Manual*, 3e, London, Sweet and Maxwell

Consent to treatment (Mental Health Act)

►Emergency treatment to save life or to prevent serious harm to the patient can (must) always be given, overriding all the safeguards below, if the patient is unable to consent to treatment (eg owing to drunkenness).

Background In general a patient must give consent for any procedure (any touching), otherwise the doctor is liable under the UK common law of battery. This means that a competent person can refuse any treatment, *however* dire the consequences. Within common law there are defences to battery other than consent: if a patient is not competent to give or withhold consent, and if treatment is in their best interests, then treatment may be undertaken under 'necessity'. The defence of 'emergency' is to allow restraint where you must act quickly to prevent the patient from harming themselves or others (or committing a crime). For example, you could restrain a patient running amok on a ward before you have a chance to assess the situation. The Mental Health Act enables treatment of someone suffering from a mental disorder *for that mental disorder* under certain circumstances (p 398) and sets down some conditions for consent for treating in certain circumstances, as follows.

Consent is required *and* a second opinion is needed (section 57) All forms of psychosurgery require this level of consent. If patients are incapable of giving informed consent or decline consent, no treatment can be given.

The Mental Health Act Commission must validate the informed consent. It does this by sending 3 members to interview the patient and review the notes. One member is a doctor (who decides if the treatment is appropriate); others are non-medical. The patient must understand the nature, purpose and likely effects of the recommended treatment for the conditions of informed consent to hold. If the patient is confused, demented, or would consent to *any* treatment, consent is not informed. Signing of an ordinary consent form is needed as well as the certificate from the Mental Health Act Commission. Although grades of informed consent are probably more realistic, the law is black and white: either the consent is informed, or it is not.

Consent is required or a second opinion (section 58)
Note: no treatment can be given to a voluntary patient without his informed consent. If the responsible medical officer (RMO) feels that electroconvulsive or drug treatment for ≥3 months is necessary, and the patient is incapable of giving informed consent, or withholds consent, these treatments may be given provided a second opinion from the Mental Health Commission states that the treatment is necessary. Section 3 of the Mental Health Act is then used. The advantage of doing this is that the patient then acquires well-defined rights for review and appeal. If informed consent is given, the RMO must sign Form 38 (as well as the ordinary consent form) stating that the patient understands the purpose, need for, and likely effects of the treatment.

Children under 16 require the same standard of informed consent from a parent or guardian for prolonged psychotropic treatment. If parents are unwilling or unable to consent, a Care Order may be necessary—under which the local authority social services department takes over responsibility for the child. It must be shown that the child's proper development or health is being avoidably prevented or neglected; or that he is exposed to a moral danger; or that he is beyond the control of his parent or guardian.

Withdrawal of consent Treatment must cease immediately, unless it is necessary to save life. If the treatment is being carried out under section 58, the RMO must contact the Mental Health Act Commission, so that the requirements of this section can be met.

The sections referred to above are those of the 1983 Mental Health Act (England and Wales)

4. Psychiatry

Autism

This neurodevelopmental disorder is, if severe, the antithesis of all that defines mental health (p 314). Prevalence up to 90/10,000 of those <16yrs old—estimates vary considerably.[1] Sex ratio: ♂:♀≈3:1). Autism is a triad of:

1 Impaired reciprocal social interaction (A symptoms).
2 Impaired imagination, associated with abnormal verbal and non-verbal communication (B symptoms).
3 Restricted repertoires of activities and interests (C symptoms).

Diagnosis of an autistic disorder depends on identifying at least 8 of the following symptoms—and these should include at least 2 'A' symptoms; 1 'B' symptom and 1 'C' symptom.[1]

Impaired reciprocal social interaction (A symptoms)

- Marked unawareness of the existence and feelings of others (eg treating a person as a piece of furniture; being oblivious to others' distress—and to their need for privacy).
- Abnormal response to being hurt (he does not come for comfort; or makes a stereotyped response, eg just saying 'Cheese, cheese, cheese').
- Impaired imitation (eg does not wave 'bye-bye').
- Abnormal play: eg solitary, or using others as mechanical aids.
- Gross impairment in making peer friendships. If he tries at all, the effort will lack the conventions of social interaction (eg reading from the telephone directory to uninterested peer).

Impaired imagination associated with abnormal verbal and non-verbal communication (B symptoms)

- No babbling, facial expressions or gestures in infancy.
- Avoids mutual gaze; no smiles when making a social approach; does not greet his parents; stiffens when held.
- Does not act adult rôles; no interest in stories; no fantasy.
- Abnormal speech production (eg echolalia, ie repetitions); idiosyncratic use of words ('Go on green riding' for 'I want a go on the swing'); misuse of pronouns ('You' instead of 'I'); irrelevances (eg starts talking of train schedules during a conversation about sport).
- Difficulty in initiating or sustaining conversations.

Poor range of activities and interests (C symptoms)

- Stereotyped movements (hand-flicking, spinning, head-banging).
- Preoccupation with parts of objects (sniffing or repetitive feeling of a textured object, spinning wheels of toys) or unusual attachments (eg to coal).
- Marked distress over changes in trivia (eg a vase's place).
- Insists on following routines in precise detail.
- Markedly narrow range of interests, eg preoccupied with lining up objects; or in amassing facts about the weather.

Causes: (Mostly unknown) Prenatal rubella, tuberous sclerosis. Concordance in monozygotic twins: ~90%.

Treatment: This is not effective. Behaviour therapy may be tried.
►*A good teacher is more helpful than a good doctor.* Special schooling may be needed (most have a low IQ). Children may learn better by overhearing, than by direct methods. Parents may gain valuable support from self-help groups.[2] Encourage parents to give more attention to the child for 'good' behaviour rather than 'bad', and to have unwavering rules for behaviour. 70% remain severely handicapped. 50% develop useful speech; 30% will develop seizures by adulthood. 15% will lead an independent life. Apply for benefits (disability living allowance if in UK).

1 L Wing 1996 BMJ i 327 2 National Autistic Society UK telephone no: 0181 830 0999

Seasonal affective disorder

. . .Lying thus in the sun one is liberated from doubts and from misgivings; it is not that problems and difficulties are resolved, it is that they are banished. The sun's radiation penetrates the mind as well as the body, anaesthetizing thought. . .[1]

Some patients find that symptoms of depression start in the winter months, and remit in spring or summer. It has been postulated that disordered secretion of the indole melatonin (*OHCM* p 568) from the pineal gland is to blame in some of these patients with 'SAD'. Melatonin, the hormone of darkness[2], is secreted by the pineal only at night—eg at 30μg/night; Evidence supporting the rôle of melatonin in depression includes the following:

- Bright light morning phototherapy (6–8am) is effective in reducing depression ratings in the winter in those with SAD. This was shown to be associated with delay in the onset of melatonin secretion.[3]
- A dose-response relationship has been shown between the amount of light administered in phototherapy and the degree of improvement in depression (as measured on Hamilton ratings). 6h/day of increased light brought about a 53% decrease in score, whereas treatments of 2h (or red-light treatment) produced only a 25% reduction. These effects were correlated with suppressed plasma melatonin concentrations at 23.00h.[4]

However, evidence in this field of research is often contradictory, and it is probably unwise to rush into recommending light therapy for all patients whose recurrent depressions start in the autumn or winter. This might have the undesirable effect of enticing such patients to book unaffordable winter holidays to exotic locations—with inevitable disappointments and recriminations.

Burnout

Signs of this syndrome of overwork-engendered emotional exhaustion are:
•Stress •Depression •Libido↓ •Insomnia •Guilt •Feeling isolated
•Apathy •Paranoia •Amnesia •Indecision •Denial •Temper tantrums

Management This is difficult. Some may respond to plans such as these:

- Diagnose and treat any depression (p 336–42 & 388–96).
- Allow time for the person to recognise that there is a problem.
- More hobbies, and more nice holidays.
- Advice from wise colleagues in the same profession (regular follow-up).
- Learn new professional skills.
- Set achievable goals in work and leisure (eg protected time with family).
- Early retirement.

1 AE Ellis 1958 & 1979 *The Rack* Penguin 2 RV Short 1993 BMJ ii 952 3 HS Yu 1993 *Melatonin Biosynthesis, Physiological Effects, and Clinical Applications*, CRC Press, Boca Raton, Florida, USA
4 F Winton 1989 *Psychol Med* **19** 585

Community care

Since the early 1980s, thousands of UK patients with mental illness have had the focus of their care moved from hospital to the community. The aim has been to save money and improve care: but, in the UK, this policy is now being partly reversed.[1] Has community care failed, or have there been successes?

Five questions keep recurring, each (ominously) prefixed by a 'Surely. . .'

1 *Surely hospitals will always be needed for severely affected people?* In general, the problem is not the severity of the mental illness, but the social context in which it occurs which determines if community care is appropriate.

2 *Surely community care, if it is done properly, will be more expensive than hospital care, where resources can be concentrated?* Not so—at least not necessarily so. Some concentration of resources *can* take place in the community, for example, in day hospitals and mental illness hostels (p 326–7). It is also true that the 'bed and breakfast' element of inpatient care is likely to be quite expensive, particularly if the running and maintenance costs associated with deploying inpatient psychiatric services are taken into account. In most studies, the cost of each type of service does not differ widely, and in some studies good community care turns out to be ~25% cheaper.[2,3]

3 *Surely there will be more homicides and suicides if disturbed patients are not kept in hospital?* It is now clear that however careful selection of patients for community care may be, this is still be a very serious problem.

4 *Surely if inpatient psychiatric beds are not available, however good the daytime team is in the community, some patients will still need somewhere to go at night?* The implication here is that the skills available in bed-and-breakfast accommodation may be inadequate at times of day when there is no other support, other than the general practitioner. Studies which have looked at this have certainly found an increase in non-hospital residential care in those selected for community care, and this increase may be as much as 280% over 5yrs.[4] In the UK, new proposals guarantee 24-hour open access to skilled help, but it is not known what pressures this will put services under.[1]

5 *Surely community care will involve a huge bureaucracy in pursuit of the unattainable goal of 100% safety?* This will be so if every patient has a lengthy care plan, and repeated risk assessments. Concern for safety may also spawn a non-therapeutic custodial relationship between health-worker and patient.[1]

Advantages reported for community care are: better social functioning, satisfaction with life, employment, and drug compliance[5]—but in randomized studies in the UK these advantages were not manifest.[6] Furthermore, trends have been repeatedly found indicating that the longer studies go on for, the harder it is to maintain the initial advantages of community care. If it is hard for teams to keep up their enthusiasm during a trial, it will probably be even harder when the trial period has ended[7]—or when team members are ill or absent. These considerations may in part explain the observation that with inadequately funded and supervised community care, patients can fail to get the services they require, and when hospitals are being run down, and a patient's condition worsens, so that 'sectioning' followed by admission becomes impossible, the patient is left in the community 'rotting with his rights on'.

1 M Marshall 1999 BMJ **i** 3 2 G Thornicroft 1998 *B J Psych* **173** 363 3 J Hoult 1984 *Acta Psy Scand* **69** 359 4 A Borland 1989 *Hosp Comm Psy* **40** 369–74 5 See *Cochrane Database of Systemic Reviews* (eg ab000270.htm) & L Stein 1980 *Arch Gen Psy* **37** 392–7 6 M Muijen 1992 BMJ **i** 749 7 P Dedman 1993 BMJ **i** 1359

Poverty and mental health

Social deprivation is positively associated with premature mortality,[1,2] and poverty makes almost *all* diseases more likely (but not Hodgkin's disease, eczema, bulimia, or melanoma). See *Health and social class*, p 463. In the UK, the numbers of homeless people ranges from 1–2 million.[3] 30–50% suffer from mental illness (~10% have schizophrenia), and most do not know where to go for help, and most have no doctor. A 3-tier strategy may help. 1 Emergency shelters 2 Transitional accommodation 3 Long-term housing.

The cost in health terms to society and the individual is enormous. Diseases and symptoms such as diarrhoea which may pass as a minor inconveniences to the well-housed may be a major hurdle for the homeless, with severe social and psychological effects. In the UK, government policy (*Working for Patients*) requires each Health Authority to determine the size and morbidity of its resident and its homeless populations. Capture-recapture techniques show that the *unobserved* population of the homeless is about twice that observed. This method of enumeration collects samples (lists) and looks for tags (duplicates) in subsequent counts, and from this determines the degree of under-counting. If all in the subsequent count are duplicates, then there is no underestimate of the original count. Statistical techniques can allow for migration in and out of the population area.[4] These studies show that psychiatric morbidity is greatest in the observed homeless populations: the implication is that the psychiatric illness makes these people more 'visible'.

In the UK, as in many other Western countries, what started out as an enlightened policy of looking after people with mental health problems in the community has resulted in large numbers of psychiatric patients living on the street in great poverty—relieved by occasional admissions to acute units. This 'revolving door' model of care has failed many patients, not least because continuity of care has been compromised.

One way to stop poverty is to pay people not to be poor—specifically not to have more than 1–2 children. In the early 1990s, the Singapore government offered poor families ^{SP}\$26,400 over 20yrs if they have ≤2 children.

In the UK the 'poverty line' weekly income is calculated on an individual basis depending on circumstances, so for an unmarried mother with 2 young children the figure is £93.85. In fact, state benefits may not amount to this sum. She will receive Income support personal allowance of £46.50 plus £15.95 per child, plus £10.25 family premium with a £5.20 single parent premium (total £93.85). Further benefits such as child benefit or maintenance will lead to a proportionate reduction in this total. From this she might typically pay £3 for water bills, £2.20 for council tax, and £10/week for fuel (in winter). In council flats there are no furnishings. Grants (eg £500) are scarce, so DoH can make a loan for this, deducted at source (eg £13/week)—so the amount some families are living on is less than £60. NB: these figures are from the min-1990s; change is frequent (freefone 0800 882200).

Note that there is no evidence that simply living in a deprived area makes a person more prone to illness and death. All the excess mortality and morbidity is explained by the person him- or herself being poor.[2] Their immediate neighbours who are not poor do not share the same risk. The implication is that targeted health care should be directed towards poor people *wherever* they live, not at poor areas.

1 P Townsend 1989 *Health & Deprivation*, London, Routledge 2 A Sloggett 1994 BMJ ii 1470
3 *Br J Psych* 1993 **162** 314–24 See also R Burridge 1993 *Unhealthy Housing: Research, Remedies and Reform* Spon/Chapman and Hall, ISBN 0-419-154410-8 4 N Retterstol 1993 *Suicide: a European Perspective*, CUP

Postnatal depression

The psychiatric and psychological phenomena of pregnancy and birth include the very common, and usually mild, 'blues'; puerperal psychosis; and postnatal depression (the risk of developing this latter is 3-fold that of those with no recent pregnancy). There are many causes, individual and social circumstances, genetic, and hormonal change (this latter 'old favourite' has now been given added veracity by a reasonably successful randomized trial of oestrogen in severely depressed postnatal patients).[1]

Natural history Reviews state that most postnatal depression resolves within 6 months, so we find ourselves thinking: "Good! Those trusty psychiatric tools of 'wait-and-see', and the passage of time will be my main tools in this illness: nothing depends critically on what I do now, to this poor depressed new mother with whom I am now confronted". NOT SO!

Consider these facts: •For the patient, 6 months is a long, long time.
- For the infant, 6 months is more than a long time: it's literally an age.
- Suicide is a waste, but for a young family, a mother's suicide is especially destructive—unthinkable, indeed, for those who have not experienced it.
- There is evidence of impaired cognition and social functioning in the offspring of mothers with postnatal depression.[2]

We therefore submit that our actions may spawn critical outcomes. So what should our actions be? The first step is to try not to be caught unawares by a major depression which apparently strikes like a bolt from the blue, but which, in reality, has been building up over time. Pregnancy and infant–motherhood is supposed to be time of unclouded joy. We professionals often collude with this view. We are always hearing ourselves saying: "Oh Mrs Salt, what a lovely baby! You must be so pleased—and you always wanted a little boy, didn't you? We are so delighted for you. . ." But what if *she* is not delighted? She hardly dares confess her traitorous thoughts that she is unaccountably sad, that she spends the nights crying, and that her exhausted days are filled with a sense of foreboding that she or some other agency will harm the child. The place to start to pre-empt these feelings is in the antenatal clinic. By addressing these issues, and, later, in the puerperium, by expressly asking after them, you give permission for the new mother to tell her woe. When this is revealed, counselling, and input from a health visitor and a psychiatrist is appropriate, as is particularly close follow-up. You may need to arrange emergency admission under the Mental Health Act: but the whole point of being prepared for postnatal depression is to avoid things getting this bad.

Pharmacology Tricyclics (p340) and progesterones are often used, but there is little evidence that they are effective.[1] Adding lithium (p 354) may help (and ECT may also be indicated). A single randomized trial ($N=61$) has concluded that transdermal oestrogen is effective in severe postnatal depression. The Edinburgh Postnatal Depression Scale (EPDS) was used to assess outcome (along with other measures). The score started off at 21.8, falling within a month to 13.3—taking some patients out of the 'major depression' category. The control group also improved over time (from 21.3 to 16.5)—but still remained severely depressed.[1] The dose régime was 3 months of transdermal 17β-(o)estradiol (200µg/day) for 3 months on its own, then with added dydrogesterone 10mg/day for 12 days each month for a further 3 months. CI: uterine, cervical or breast neoplasia; previous thrombo-embolism or thrombophlebitis—and breast-feeding.

As ever, we recommend caution in applying results of a single trial. The key issues are prevention, support, and frequent follow-up, with admission (with the baby) as needed. Before starting oestrogens, try to get a joint decision, with the family, the health visitor, the psychiatrist, and the general practitioner verified by your local drug information service.

1 AJP Gregoire 1996 *Lancet* F**347** 930 2 EM Cummings 1994 *J Child Psychol Psychiat* **35** 73–112

4. Psychiatry

5. General practice

Relevant pages in other chapters ► *Every page in all chapters*. All diseases are relevant. This is a key feature of general practice, which is the axis around which all our medical events revolve, every day drawing millions of patients to it before scattering a few handfuls to every corner of the medical establishment. Only in general practice is the full gamut of what can go wrong with people's lives made manifest. Because of the huge and undefined range of general practice, it has been said (not just by GPs themselves) that the general practitioner needs to be the most comprehensively educated of any kind of doctor.[1]

1 D Hill *Psychiatry in Medicine, Retrospect and Prospect*, London, Nuffield Provincial Hospitals Trust

Index on prevention

Introduction

General practice is not a specialty in the usual sense, and GPs make much of being the last of the true generalists in medicine (they were also the first). They are specialists in their patients, rather than in disease—having no special and unique knowledge of disease (except for disease in its earliest stages), and having no unique treatments. They can answer questions like '*Why doesn't Miss Phelps ever attend the hospital antenatal clinic? What would have to change for her to do so?*' There are few medical instances in which GPs are in a position to offer more skill and expertise than all other doctors—but there are many circumstances when the GP's understanding of his patient is what counts, and for which no amount of expertise can ever be a substitute. So when, for example, Miss Phelps's baby dies, to whom does she turn in her distress? She is not a medical problem; she is not an obstetric problem; she is not even a psychiatric problem—she is Miss Phelps. And the doctor who specializes in Miss Phelps is (or ought to be) her GP. He is the one who knows what to do and what to say; when to be quiet and when to explain; and when to appear and when to disappear, humbled as he is by having witnessed a wealth of such grief.

Combined with *knowledge of the patient*, and *knowledge of disease in its earliest phases*, there is a third component which contributes strongly to general practice: the *ability to diagnose health*—taking into account all the definitions of health on p 414. If a patient is asking 'Am I well, or could I have cancer' the doctor who is always responding by saying '. . . Well, I'm not sure. . . let's do one more test. . . ' is sometimes a bad doctor, and always an expensive one. Some doctors have the gift of appraising a patient, and knowing almost instinctively whether to treat now, or investigate, or refer, or reassure. Nowhere is this skill more apparent than in general practice—and this instinctive skill is born of countless contacts with patients from all walks of life, with diseases affecting any organ of the body or mind. A chest physician may tell you that your lungs are healthy, but if, on your way out, you say "Oh, and I've also got this pain in my leg. . ."—then he may feel out of his territory. He thought he was sending his patient away rejoicing in his health, but then one new symptom undermines this, and he is likely to end up saying "Go and see your GP". It is then up to the GP to reassure, treat, or to orchestrate the deployment of all the many sophistications of technological medicine.

Even if all our scientists had unlimited abilities and facilities, there would still be a limit to technological medicine. Even if we could turn the whole world into a hospital so skilled as to be able to manipulate the totality of the *milieu intérieur* there would still be a vast abyss between the possibility of health and its attainment. On the other side of the abyss is the patient, surrounded by unknown (but not unknowable) myths, hopes, fears, ideas, expectations and fantasies directing him away from the very things that could help him most. It is the GP's rôle to bridge this abyss, not so much to haul the patient to safety, but rather to be the platform on which the patient crosses of his own (enlightened) free will. In bridging this gap, the GP needs sure foundations on both of its sides, and this is the great challenge of general practice—to foster in oneself an equal love of, and an excellence in, both the technological and the personal realm.

Although general practice is not a specialty in the usual sense, it *is* a discipline, as it creates and publishes original material about its sphere of activity in peer-reviewed journals (eg *British Journal of General Practice* and *Journal of Family Practice,* which are among the top 5 world-class medical journals related to a specific discipline, as ranked by citations and immediacy).[1] Because these journals are the lifeblood at the scientific heart of the discipline, they are not necessarily an easy read—but they do repay careful study.

1 D Pereira Gray 1997 *British Journal of General Practice* (formerly *J Roy College Gen Pract* **47** 139)

Fame, fortune, medicine, and art

Let us start with an elementary observation: *there are no famous living doctors*; indeed *there are no famous dead doctors*. The only famous doctors who are household names are those immortalized in literature—for example, Dr Watson, Dr Frankenstein, and Dr Faustus. Hereby we demonstrate the power of the written word. When we curl up in an armchair and read for pleasure, we open the portals of our minds because we are alone. While we are reading, there is, it seems, no point in dissembling. We confront our subject matter with a steady eye because we believe, that, while reading to ourselves, we cannot be judged. Then, suddenly, when we are at our most open and defenceless, literature takes us by the throat—and that eye which was so steady and confident a few minutes ago is now perhaps misting over, or our heart is missing a beat, or our skin is covered in a goose-flesh more papular than ever a Siberian winter produced. Once we have been on earth for a few decades, not much in our mundane world sends shivers down our spines, but the power of worlds of literature and art to do this ever grows.

There are just a few doctors fortunate enough to enjoy celebrity: Conan Doyle, William Carlos Williams, Somerset Maugham, and Chekhov—all are artists. What about Freud? Here is the exception which proves the rule—proves in the sense of testing, for he is not really an exception. We can accept him among the great only in so far as we view his oeuvre as an artistic oeuvre, rather than as a scientific one. Science has got on perfectly well for years without Freud, but, as art, his work and insights will survive: and survival, as George Bernard Shaw pointed out, is the only test of greatness.

The reason for the ascendancy of art over science is simple. We scientists, in our humble way, are only interested in explaining reality. Artists are good at explaining reality too: but they also *create* it. Our most powerful impressions are produced not by simple sensations but by the association of ideas. It is a pre-eminent feature of the human mind that it revels in seeing something as, or through, something else: life refracted through experience—light refracted through jewels, or a walk through the woods transmuted into a Pastoral Symphony. Ours is a world of metaphor, fantasy, and deceit. Although it may be true to say that all the best pleasures are sensory, it is all the more true to state that sensory pleasures never last very long—which is why humankind does not spend *all* its time eating and making love.

What has all this to do with the day-to-day practice of medicine? The answer lies in the word 'defenceless' above. When we read alone and for pleasure, our defences are down—and we hide nothing from the great characters of fiction. In our consulting rooms, and on the ward, we so often do our best to hide everything, beneath the white coat, or the avuncular bedside manner. So often, a professional detachment is all that is left after all those years inured to the foibles, fallacies and frictions of our patients' tragic lives. It is at the point where art and medicine collide, that doctors can re-attach themselves to the human race and re-feel those emotions which motivate or terrify our patients. We all have an Achilles heel: that part of our inner self which was not rendered forever invulnerable to mortal cares when we were dipped in the waters of the river Styx as it flowed down the wards of our first disillusion. Art and literature, among other things, may enable this Achilles heel to be the means of our survival as thinking, sentient beings, capable of maintaining a sympathetic sensibility to our patients.

The American way of dealing with these issues is to create Professors of Literature-in-Medicine and to conjure with concepts such as *the patient as text*, and at least one-third of American medical schools do courses in literature in an attempt to inculcate ethical reasoning and speculation. Our way, here in Britain, is a bit different, in that we try not to hive off these issues to some special course in medical literature but to demonstrate, albeit imperfectly, in our writings and in our practice of medicine, that *every* contact with patients has an ethical and artistic dimension, as well as a technical one. But the aims are the same, and both deserve to flourish.

Some definitions and measures of health

Primary care and distributive justice The WHO Alma-Ata statement declares that primary care should 'be made universally accessible to individuals and families in the community, by means acceptable to them, through their full participation, and at the cost that the community and country can afford to maintain in the spirit of self-reliance. . . [and] addresses the main health problems in the community, providing promotive, preventative, curative and rehabilitative services accordingly.' Factors affecting access to health include finance, ideology, and education.

4 GP job descriptions •To clear the waiting room *efficiently* (*kindly* if possible).
- To deal with the realities of patients as you find them (eg loneliness, addiction, poverty, and mental ill-health) rather than ideal patients (eg interesting diagnostic problems leading to technically brilliant cures).
- To be skilled in: prioritization; delegation; health-need measurement; rationing; purchasing/delivery of primary healthcare; time- and staff-management.
- To give healthcare to people irrespective of age, sex, illness or social status. To make early diagnoses, framed in physical, psychological, and social terms. To make initial decisions about all problems presented or unearthed. To arrange continuing management of chronic, recurrent, or terminal illness. To practise in co-operation with other colleagues, medical and non-medical. To treat, prevent, and educate to promote health of patients and their families, while reconciling professional responsibility to the community.

Health 4 definitions to compare: Health is: **I** The absence of disease.
II A state of complete physical, mental, and social wellbeing (WHO definition).
III A process of adaptation, to changing environments, to growing up and ageing, to healing when damaged, to suffering, and death. Health embraces the future [so] includes anguish and the inner resources to live with it.[1]
IV Any process enabling the giving or promoting of life.
V 'Health is whatever works, and for as long'.[2]

All the above have limitations, but I and IV seem least counter-intuitive. Consider the following: •Was Charles I healthy as he laid his head on the executioner's block? •What about a priest in the act of losing his celibacy? •Can a heart with a prosthetic valve which is gradually wearing out be healthy? •Was Ghandi healthy at the end of a hunger strike? •Can animals or babies be healthy? •What about death in childbirth? 'Answers' below:

Healthy according to definition:

	I	II	III	IV	V
King Charles on the scaffold	yes	no	yes	yes	no
Fasting Ghandi	yes	no	yes	yes	yes
Fingerless old person	yes	no	yes	yes	no
Babies and animals	yes	yes	no	yes	yes
Heart with failing valve	no	no	no	yes	yes
Priest losing his celibacy	yes	no	yes	yes	yes
Death in childbirth	no	no	yes	yes	yes

Measures of health Scores on the health survey Short Form 36 (SF36) are reproducible and quantifiable, related to patients' clinical state, the GP's decision to refer, and GP's views on severity. It is valid when combined with a patient-generated index of quality of life (which asks patients to name the 5 most important activities/areas affected by their condition, and to value importance of improvements to them) and a daily time trade-off calculation (how much time would you give up to be in perfect health?). By combining instruments, defects in one can be mitigated (eg the SF36 asks if health limits your ability to walk a mile—irrelevant if the patient does not need or want to walk much). *Health need* is the difference between the state now and a goal. Needs may be ranked by the distances between states and goals. Health indicators measure whether needs are met. Abortion rates can be used to measure the need for sex education. Surveys may measure health, but not needs. Practical guides to ascertaining needs in primary care are now available.[3]

1 I Illich 1976 & 1995 *Medical Nemesis*, Boyars 2 John Stone 1980 *In All This Rain* Louisiana Univ Press 3 J Wilkinson 1998 BMJ i 1524 (***5 stages:*** collecting GP data; hospital data; public involvement; postal surveys; collating sources)

What are the determinants of health?

The answer is ***wealth***. With wealth comes more stable political systems, and these are what are necessary for literacy and education to flourish, which in turn leads to easy access to clean water (the key issue, as more than 1 billion people have no access to clean water[1]), and the possibility of developing equitable health delivery systems.

A consensus is emerging in some public health units in the UK on what have been the most important influences on health in the last 20 years.[2]

- Improvements in living standards from greater disposable income.
- Improvements in the environment, eg housing and road safety.
- Reduction in tobacco use (but the young continue to take up smoking).
- Improvement in education and communication.
- Better, more effective health services, with easier access to them.

Other influences include nutritional improvement, smaller families, exercise, community self-help, and the prevention of HIV infection.

Future determinants of health are thought to rest on:

- Reducing inequalities in access to health care, and in its content.
- Reducing unemployment (a potent cause of ill health, see p 406).
- Decline in tobacco consumption in all age groups.
- Better health services with more effective, more acceptable treatments.
- Education capable of influencing behaviour so that exposure to identified risk factors is reduced.
- Better protection of the environment, and better housing.
- Applying existing knowledge in a better, more systematic, way.
- Introducing a more patient-centred style of health care, in which patients are not the passive recipients of care, but well-educated partners in the struggle against disease and its causes.

1 J Mackay 1993 *The State of Health*, ISBN 0-671-71147-4   2 R Bhopal 1994 BMJ ii 1156

Primary health care

The philosophy of primary health care Primary medical care is the system of care used by people as their first contact with health services. Where needed, referrals are made (eg in ~10% of UK patients) to centres of secondary care—usually district hospitals. Further referral may be necessary to regional 'super-specialists', so constituting tertiary medical care. This seductively simple model of medical provision misses out entirely on the cornerstone of primary health care—the responsibilities that individuals and families have for their own physical and mental wellbeing. ►*Up to 90% of all health problems are taken care of outside the official health care system.* Unless individuals and families act on their own initiative to promote their health, no amount of medical care is going to make them healthy; coronary artery bypass grafting may be helpful, but it is no substitute for families taking the initiative in promoting their own health by trying to live sensibly (eg *vis-à-vis* diet and smoking) and by learning to look after their own health. In fostering and enlightening this sense of initiative, a large number of groups are involved—not just doctors but also teachers, health educators, politicians and, above all, the families themselves. So in assessing how good a community is at primary health care, one needs to look not just at medical care, but also at social, political, and cultural aspects as well. One must ask questions such as: 'Is society making it easy for individuals to choose a healthy lifestyle?' and 'How is society promulgating health education?' and 'When does this education become indoctrination?'

Primary health care defined as a set of activities
• Providing safe food and water. • Ensuring freedom from want. • The basic treatment of illness. • Provision of necessary drugs. • Preventive care throughout the lifecycle (p 426).

Primary health care defined as a strategy. No country in the world is rich enough to provide its citizens with everything that medical care can offer. This fact pinpoints the need for the efficient use of limited resources—and this presupposes an effective system of primary health care. To be effective, this must be accessible; relevant to the population's needs; properly integrated; have full community participation; be cost-effective, and characterized by collaboration between sectors of society.

Barriers to primary health care
- People who are rendered helpless and hopeless by the great scourges of our time: unemployment, poverty, and family strife.
- Professionals who want to monopolize and medicalize health.
- Nations which are keener to take up arms than to vaccinate them.
- A world which behaves as if it does not know the meaning of social justice and equality, and in which rich and poor fail to share common objectives—or simply fail to share anything.

Some facts • 90% of ill health episodes reported to the NHS are handled in general practice.
- GP services account for < 10% of the cost of the NHS.
- The number of unrestricted principals in the UK is rising (now 35,675) with 1653 GP registrars, and 755 assistants. Supporting staff: ~63,000 whole-time equivalents (in England & Wales; see http://www.rcgp.org.uk).

5. General practice

The primary health care team

Whenever a task can be successfully delegated, delegate it. The antithesis is: *If you want a job done properly, do it yourself.* Nature favours the first maxim: when we die all our tasks are either forgotten or delegated, often by default. So the question is not *whether* to delegate, but *when*, and *to whom*. The principle of team work is: *No member is indispensable; all can contribute.*

Doctors As general practice develops it becomes less true that all doctors are 'totipotent'—ie equally able to do any task. Within any group practice, large or small, rôles can complement each other. Some may specialize in a topic or a procedure, others may lead in information technology, and others see to staff relationships, management, or preventive initiatives. Other rôles include skills in purchasing care (p 466) and practice research. A good question for any partnership to ask itself is what is its range of skills, and is postgraduate training being arranged to fill in any lacunae? These areas of expertise are helpful in furthering a career in general practice[1] and need not undermine the central rôle of the GP as a generalist.

The community (district) nurse She is usually employed by the local health authority and attached to a practice or to a sector. Sectorization has the advantage of making all her many home visits near to each other but has the disadvantage that she has to relate to many GPs. Her activities include visits to post-op patients for dressings and the removal of sutures, dressing leg ulcers, and giving 'all care' to the elderly housebound, giving injections (eg to blind diabetic patients), and supplying incontinence and other aids. Male nurses may be available for catheterizations.

The community midwife Conducts her own antenatal classes and clinics—often with a GP next door, so that they can advise each other about difficulties as they arise. She will also visit at home. Many do planned home deliveries (where appropriate) and all will do so in emergency. She has a statutory obligation to visit in the puerperium for the first 10 days (she has right of access). At 10 days the health visitor takes over (p 466).

The health visitor She has a nursing and midwifery background, and has a further qualification in health visiting. Rôles: developmental testing of children; advice on immunizations, breast feeding, minor illness in children, and handicap; advice to adults about healthy eating and giving up smoking; implementing the strategies of the health education officer (p 438), screening of the elderly in their homes, bereavement visits.

The practice nurse is employed by GPs (some of her salary may be reimbursed by health authorities. Activities include *tests* (urine, taking blood, audiometry, ECGs, peak flow); *advice* (eg about diets); treatment—eg ear syringing (93% of nurses), injections (93%), BP (52%), UTI (30%), otitis media (19%), asthma (16%); *prevention* and *audit*—eg immunizations, BP, cervical smears and family planning (eg if she holds the English National Board Certificate of Competence[2]); *chronic disease management* (diabetes/asthma clinic, chaperoning, IUCD insertion). *Nurse practitioners* have an extended diagnostic rôle as trained by the GP—if happy to take extra responsibility.

Receptionists, secretaries, practice managers These are employed by GPs and salaries are reimbursed as above. Just because they are 'non-medical' it does not follow that they do no medicine—eg a depressed patient may find quiet times to come in and have a chat with a receptionist, and may find this better than official visits. Receptionists may also be trained to take blood, test urines, do blood pressures, capillary glucose, ECGs, or audits.

Others: Social worker, psychologist, counsellor or facilitator (to encourage preventive activities), physiotherapist. *Beyond the surgery:* Community pharmacists, health education officers (p 438), and community physicians.

1 S Handysides 1994 BMJ i 253 2 S Haslett 1987 *J Roy Col Gen Prac* 37 561

Single-handed and small practices

In the UK, much of the progress in general practice over the recent past has evolved in the context of group practice and the primary health care team—the credo of modern-day doctoring. Single-handedness puts a question mark over the primacy and validity of these ideas. The benefits of highly ordered, management-led, high-investment, team-based general practice are real and not to be gainsaid. But at what price have these benefits been bought? Can small be beautiful?—and what this does concept mean for health care the world over? Let us start with the observation that general practice is about people. Their illnesses are the incidental accidents, and their deaths the only certainties which mark the impingement of these individuals on our general practice nights and days. These contacts in the night are, for the larger practices, usually boring or worse. There is no before or after: just a job to be done. For the single-handed GP doing more of his or her own visiting, these occasions may also be boring—initially. But the utility and the interest inherent in these visits can, with continuity of care, stretch over the decades, as this example illustrates. One of us (JML) was called late to an an unrousable, sweating 60-year-old man, whom we admitted to hospital with suspected septicaemia—which, years later, turned out to be the presenting symptom of an occult, indolent malignancy. We looked after him until his death at home. The continuity of care made the job interesting for us, not the clinical details. But the continuity does not stop at the end of one life. Now, whenever we see his wife, on however trivial or grave a problem, we have this shared bond. Recently she refused hospital admission for pneumonia, and the doctor could use this shared bond to induce her, over 24 hours, to change her mind. Of course, doctors in large groups will be able to tell of similar instances. Our point here is simply that these stories are more common, the more personal your care.

The dangers of exhaustion and isolation in single-handed practice are real, but they are usually pointed out by people who are thinking about isolation from one's colleagues. (How many partnerships are only partnerships on paper, and conceal or exemplify worse things than isolation?) The single-handed doctor is more likely to compensate for isolation from colleagues by identifying more with his or her patients.

As one GP has commented '. . . I am now about to start a day of single-handed general practice as my partner is away. The day is unplanned, with no appointments. People just turn up, bringing their infarcts, their sorrows, their trivia, and their life events to me. Some of the people who will come have not yet even fallen ill. There are the coronary artery plaques on the point of rupturing, the dizziness before the fall, the hallucination before its enactment, and someone is now writing a note to explain the impending suicide or the fact that they are leaving home forever, and taking the kids with them. All this is in the future; but for now, none of this has happened yet. I am completely up to date, and I command my general practice sitting behind an empty desk. I saw the last person who wanted to see me yesterday. There is no waiting list. Just the unknown. And what of the concept of the primary health care team? Can it really be called a team when I own the premises, hire most of the staff, pay them their wages, draw up their job description, and stipulate the bounds of their practice? It is certainly not an *equal* partnership. But when the patient's dizziness *does* lead to the fall in the village shop, as it did yesterday, I will be on hand to patch up the old lady, and the receptionist will kindly finish off the patient's shopping for her, and escort her home. We think that the price of a personal service is well worth paying.'

Time and the general practitioner

How do general practitioners spend their time? A typical GP with a list of ≤2000 (mean=1902) patients of whom ~15% are over 65yrs might see 50 patients in a day with 5 home visits (mean=9745 consultations/GP/yr costing ~£13 each). The major categories of care are for self-limiting illnesses (65% of consultations), chronic illness (20%), and acute major illness (15%). The most common conditions are listed below as rates/100,000 patients/yr derived from painstaking, validated Read-coded data in representative practices of a typical UK county (note that the idea of drawing health purchasing conclusions from some idealized 'typical' practice is flawed: there will be very few typical practices, and, like Tolstoy's unhappy families, each atypical practice is atypical in its own particular way[1]).

Infections/infestations	♂: 11,194	♀: 13,924
Neoplasms	♂: 2,473	♀: 3,695
Endocrine/nutrition/metabolic	♂: 3,346	♀: 4,326
Blood diseases	♂: 617	♀: 1,609
Mental disorders	♂: 5,440	♀: 8,442
Neurological/sense organ diseases	♂: 16,172	♀: 19,305
Circulatory diseases	♂: 10,359	♀: 12,902
Respiratory diseases	♂: 24,708	♀: 29,563
Digestive diseases	♂: 6,806	♀: 8,229
Genitourinary diseases	♂: 3,657	♀: 15,654
Pregnancy/childbirth/puerperium	♂: 0	♀: 1,467
Skin/subcutaneous diseases	♂: 12,653	♀: 15,817
Musculoskeletal/connective tissue	♂: 13,736	♀: 18,120
Congenital anomalies	♂: 472	♀: 444
Perinatal conditions	♂: 59	♀: 86
Symptoms/signs/ill-defined	♂: 25,719	♀: 38,373
Injury and poisoning	♂: 13,810	♀: 12,605

Time and the consultation ►*Does heavy demand produce short consultations, or do short consultations produce heavy demand by failing to meet patients' needs?* GPs' average consultation time is ~7mins (with some consultations lasting ~½h). This seems vey short, but remember that over a yearthe average time spent with each patient is nearer one hour. The consultation time influences the degree of patient satisfaction,[2] and may influence the consultation rate (2.5–6/patient/yr), with lower return visit rates for longer consultations, (not shown in all studies)[3], and lower rates of prescription issue (especially antibiotics), and more preventive activities occurring. Mean face-to-face consultation time is 8min for 10min appointments but only 9.2min for 15min appointments suggesting extra time may not be well used by doctors when booking interval exceeds 10min.[3] Running late is stressful for doctors[3] (and patients): it is easier keeping to time for 10min (rather than shorter) bookings. (Why have appointments at all, since balloted patients prefer non-appointments, and, although they reduce waiting times, exasperation is increased as appointments foster high expectations?)
Other factors which increase (↑) or decrease (↓) consultation rates:

- List size (↑,↓), and having personal lists (↓ by 7%).
- Not prescribing for minor ailments—see p 458 (?↓)
- New patients (first year), and patients over 65yrs (↑).
- Time of year (epidemics), geography, and social setting (↓,↑).
- If the GP is extrovert he recalls more, and his rate is higher than others (eg 6/yr *vs* 2/yr). GP age and sex also influences rates.
- High latitudes—within UK (↑). The South-East has lowest rates.
- Social deprivation (↑) and morbidity (↑). Rates fell in the 1960s–70s, perhaps because the burden of respiratory disease lessened.
- Preventive activities (↑). Non-attenders are now invited to clinics.

There is good evidence for the Howie hypothesis that average time of consultations is a valid and measurable marker of quality of care.[2] ►See p 459.

1 N Pearson 1996 BMJ i 1517 2 *Anna Karénina* by Leo Tolstoy starts: 'All happy families resemble one another, but each unhappy family is unhappy in its own way...' 2 PJ Howie 1997 RCGP *Occasional Paper* 75

Classification and the James Read codes

The problem: my secretary in Worthing wants to find out from your secretary in Bali whether you are seeing more people with myocardial infarction this year compared with last year. She looks through your cherished manual system and does not find very much, because you usually code myocardial infarction as MI, or coronary thrombosis, or acute MI, or acute coronary insufficiency. She concludes that myocardial infarction is very rare in Bali, and advises all her friends to move there at once. How can a mass exodus be prevented? The first step is to produce a database of *preferred terms* (MI=G32) and their *true synonyms* (a dash followed by a synonym code, eg G30–2), along with *misnomers, obsolete terms* (asterisked in Read 3.1) and *homonyms*—whose meaning depends on context—eg 'section', which is legal to psychiatrists, uterine to obstetricians, and frozen to pathologists.

A system which aims to code general practice must be: *comprehensive, computerized, hierarchical, cross-referenced, dynamic*, and *multi-axial*.

Comprehensive

History/symptoms	Operative procedures	Education
Examination/signs	Drugs and appliances	Administration
Diagnosis	Psychotherapy	Health status facts
Diagnostic procedures	Physical treatments	Occupation/social milieu
Preventive procedures	Alternative therapy	Diagnostic related groups
	Other treatments	Natural language usage

It must facilitate transfer of information between primary, secondary, and tertiary care, and be easy to use by clinical staff, researchers and planners.

Hierarchical Read uses stepwise ranking of classes into subclasses so that it is easy to quantify all operations (7. . . .), all appendix operations (770. .), and all emergency excisions of a normal appendix (77002). There is a *concept* (operations), *subclasses* of this, and a *terminal class*. The code is *alphanumeric* (0–9; A–Z; a–z—with i and o excluded to avoid confusion with I and 0, so there are 58 options at each junction in each of the 5 levels of code hierarchy). So there are 656,356,768 (58^5) codes available (enough for all diseases but not for every symptom cluster), and all descriptions are reduced to 5 easily stored and retrieved digits or letters.

Dynamic 656,356,768 codes offers enough *redundancy* to accommodate new ideas. Our own synaptic connexity confers *unlimited* redundancy. This book has 2 kinds of *limited* redundancy: the blank pages offer a strictly limited redundancy, so that a few new ideas can be accommodated in the right place, and a less strictly limited redundancy is provided by the addition of new pages in the wrong place at the end of the text. The Read codes are limited in theory, but in practice almost infinitely expandable (ie dynamic).

Cross-referenced Read codes aim to be superset of all common classificatory systems (ICD-9; ICD-9-CM; ICD-10; OPCS-4, CPT-4, *BNF*), and at least as detailed as any, and to be compatible with them all. *Internal mapping* allows automatic grouping of DRGs (diagnostic related groups) from clinical data.

Multi-axial Read *v*3.1 is partly multi-axial in that each code remains a unique identifier but no longer acts as a fixed address within a branching hierarchy. Relational database techniques are used, so that meningococcal meningitis appears as a subset both of bacterial meningitis, and of meningococcal disease. There exist core terms with any number of linked near-synonyms, and linked qualifiers, such as *Right/Left*, or *Severe/Mild*.

So, despite conceptual flaws, and practical limitations and omissions, Read codes are becoming *the* standard for data recording and exchange.

The consultation

'The essential unit of medical practice is the occasion when in the intimacy of the consulting room or the sick room, a person who is ill, or believes himself to be ill, seeks the advice of a doctor whom he trusts. This is a consultation and all else in medicine derives from it.' When medical errors occur, the reason usually lies in a failure of some process of the consultation. We must acquire flair for telling which part of which model is vital at any time, so that in busy surgeries with urgent visits mounting up, both the doctor and his or her patients can survive.

A medical model This is a way of describing what happens in a consultation in purely medical terms: History → examination → investigation → diagnosis → treatment → follow-up.

A task-orientated model[2] This comprises 7 stages:

1 Define the reasons for the patient's attendance in social, psychological, and physical dimensions. Elucidate the nature, history, cause, and effects of the stated problems, along with the patient's ideas, concerns and expectations.
2 Consider other problems and at-risk factors (eg smoking).
3 Choose appropriate action (or inaction) for each problem.
4 Share understanding of the problems with the patient.
5 Involve the patient in his own management, and encourage him to accept responsibilty for promoting his own health.
6 Use time and resources appropriately.
7 Establish or consolidate a good relationship with the patient.

How to achieve these aims is not stated. Presumably healing is amenable to analysis, but such analyses have yet to be propounded.

The problem-solving model Problem stated → problem examined → problem defined → problem agreed. Solutions generated → solutions examined → solutions selected → solutions agreed.

The Stott and Davis model[3]

Management of the presenting problems	Modification of help-seeking behaviour
Management of continuing problems	Opportunistic health promotion

A hypothesis-testing model Information is collected and its validity is ascertained by generating and testing hypotheses.

Goal models (ie ends matter, not means) Aim to:

- Cure; comfort; calm; counsel; prevent; anticipate; explain.
- Enable the patient to put himself back in control of his life.
- Manipulate society to the patient's advantage.
- Facilitate change where change is what the patient desires.
- Increase patients' stature—by tapping the sources of richness in their lives, so freeing them from the shadow of insoluble problems.

In consultations that are going wrong, ask yourself:[4]
'Am I granting as much space to the patient's agenda as to mine?'
'Have I discovered his hopes and expectations—and his fears?'
'Am I negotiating openly with the patient over our clashing ideas?'
'What are my feelings, and how can they be used positively?'
Try saying: 'Things aren't going very well. Can we start again?'

1 J Spence 1960 *The Purpose & Practice of Medicine*, OUP 2 D Pendleton 1983 *Doctor Patient Communication*, Academic Press 3 *J Roy Col Gen Pr* 1979 **29** 201 4 J Middleton 1989 *J Roy Col Gen Pr* **39** 383

Unconscious consultations and decision analysis

We do not refer here to those consultations, after a night call, when patients fail to register *at all* in our consciouness—the *automatic stimulus-and-response medicine* whereby a patient offers their upper arm, and we unconsciously respond by applying the sphygmomanometer cuff—or, sometimes getting it wrong, to our later consternation, when we have to explain why we gave a tetanus injection, rather than the expected blood pressure check.

What we want to examine here is that mental set and 'perceptual filter' which determines the outcome of consultations. When decision-analysts first started work observing consultations they were amazed at the number of decisions per minute, and the wide range of possible outcomes, such as 'no action—see again next week' or 'blue-light ambulance trip direct to tertiary referral centre' or 'refer to nurse for ECG' or 'prescribe X, Y, and Z, and stop Q in a week if the blood-level is such-and-such'. The average decision-analyst is disorientated by the sheer pace and apparent effortlessness of these decisions—so much so that doctors were often suspected of choosing these outcomes almost randomly, until the idea of a 'perceptual filter' was developed.

The perceptual filter[1] This is the internal architecture of our mind—unique to each doctor—into which we receive the patient's history. It comprises:

- Our unconscious mental set (*tired/uninterested* to *alert, engaged, responsive*).
- Our entire education, from school to last night's postgraduate lecture.
- The sum of all our encounters with patients. Ignore the fact that we can recall very few of these: this does not stop them influencing us strongly: does the rock recall each of those many, many waves which have sculpted it into extraordinary shapes, or which have entirely worn it away?
- Our past specific, personal experience with this particular patient.
- Our past specific, personal experience with the disease(s) in question.
- Non-personal *subjective* (eg 'endocarditis is the most dangerous and stealthy disease we know. . .') or *objective* ideas (eg evidence-based medicine, p 433).

The mind's working space—its random access memory (RAM)[2] The perceptual filter achieves nothing on its own. What is needed is: interpretation, rearrangement, comparison, and planning of executive action. ▶ *The abilities of our mental working space are determined by the number of items of data that can be integrated into a decision.* There is evidence[3] that this vital number is, for us, if not for computers, ~3 to 8 (this is the number of factors that can be considered *simultaneously*: like a juggler, you may have a hundred balls, but you can only keep 8 in the air at once). So, in trying to decide whether to start antidepressants, I might weigh the depression's severity (eg early waking with poor appetite and concentration), the patient's past omnivorous attitude to her pills (3 past overdoses), her expectations about treatment, the disadvantages of remaining depressed (eg child abuse), and knowledge that beating depression is a UK 'Health of the Nation' target. There may be just room enough in my 'RAM' to take in to account evidence-based medicine on whether SSRIs (p 341) are likely to lead to deaths from overdose. The interesting experimental point here is that if we overload our 'RAM' in the consultation by recourse to a drawer full of guidelines, or unfiltered information—eg looking things up in an unstructured textbook, performance may decline.[3]

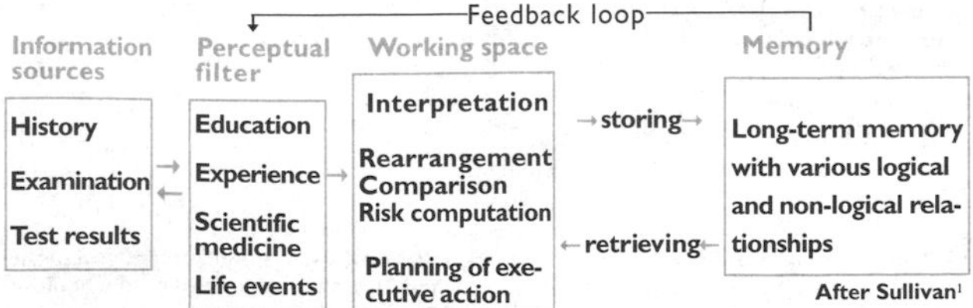

After Sullivan[1]

1 F Sullivan 1996 *Lancet* **348** 841 2 A Johnstone *Int J Sci Ed* **15** 663 3 C Vleuten 1995 *Lancet* **345** 1032

Consultation analysis

It is a sad fact that we lose some of our innate skills in communicating while at medical school. Consultation analysis aims to revive and extend this art, and we known it brings permanent improvement in those who participate. But do not conclude from this that research into the perceptible surface of behaviour can ever fully show us what is happening in the consultation.[1,2]

Methods The first step is to gain the patient's consent. The method which gives the most information and the most scope for learning employs an observer/director sitting behind a 2-way mirror, who can pass verbal instructions to the doctor through an earphone which is worn unobtrusively. The activity is videotaped for later analysis. By directing the verbal and non-verbal behaviour, the observer can demonstrate the potential of a consultation in ways that the doctor may not have imagined possible. Other methods include simple videotaping, audiotaping, and joint consultations, in which the second doctor either participates in or observes the first doctor's consultations.

Consultation analysis is likely to be a somewhat threatening activity, so rules have been evolved to minimize this.[3] For example, facts are discussed before opinions, the consulting doctor says what he did well, and then the group discusses what he did well. Then the consulting doctor says what he thinks he could have done better, and finally the group says what he could have done better. In practice, these constraints are occasionally stultifying, but it is better to be stultified than hurt.

Mapping the consultation and scoring its effectiveness In the consultation mapped below, the patient's inferior myocardial infarction (sudden chest pains on swallowing hot fluids) was mistaken by the doctor (JML) for indigestion, illustrating that there is no point in being a good communicator if you communicate the wrong message. It also shows how misleading it is to add the scores (50/84, but the patient nearly died).

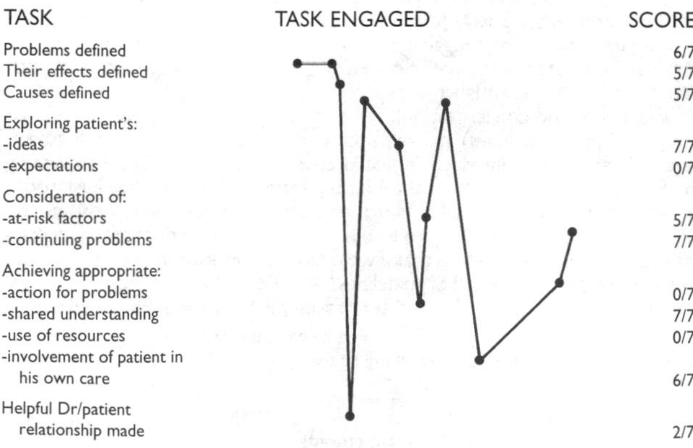

1 J Skelton 1999 *Lancet* **353** 108. This paper uses concordances of serial consultations to investigate such things as the play of power in doctor/patient relationships, and shows that the old schools of behaviour-based and meaning-based analysis need not be mutually antagonistic. **2** N Chomsky 1965 *Aspects of the Theory of Syntax*, Cambridge. **3** D Pendleton 1984 *The Consultation*, OUP

On the impossibility of being a good a doctor

Here is a list of some of the things pundits tell us we should be doing when we meet patients[1,2] (don't get depressed yet: we promise there *is* a solution to prevent any mounting feelings of inadequacy):

1 Listen to the history without interrupting or taking control of the agenda (how often are we guilty of indicating to the patient: "don't talk to me when I am interrupting you?").
2 Examine the patient thoroughly (a nonsensical idea, or at least, so it would seem to the average patient with sciatica when you ask them to name the parts of a clock, or to pronounce "The British Constitution").
3 Arrange cost-effective investigation (via a trip to the library if needed).
4 Formulate a differential diagnosis in social, psychological, and physical terms (a famous triad, no doubt, but why exclude spiritual, allegorical, materialistic, metaphysical and poetic dimensions of the consultation?).
5 Explain the diagnosis to the patient in simple terms (then re-explain it all to relatives waiting anxiously outside, and then try re-explaining it to the computer in terms *it* understands—ie 5-digit Read codes, p 421).
6 Consider additional problems and risk-factors for promoting health.
7 List all the treatment options, and seek out relevant systematic reviews, guidelines, clinical trials etc (evidence-based bedside medicine).
8 Incorporate the patient's view on the balance of risks and benefits, harmonizing his view of priorities, with your own assessment of urgency.
9 Arrange follow-up and communicate with all of the healthcare team.
10 Arrange for the purchase of all necessary care, weighing up cost implications both for your other patients and the whole community, being prepared to be held accountable for your actions and inactions, and for the efficient use of resources—with recourse to justifications based on explicit criteria, and the principles of autonomy, non-maleficence, beneficence and distributive justice.

The alternative Look the patient in the eye. Look the disease in the eye, and then do you best.

The synthesis The alternative looks promising—even attractive, when compared to the ten impossibilities above. But note that the alternative only looks attractive because it is vague. "Do your best" is not very helpful advice—and once we start unpacking this "best" we start to get a list like the ten impossibilities. So. . . the answer is to rejoice in the fact that we are members of a profession where top marks go to the person who knows what *should* be done, not simply what *can* be done. In other words, we can rely on our own instinctive flair and judgement to decide which, if any, of the ten impossibilities we should address in any given consultation.[3] What we cannot leave to our own instinct is the furnishing of our mind so that, should the need arise, we are *equally confident* in negotiating our way around *any* of the ten obstacles above.

1 Stott & Davis *J Roy Col Gen Prac* 1979 **29** 201 2 T Greenhalgh 1996 BMJ **ii** 957 3 Professor Cottard's approach in M Proust *Rememberance of Things Past*, vol 1 page 536 (Chatto & Windus, 1[e])

Prevention

▶In all disease the goal is prevention. This is not to say that preventive activities are without side-effects. Classification: preventing a disease (eg by vaccination) is *primary prevention*. Controlling disease in an early form (eg carcinoma *in situ*) is *secondary prevention*. Preventing complications in those already symptomatic is *tertiary prevention*.

Prevention through the human life cycle Pre-conception (p 94). Is she using folic acid supplements? Is she rubella immune? If not, vaccinate (p 214—ensure effective contraception for 3 months after vaccination. Is she diabetic? If so, optimize glycaemic control as early as possible (p 156).

The child: Vaccination (p 208); safety lessons; developmental tests (p 288).

Preventing myocardial infarction: Cigarette smoking trebles the risk above the rate for men who have never smoked. A systolic BP >148mmHg (40% of men) doubles the risk, and if the serum cholesterol is in the top fifth of the observed range, the risk trebles. Helping to stop smoking, and treating marked arterial hypertension (*OHCM* p 302) and hyperlipidaemia (*OHCM* p 566) are the chief interventions (p 452). In America, intensive dietary advice is recommended for those in the top ¼ of the distribution of cholesterol values (this would include 50% of all British men), using drugs for those in the top 10th who do not respond to diet alone. The UK government recommends reductions in total fat and saturated fat to 35% and 15%, respectively, of total energy. GPs and practice nurses have a central rôle in preventing cardiac deaths, eg by identifying and reducing risks in young, first degree relatives of those who have had early coronary events (<50yrs), screening for hypertension, and encouraging less smoking. The fact that the optimum diet for reducing mortality has yet to be declared does not justify inaction with regard to the above preventative measures.

Preventing deaths from breast cancer: Education and self-examination. Well-woman clinics. Mammography (using negligible radiation)—cancer pick-up rate: 5 per 1000 'healthy' women screened. Yearly 2-view mammograms in postmenopausal women might reduce mortality by 40%—but the price is the serious but needless alarm caused: there are ~10 false +ve mammograms for each true +ve result. The UK national health service offers 3-yearly single views to those between 55 and 64 years old (older women may be screened if they want, but are not sent for).

Prevention in the reproductive years (p 432): Safer sex education starting in adolescence (teaching to use condoms need not increase rates of sexual activity[1]); family planning (p 60–8), antenatal/prenatal care (p 94, eg folic acid), screening for cervical cancer (p 34), blood pressure, rubella serology.

Preventing oxidative damage by free radicals:[1] Antioxidants such as vitamins E and C, carotenoids, flavenoids, and selenium (*OHCM* p 644) are found in diets rich in fruits, vegetables, grains, and nuts—and are thought to protect from cardiovascular diseases (*OHCM* p 277: free radical action on LDL is central to atherogenesis), diabetes mellitus, cancer, and Alzheimer's disease (see p 352 for the effects of ginkgo biloba—extracted from the maidenhair tree).[2]

Old age and prevention: 'Keep fit', pre-retirement lessons, bereavement counselling visits from the health visitor may help in preventing disease. HRT (p18) also has a central rôle. But the main aim is to adopt the measures outlined above to ensure that there is an old age in which to prevent disease.

Side-effects No intervention is without possible side-effects (eg those of antihypertensives), and when carried out in large populations the problems may outweigh the benefits.

Smoking and prevention: p 452. Seat belts and prevention: p 678. For a fuller list of preventable conditions, see p 411.

1 *Lancet* **349** 1997 1189 2 P Le Bars 1998 *E-BM* **2** 80

5. General practice

Barriers to prevention

Cognitive barriers (See opposite.) When, if ever, we contemplate cataclysmic, but preventable, ill health in ourselves, we may either believe that '*It won't happen to me*' or we deliberately dare fate to *make* it happen to us. To some people, over-zealous and sanctimonious-sounding hectoring from bodies such as the UK Health Education Authority creates barriers to prevention, inciting anger and rejection by those who resent their taxes being spent by some State Nanny who assumes that all her charges are 'backward 5-year-olds' who cannot be trusted to think for themselves.[1] So people are now proud to announce that '. . . I eat everything, as much butter and fried foods as I can get. . . I smoke 40–60 cigarettes a day. . . To eat cornflakes, you've got to have sugar on them, and lots of cream, otherwise there is no point in eating them. . . As long as you keep smoking cigarettes, and drink plenty of whisky, you'll go on for ever.'

Psychological barriers All of us at times are prone to promote our own destruction as keenly as we promote our own survival. Knowing that alcohol may bring about our own destruction gives the substance a certain appeal, when we are in certain frames of mind—particularly if we do not know the sordid details of what death by alcohol entails. It provides an alluring means of escape without entailing too headlong a rush into the seductive arms of death. Gambling and taking risks is all part of this ethos.

Logistic barriers A general practice needs to be highly organized to be in a state of perpetual readiness to answer questions like 'Who has not had their blood pressure checked for 5 years'? or 'Who has not turned up to their request to attend for screening'? or 'Who has stopped sending in for their repeat prescriptions for antihypertensives?' On a different front, providing a sequence of working fridges in the distribution of vaccines to rural tropical areas poses major logistic problems.

Political barriers It is not unknown for governments to back out silently of preventive obligations as if influenced by pressure groups who would lose if prevention were successful. Some countries are keener to buy tanks than vaccines.

Ethical barriers If child benefits were available only to those children who had had whooping cough vaccine, much whooping cough would be prevented. This approach is not popular.

Financial barriers A practice may have to pay for extra staff to run an effective screening programme. Coronary artery bypass grafts may prevent some consequences of ischaemic heart disease, but they are too expensive to use on everybody whom they might benefit.

Motivation barriers As we rush out of morning surgery to attend the latest 'coronary' we use up energy which might have been spent on studying patients' notes in the evening to screen to prevent the next one. Changing from a crisis-led work pattern to strategic prevention is one way that practice nurses can lead the way. There is some evidence that they are particularly successful at the meticulous, repetitive tasks on which all good prevention depends.

1 B Levin & P Barthrop 1990 *The Times* 11/8/90 page 10 column 3

Metaphysics at the bedside—and the world's worst patient

We often find ourselves sitting on beds trying to persuade wayward people to courses of preventive action which will clearly benefit them, usually at some distant time in the future. We think this very clarity should be enough to persuade the person to act. But, as we dismally stamp our feet on the bare boards of our impatience, we resign ourselves to the fact that action will not follow. Why is this so often the case?

The first person to know the answer to this question was the world's worst patient and our own greatest poet: great not because of his mastery of his world, but because, as the world used him, often cruelly, and as his London doctors gave him up as a hopeless addict, he took on all our petty confusions and made them human, compelling, and universal. Samuel Taylor Coleridge answers our question in this way:

'To love our future Self is almost as hard as to love our Neighbour—it is indeed only a difference of Space & Time. My Neighbour is my other Self, 'othered' by Space—my old age is to my youth and other Self, 'othered' by Time...' See *Coleridge* ii p225, R Holmes

By being consumed by the fires of his addictions this poor poet became the burning wick in the lamp we now use to illuminate our patients' frailties.

Screening

This entails systematic testing of a population, or a sub-group for signs of illness—which may be of established disease (pre-symptomatic, eg small breast cancers), or symptomatic (eg unreported hearing loss in the elderly).

Modified Wilson criteria for screening (1–10 spells iatrogenic):

1. The condition screened for should be an important one.
2. There should be an acceptable treatment for the disease.
3. Diagnostic and treatment facilities should be available.
4. A recognizable latent or early symptomatic stage is required.
5. Opinions on who to treat as patients must be agreed.
6. The test must be of *high discriminatory power* (see below), *valid* (measuring what it purports to measure, not surrogate markers which might not correlate with reality) and be *reproducible*—with safety guaranteed.
7. The examination must be acceptable to the patient.
8. The untreated natural history of the disease must be known.
9. A simple inexpensive test should be all that is required.
10. Screening must be continuous (ie not a 'one-off' affair).

Summary: screening tests must be cost-effective.

Informed consent: Rees' rule Before offering screening, there is a duty to quantify for patients their chance of being disadvantaged by it—from anxiety (may be devastating, eg while waiting for a false +ve result to be sorted out) and the effects of subsequent tests (eg bleeding after biopsy following an abnormal cervical smear), as well as the chances of benefit.

Comparing a test with some 'gold standard'		Patients with condition	Patients without condition
TEST RESULT	Subjects appear to have the condition	True +ve (a)	False +ve (b)
	Subjects appear not to have condition	False –ve (c)	True –ve (d)

Sensitivity: How reliably is the test +ve in the disease? a/a+c
Specificity: How reliably is the test –ve in health? d/d+b

Examples of effective screening	**Unproven/ineffective screening***
Cervical smears (if >20yrs, p 34)	Mental test score (dementia, p 352)
Mammography (after menopause)	Urine tests (diabetes; kidney disease)
Finding smokers (+quitting advice)	Antenatal procedures (p 95)
Looking for malignant hypertension	Elderly visiting to detect disease

Why screen in general practice? If screening is to be done at all, it makes economic sense to do it in general practice. In the UK ≥1 million people see GPs each weekday, providing great facilities for 'case-finding' (90% of patients consult over a 5-yr period). Provided the GP's records are adequate, the remaining 10% may then be sent appointments to attend for special screening sessions—eg at the well-woman clinic (p 432). Private clinics do limited work, eg in screening for cervical cancer, but there is no evidence that their multiphasic biochemical analyses are effective procedures.

*There is evidence that some screening causes morbidity (mortality-awareness and hypochondriasis↑)—so why is screening promulgated? One reason is that it is easier for governments to be optimistic than to be rigorous.

Problems with screening

All these have affected UK screening programmes, reducing their benefit.

1 Those most at risk do not present for screening, thus increasing the gap between the healthy and the unhealthy—the *inverse care law*.
2 The 'worried well' overload services by seeking repeat screening.
3 Services for investigating those testing positive are inadequate.
4 Those who are false positives suffer stress while awaiting investigation, and remain anxious about their health despite reassurance.
5 A negative result may be regarded as a licence to take risks.
6 True positives, though treated, may begin to see themselves as of lower worth than hitherto.

►Remember: with some screening programmes of dubious value, *it may be healthier not to know*: see *OHCM* p 654.

General practitioner and shared-care clinics

Examples of mini-clinics which are conducted in general practice

- Well-woman/well-man clinic
- Elderly 'non-attending' patients
- Giving-up-smoking clinic (p 452)
- Joint outreach clinics with a consultant who shares care (eg orthopaedics)
- Antenatal clinic
- Hypertension clinic
- Citizen's advice clinic
- Diabetes mellitus clinic
- Asthma clinic

Advantages of mini-clinics

- Easy to keep to management protocol
- Check-lists prevent omissions
- Co-operation cards allow shared care
- Flow-charts to identify trends
- Help from specialist practice nurse
- Fewer referrals to outpatients (↓by 20%)
- Better co-operation with hospitals
- GPs can improve their clinical skills[1]
- Focused dialogue with on-site specialist *does* improve treatment and referrals[1]

Disadvantages

- Extra time needed
- Extra training needed
- Not holistic
- Not flexible
- Value often unproven
- Access to hospital technology↓
- Travelling time by consultants to outreach clinics is wasteful

It is likely that starting a clinic is a good (but not the only) method of implementing the advantages above. The main disadvantage is the temptation for doctors to manage the disease, and to forget about the patient who suffers it: 'I've had enough, doctor. I want to kill myself.' 'Yes, well, your blood sugar is not too bad. Any spells of hypoglycaemia recently?'

Some activities in a well-woman clinic

- Cervical smear and breast examination
- Breast examination/mammography
- Pre-conception counselling (p 94)
- Antenatal and postnatal care
- Rubella and tetanus* vaccination
- Smoking and alcohol advice*
- Safer sex advice for HIV*
- Family planning/sterilization*
- Diet and weight* (OHCM p 490)
- Blood pressure*
- Discussion of HRT issues

Breast examination and teaching breast self-examination in well-woman clinics

There is disagreement about whether this is desirable, and, if so, whether we can delegate this to nurses. Some (but not all) studies report that cancers in those having this protocol are detected earlier, with improved survival curves, compared with mammography alone.[2] But UK DoH advice is against breast palpation in asymptomatic women, even if on the Pill or HRT.[3] *Data Sheets* are bound to be cautious, and they *do* recommend such examinations. The DoH says breast examinations should not be delegated to nurses, but in some practices it may *only* be nurses whom women find acceptable—and doctors are frequently too busy: so validating nurse training is a key issue.

Well-men It is paradoxical that well-woman clinics are more popular than well-man clinics, since women live longer than men and are more frequent attenders at the surgery (where they make ideal candidates for opportunistic screening). Nurses can do all the well-woman activities *starred above in well-man clinics. One such clinic yielded ≥25% obese; 14% with sustained diastolic BP ≥100mmHg; 66% needing tetanus vaccination; and 29% needing smoking advice. See the OXCHECK study, p 439.

A diabetic mini-clinic ►*Education is the single most important activity.* The GP and the patients educate each other. Advantages over hospital clinics: the patient sees the same doctor every time; weekly (or more frequent) appointments are possible during periods of difficult control; telephone advice is easily available. Mini-clinics are cheaper than outpatient clinics. Even young insulin-dependent diabetics can be managed *wholly* in the mini-clinic from the time of presentation (with extra appointments, as necessary) provided there is no overt ketoacidosis. There are dangers in adhering too closely to protocols (p 434). However, the vital test is retinal photography or dilating the pupil for fundoscopy (p 476 & p 508). The other important areas are diet, blood pressure control, smoking advice and round-the-clock blood glucose monitoring, with checks on U&E and Hb_{A1c}.
Liaison with community based consultant-services: May prevent hospital admission.

1 W Vierhout 1995 *Lancet* **346** 990 2 Y Kokoe 1998 *Onc Rep* **5** 151 3 Chief Med. Officer 1998 *Update* **18** 6

Evidence-based medicine (E-BM)[1]

This is the conscientious and judicious use of current best evidence from clinical care research in the management of individual patients.

The problem 2,000,000 papers are published each year. Patients may benefit directly from a tiny fraction of these papers. How do we find them?

A partial solution 50 journals are scanned not by experts in neonatal nephrology or the left nostril, but by searchers trained to spot papers which have a direct message for practice, and meet predefined criteria of rigour (below). Summaries are then published in *Evidence-based Medicine*.[2]
Questions used to evaluate papers: **1** Are the results *valid*? (Randomized? Blinded? Were all patients accounted for who entered the trial? Was follow-up complete? Were the groups similar at the start? Were the groups treated equally, apart from the experimental intervention?) **2** What *are* the results? (How large was the treatment effect? How precise was the treatment effect?) **3** Will the results help *my* patients (cost–benefit sum).[1]

Problems with the solution *The concept of scientific rigour is opaque.* What do we want? The science, the rigour, the truth, or what will be most useful to our patients? These may overlap, but they are not the same.

- Will the best be the enemy of the good? Are useful papers rejected due to some blemish? Answer: *all* evidence needs appraising (often impossible!).
- By reformulating patients in terms of answerable questions, E-BM risks missing the point of the patient's consultation. He might simply want to express his fears, rather than be used as a substrate for an intellectual exercise.
- Is the standard the same for the evidence for *all* changes to our practice? For example, we might want to avoid prescribing drug X for constipation if there is the slimmest chance that it might cause colon cancer. There are many other drugs to choose from. We might require far more robust evidence than a remote chance to persuade us to do something rather counter-intuitive, such as giving heparin in DIC. How robust does the data need to be? There is no science to tell us the answer to this: we decide off the top of our head (albeit a wise head, we hope).
- EBM is a lucky dip if gathering *all* the evidence on a topic proves impossible.[3]
- What about letters columns? It may be years before fatal flaws are aired.
- There is a danger that by always asking 'What is the evidence...' we will divert resources from hard-to-prove activities (which may be very valuable) to easy-to-prove services. An example might be physiotherapy for cerebral palsy. The unique personal attributes of the therapist may be as important as the objective regimen: she is impossible to quantify. It is a much easier management decision to transfer resources to some easy-to-quantify activity, eg neonatal screening for cystic fibrosis.
- Evidence-based medicine can never be always up to date. Reworking meta-analyses in the light of new trials takes time—if it is ever done at all.

Advantages of evidence-based medicine
- It improves our reading habits.
- It leads us to ask questions, and then to be sceptical of the answers.
- As taxpayers, we should like it (wasteful practices can be abandoned).
- Evidence-based medicine presupposes that we keep up to date, and makes it worthwhile to take trips around the perimeter of our knowledge.
- Evidence-based medicine opens decision-making processes to patients.

Conclusion There is little doubt that, *where available*, evidence-based medicine can be better than what it is superseding. It may not have as much impact as we hope, as gaining unimpeachable evidence is time-consuming and expensive, and perhaps impossible. Despite these caveats, evidence-based medicine is one of the most exciting recent medical developments. Let's all join in by subscribing to ideals and its journal.

1 F Davidoff 1995 BMJ **i** 1085 and W Rosenberg 1995 BMJ **i** 1122 & **ii** 259 **2** *Evidence-based Medicine* BMA, Journal dept, PO box 299, London tel. 0171 383 6270. See L Ridsdale *Evidence-based General Practice:*, ISBN 0 7020 1611 X & A Miles 1995 *Effective Clinical Practice*, Blackwell **3** R Horton 1999 *Lancet* **353** 164

Protocols and guidelines

► Freedom from only doing ordained tasks is essential for mental health.
► Beware accepting even the most enticing protocol without asking yourself if it will affect your sympathy at the bedside. Other questions:

- Has the protocol been *evaluated* by someone who is not its author?
- What is its *objective* (cost-containment, conformity, or care-enhancement?).

Sympathy is a delicate flower which has often withered before the end of morning surgery; it is also the elusive harmony which makes clinical medicine hum. If your new protocol says that you must do 10 things to Mrs James who happens to have diabetes, both of you may become inconsolably irritated by item 5: the doctor is running out time, and the patient is running out of goodwill. She is really worrying about her husband's dementia, having long-since stopped worrying about her own illnesses. She does not really mind being assailed by lights, forks, stix and lancets, if this is the price that must be paid for a portion of her doctor's sympathy. But if she finds that this sympathy has withered, who knows what her feelings may be, and how she will view her doctor?

Guidelines are perceived as friendly, if flexible[1] and allowing for the frailties of clinical science as it meets reality at the bedside; they can also be interactive, if instituted in a computerized record during the consultation.[1] Protocols, particularly if they have been handed down from some supposedly higher authority, have a reputation for being strict, sinister, and ultimately stultifying instruments for thought-control. How well do these stereotypes stand up in practice? It is known that doctors working in highly regulated environments with strict protocols perform suboptimally.[2,3,4] It is also worth noting that very few laws are flexible: those which are, are dangerous because they invite abuse. (All men are equal, but. . .). But what laws *can* do is to state when they do not apply. This does not necessarily make them mere guidelines. You could say, for example, that patients have a right to be asked if they want to participate in a protocol, and if they do, that it should be done properly. But what if it is the child's birthday today, and he really does not want to have his finger pricked for a blood glucose test, but he is most willing to go along with all other aspects of a protocol? If you are flexible, the price may be ketoacidosis after the party. Herein lies the central paradox of protocols. They are designed to remove the many indefensible inconsistencies found in clinical medicine, yet the protocols depend on the individual doctor's own flair and instinctive judgement to be applied in the best way.

Perhaps the best approach is to welcome the good protocols, and develop some sort of meta-protocol which should be answered whenever (or almost whenever) such protocols are not adhered to. Why did you not adhere to the protocol? Please tick the appropriate box. ❑My own convenience. ❑The patient's stated wish. ❑The patient's stated wish after being given full information. ❑The protocol is contraindicated in this case because my instinctive flair and judgement tells me so.

In conclusion, each protocol should come with a comment on the likely effect on the doctor's sympathy; how often, on average, one would expect the protocol not to be adhered to; and what resources and time will be required to implement the protocol and its matching meta-protocol. There should also be a statement about each element of the protocol, and just what benefit it is likely to confer—not on the ideal patient, but on the ones likely to be found in the population being offered the protocol. If a protocol does not come with these safety features, beware it, unless, that is, you have invented it yourself—for your own protocols will always have a special status, being infallible, ingenious and innocuous.

1 C Watkins 1999 BJGP **49** 11 & I Purves 1992 BMJ **ii** 1364 **2** T O'Dowd 1991 BMJ **ii** 450 **3** S Shortell 1988 NEJM **318** 1100 **4** A Nicoll 1986 *Lancet* **i** 606 3 See *Clinical Guidelines* RCGP Occasional P 58 1992, J Grimshaw 1993 *Lancet* **342** 1317 & Clinical Resource & Audit Group 1993 *Clinical Guidelines*, Scottish Office

The placebo effect

Placebo effects are very powerful and are important not just in research, but also in demonstrating to us how our demeanour may be just as important as the drugs we give. It is often said that if two obstetric units (for instance) do things quite differently (eg for or against artificial rupture of the membranes) then if one unit is vindicated by research, the other unit must be wrong. This need not follow—not just because the population served by the 'errant' unit may be different. The errant unit may believe it is a centre of excellence, and its staff may rupture membranes with joy in their hearts, knowing they are fulfilling their destiny as the best obstetric unit bar none. This feeling may communicate itself to labouring mothers, who, due to an interaction between communication, beliefs, cognition, and contractility, have their babies with few complications—so much so, that if the unit went over to the 'correct' method, their results might come to mirror their plummeting self-confidence. (This is an important reason for the failure of imposed protocols which look good on paper: see p 434.) Research in this area is very difficult to do, because you cannot easily control for 'joy in the heart'—but with care it can be systematically analysed: in a placebo-controlled study of antihypertensives the partners of the enthusiastic doctor broke the code, and told him that his experimental treatment appeared similar to existing treatments without telling him who was having the active drug, and who was having the placebo. ►From this point, there was an immediate, marked increase in BP in both groups, although the difference between the drug and the placebo was maintained.[1] What we believe and how we behave really do matter—sometimes more than the drugs we use.

The mechanism for the placebo effect is disputed. It is not the case that there is a 'placebo-responsive' personality. Anxiety reduction is important, and endorphins may play a part.

From the above it should not be assumed that we should give placebos to all our patients, and be enthusiastic about their likely effects. Most of this book is founded on the precept that we should be honest and straightforward with our patients. Nevertheless, it may often be unwise to share too many of our doubts with our patients—as demonstrated by the GP who randomly assigned his consulting style in those with apparently minor illness to a 'positive encounter' or a 'negative encounter'. In the former, patients were given a diagnosis and told they would be better in a few days, the latter group were told that it was not certain what the matter was. Just over ⅓ of the patients having negative encounters got better in 2 weeks, but over ⅔ of the positive group did so.

Nocebo effects Pharmacists are in the habit of 'leafleting' customers with long lists of their drugs' side-effects, which, like Voodoo death, may become self-fulfilling prophesies. When one of the authors (JML) gives diamorphine IV to patients having a myocardial infarction, he says in a loud voice 'Your pain will end now' (maximizes placebo effect)—and, in a very quiet voice to the spouse, 'Get a bowl: he may be sick.'—to avoid the reverse 'nocebo' effect. We tend not to tell patients about side-effects such as impotence, justifying this dishonesty on the grounds that in such a sensitive area, the mere mention of impotence will bring it about. Central to this debate is the question of how paternalistic we should be. We do not know the answer, but simply recommend getting to know individual patients well, and having a flexible approach: in doing so we may occasionally strike the right balance.

1 JA Turner 1994 *JAMA* **271** 1609-13 See also VM Oh 1994 *BMJ* **ii** 69

Ethnic matters

How to avoid offending Western manners This is not just a question of 'please', 'thank you', 'after you', and 'I'd love to. . .' rather than 'I don't mind if I do. . .' with feigned enthusiasm—Westerners are notoriously sensitive to gaze and mutual gaze: not enough, and they think you are shifty; too much, and you are making unwelcome advances; the same goes with interpersonal distance: if you get too close, invasion is threatened.

How to avoid offending Eastern manners •Avoid prolonged eye contact and loud speech—which can indicate lack of respect.
- Control your gesticulations (the 'thumbs up' sign, for example, may be considered very rude).
- Do not expect an Afro-Asian to answer intimate questions, without first explaining about confidentiality.
- A psychiatric referral may destroy eligibility for marriage.

Hindu names •First names are often male and female, but middle names always denote sex. •First (eg Lalita) and middle (eg Devi) names are often written together (Lalitadevi). •When asked his name a Hindu is likely to give only his first 2 names, withholding his family name, to be polite. This can cause great confusion with receptionists, and duplication of notes.

Sikh names Few Sikhs have a family name. Singh and Kaur indicate only sex and religion, so that extra identification is needed on the notes (use the father's or husband's name also).

Muslim names Sometimes the last name is not a family name, and the first name is not the personal name. There may be no shared family name. The first name is often religious (eg Mohammed). Common female second names are Banu, Begum, Bi, Bibi, and Sultana. They are of as little help in identification as the title Ms is in UK names, but because they are given as second names they are often used for filing purposes (so other family members should be entered as well, to give extra identification).

Clinical phenomena •Centile charts make normal Bangladeshi, South Indian and Chinese babies seem small (below 3rd centile).
- Bilateral cervical and inguinal lymphadenopathy may be normal in Asian and African children (or it may indicate TB).
- Genetic diseases may be common, eg glucose-6-phosphate dehydrogenase ↓ (sex-linked recessive), sickle-cell anaemia in Africans and West Indians; haemoglobin E disease in Chinese.
- Unusual malignancies (oesophagus in Japan, tongue from betel nuts).
- The cow is sacred to Hindus—so do not offer beef insulin (or pork insulin to those of Jewish or Islamic religions).
- Some Asians will consider measles to be a curse from the Goddess Mata and will opt for an offering in the temple, rather than a visit to the GP.
- Some Muslims will avoid all alcohol (so do not offer tonics).
- Taking drugs may be a problem for Muslims during Ramadan.

Muslims and death (Muslims are the largest non-christian UK sect).
- Religious observance requires prompt burial, not cremation.
- Washing and shrouding is an important ceremony done by respected elders of the same sex (they should be immunized against Hepatitis B).
- The dead body is sacred, and never abandoned by relatives; so it is rare for undertakers to be involved. The body may be moved in a family van.
- Bereavement lasts for 3 days, during which prayers in the home are said almost continuously. The wife is expected to stay at home for up to 4½ months after death of a spouse. Plain, but not black clothes are worn.
- Shoes are to be taken off before entering the house of the dead.
- Transplantation may be fine for Arab, but not Indian Muslims (the latter may allow corneas; bone marrow does not count as a transplant).

1 AR Gatrad 1994 *BMJ* ii 521

Language, interpretation, and health[1]

Dislocation, globalization, migration, refugee numbers, and war have all conspired to separate doctors and patients linguistically. 90 million people now live outside their country of birth. Heterogeneous populations need heterogeneous methods of health-orientated communication—in many languages. All too often interpreters, if available at all, are only on hand during office hours. Friends and relatives may be available, but confidentiality issues are important. When a child interprets for his mother's mortal illness, many other unknowable issues are raised.

Alternatives include telephone interpretation (ideally with a hands-off conference telephone). Although non-verbal signs are lost, do not underestimate the value of these measures. Whenever needed, ask for these services from Health Authorities—and then the services are more likely to be in place, and the wheels well-oiled when the real emergency arises.

1 Paramjit Gill 1998 BMJ i 1476

Health education

What is education?—four incomplete answers

- Education is the system used for passing down, from one generation to the next, society's values, attitudes, and culture. Thus are crime, duplicity and double standards (and, on a good day, idealism) perpetuated in a kind of cultural inheritance.
- Education is an activity carried out on ignoramuses by people who think they know better.
- Education is about changing people. It usually ends up implying 'change your ways . . . or else.' The most extreme form of education is prison.[1]
- Education performed on one mind by another, under duress, is indoctrination. Indoctrination has its uses. Its value is measured by its propensity to encourage *self-education*, through, for example, travel, reading, or dialogue. Self-education is the food of the mind: the procedure by which we can touch the great minds of the dead and know we are not alone in all our confusions and questionings. By standing on their shoulders we can find a new view of our world—sometimes, even, new worlds to view.

Health education messages To be effective, they must be specific and direct. Eg in getting people to sign on for help for drinking problems, it is of little use saying 'If you don't stop drinking you'll get these diseases. . .' (only ~25% respond); saying 'Signing on is good for you because of these benefits. . .' (~50% respond); saying 'If you don't sign here, you've had it. . .' brings the biggest response. A certain amount of 'fear' in the message is not bad: in enlisting patients for a tetanus vaccine a 'low fear' message gets a 30% response, while a more fear gets a 60%. Optimum messages must be very specific about dates, times and places of help. Too high a level of fear is counter-productive. A gruesome film about the worst effects of caries produces petrified immobility, not self-help or trips to dentists.

The messenger Peers may be better than authority-figures (eg in stop smoking messages). A message about breast feeding will come best from a mother. However, if the issues are not well understood, authority may be helpful (the *BMJ* is more effective than *Woman's Own* in suggesting to mothers that a new formulation of aspirin should not be taken).

Changing attitudes The following paradigm holds sway: **Knowledge → Attitudes → Intentions → Behaviour**. As the Chinese thought reformers knew so well, attitude changes depend on a high level of emotional involvement. In questions of belief, as in so many other questions, emotion trumps reason '. . .*people don't demand that a thing be reasonable if their emotions are touched. Lovers aren't reasonable, are they?*. .'[2] Only resort to applying reason to attitudes if emotions are too hot to handle. NB: the arrows in the model above may be reversed: if our behaviour is inconsistent with our ideas (cognitive dissonance) it is often our ideas, not our behaviour which change.

The health education officer (health authority) These are likely to have a nursing, teaching or health visiting background. They may have a postgraduate diploma in health education. There are ~300 in England and Wales. A team may comprise a technician and a graphic artist, as well as clerical staff. One rôle is to give information and Health Education Authority leaflets. They also liaise with health visitors and the district medical officer, as well as engaging in planning and research.

Examples of health education at work •Education about 'safer sex' and the prevention of AIDS. •Leaflets and tape/slide programmes can (slightly) increase knowledge of breast self-examination (which is associated with smaller tumours and less spread in those presenting with breast cancer).

Health promotion by nurses Nurses are the experts in this field[3]—but even they are not very effective in reducing coronary risk. In the community-based OXCHECK randomized trial (*N*=6124, aged 35–64) serum cholesterol fell by only 0.08–0.2mmol/L—and there was no significant difference in rates of giving up smoking, or in body mass index. Systolic (and diastolic) BP fell by ~2.5% in the intervention group receiving dietary and life-style advice.[4] Blanket health promotion may not be a complete waste of resources, but it is certainly expensive for rather limited gains. Slightly more optimistic results were obtained by the *Family Heart Study Group*[5]

The conclusion may be that energies are best spent on those with highest risk as determined in routine consultations by a few 'simple questions' about smoking, family history, etc. One trouble is that these questions are not always innocuous. It is not necessarily a good thing to bring up 'strokes and heart attacks in the family' in, for example, consultations about tension headaches. OXCHECK is not the last word—and there is some evidence that if lipid-lowering drugs were used very much more extensively, cholesterol (and cardiac events) could fall by up to 30%.

1 P Theroux *Down the Yangtze*, Penguin ISBN 0-14-600032-3, page 35-6 2 Graham Greene 1951 *The End Of the Affair*, page 115, Heinemann 3 JL Curzio 1990 *J Hum Hyperten* 4 665 4 OXCHECK 1994 BMJ i 308 & 1995 BMJ i 1099 5 1994 BMJ i 313

Patient groups

Mother-and-baby groups These are best set up in the first weeks after the birth of four or five babies. The health visitor encourages the group to form. A doctor may attend the group—regularly to start with, then less often as the group becomes self-sufficient. After a year or two a large practice will have a number of groups running. One aim is to increase motivation (through discussion) to enhance the uptake of health education and preventative medicine. Another aim is to ease the stresses involved in becoming a responsible parent by providing a social support network. A mother, noting for the first time her beautiful baby's ability to hate, to destroy and to hurt, may find it a relief to know that other babies are much the same.

Patient participation groups ▶Working *with* your patients is as important as working *for* them. The health care team meets with patients' representatives to discuss some of the following:[1]

- Dealing with complaints (less adversarial than with formal methods).
- Harmonizing the 'consumer's' and the 'provider's' aims.
- Feedback to aid planning, implementation and evaluation of services.
- Identifying unmet needs (eg among the isolated elderly).
- Improving links between the practice and other helpers.
- Health promotion in the light of local beliefs (p 416).
- Pressurizing health authorities over inadequate services.

Owing to lack of interest, or to there being no clear leader or task, up to 25% of groups have closed. The complaint that participation mechanisms lead to tokenism (ie the democratic ideal has been exercised, but what has been created is just a platform for validating the *status quo*) does not turn out to be the case when a patient group has power over funds which it has raised. Here, our experience is that analysis may be penetrating and decision swift, in a way which makes even the best-run health authorities look pedestrian.

The patients' association This group represents and furthers the interests of patients by giving assistance, advice, and information. It aims to promote understanding between patients and the medical world. Publications: Patient Voice and a directory of self-help organizations. See also the *Contact-a-Family* Directory.[2]

Self-help organizations Many thousands of these groups have been set up all over the world for sufferers of specific rare or common diseases. They offer information, companionship, comfort and a life-line to patients and their families, eg for sharing techniques and self-remedies. A danger is that they share nightmares as well, for example, unnecessarily graphic descriptions of their children dying of cystic fibrosis may be spread, causing unneeded despondency. They raise funds for research, providing a 'welcome alternative to the expensive services of professionals'. Full directories exist.[3,4]

Community health councils These are independent monitors of health services. A member may be taken along by a patient to hearings of complaints made against doctors held by health authority service committees.

1 HD Chase 1993 *Br J Gen Prac* **43** 341 2 A Brownlea 1987 *Soc Sci Med* **25** 605 3 CaF Directory 1991 (tel. 0171 383 3555) ISSN 0964 0703 4 Room 33, 18 Charing Cross Road, London WC2H OHR (tel. UK 0171 240 0671)

5. General practice

Dying at home

'We are compelled to admit that our best efforts sometimes fail to keep loved ones on this side of the Jordan. What a great thing it is in such cases as baffle all our skill and defy our every effort, when we can so mitigate suffering as to make the passage a comparatively smooth one.'*

The UK death rate is ~12/1000/yr, or ~30 deaths/GP/yr. 65% die in hospital, 10% die in hospices, public places, or on the street, and 25% die at home. Of these deaths at home over half will be sudden. In the remainder, the GP has a central rôle to play in enabling the patient to die a dignified death in the way that he or she chooses. Pain relief and symptom control are the central preoccupations of death in hospices, where death has already been somewhat medicalized, but in those who choose to die at home there often runs a fierce streak of independence, so that their main aim is to carry on with the activities of normal living—come what may. This may cause distress to relatives who feel that the dying person is putting up with unnecessary pain. An open discussion is often helpful in harmonizing the family's aims. The important step is to find out what a patient wants, and then to enable him to do it, being aware that his aims may change over time. The next step is to find out about his hopes and fears and how they interact with those of the family.

Pain ▶See *OHCM* p 688: *diagnose each pain*. Bone pain will need opiates, ± NSAIDs, eg naproxen 250mg/8h PO pc or prednisolone 5mg/8h PO; pain from constipation responds to laxatives or enemas. Document each pain's response to treatment. Morphine (oral) is given eg every 4h. Strength examples (/5ml): 10mg, 30mg, 100mg. Once the daily dose which controls pain is known, consider giving the same 24h dose as slow release tablets every 12h (eg MST® 5, 10, 15, 30, 60, 100 or 200mg). Take the first MST tablet 4h after the last dose of morphine solution. (Starting dose of MST in children: 200–800µg/kg/12h PO.) If pain breaks through, give extra morphine solution, and ↑MST at the next dose (don't give more than twice daily to avoid pharmacodynamic confusion). If the patient cannot swallow, use diamorphine SC, at ½ the daily oral morphine dose, given eg divided into 4-hourly injections or via a pump. Laxatives ± antiemetics will be needed.

Help •Family •Community nurse •Hospice •Friends/neighbours •Night nurses •GP/health visitor •CRUSE[1] •Pain clinic

Bereavement is the process of adapting to a loss, which is causing sorrow. ***Mourning*** is the active evocation of that loss, which may take a formal, ritualistic and dignified style, or be personal and idiosyncratic. ***Lamentation*** is the vocal outpouring of grief at its cusp, with wailing, lachrymation, or verbal expressions uttered from the depths of despair. ***Grief*** has components of all these, but its defining feature is the sense of irreversible personal loss. ▶*There is in this world in which everything wears out, everything perishes, one thing that crumbles into dust, that destroys itself still more completely, leaving behind still fewer traces of itself than Beauty: namely Grief.*[2]

The normal grieving process: Numbness → denial → yearning → depression → guilt/ aggression → reintegration. This process may take years. The process may become pathological if major depression (p 336) is precipitated. An extended example of this is described on p 388–396. It is often tempting for us to try and 'do something' by prescribing psychotropics, but it is known that most bereaved people do not want this, and there is no evidence that drugs reduce problems. Sympathy and helping the patient to shed tears is probably the most valuable approach, especially when losses are covert or hard to acknowledge.[3] Counselling after bereavement is effective.

After bereavement, risk of death in the spouse rises in the first 6 months (men) or in the second year (women). Men and the younger bereaved are at greatest risk.[4] It is not known whether this is due to shared unfavourable environments or to psychological causes (eg mediated by the immune system). The main causes of death are vascular, cancer, accidents and suicide.

Activities which we should try to avoid[5]

- Distancing tactics: 'Everyone feels upset when there is bad news, but you'll soon get used to it.'
- False reassurance: 'I am sure you will feel better; we have good anti-emetics these days.'
- Selective attention: 'What is going to happen to me? I'm beginning to think I'm not going to get better this time. The pain in my hip is getting worse.' Doctor: 'Tell me more about your hip.'

Breaking bad news

There are at least 6 central activities to the breaking of bad news.[6]

1 Choosing a quiet place where you will not be disturbed.
2 Finding out what the patient already knows or surmises.
3 Finding out how much the person wants to know. You can be surprisingly direct about this. 'Are you the sort of person who, if anything were amiss, would want to know all the details?'
4 Sharing information about diagnosis, treatments, prognosis, and specifically listing supporting people (eg nurses) and institutions (eg hospices). Try asking 'Is there anything else you want me to explain?'
5 Be responsive, and recognize the patient's feelings.
6 Planning and follow-through. The most important thing here is to leave the patient with the strong impression that, come what may, you are with him or her *whatever*, and that this unwritten contract will not be broken.

*Professor Kirk, Papers on Health, Edinburgh 1894 1 CRUSE (help for the bereaved: tel 1081 332 7227. 2 M Proust 1925 *Albertine Disparue.* NB: Proust's view is clear enough for grief surviving down generations–which it does not. But what of one person's grief? Surely this can last a lifetime, and Proust is wrong? No: we must assume that Proust had in mind an image from Gérard de Nerval (whom he rated very highly) who describes great grief as being carved into us, not like lettering on stone, which may be worn away by time, but like those initials we carve into the bark of a living tree. As the tree grows, the lettering sinks ever deeper, so that it may, apparently, to the casual observer, disappear, but really it has been embodied, internalized, and taken up into the inner life of the organism and distributed even to its fingertips (*see* Richard Holmes' on Gérard de Nerval in *Footsteps* 1996 HarperCollins, p222). 3 C Parkes 1998 BMJ i 1521 4 B McAvoy 1986 BMJ ii 835 5 P Maguire 1985 BMJ ii 1711 6 R Buckman 1992 *How to Break Bad News*, PaperMac

Useful agents in terminal care*

Pain *Remember that pain has physical, emotional and spiritual componants: all aspects need to be addressed. Diagnose and monitor each pain separately. Opiates:* Diamorphine PO: 2mg≈3mg morphine. SC: 1mg diamorphine≈1.5mg morphine. Sustained release morphine is available, eg MST-30® (30–100mg/12h PO) or MXL (lasts 24h). *Syringe drivers* or *suppositories* can be used when *dysphagia* or *vomiting* make oral drugs useless, eg oxycodone 30mg suppositories (eg 30mg/8h, ≈30mg morphine). If crystallization occurs with drugs mixed in syringe drivers, either increase the dilution, or use 2 syringe drivers. *Transdermal patches* are also useful, eg fentanyl (Durogesic® patches last 72h: typical starting dose for someone needing the equivalent of 90mg morphine/day would be one Durogesic-25® patch (the 25 means 25μg fentanyl/h; $50^{\approx 135\text{–}224\text{mg MST}}$, $75^{\approx 225\text{–}314\text{mg MST}}$ and $100^{\approx 315\text{–}404\text{mg MST}}$ patches are also available). Use non-irritated, non-irradiated, non-hairy skin on the torso or upper arm; remove after 72h and replace by another patch at a different site. *Non-opiate analgesia* may especially help *bone pain* (ibuprofen 400mg/8h PO or diclofenac + misoprostol, as Arthrotec®, 1 tablet/12h PO.) Pamidronate may also relieve pain from bony secondaries (OHCM p 644). *Nerve destruction pain:* Amitriptyline 25–50mg PO at night ± clonazepam 0.5–1mg/24h PO nocte, increased slowly to 1–2mg/8h. *Resistant pain*—Nerve blocks are useful.

Gut symptoms *Diarrhoea (post radiotherapy):* Low residue diets.
Constipation: Co-danthramer (forte) capsules or liquid ± bisacodyl 5–10mg nocte.
Gastric irritation eg associated with gastric carcinoma—H_2 antagonists (eg cimetidine 400mg/12h PO or proton pump inhibitors (omeprazole).
Itch in jaundice—Cholestyramine 4g/6h PO (1h after other drugs).
Pain with dysphagia or *vomiting:* Buprenorphine sublingual 0.2–0.4mg/8h. Not a pure agonist. 'Ceiling' effects negate dose increases. Hence alternative is oxycodone 30mg suppositories, eg 30mg/8h (=30mg morphine).
Foul rectal discharges—Betadine vaginal gel®.
Vomiting Cyclizine 50–150mg/4–8h PO, PR, IM, SC. Prochlorperazine suppositories: 25mg/12h. Haloperidol (p 360) 5–10mg PO. *If from inoperable GI obstruction,* try hyoscine hydrobromide 0.4–0.8mg sc/8h or 0.3mg sublingual. Octreotide, max 600μg/24h via a syringe driver may remove the need for palliative surgery, IVIs and NGTs. *If from gastric stasis:* Metoclopramide 10mg/8h PO or SC. If this fails, try domperidone 60mg/8h rectally.

Lung symptoms *Pleural effusion:* Thoracocentesis (bleomycin pleurodesis).
Air hunger: Chlorpromazine (eg 12.5mg IV, 25mg suppository).
Bronchial rattles: Hyoscine (as above) 0.4–0.8mg/8h SC or 0.3mg sublingual.
Dyspnoea: (hypoxic)—Table fans ± supplemental humidified oxygen.
Haemoptisis: Diamorphine, above, IV if massive.
Pleural pain: Intercostal nerve blocks may bring lasting relief.

Cardiovascular symptoms *Distension from ascites* often causes distressing symptoms. Try spironolactone 100mg/12h PO + bumetanide 1mg/24h PO.

Genitourinary symptoms *Foul vaginal discharges:* Betadine vaginal gel®.
Massive bladder bleeding—Alum irrigation (1%) by catheter (in hospital).

Psychological symptoms *Agitation*—Try diazepam 10mg suppositories (eg 10mg/8h), or haloperidol (p 360) 5–10mg PO (may help nightmares, hallucinations and vomiting too). Midazolam may be used in syringe drivers (eg 5–10mg/24h)—or methotrimeprazine (Nozinan®) 12.5–50mg IM stat or 25–200mg/24h SC via a syringe driver.
Appetite low, or headache due to ↑ICP—Steroids; most useful is dexamethosone, eg 4mg/12–24h PO to stimulate appetite, reduce ICP, and in some patients induce a satisfactory sense of euphoria.

Others—*Coated tongues* may be cleaned by 6% hydrogen peroxide, chewing pineapple chunks to release proteolytic enzmes, sucking on ice or butter.
Superior vena cava or *bronchial obstruction, or lymphangitis carcinomatosa*—Steroids; dexamethasone is most useful: give 8mg IV stat. Tabs are 2mg (≈15mg prednisolone) NB: dexamethasone given at night can prevent sleep.

*UK patients and relatives may get much support via BACUP (British Association of Cancer United Patients, 3 Bath Place, Rivington St, London, EC2A 3JR, tel. 0171 613 2121). In the UK, *Social Services* have a vital rôle in fast-tracking applications from financial help in the form of the *Disability Living allowance*, and the *Attendance Allowance*, once the prognosis is <6 months. See p 462–3.

Principal sources: GW Hanks 1996 BMJ **i** 823–26; BNF 1997 *Prescribing in Palliative Care* (ch 1); D Doyle 1994 *Oxford Textbook of Palliative Medicine*; P Kay 1994 A–Z *of Hospice and Palliative Medicine*; *MJ Baines* Annals Acad Med **23** 178–82 ***Acknowledgement:*** This page owes much to Dr Tim Wiggan.

Records and computers

►We cannot make ourselves better people by using a system or a machine: reflection, dialogue, and action are more likely routes to self-improvement. ►It is the care and interest a doctor takes in his records that matters, not the details of the particular system employed.

Problem-orientated records—*List problems as 'active' or 'inactive'* Eg 'breathlessness' (not '?bronchitis'—or 'Down's syndrome', which may be unproblematic to the individual, but a problem to us 'normals', who do not like disability: so often such a patient's *real* problem is that *we* have a problem).
Subjective interpretation: How the patient and/or carer sees the problems.
Objective: Physical examination and results of tests (not always objective!).
Assessment: Social, psychological and physical interpretation.
Plan: Do the following tests. . .' or 'Wait on events'; treatment: eg 'Start psychotherapy' and explanation—note what the patient has been told.

French Weir system This uses health authority cards (free to all UK GPs):
FP5: This is the record of immunizations.
FP9A: Pink (male) PMH summary card. Use for both sexes.
FP9B: Blue (female) summary card is used as a drug card. These are placed in front of the continuation cards (FP7), which are kept in time order by a treasury tag. A second treasury tag orders hospital letters.

Computers Computers gained acceptance by UK GPs as they made it easier to perform and monitor repeat prescribing, and to fulfil NHS requirements (elderly health checks; prevention targets). Increasingly they are used for:

- Faster communication with laboratory and hospital (Read codes, p 421).
- Better and *more* preventive care, not just in theory, but in practice (eg 8–18% more vaccinations in consultations with a computer on the desk, more BP measurements, with a ~5mmHg fall in BP in those with hypertension; the price is longer consultations—by 48–90sec).◄1►
- Audit: eg computerized record of everyone's BP and vaccinations.
- Prescribing: computers save money (8%) by making generic prescribing easy. They are more likely to be associated with complete records (95% *vs* 42%). The electronic *BNF* allows simultaneous viewing of various sections, and 'hot-links' to drug interactions. Computer-assisted prescribing linked to Read codes (eg PRODIGY) can aid prescribing, and aims to improve quality by automatically linking prescribing to practice-modifiable guidelines.[2]
- To can send letters to patients, eg in the light of new drug information.
- Integration of data from multiple sources—eg drug interactions.
- Quick exploration of hypotheses. (Do I see more depression in winter?)
- Assessing eligibility for social security benefits.
- Rule-based systems/neural networks (p 35)—is this ECG/smear abnormal?
- Keeping up-to-date, decision support and evidence-based medicine, eg the Internet,* and the *Oxford Clinical Mentor*,[3,4] the latter uses this text, *OHCM*, and the *Oxford Handbook of Clinical Rarities*. This database is updated monthly by modem and contains >25,000 key-worded facts connected by an intelligent indexing system—linked to the medical record via the Read classification (p 421) to enable explanation of apparently unrelated or obscure signs, symptoms and results, eg chest pain, depression, MCV↑ and melaena are explained by alcoholism, with 'postulates' of related trauma (fractured ribs) or cardiomyopathy—both known associations of alcoholism.

NB: there are big problems in realizing the potential of computers: see p 447.

◄1►F Sullivan *E-BM* **1** 96 **2** I Purves 1998 *JRCGP* **48** 1552; M Johnston 1994 *Arch Int Med* **120** 135
3 Oxford Clinical *Mentor*–from OUP, tel. +44 (0)1865 242913/EMIS, tel. +44 (0)1132 582454/01132 591122
4 *BMJ* 1993 ii 679 *Eg Global health http://www.pitt.edu/HOME/GHNet/GHNet.html

Paperless medical enterprises?

We have been recording our interactions with patients using computers for a decade—not long in the history of medicine, but at least 4 generations in the world of computers. We have also been using computers for other activities. We use a sophisticated networked system when we shop (credit cards), bank, and write using typesetting software rather than 1000 hot metal workers. From these vantage points we look back to the age of DOS (Microsoft's old *Disk Operating System*) and other embryonic operating systems as if to a past ice age. Why is medical computing still stuck in this ice age? The reason is that we have not been very good at capturing the consultation in electronic form, and the benefits of doing so are not very great—ie not enough to drive development. Unlike banking, where computers bring sufficient advantages to warrant investment so that systems *have* to work efficiently, in medical computing this imperative is absent. So, unfortunately, 90% of UK GPs use both manual and electronic records.

The coding systems for capturing consultations do not work. It's probably not their fault. In the daily tussle of trying to reduce Mrs Salt (*OHCM* p 478) to a 5-digit code, we can lose what we are trying to record. We are asking too much of the codes: to speed data entry, aid audit, decision support, planning, and delineating and communicating human predicaments.

This is not like banking or typesetting a document: it is ultimately a philosophical, biographical and poetic enterprise. We cannot expect a coding system to do all this, and free text does not work very well either. We often end up requiring 2 systems if one of them is electronic. What we put in the electronic record is coded detail, using a shoehorn to force-fit an incongruent match. If we want to know a bit more of the real truth, we have to look in the physical record. Medical computing will not fly until double data entry is a thing of the past—but this cannot be as there is no good, *quick* electronic way of dealing with ECGs, diagrams, old hospital letters, slowly dawning possibilities, subtle uncertainties, and verbatim examples of patients' problems using their own words. What should we do? Give up the unequal struggle? There is a real danger of this. Computers are no longer new. We do not now come to them with a forgiving frame of mind welcoming a new medium to explore, but in the cynical knowledge that compromise and frustration is just round the corner. So to someone who says "Let's put our efforts into a *single* system, but a manual one", we no longer answer from conviction, but from the point of view of "We could hardly fulfil our terms-of-service requirements if we did this". So we limp on. But it's not quite this bad: we have written as if the old system was reasonably OK, if pedestrian. But anyone who has come to an unfamiliar, complicated patient described in a manual system will know how difficult it is to get simple information from the notes. Has the patient ever had codeine, or penicillamine, before? This might take half an hour of textual analysis, which is why few of us ever used to bother than do more than ask the patient (not a bad solution when all else fails).

Now computerized medical environments take the ease of answering this sort of question for granted—and herein lies the problem. Our greed for ever more fancy programs and the runaway success of computing applications in a few simple environments leads us to be over-critical and so pessimistic about our own not-so-simple computer environment. Using a manual system presupposes being able to read and write efficiently. These skills needed years of teaching and practice, starting at an ideal, formative age. This enables us to read, write, talk, and listen all at the same time—which is how most manual records get written, ie in time that isn't there. Real-time computerized data capture needs its own allotted time *at the moment*. But we are not so very far from easier data entry: graphical user interfaces, pen systems for writing on the screen combined with the will to make more space for training may yet bring us out of the ice age.

Audit—two schools of thought

Audit has various meanings. To health authorities it means checking up that we are fulfilling our terms of service, and advising on cost-effective use of resources via its increasingly powerful supervising financial auditor and its Medical Audit Advisory Group. Here, audit is unrelated to education, and has only a tenuous link with quality. Academically and professionally audit means quality control by counting and measurement; it merges with research,[1] but is usually more about aims and changing behaviour, whereas research aims to reveal new facts, theories or relationships. Audit means asking questions like: 'Have we any agreed aims in medical practice?' and 'Are we falling short of these aims?' and 'What can we do to improve performance?' The process of audit can be divided into 6 stages.[2] These are illustrated below, using a practice that wants to know whether something more formal than their ad hoc methods of summarizing notes is needed.

1 **Aim (ie choice of topic)** This might be to have all important information about a patient immediately available in an accessible form.

2 **Setting standards** The practice may decide that notes must be in chronological order, fat notes should have a summary card, and patients on long-term treatment should have a treatment card.

3 **Observing current practice** The practice manager arranges a random sample of the notes for 'quality control' analysis.

4 **Compare performance with targets** A record is made of the proportion of notes in chronological order, and whether summary cards are used.

5 **Implementing changes** If some notes analysed are not up to standard, a method is be devised to achieve this. For example, practice staff could place notes in chronological order, and each doctor could aim to summarize a certain number per day to complete the job in a specified time.

6 **Evaluation** Have the plans worked? A later random sample is analysed. This last element is of some importance, as it prevents us deluding ourselves that our present strategies are necessarily effective.

As demonstrated above, other people's audit exercises are very boring. It is only when a practice engages in audit itself that interest is aroused, and it can become quite satisfying to watch one's practice develop through a series of audits. Once an age–sex register exists, or the practice is computerized, it is possible to do audits on many aspects of care, to answer questions such as 'Is our care of diabetics adequate? Would a mini-clinic be effective? Are all our fertile female patients rubella-immune?

Notice that the practice manager can have a central rôle in running an audit exercise—eg by relieving doctors of the burden of data collection, and is able to communicate the results of the audit in a practice's annual report, along with less formal audits of the consultation and home visits rates, referrals to hospital and whatever else the practice does.

Possible dangers of audit (No intervention is without side-effects.)

- It takes time away from eye-to-eye contact with patients.
- In becoming the province of professional enthusiasts, it can alienate some practice members, who can then ignore the results of the audit.
- There is no guarantee that audit will improve outcomes.
- It may limit our horizons—from the consideration of the vast imponderables of our patients' lives in a world of death, decay, and rebirth—to a preoccupation with attaining tiny, specific, and very limited goals.
- Some doctors fear that in espousing audit they risk transforming themselves from approachable but rather bumbling carers and curers who perhaps don't know *exactly* where they are going, into minor administrative prophets, with too much of a gleam in their eyes and zeal in their hearts.

1 IK Crombie 1993 *Audit Handbook* Wiley, ISBN 0-471-93766-5 2 M Lawrence 1994 BMJ ii 513

Peer review during a practice visit

GPs ask other GPs to place them somewhere between 2 opposed views:[1]

1 Professional values	
He balances his own convenience against that of his patients, keeping the interest of the wider community in mind.	He puts his own convenience above the needs of patients, having no concern for wider responsibilities.
He believes in the importance of the continuity of care, and gives as personal and comprehensive a service as possible.	He does not think continuity matters. He delegates too much; clinical interests are dominated by hobby horses.
He subjects his work to critical self-scrutiny and review by colleagues. He enjoys being a GP and he accepts the obligation to maintain his own health.	He is complacent about his work and never reviews it. He has become defeated or drives himself excessively.
2 Accessibility	
It is easy to see him quickly if needed.	You cannot see him quickly.
He does not keep patients and staff waiting unnecessarily.	The doctor is regularly late for appointments.
3 Clinical competence	
He consistently gives evidence of taking relevant histories, and appears to listen to what his patient says.	He fails to elicit histories appearing not to listen to what the patient is saying.
His use of drugs is appropriate.	Prescribing is inappropriate
4 Ability to communicate	
He creates a calm, receptive atmosphere encourages patients to talk freely	No communication with patient in defining the reasons for the patient's attendance.
Regular meetings take place with other members of the health care team. He encourages a free exchange of ideas.	He discourages talk among the team. He is insensitive, misunderstanding their rôles.

There are ~70 such statements in the RCGP document (as well as much else), and the main difficulty is not what the scheme leaves out (eg cost containment), but that it is so thorough that some might quail before so much goodness-in-theory because of what actually happens in practice. If this is the case, the best plan is to buy the College document, but only to read it in very short bursts until one's practice gradually comes into shape—when the whole document can be read without inducing a fit of despair about one's own performance.

1 *What sort of Doctor? J Roy Col Gen Prac* 1985 Report 23

Under- and over-performing doctors

It would be very nice for the public and the 'leaders' of our profession if there were a small number of under-performing doctors who could be easily identified and retrained, or, failing this, struck off. Things are rarely so simple, and we may have to accept that, for many reasons, including chance, training, and resilience, the performance of *all doctors* will, at times, be, or appear to be suboptimal. If all doctors were the same, and there was a valid yardstick for measuring quality (a big 'if'), then there would be, by chance, a large under-performing group, with a corresponding apparently 'over-performing' group. Anyone assessing performance data needs to take into account these questions:

What counts as data? Usually only what can be *quantified. Quality* is different.
Is the data stratified for risk? Doctors' case-mixes can vary markedly.
Has our personal data's accuracy been validated? Data entry is often unreliable.
Has the accuracy of the data we are being compared with been validated?
Could the differences between our data and others have arisen by chance? This is the most revealing question. Imagine a thought-experiment in which 4 equal doctors use different strategies for predicting whether a tossed coin will land heads or tails. One always chooses heads, one always chooses tails, and the other two alternate their choices out of synchrony with each other. When I did this experiment for a pre-decided 14 throws each (56 throws in total), the best doctor only had 2 errors, whereas the worse had 7 errors—over 3 times the rate for post-operative deaths (or whatever). The public would demand that this doctor be retrained or struck off, and the General Medical Council might feel obliged to comply, simply to keep public confidence (it is under great pressure to 'do something'). So must we all be prepared to be sacrificial lambs? The answer is *Yes*, but there are certain steps that can be taken to mitigate our own and our patients' risk-exposure.

- When we encounter doctors who are clarly under-performing (eg due to addictions) we must speak out. This will encourage belief in the system.
- For statistical reasons any series with <16 failures might be best ignored. Such series simply do not have enough power to detect real effects.[1]
- We must strive to be both kind and honest with our patients. The best response to 'I'd like a home-delivery' might be to say 'I haven't done one for 5 years—and that one went wrong: are you sure you want my services?'—rather than 'the UK perinatal death-rate is the same for home and hospital'.
- It might be the case that, contrary to the GMC, we should *not* always be on the look-out for colleagues who might be under-performing so that we can report them to the proper authorities: rather we should be encouraging an atmosphere of mutual support and trust—the sort of environment in which doctors feel safe to say 'all my cases of X seem to be going wrong—can anyone think why?' To stop this trust turning into crony-ism we must be prepared to engage in, or be subjected to, audit (p 448). The alternative is for clinicians to develop into secret police, informers, and counter-informers. No one would benefit from this. We note that malicious informing is not an isolated occurrence in the UK;[2] 80% of those suspended for presumed under-performance are exonerated, but few return to their previous job owing to the stresses enquiries always engender.

Typical areas in which doctors are seen to be under-performing

Local Medical Committees (LMCs), Community Health Councils, and NHS commissioners have all been systematically questioned about doctors whose performance they are reviewing. In the case of LMCs, for example, clinical skills were the chief worry, followed, in order, by communication problems, management problems, prescribing problems, and record-keeping problems. Health authorities had more concern over referral patterns.[3]

1 CRAM (cumulative risk-adjusted mortality/morbidity) has been devised for giving valid estimates of risks of procedures, provided there have been at least 16 failures—see J Poloniecki *BMJ* i 1998 1734 & *ibid* 1697 2 Anon 1998 *BMJ* i 1756–7 3 G Taylor 1998 *BMJ* i 1705

Patient satisfaction

►*The patient is the nearest thing we have to an infallible judge of what constitutes good medicine.* In summary, what patients mostly want is a *personal service* from a *sympathetic* doctor who is *nearby* and *easy to get to see*. Satisfaction is one of the few measures of *outcome* (not *process*) which is fairly easy to measure, eg by questionnaire agreement with these 13 statements (*Baker's dozen*[1]).

Satisfaction

1 I am totally satisfied with my visit to this doctor.
2 Some things about my visit to the doctor could have been better.
3 I am not completely satisfied with my visit to the doctor.

Professional care

4 This doctor examined me very thoroughly.
5 This doctor told me everything about my treatment.
6 I thought this doctor took notice of me as a person.
7 I will follow the doctor's advice because I think he/she is right.
8 I understand my illness much better after seeing this doctor.

Relationships

9 This doctor knows all about me.
10 I felt this doctor really knew what I was thinking.
11 I felt able to tell this doctor about very personal things.

Perceived time

12 The time I was allowed with the doctor was not long enough to deal with everything I wanted.
13 I wish I could have spent a bit longer with the doctor.

Why do patients change their doctor? The most common reasons are that either the patient has moved, or the doctor has retired or is perceived to be too far away. There are additional reasons:[2]

Patient needs:		*Organizational problems:*		*Problems with doctor:*	
One doctor for all the family	5%	Long waits	13%	Lost confidence in	21%
Want woman doctor	4%	No continuity of care	6%	Dr not interested	10%
Want alternative medicine	2%	Rude receptionist	6%	Rude doctor	10%
Obstetric needs	1%	Appointments wanted	1%	Prescriptions criticized	5%
		Open surgeries wanted	1%	Doctor too hurried	4%
		Other staff rude	1%	Visits problematic	4%
				Communication poor	4%
				Referral problem	2%

A USA study found that a *participatory decision making style* leads to patient satisfaction. Participation was found to depend, in part, on the *degree of autonomy* perceived to be enjoyed by the GP, and on the volume of work.[3]

Another approach to gaining satisfaction is to agree and publish standards of care that patients can expect, along with performance figures for how nearly these standards are achieved in practice. This is the philosophy behind the UK government-led *Patient's Charter* and the British Standards kitemark BS5750—the aims of which are to:

- Set standards, eg by agreement with patient participation groups (p 440).
- Monitor progress towards these standards, and publish progress locally.
- Provide information about how services are organized. Maximize choice.
- Let users know who is in charge of what, and what their rôles are.
- Explain to users what is done when things go wrong, and how services are improved, and what the complaints procedure is.
- Show that taxpayers' money is being used efficiently.
- Demonstrate customer satisfaction.

This culture has proved alien to most GPs, perhaps owing to a very necessary preoccupation with illness and its curing, rather than service, and its glorification.

1 R Baker 1990 *B J Gen Prac* 487 & 1996 601 2 B Billinghurst 1993 *Ibid* 43 336 3 S Kaplan 1996 *An Int Med* **124** 497

Stopping smoking tobacco[1]

Epidemiologists estimate that ~50% of smokers will die of smoking if they do not give up—and it is not the case that they only lose a few years: a quarter of a century is more likely for those dying between the ages of 35 and 69. Stopping smoking diminishes the excess risk from tobacco, so that after 10–15yrs the risk of lung cancer effectively reverts to that of lifelong non-smokers. A similar, but quicker diminution of excess risk (↓ by ~50% in the first year) is found for deaths from coronary artery disease and, to a lesser extent, risk of stroke.[2] ►*60% of smokers want to give up.*

Annual UK health costs of smoking •GP consultations: £89 million •GP prescriptions: £52 million •Hospital episodes: £470 million

Advantages of stopping smoking Saving of life (110,000/yr in UK).
- Larger babies (smokers' babies weigh on average 250g less than expected, and their physical and mental development may be impaired).
- Less bronchitis (accounts for millions of lost working days).
- Less risk from the Pill: cardiovascular risk↑ ×20 if uses >30 cigarettes/day.
- Less risk from passive smoking (cot deaths, bronchitis, lung cancers).
- Return of the sense of taste and smell.

Helping people quit (AAAA= ask, advise, assist, arrange follow-up.)[1]
- Ask about smoking in all consultations, not just those on smoking-related diseases (be subtle; patients won't listen if you do not share agendas).
- Advise according to need. Ensure that advice is congruent with beliefs about smoking. Concentrate on the benefits of giving up (as above).
- Assist in practical ways, eg:
  - Invite the patient to choose a date (when there will be few stresses) on which he or she will become a non-smoker.
  - Suggest that he throws away all smoking accessories (cigarettes, pipes, ash trays, lighters, matches) in advance.
  - Inform friends of the new change.
  - Try offering nicotine patches *and* spray (or gum, chew intermittently to limit nicotine release; ≥ten 2mg sticks may be needed/day). Adding a spray (0.5mg/dose) to patches ↑quitting from ~11% to 27.[3] To counter cravings, the spray may be used for ≤7 months once regular patches are stopped—eg after 5 months' use. A dose increase at 1 week is helpful for some who are in difficulties.[4] NB: gum may be better than patches in those most addicted (eg craving on waking).[4] Giving additional detailed written advice offers no added benefit to simple advice from nurses.
- Arrange follow-up. This shows you are commited to your patient.[5]

For those who do not want to give up Give them a health education leaflet, record this fact in the record, and try again later.

Cigarette smoking is declining in older adults, but increasing among the young, particularly in the developing world. ►In the UK, ~450 children start smoking per day; and ¼ of school leavers smoke regularly.[6] Numbers are rising. This has prompted the Health Education Council's family smoking education project for schools.

Every health 'outlet' should have a policy on promoting non-smoking, and offering practical advice: primary health care teams; hospitals; midwives; pharmacies—and also, perhaps, schools and employing authorities. Health commissioners also need to promote knowledge and training in this area.[1]

1 Smoking Cessation Guidelines (M Raw) 1999 BMJ i 182 2 SG Wannamethee 1996 E-BM 1 95 3 T Blondal 1999 BMJ i 285 4 M Russell 1993 BMJ i 1308 5 M Russell 1979 BMJ ii 231

5. General practice

Reducing alcohol intake

With the toll that excess alcohol takes in terms of personal misery and the national purse (>£1600 million/yr in the UK), the need to reduce alcohol intake should rank as one of the leading aims of preventive care. The reason why alcohol is not at the top of the agenda is not just that doctors are so fond of it (the profession has three times the national rate of cirrhosis), but because there is a powerful and pervasive lobby which ensures that alcohol is cheaper (in relative terms) and more readily available than ever before—so that its use on an individually moderate scale arouses no comment. It is assumed to be safe, provided one is not actually an alcoholic. However, it is more helpful to view alcohol risks and benefits as a spectrum (see the French Paradox, *OHCM* p 482 for the *benefits* of alcohol). Problems are listed on p 363. A strategy to reduce the bad effects of alcohol in your patients:

- Whenever a patient presents with symptoms or signs related to alcohol, be sure to ask in detail about consumption.
- Question any patient with 'alerting factors'—accidents, driving offences, child neglect, assault, attempted suicide, depression, obesity.
- Question all remaining patients (not infants) as they register, consult or attend for any health check.

Helping people to cut down • Take more non-alcoholic drinks.

- Limit your drinking to social occasions—and learn to sip, not gulp.
- Reduce the frequency of sips, eg by shadowing a slow drinker in the group. Don't pick up your glass until he does (and don't hold your glass for long: put it down to avoid unconscious sipping).
- Don't buy yourself a drink when it is your turn to buy a drinks' round.
- Reduce the period of drinking—go out to the pub later.
- Take 'days of rest' when no alcohol is drunk.
- Learn graceful ways of refusing: 'No more for me please, I expect I'll have to drive Jack home' or 'I'm seeing what it's like to cut down.'

Maintaining reduced drinking • Agree goals with the patient.

- Suggest he keeps an alcohol diary in which he records all drinking.
- Teach him to estimate his alcohol intake (u/week, see below).
- Consider an 'Alcohol Card' in the notes to show: units/week; pattern of drinking; reasons for misuse; each alcohol-related problem (and whether a solution has been agreed and action implemented); job record; family events; biochemical markers (GGT, MCV); weight.
- Give feedback about how he is doing—eg if GGT (γ-glutamyl transpeptidase) falls are discussed at feedback, there is much lower mortality, morbidity and hospitalization compared with randomized control subjects.[1]
- Include the family in plans for ongoing alcohol reduction. Agree a system of 'rewards' for sobriety.
- Group therapy, self-help groups, disulfiram, local councils on alcohol, community alcohol teams and treatment units may also help (p 363).

Setting limits for low-risk drinking eg ≤20u/week if ♂; ≤ 15u/week if ♀—there are no absolutes: risk is a continuum. NB: higher limits are proposed, on scant evidence[1] (eg 4u/day for men and 3 for women). One unit is 9g ethanol, ie 1 measure of spirits, 1 glass of wine, or a pint of beer.[2,3] ►*Primary care is a good setting for prevention*: intervention leads to less alcohol consumption by ~15%, reducing the proportion of heavy drinkers by 20%—at one-twentieth the cost of specialist services.[4] There is no evidence that GP intervention has to include more time-consuming advice such as compressed cognitive/behavioural strategies.[5,6] Simple advice works fine as judged by falling GGT levels—at least for men. After interventions, women may report drinking less, but this is not reflected in a falling GTT.[5]

1 M Marmont 1995 *Lancet* **346** 1643 2 R Doll 1994 **ii** BMJ 911 3 J Gaziano 1995 BMJ **ii** 3 4 J Volpicelli 1995 *Lancet* **i** 456 5 P Anderson 1991 BMJ **i** 766 6 P Anderson 1993 *Br J Gen Prac* **43** 386

5. General practice

Alternative and holistic medicine

Alternative (complementary/fringe/non-orthodox) medicine

These terms are used to describe therapies which are not included in conventional medical/paramedical training—although an increasing number are being subjected to rigorous assessment in double-blind, randomized trials.[1]

Some are the orthodoxies of a different time (eg *herbalism*) or place (the *Ayurvedic medicine* of India), some are mainly diagnostic techniques (*iridology*), some mainly therapeutic (*aromatherapy*). Some doctors are suspicious of unorthodox medicine, and feel that its practitioners should not be 'let loose' on patients. However, in many places the legal position is that, however unorthodox a practitioner's treatment may be, he or she cannot be convicted of unethical practice in the absence of demonstrable harm to patients.[2]

Many patients (an estimated 5 million annually in UK) consult alternative practitioners, usually as a supplement to orthodox treatment and for a limited range of problems—predominantly musculoskeletal. Many will feel unable to tell their doctor.

Modern medicine is criticized (both from within and from without) for sacrificing humanity to technology, and with little benefit for many patients. In contrast to the orthodox doctor, alternative practitioners may be seen as taking time to listen, laying on hands rather than instruments, and giving medicines free (not always!) from side-effects.

Many alternative therapies seem scientifically implausible, and controlled trials are difficult to design, as treatment is often individualized and the rôle of the therapist crucial. However, the same comments could be made of much of orthodox practice. GPs are showing increasing interest in what their rivals are offering, and some incorporate alternative therapies into their armamentarium. Some of the therapies commonly available to patients are briefly described below.

Acupuncture: Traditionally used to treat a wide range of conditions, acupuncture is increasingly employed in orthodox practice for pain relief, control of nausea and treatment of addiction. For these, endorphin release provides a scientific rationale.

Homeopathy: This is based on the principles that like cures like, and that remedies are made more efficacious ('potentiated') by infinite dilution. NHS GPs may prescribe homeopathic remedies on an FP10. Randomized trials suggests real (small) benefits, eg in asthma, but nobody knows if the reason *why* they are effective is 'like cures like'.[3,4]

Manipulative therapies (osteopathy and chiropracty): These are widely used and of proven benefit in musculoskeletal problems, but some use them to treat more general conditions such as asthma.[5]

Clinical ecology Starting from the fact that atmospheric pollutants, toxins and xenobiotic chemicals (from other organisms) are known to be harmful, a system is built up around techniques (using intradermal injections) for provoking and neutralizing symptoms related to foods.[1,5]

Holistic medicine[5] The holistic approach means taking a broad view: of the patient as a whole person, of the rôle of the therapist, of the therapies used. The patient's autonomy is encouraged through patient involvement in decision-making and nurturing of self-reliance. Specialism does not exclude holism; nephrologists can be as holistic as naturopaths. As shown on p 422, most models of the GP consultation are based on a patient-centred approach which is essentially holistic. Compare the sequence 'bronchitis → antibiotic' with 'bronchitis → smoker → stressed → redundancy-counselling → ?antibiotic'.

1 http://altmed.od.nih.gov/oam 2 K Mumby 1993 BMJ ii 1055 3 D Reilly 1994 *Lancet* 344 1601 4 1991 BMJ i 316
5 W King 1988 *Otolaryngol Head Neck Surg* 99 263 & 272 5 P Pietroni 1988 *Primary Care* p 114 Heinemann

Living dangerously

Ten years ago a patient had a seminoma treated, apparently successfully, in a well-known London hospital, to which he had been referred from his distant Sussex village. In the year that follow-up stopped, the patient had a major myocardial infarction—again, followed by an apparently reasonable recovery. But the patient became morbid, self-centred and depressed, perhaps because of the dawning appreciation of his mortality, his residual breathlessness, and his inability to carry out his hobby of carpentry. His GP tried hard to cheer him up, and rehabilitate him by encouraging exercise, sex, a positive self-image, and alternative hobbies. Rehabilitation was almost working when he began to develop headaches and kept asking forlornly whether these were a sign that his cancer had spread to his brain. There were no signs of recurrent tumour or raised intracranial pressure. His GP appreciated that there *was* a chance that the tumour was resurfacing, but judged that starting a pointless chain of investigations would be disastrous to the patient's mental health. So instead of arranging CT scans the GP interpreted the patient's forlorn question for him, saying that he was only asking questions like this because he was in a negative frame of mind, and the patient and his GP developed strategies to avoid negative cognitions, in co-operation with the local consultant who had helped to look after his myocardial infarction. The headaches improved, and the pressure to investigate was resisted.

Had a CT scan been done, it would by no means have achieved reassurance if it was negative—in the patient's frame of mind he would be all too willing to ask if the CT scan is 100% reliable, and then to request some other test in addition, and so on, until illness had become a major preoccupation. So in this case, it was rational for the doctor to live dangerously, take risks, and be prepared to take the blame if things had gone wrong.

How do we cope with and thrive on uncertainty? The first step is to get away from the idea that if you do not do all you can to reduce uncertainty, you are somehow being lazy. (The reverse may be true.) The next step is to share the uncertainty with a colleague—to see if he or she agrees with your judgment. From the medicolegal viewpoint it is wise to document your thought processes. Another caution is to follow in the steps of those adventurous but wise mountaineers who never plan a route without also planning an escape route: in the medical sense, this means the triad of follow-up, the taking of the family into one's confidence, and honest reflection on the chances of error and the chances of detecting it. This means that, as far as possible, you will get early warning of error, and then be able to adjust your therapeutic approach in line with the way the illness unfolds.

Minor illness

Many people with apparently minor illnesses visit their GPs, although GPs do not have a sufficient monopoly of this to justify being called 'triviologists'. Most minor illnesses are dealt with from a disease point of view, in the relevant chapter in which they occur. Here, the concern is with the study of minor illness itself, and in this context much minor illness does not come to the general practitioner: only *people* come to general practitioners, and it may not be known for some time whether the symptoms are serious or minor (minor to whom?). A GP may not want to spend all his time on minor conditions, but this may become almost unavoidable if he issues a prescription for such complaints. This reinforces attendance at the surgery, as a proportion of patients will come to assume that a prescription is necessary. In current practice, GPs rate about 14% of their consultations as being for minor illness (mild gastroenteritis, upper respiratory problems, presumed viral infections, 'flu, and childhood exanthemata).[1] More than 80% are likely to receive a prescription, and >10% are asked to return for a further consultation. Why does this great investment of time and money occur? Desire to please, genuine concern, prescribing to end a consultation, and therapeutic uncertainty may all play a part. Positive correlations with low prescribing rates include a young doctor, practising in affluent areas and long consultation times. Patients in social classes I and II are more likely to get a home visit for minor ailments than those in other social classes. Membership of the Royal College of General Practitioners does not influence prescribing rates.[1] Not everyone wants to reduce prescribing, but advice is available for those who do:[2]

- Using a self-care manual explaining about minor illness.[3]
- Using self-medication (eg paracetamol for fever).
- Using the larder (eg lemon and honey for sore throats).
- Using time (eg pink ear drums[4]—follow-up).
- Using granny (a more experienced member of the family).
- Pre-empting the patient's request for antibiotics (eg for a sore throat), eg: 'I'll need to examine your throat to see if you need an antibiotic, but first let me ask you some questions. . . From what you say, it sounds as if you are going to get over this on your own, but let me have a look to see.' [GP inspects to exclude a quinsy.] 'Yes, I think you'll get over this on your own. Is that all right?'

1 C Whitehouse 1985 *J Roy Col Gen Prac* **35** 581 **2** G Marsh 1977 BMJ **ii** 1267
3 D Morrell 1980 BMJ **i** 769 **4** D Brooks 1983 *Update* **26** 1961–4

Empowering patients

Any illness, minor or otherwise, is an opportunity to empower patients. Use the time to enable patients to improve their ability to:

- Cope with life
- Understand their illness.
- Cope with specific illnesses.
- Feel able to keep themselves healthy.
- Feel confident on handling health issues.
- Be confident about the ability to help themselves.

We know that time spent this way improves patient satisfaction and clinical outcome.[1,2]

1 P Howie 1997 RCGP *Occasional Paper* 75 **2** Headache Study Group 1986 *Headache* **26** 285

Prescribing and compliance ('concordance')

On any day ~60% of people take drugs, only half of which are prescribed. The others are sold over the counter (OTC). The commonest OTCs are analgesics, cough medicines and vitamins; for prescribed drugs the common groups are CNS and cardiovascular drugs, and antibiotics. On average, 6–7 NHS prescriptions are issued/person/year (21 in Italy and 11 in France).

GPs account for 75% of NHS annual prescribing costs (>£2000 million, or ~10% of the total cost of the NHS), although many of these 'GP drugs' will have been initiated in hospital. The cost of these prescriptions has risen by a factor of ~5 since 1949 (after allowance for inflation) and is ~£100,000/GP/year. Positive correlations with low prescribing rates include a young doctor, practising in an affluent area, and a longer consultation time (>7 min). The reason for this may be that if extra time is spent with the patient, more explanation about minor ailments (p 458) may be given, so that a patient's expectation for a prescription is replaced by enlightened self-awareness.

General practice formularies The aim is to reduce the drug 'bill' and to make prescribing more effective, by producing an agreed list of favoured drugs. This voluntary restriction can work in tandem with compulsory NHS restricted lists, and lead to substantial savings[1] (eg 18%). The UK DoH recommends development at individual practice level but this time-consuming task may be better achieved by adapting an existing local formulary.[2] Unless you wish to reinvent the wheel, this would seem excellent advice.

Dispensing doctors In rural areas where there is no chemist's shop GPs are allowed to dispense to their patients. Their annual prescribing rate can be as low as 70% of their non-dispensing fellow GPs.

Compliance (Does the patient take the medicine?)

► *There is no point in being a brilliant diagnostician if nobody can be persuaded to take your treatments.*

Even in life-threatening conditions, compliance is a major problem occurring in up to 56% of patients (eg adolescents with acute lymphatic leukaemia). The following have been found to be associated with increased compliance:

- Being able to identify with a personal doctor.
- Patient's overall satisfaction with the doctor.
- Simple therapeutic regimens.
- Supplementary written information[3] (use short words—Flesch formula >70, *OHCM* p 3).
- Longer consultation times or prescribing on home visits.
- Prescribing in association with giving health education.
- Continuity of care by the GP.
- Short waiting time for appointments.
- The encouragement of self-monitoring by the patient.
- Belief in the efficacy of the treatment.

Monitoring compliance: Monitoring plasma drug levels is the most reliable way of doing this, but it is cheaper to ask patients to return with their tablets, so that you can count them—or, better still, establish a basis of trust so that the patient can check for him- or herself.

1 *Drug Ther Bul* 1991 **29** 25   2 P Green 1985 *J Roy Col Gen Prac* **35** 570–2   3 P Ley 1976 in *Communications Between Doctors and Patients*, Ed A Bennett, OUP

5. General practice

Social matters[1]

Unemployment in families 50% of children in care have parents who are unemployed. UK data show an association between child deaths and unemployment, lower social class and overcrowding. Babies whose fathers are employed are heavier at birth (by 150g) than unemployed fathers' babies, after adjusting for other factors. Accidents and infection are more rife among children of the unemployed compared with carefully selected controls, and their mothers may be more prone to depression. As unemployment rises, so does child abuse. Other factors identified with this rise are marital discord, debt, and parents' lack of self-esteem, as affected families reveal: 'When he lost his job he went bonkers. He changed completely. He became depressed and snappy. Frustrated.'

Marital breakdown heads the list of problems of women in general practice with neurosis, and comes second (to employment difficulties) in men, and is a leading factor in >60% of suicide attempts. In the USA divorced males have the highest rates of mortality. The greater incidence of cardiac deaths is most marked in young divorced males. Being divorced and a non-smoker is nearly as dangerous as smoking a pack a day and staying married.[3] Marital harmony (eg cuddling) protects from cardiac death, as shown in one prospective study of 10,000 Israeli hearts.

UK social security benefits[4] *The elderly:* If the only source of income is the pension, it may well be worthwhile applying for income support (formerly supplementary benefit). This provides a basic personal allowance ± a premium (eg £39.85/wk if <25yrs or £50.35 if >25yrs) depending on needs arising out of old age, sickness, disability (or family responsibilities).

The disabled child premium is for a child who is registered blind or who is receiving an attendance or mobility allowance.

The disability premium (£21.45/wk) is for claimants or partners receiving income support, attendance or invalid care allowance, or the severe disablement allowance. It is payable if the claimant (not the carer) has not worked because of ill health for 28 weeks.

The severe disability premium (£38.50/wk) is for those receiving an attendance allowance, if no one is receiving invalid care allowance for looking after him or her and he or she is living alone (defined by DoSS).

This system of a basic allowance plus premiums is used for calculating housing benefit for those who are not entitled to income support. No housing benefit is due if the claimant has more than £16,000 in savings.

Families: If the breadwinner is low paid, family credit may help (doesn't need repaying), as may a loan from the cash-limited social fund for buying essential equipment. Family credit (average value £25/week) is a tax-free cash payment to families in which the breadwinner works for ≥16h/week. Those earning ≤£110–£170/week may be eligible (depending on number of children and savings, which may be up to £8000).

The disability living allowance: This is a tax-free benefit, not affected by earnings or savings, for people <65yrs old, and is divided into two components. The *Care* component for those needing help with washing, dressing, toilet and (if >16yrs) preparing main meals. This can be claimed even if no-one is actually giving the care (£51.30 high rate, £34.30 middle, £13.60 low). The *Mobility* component is for those aged ≥5yrs who have difficulty walking, or who need help to ensure that walking is not dangerous (unsafe or disorientated patient)—it is £35.85 high rate; £13.60 low). There are special rules for those with terminal illness (<6 months to live) to ensure prompt payment. These require a care worker, often the GP, to complete a DS1500 form (for which a fee may be claimed by the doctor).

The attendance allowance: This is tax-free weekly benefit for people aged 65 or over who need help with personal care because of illness or disability. This is payable to the person needing attending to, and not the person attending. Depending on the disability, the weekly rate is either £34.30 or £51.30. All applications are made to Social Security (freefone 0800 882200).

Health and social class

Throughout human history there have been inequalities in the health of classes and populations, caused by social factors. With the introduction of the British National Health Service, with its ideal of equal access to medical care for all groups in society it was assumed that differences in the health of different social (occupational) classes would be eliminated. We now know that this has not happened, and this has been amply documented in various reports such as the *Black Report (Inequalities in Health)* and the *Health Divide*.

Registrar General's scale of 5 social or occupational classes

Class I	Professional	eg lawyer, doctor, accountant
Class II	Intermediate	eg teacher, nurse, manager
Class III^{N}	Skilled non-manual	eg typist, shop assistant
Class III^{M}	Skilled manual	eg miner, bus-driver, cook
Class IV	Partly skilled (manual)	eg farmworker, bus-conductor, or packer
Class V	Unskilled manual	eg cleaner, labourer

There is a remarkable concurrence of evidence concerning the factor by which mortality rates are higher in social class V compared with those of social class I (with regular gradations between). For stillbirths, perinatal deaths, infant deaths, deaths in men aged 15–64 and women aged 20–59 this factor is respectively 1.8, 2, 2.1, 2, and 1.95[1] The same sort of factors hold true for specific diseases such as the standardized mortality ratios (SMR) from lung carcinoma (1.98), coronary heart disease (1.3) and cerebrovascular disease (1.9). Only malignant melanoma, anorexia/bulimia nervosa, eczema, and Hodgkin's disease in early adulthood show a reverse ('disease of affluence') trend. Note: the SMR is the ratio of mortality rates in one class compared with the average for the whole population. The whole population has a SMR of 1.00.

There is more emotional stress and chronic ill health in the 'lower' occupational classes. Furthermore, people who own their own homes have less ill health than private tenants, especially if they live in residential retirement areas.

Within occupations the effect of social class is seen in a 'purer' way than when groups of many occupations are compared: in a study of >17,000 Whitehall civil servants there was a greater than 3-fold difference in mortality from all causes of death (except genitourinary diseases) comparing those in high grades with those in low grades. Similarly in the army there is a 5-fold difference in mortality rates from heart disease between the highest and the lowest ranks.

It has been pointed out that being ill makes a person 'descend' the social scale, but it is estimated that this effect is not large enough to account for the observed differences between classes. It is much more likely that the differences are due to factors such as smoking behaviour, education, marital status, poverty and overcrowding.

Purchasers and providers

Two sets of contrasting principles ►He who pays the piper, calls the tune. ►Priceless therapeutic assets cannot be bought or sold: these include compassion, continuity of care and commitment. ►My job is to spend, spend, spend, until all my patients are healthy. ►The job of the Treasury is to squeeze, squeeze, squeeze, until all spending is minimized. (The clarity of this dichotomy becomes turbid when the doctor is asked to do the squeezing.)

Never just ask how good a structure is without also asking how good it is at transforming itself: that which cannot transform, dies. The UK National Health Service is the largest employer in the Western world and for years the search has been on to find ways to control and transform this dear, mighty thing. The purchaser-provider split is the most powerful lever yet developed for this purpose. *Purchasers* commission care by drawing up contracts with competing *providers*, who deliver the care. In England, purchasers may be Health Authorities or autonomous budget-holding Primary Care Groups (which are run by a board comprizing a majority of GPs but also nurses, social workers and lay members etc). The better the provider delivers secondary care (do *not* pause to ask what 'better' means: speculation on this point might ruin the argument) the more likely they are to get the contract next year. The catch is that all the extra effort the provider makes to out-perform a contract this year will be assumed and taken for granted next year. The same may hold true if purchasing is used for the imposition of guidelines ('evidence-based purchasing').[1] What has been created is a treadmill which goes faster and faster, while taking less and less account of individual patients' and doctors' legitimate but varying needs. Unless the market is rigged, natural selection ensures that the fittest and fastest providers survive. Patients and taxpayers benefit—until the point where cynicism and exhaustion set in. There is no evidence that once the purchaser–provider path is chosen, then cynicism and exhaustion *inevitably* follow, and there is evidence at local level that benefits accrue, and services become more tuned to consumers' desires. (Consumers are not infallible judges of what constitutes health—but they are the best judges we have.)

Controlling change—from on top: an example from maternity[2]

1 Government sets up an expert group to change a specific area—eg maternity, containing mothers, midwives, ministers, obstetricians and general practitioners (these are jokers in the pack, because they are simultaneously consumers, purchasers *and* providers).
2 Issuing of objectives and indicators of success—eg by 5 years:
   - She should have a named midwife to ensure continuity of care.
   - Women should be able to choose their place of delivery (98% are in consultant units, but surveys show 72% wanted other options—22% saying they would like the choice of home birth). Every effort must be made to achieve the outcome that she believes is best for her baby and herself.
   - ≥75% of women should know the person who is to deliver them in labour.
   - Midwives should have direct access to some beds in all maternity units.
   - ≥30% of women should have a midwife as the lead professional.
   - ≥30% of admitted deliveries to be admitted under midwife management.
3 The group's attractive-looking report is issued[2] (using taxpayers' money) to all groups and personnel involved (except mothers).
4 Debate is stimulated, and progress is reviewed.

The anatomy of change Ideals (woman-centred care)→Specific policy objective (all women to have the chance to discuss their care)→Purchasers' action point (set up maternity services liaison committee with lay chairperson)→Providers' action point (provide link-workers, and advocacy schemes for women whose first language is not English).

Controlling change—from grass-roots upwards Example: GP buying on-the-spot (in-house) consultant services for their patients (p 470).

1 M McKee 1995 BMJ i 101 2 DoH 1993 *Changing Childbirth*, HMSO, London, ISBN 0 11 321623 8

Referral statistics

Understanding the intricacies of purcasing health care depends on understanding referral patterns. UK GPs are obliged to give Health Authorities details of hospital referrals. There is the implication that some GPs over-refer, and waste hospital resources. What is the evidence for this? Why is there a 4-fold difference in referral rates between GPs?

If high-referring GPs refer unnecessarily, then the proportion of their referrals resulting in admission should be smaller than that of practices of similar size with low-referring GPs. Usually, this is not the case. Those with high-referral rates have high admission rates. How far does this relation hold? If I refer an ever-increasing number of my patients to a geriatric clinic, must a time come when admissions level off? The idea of a 'levelling-off effect' is important. If the consultant's actions are 'correct', and the GP's expectation as to the outcome of referral are uniform (probably never true) then when a levelling-off effect is observed, it may be true that the *average* referral rate is optimal, and that low-referrers are depriving patients, and high-referrers are wasting resources. In fact, levelling-off effects are rarely found—except in general surgery. What are we to conclude from most of the other specialties where no levelling-off effect is observed? Perhaps specialists admit a fixed proportion of patients referred to them. There is some evidence that this is true for ENT consultants and tonsillectomy. Another possibility is the Coulter–Seagroatt McPherson hypothesis that consultants have a threshold of severity for admission (eg a claudication distance of 50 metres) and even the majority of patients from the high-referrers fulfil this criterion. In this case (assuming the consultant is right), even the high-referrers are not referring enough. This may be true for all forms of angiography, for example. However, if the consultant is over-enthusiastic, and over-optimistic about the benefits of treatment, then the lower referrers are to be applauded for limiting the excesses of the consultant.

Overall, referral rates are no more variable than admission rates, even among populations with similar morbidities. The reason is probably that there is still a great deal of uncertainty underlying very many clinical decisions. We don't know who should have knee replacements, coronary angiography, cholecystectomy, aneurysm surgery, transplants, or grommets.

►There is no known relationship between high or low referral rates and quality of care. Here are 3 cautions in interpreting referrals:

1 Individual list size should not be used as a denominator, as it takes no account of differing workloads within a practice. Consultations per year would be a better denominator.
2 If doctors within the practice have special interests, these must be taken into account in comparing referral patterns.
3 Years of data are needed to compare referrals to rarely-used units.

Fitness to drive[1] (Ordinary UK licences only)

Ordinary UK driving licences issued by the DVLA (Driver & Vehicle Licensing Agency) are inscribed *'You are required by law to inform Drivers Medical Branch, DVLA, Swansea SA99 1AT at once if you have any disability (either physical or medical condition), which is, or may become likely to affect your fitness as a driver, unless you do not expect it to last more than three months.'* It is the responsibility of the driver to inform the DVLA. It is the reponsibility of their doctors to advise patients that medical conditions (and drugs) may affect their ability to drive and for which conditions patients should inform the DVLA. Drivers should also inform their insurance company of any condition disclosed to the DVLA. ▶If in doubt, ask your defence union.

Cardiovascular conditions People should not drive: •Within 1 month of uncomplicated myocardial infarction: there is no need to inform the DVLA.

- Within 1 month of angioplasty, pacemaker, heart valve/artery surgery, 2 months of heart ± lung transplant.* (* = inform DVLA.) Defibrillating pacemakers or implanted anti-tachycardia devices preclude future driving.
- Angina provoked by driving.*
- Symptomatic arrythmia/bradycardia.* Asymptomatic atrial fibrillation is OK.
- If medication reduces alertness, or causes vertigo or faintness.
- If unexplained syncope, acquired complete or 2° heart block.*

Diabetes All on *oral hypoglycaemics* or *insulin* must inform DVLA. If insulin-treated, drivers must demonstrate satisfactory control, and must recognize the onset of any hypoglycaemia—the main risk. Check that vision conforms to required standard (above). Advise avoid driving if hypoglycaemic risk ↑ (eg meal delay; or after excess exercise). Carry rapidly absorbed sugar in vehicle and stop, turn off ignition and eat it if any warning signs. A card should be carried to say which medications they are using to aid with resuscitation if needed. If an accident is due to hypoglycaemia a diabetic driver may be charged with driving under the influence of drugs.

CNS disorders Disabling giddiness, vertigo, and problems with movements preclude driving. DVLA need to know about unexplained blackouts, multiple sclerosis, Parkinson's (any 'freezing' or on–off effects), motor neurone disease, recurrent TIAs and strokes. In the latter the licence is usually withheld for 3 months depending on an examination by an independent doctor, and sometimes a driving test. Those with dementia should only drive if the condition is mild (do not rely on armchair judgements: on-the-road trials are better). Encourage relatives to contact DVLA if a dementing relative should not be driving. GPs may desire to breach confidentiality (the GMC approves) and inform DVLA of demented or psychotic patients (tel. 01792 783686). Many elderly drivers (~1 in 3) who die in accidents are found to have Alzheimer's.

For post-op driving in those with with brain tumours, see reference 1.

Epilepsy and brain surgery: A licence may be granted if:

1 Free from attack for 1 year prior to licence validity date—or

2 For previous 3 years attacks only occur during sleep.

All drivers developing epilepsy must inform DVLA. Those with a single fit, their first fit during sleep, brain surgery, intracranial haematoma removal, or depressed skull fracture must usually wait one attack-free year before driving. If a first attack has been diagnosed and the person has persistent 3-per-second spike and wave activity on the EEG they are still regarded as suffering from epilepsy and are precluded from driving. Epileptic drug withdrawal risks a 40% seizure rate in the first year. Those wishing to withdraw from medication should cease driving from the beginning of withdrawal and not recommence until 6 months after treatment has ceased.

For *flying with medical conditions*, see our electronic version (details, p 466).

1 D Taylor 1995 *Medical Aspects of Fitness to Drive,* Medical Commision on Accident Prevention, 35 Lincoln's Inn Fields, London WC2A & DVLA 1993 *Guide to Current Medical Standards of Fitness to Drive* 2 Lancet 1997 **349** 1143 3 IATA 1994 *Passenger Services Conf Resol Man* 14e. 3 *Drug Ther Bul* 1996 **34** 30

What general conditions make driving illegal?

Driving is prohibited if:
- Severe mental disorder (including severe mental impairment).
- Severe behavioural disorders.
- Alcohol dependency (including inability to refrain from drink driving).
- Drug abuse and dependency.
- Psychotic medication taken in quantities to impair driving ability.

Vision Acuity (± spectacles) should be sufficient to read a 79.4mm-high number plate at 20.5 metres (~6/10 on Snellen chart).
- Monocular vision is allowed only if the visual field is full.
- Binocular field of vision must be >120°.
- Diplopia is not allowable unless *mild* and *correctable (eg by an eye patch)*.

Drugs Driving, or being in charge of a vehicle when under the influence (including side-effect) of a drug is an offence under the Road Traffic Act 1988. Many drugs affect alertness and driving ability (check *Data sheets*), and many are potentiated by alcohol so warn patients not to drive until they are sure of side-effects, not to drink and drive, not to drive if feeling unwell, and never to drive within 48h of a general anaesthetic.

Tiredness and the chronic fatigue syndrome[1]

'Tired all the time' The cause of this frequent complaint is usually emotional distress, but it may signify anything from acute leukaemia to sexual dysfunction. Tiredness is an acceptable ticket of entry to the GP's surgery. Once there, there is a danger that doctor and patient may collude in establishing a physical cause, rather than explore difficult emotional territory—arranging or having a hysterectomy for menorrhagia may be much easier than dissecting out the strands of family breakdown.

Physical symptoms, drug and alcohol habit, job, family relations, life events, hopes and fears need exploring. Just inviting consideration of these may clarify for her (♀/♂ ≈ 3) the cause of her symptoms, though some may need to see the weight of their stress reflected back to them by the doctor, or need permission to admit to feelings, or wish for reassurance of normal blood tests before accepting a psychosocial diagnosis.

In one careful GP-based study[1] blood tests contributed to management in only 9% of patients, who mostly had anaemia, hypothyroidism, infections (eg glandular fever), diabetes mellitus or carcinomatosis. Most of the rest had emotional distress. Only 1 in 400 episodes of fatigue lead to a GP consultation, and only 2% of these lead on to secondary care.

Prognosis: This is better if there is no past history of emotional problems and if the fatigue has lasted less than 3 months.

Post-viral fatigue A variable period of debilitation is common after viral infections, notably 'flu and Epstein–Barr virus, with spontaneous, if slow, recovery. The name is sometimes used for the chronic fatigue syndrome.

Chronic fatigue syndrome (Miscalled myalgic encephalomyelitis, or ME: it is neither a myalgia nor an encephalitis). As with previous outbreaks of fatigue, it is debated whether the pathology lies in the moral or the muscle fibre—or the brain. Symptoms include myalgia (studies of muscle function are consistently normal), malaise, weakness, poor concentration/memory. They may find it hard to find the right word in speech. A study in neuroendocrine function suggests subtly deranged cerebral function[2]—but this may turn out to be another unrepeatable finding in this elusive condition. Most patients fulfil the criteria for a psychiatric disease, but is this cause or the effect of the condition? Evidence suggesting an important rôle for viral infection or persistence is far from convincing.

Tests/examinations rarely help, but exclude other diagnoses—but consider depression, poisoning and hysteria—and then reassure. Check FBC, ESR, U&E, LFT, TFT. Consider autoantibody screen, creatine kinase, and blood culture.

Treatment None is specific—and chronicity is common. Aim for a therapeutic alliance with your patient. Our chief aim must be to prevent somatic fixation: the strongest predictor of a poor prognosis is a fixed belief that symptoms are due to only to physical causes.[3] Allow non-threatening discussion about psychological issues, keeping an open mind on aetiology. Make it clear that psychological symptoms are not the same as malingering—instead, suggest that what starts as an illness may not be what keeps it going. Psychological factors affect the outcome of many illnesses: why should this be different? Cautious increases in levels of activity are recommended (not quite the same as 'take more exercise'), to maintain muscle function, and improve confidence. Be sure to treat any associated anxiety/depression (p 388–96). Address family and work problems. Talking with similarly afflicted peers sounds sensible, but there is a suggestion that this may prolong symptoms.[3] Some have benefited from cognitive therapy (p 370; p 388–96). Slow recovery is the norm.

1 S Wesseley 1997 *Chronic Fatigue & its syndromes* OUP 2 L Ridsdale 1993 BMJ ii 103 & *ibid* 1992 1010
3 Wilson *et al* 1994 BMJ i 756

5. General practice

Managing obesity

The hypothalamus with its 40-or-so neurotransmitters regulates appetite and energy balance, by integrating hormonal, neural and peripheral messages (eg concerning gut distension). Neuropeptide Y is a transmitter stimulating feeding, and suppressing the sympathetic nervous system (thus reducing energy expenditure). Other transmitters increase the release of serotonin and noradrenaline from nerve terminals, and act as mediators of satiety, as does peripherally produced cholecystokinin. Animal models show that highly palatable foods lead to obesity, limited by 'futile thermogenesis'—a metabolic cycling achieved by genetically controlled uncoupling oxidative phosphorylation in mitochondria. Genes for uncoupling proteins have been cloned, and may lead to novel treatments for obesity. Other agents under review are sibutramine (inhibits serotonin and noradrenaline reuptake) and orlistat, a pancreatic lipase inhibitor (see below[1] for details). *Desirable weight:* See opposite. A guide to ↑intra-abdominal fat (correlates best with obesity's problems) is a waist >94cm in men.[2] ~1/3 of a GP's list is are overweight by this criterion: *the richer a society, the more prevalent is obesity.* Despite 33,000 publications on obesity and spending $33 billion/yr (USA), there are no good, *well-tried* non-surgical techniques for long-term *maintained* weight loss. *Prevention by education* can work, eg in school, and may be the best way forward.

Obesity (BMI >30) shortens life, aggravates diabetes, gout, osteoarthrosis, heartburn, hypertension, hyperlipidaemia, sleep apnoea, and venous thrombosis. Weight loss in the obese lowers BP, diminishes osteoarthrosis of weight bearing joints, and restores life expectancy to normal.

Excess weight in obesity consists of 75% fat (energy value 9000kcal/kg) and 25% other tissues—fat free mass, FFM, (water, protein and glycogen—energy value 1000kcal/kg) so each kg of excess weight ≈ 7000 kcalories of stored energy. Weight is lost by creating a –ve energy balance. With modest energy deficit (intake 500–1000kcal/24h) fat : FFM loss is 3:1 and weight loss of 0.5–1kg/week should occur. With very low calorie diets (<330kcal/24h) FFM loss is higher and weight loss more rapid. Physical activity accounts for 20% of energy expenditure so exercise contributes much less to weight loss than cutting intake—but regular aerobic exercise (>5h/week) can contribute to weight maintenance in the moderately, but not severely obese.

Dietery considerations •Ask patients to keep a diary of foods eaten.
- Aim for realistic loss (< 1 kg/week for 1000kcal per day's diet).
- Regular (weekly) weighing to watch trends.
- Consider weighing food to calculate calorie intake to prevent 'cheating'.
- Groups such as Weight Watchers[3] can be very useful motivating forces.
- Aim to re-educate eating habits to maintain reduced weight.
- Ensure that the diet is nutritious. ►See the *Healthy Diet, OHCM* p 482.

Very Low Calorie Diets (VLCDs) give 400kcal/24h with 40g protein/24h for women, 500kcal/24h and 50g protein/24h for men, and women >173cm. 2 pints of skimmed milk with bran for bulk and unlimited calorie-free drinks gives the former, 3 pints the latter. All should take 200mg ferrous sulfate and one multivitamin tablet/24h. This is cheaper than commercial VLCDs. As excess fat free mass is lost, use for >4 weeks needs medical supervision.

Appetite suppressant drugs are not advised as tolerance develops and weight rises on stopping drugs. Bulk-forming drugs are ineffective.

Surgery is reserved for the morbidly obese (BMI >40; or >35 with associated cardiovascular risk factors[1]). Gastric bypass results in more weight loss than gastroplasty. Both result in sustained weight loss. Side-effects: dumping (*OHCM* p 164) and vitamin or mineral deficiency.

1 *Drug Ther Bul* 1998 **36** 89; **Orlistat** is licensed for ≤2yrs use in those with BMI >28kg + associated risk factors who have shown weight↓ on a diet (which must be continued). SE: (little is absorbed) oily faecal incontinence/spotting, flatus, urgency. CI: malabsorption. Dose: eg 120mg with a meal (up to 3/day, =£560/yr); stop after 12 wks if wt loss <5% **2** D Pounder 1998 *BMJ* **i** 1428 **3** tel[UK]: 0181 491 1929

Weights and heights

Men Height			Acceptable weight range					Overweight			Obese		
cm	ft	in	kg	st	lb	– st	lb	kg	st	lb	kg	st	lb
158	5	2	44–64	6	13	– 10	1	70	11	0	77	12	2
160	5	3	44–65	6	13	– 10	3	72	11	5	78	12	4
162	5	4	46–66	7	3	– 10	6	73	11	7	79	12	6
164	5	4	47–67	7	6	– 10	8	74	11	9	80	12	8
166	5	5	48–69	7	8	– 10	12	76	12	0	83	13	1
168	5	6	49–71	7	10	– 11	3	78	12	4	85	13	5
170	5	7	51–73	8	0	– 11	7	80	12	8	88	13	12
172	5	8	52–74	8	3	– 11	9	81	12	11	89	14	0
174	5	9	53–75	8	5	– 11	11	83	13	1	90	14	2
176	5	9	54–77	8	7	– 12	2	85	13	5	92	14	7
178	5	10	55–79	8	9	– 12	6	87	13	10	95	14	13
180	5	11	58–80	9	2	– 12	8	88	13	12	96	15	2
182	6	0	59–82	9	4	– 12	13	90	14	2	98	15	6
184	6	0	60–84	9	6	– 13	3	92	14	7	101	15	13
186	6	1	62–86	9	11	– 13	8	95	14	13	103	16	3
188	6	2	64–88	10	1	– 13	12	97	15	4	106	16	10
190	6	3	66–90	10	6	– 14	2	99	15	8	108	17	0
192	6	3	68–93	10	10	– 14	9	102	16	1	112	17	9

Women			Acceptable weight range					Overweight			Obese		
cm	ft	in	kg	st	lb	– st	lb	kg	st	lb	kg	st	lb
148	4	10	37–53	5	12	– 8	5	58	9	2	64	10	1
150	4	11	37–54	5	12	– 8	7	59	9	4	65	10	3
152	5	0	38–55	6	0	– 8	9	61	9	8	66	10	6
154	5	1	39–57	6	2	– 9	0	63	9	13	68	10	10
156	5	1	39–58	6	2	– 9	2	64	10	1	70	11	0
158	5	2	40–58	6	4	– 9	2	64	10	1	70	11	0
160	5	3	41–59	6	6	– 9	4	65	10	3	71	11	3
162	5	4	42–61	6	9	– 9	8	67	10	8	73	11	7
164	5	5	43–62	6	11	– 9	11	68	10	10	74	11	9
166	5	5	44–64	6	13	– 10	1	70	11	0	77	12	2
168	5	6	45–65	7	11	– 10	3	72	11	5	78	12	4
170	5	7	45–66	7	11	– 10	6	73	11	7	79	12	6
172	5	8	46–67	7	3	– 10	8	74	11	9	80	12	8
174	5	9	48–69	7	8	– 10	12	76	12	0	83	13	1
176	5	9	49–70	7	10	– 11	0	77	12	2	84	13	3
178	5	10	51–72	8	0	– 11	5	79	12	6	86	13	8
180	5	11	52–72	8	3	– 11	9	81	12	11	89	14	0

Figures from Fogarty table but taking account of extended lower range suggested by 1979 Build study. Overweight = 110–119%; obese = >120% upper acceptable limit. *Desirable weight* for adults is defined by the body mass index (BMI), W/H^2, where W is body weight (kg) and H is height (metres); mortality is lowest for BMIs of 20–25.

Seven (Mayo Clinic) questions for weight-loss programmes to answer

1 Is there proof that it works (ask for evidence of long-term results)?
2 Any qualified dietitian or specialist in behaviour modification employed?
3 Is the recommended intake nutritionally balanced?
4 Does the patient have to buy special products?
5 Will the patient receive advice on starting safe, moderate exercise?
6 How will the programme reward and monitor progress?
7 Is there support and follow-up for after the formal programme ends?

Healing

Since neolithic times, healing has had a central place in our culture, and has long been recognized as 'mor bettir and mor precious þan any medicyne'.[1] Recently medicines have improved greatly, so that the rôle of doctors as the purveyor of medicines has eclipsed their more ancient rôles. We all recognize the limits of our rôle as prescribers, and we would all like to heal more and engage in repetitive tasks less often. But what, we might ask, *is* healing? How is it different for from curing? Healing is, at one level, something mysterious that happens to wounds,[2] involving inflammation → granulocyte, macrophage, and platelet activation → release of platelet-derived growth factor and transforming growth factors α and β → neovascular growth → fibroblast-mediated contraction → proteoglycans and collagen synthesis, lysis, and remodelling.

On another level, healing involves transforming through communication—a kind of hands-on hypnosis. We can cure with scalpels and needles, but these are not instruments of communication. Here is a serendipitous example of healing (an all too rare event in our own practice). On a rainy February evening, after a long surgery, I visited a stooped old man at the fag-end of life, with something the matter with his lung. 'I suppose it's rotting, like the rest of me—it's gradually dying.' I reply: 'Do you think you're dying?' 'Aren't we all?' 'Green and dying' I reply for some reason, half remembering a poem by Dylan Thomas. The patient looks mystified: he thinks he misheard, and asks me to repeat. 'Green *and* dying' I say, feeling rather stupid. There is a pause, and then he rises to his full height, puffs out his chest, and completes, in a magnificent baritone, the lines: '. . . Time held me green and dying, though I sang in my chains like the sea.'[3] By chance I had revealed a new meaning to a favourite poem of his which perhaps he thought was about childhood, not the rigours of his old age. Both our eyes shone more brightly as we passed on to the more prosaic aspects of the visit. This illustrates the nature of healing: its unpredictability, its ability to allow us to rise to our full height, to sing, rather than mumble, and how externally nothing may be changed by healing—just our internal landscape, transformed by a moment of illumination. It also shows how healing depends on communication, and how it is bound up with art. Healing may be mysterious, but it is not rare. We have so often kissed the grazed knees of our daughters that we expect the healing balm of kisses to wear out, but, while they are young, it never will, because children know how to receive but not how to doubt, and the kiss is the paradigm of healing: contact between two humans, wordless service of the lips, which the sterile advice of a microbiologist would never condone, an activity for which there is no Read code, and which we know as healing.

The bread and butter of our work comprises the sifting of symptoms, deciding what is wrong, and prescribing treatment—all tasks which, according to an historic prediction by no less a personage than the editor of the *Lancet* are destined for delegation to microchips.[4] This implies that our chief rôle will be as healers and teachers. There is much to be said for the idea that we should throw away the paraphernalia of mechanistic medicine, our formularies, our computers, and our audits—and insist on returning our primordial rôle. We should, perhaps, pay more than lip-service to our daughter's view of general practice, revealed when she wanted one of us to return home promptly for a family outing, when she said 'Can't you just kiss them all a bit faster, and come home quickly today?'

No doubt there will always be some way to go before healing, the central ideal of medicine, becomes its central activity. After all, the last thing any of us wants, when struck down by appendicitis, is a poet or a healer—but last things will always retain their power to set us thinking.

1 Anon ~1400 *Secreta Secret*. Gov. Lordsh. EETS 66 & OED 1ed **V** page 152 col 1 **2** *Oxford Textbook of Surgery* 1e 1994 page 5, OUP **3** Dylan Thomas *Fern Hill* **4** *Lancet* Ed 1995 **345** 1126

6. Ophthalmology

Looking at words

Accommodation The active changing of lens shape to focus near objects.
Acuity A measure of how well the eye sees a small or distant object.
Amblyopia Reduced acuity which is not from an anatomic optic defect.
Amsler grid Test chart of intersecting lines used for screening for macular disease. Lines will appear wavy and squares distorted to those with macular disease.
Anisocoria Unequal pupil size.
Anisometropia Having different refractive errors in each eye.
Aphakia The state of having no lens (eg removed because of cataract).
Blepharitis Inflamed lids.
Canthus The medial or lateral angle made by the open lids.
Chemosis Oedema of the conjunctiva.
Choroid Vascular coat between the retina and the outer scleral coat.
Ciliary body Portion of uvea (uveal tract) between iris and choroid, containing the ciliary processes and ciliary muscle (for accommodation).
Conjunctiva Mucous membrane on anterior sclera & posterior lid aspect.
Cycloplegia Ciliary muscle paralysis preventing accommodation.
Dacryocystitis Inflammation of the lacrimal sac.
Dioptre Units for measuring refractive power of lenses.
Ectropion The lids evert (especially lower lid).
Entropion The lids invert (so that the lashes may irritate the eyeball).
Epiphora Passive overflow of tears on to the cheek.
Fornix Where bulbar (scleral) and palpebral (lid) conjunctivae meet.
Fovea The tiny, vital, cone-rich area of retina capable of 6/6 vision.
Fundus That part of retina normally visible through the ophthalmoscope.
Keratoconus The cornea is shaped like a cone. See p 520.
Keratomalacia The cornea is softened.
Limbus The annular border between clear cornea and opaque sclera.
Macula Rim of avascular retina surrounding the fovea.
Miotic An agent causing pupil constriction (eg pilocarpine).
Mydriatic An agent causing pupil dilatation (eg tropicamide).
Near point Where the eye is looking when maximally accommodated.
Papillitis Inflammation of the optic nerve head.
Optic cup The cup like depression in the centre of the optic disc (p 503).
Optic disc The portion of optic nerve seen ophthalmoscopically in the fundus of the eye.
Presbyopia Age-related reduced near acuity from failing accommodation.
Pterygium Wing-shaped degenerative conjunctival condition encroaching on the cornea.
Ptosis Drooping lids
Refraction Ray deviation on passing through media of different density; OR determining refractive errors, and correcting them with lenses.
Retinal detachment The sensory retina separates from the pigmented epithelial layer of retina.
Sclera The whites of the eyes starting from the corneal perimeter.
Scotoma A defect causing a part of the field of view to go missing.
Slit lamp A device which illuminates and magnifies structures in the eye.
Strabismus (squint) Eyes deviate (they are not looking at the same thing).
Tarsorrhaphy A surgical procedure for uniting upper and lower lids.
Tonometer A device for measuring intraocular pressure.
Uvea Iris, ciliary body and choroid.
Vitreous Jelly-like substance filling the globe behind the lens.
Vitrectomy Surgical removal of vitreous.

Examination of the eye

The history indicates the part of the examination to focus on. Asking about trauma, symptoms of pain *vs* irritation, loss of vision, and pattern and speed of onset, give vital diagnostic clues. To assess the retina and optic nerve (nerve of vision), test acuity, visual field and colour vision (p 517).

Visual acuity This is a measure of central (macular) vision. Always test acuity carefully as loss of acuity is a grave sign. Record it accurately, especially in a patient with eye injury. Examine the right eye first. Sit the patient at the required distance from the Snellen chart (traditionally 6 metres, but charts are available for the much more convenient 3 metres). Obscure the left eye with an 'eye paddle', not *pressed* against the right eye—simply enough to *occlude* the visual access. Card is an alternative (more reliable than peepable-through fingers). Read the Snellen chart from the top using the right eye. Then, test acuity of left eye. Use glasses if worn. The last line completed accurately indicates the acuity for distant vision.

The chart is designed so that the top line can be read by someone with normal vision at 60 metres, the next at 36 metres, the next at 24, the next at 18, the next at 12, the next at 9, and the next at 6 metres. Acuity is recorded as 6/60, 6/36, 6/24, 6/18, 6/12, 6/9, 6/6 to indicate the last line accurately read (6/6 vision is normal). For acuities of worse than 6/60 the patient can be brought forward to 5, 4, 3, 2 and 1 metre from the chart to read the top line. If he can read it then acuity is expressed as that distance, eg 5/60, 4/60, 3/60, 2/60 or 1/60. If the vision is below 1/60 ask the patient to count your fingers at ½ metre distance. This is recorded as CF (count fingers). If they cannot count your fingers move your hand in front of the eye at ¼ metre distance. If the patient can appreciate that your hand moves, record HM (hand movement). If the patient cannot appreciate hand movement, dim the light in the examination room and shine a torch light into the eye. If the patient perceives light, record PL. If there is no perception, record 'no PL' (the eye is blind). NB: in practice, if nothing on the Snellen chart can be read, it is common to go straight to finger counting.

If the patient sees less than 6/6 with or without glasses, examine again with a pin-hole in front of the eye. A narrow beam of light then enters the eye eliminating the need to focus a beam. If the patient has only refractive error, there will be an improvement in vision as seen through the pin-hole. This is an important test as it eliminates ocular pathology as a cause of reduced acuity. (Make a pin-hole with a 22G needle in a 10 × 10cm opaque card; check that you can see through the hole before giving it to the patient.)

If patients >40 years old complain of near-vision blurring, the cause may be presbyopia (p 490). Test near vision using a near vision testing card (p 478). If the patient can read N5 at 30cm, near vision is normal.

Visual field This is the area that can be seen with both eyes without shifting gaze. The uni-ocular field is smaller than the binocular field. When assessing for visual field defects establish whether the defect affects only one eye or both, whether there are clear boundaries to the defect, if the boundaries lie in the vertical or horizontal meridians, and to what degree acuity is affected. For confrontation tests see p 492.

External examination: *Lids:* They should be symmetrical and retract normally on upward gaze (abnormal in dysthyroid disease). Note ptosis (p 480), spasm, inflammation or swellings (p 480).

Conjunctiva: Look for inflammation (if circumcorneal, suspect anterior uveitis; injection away from the cornea and on the tarsal surfaces suggests conjunctivitis; focal injection adjacent to the cornea 'points' to a problem on the cornea). Is there discharge, follicles or cobblestone patterns on tarsal conjunctiva of upper lid, or any subconjunctival haemorrhage (p 496)?

Cornea: Examine with a torch for opacity, abrasion, ulcer (the latter two stain green with 1% fluorescein), or oedema.

Anterior chamber: It is filled with clear aqueous humor but can be cloudy in anterior uveitis (p 494), may have sterile pus (hypopyon) with corneal ulcer, or blood (hyphaema) after injury.

Pupils should be equal, reacting to light and accommodation (PERLA). They are small and irregular in anterior uveitis, dilated and fixed in acute glaucoma (p 494). For other pupillary abnormalities see p 488.

Lens: When the lens is normal the pupil appears black. With mature cataract it may appear white.

Extraocular movements It is vital to examine these in those with diplopia. Ask the patient to watch a pencil move diagonally: up left; up right; down left; down right; horizontally left; horizontally right. Ask which movement provokes most diplopia, and when looking in that direction, block each eye in turn and ask which one sees the *outer* image: that is the eye which is malfunctioning. NB: avoid extremes of movement as inability to maintain fixation stimulates nystagmus. For eye movements and squint see p 486.

Ophthalmoscopy This helps detect pathology in the lens, vitreous and retina. Start with high + numbers (usually marked in red on the dial). To examine the lens and the vitreous focus the beam of the ophthalmoscope at the pupil at ~1 metre from the eye. In the normal eye there is a red glow from the choroid (the red reflex). Any lens opacity (cataract) will be seen as a black pattern obstructing the red reflex. Blood or loose floaters in the vitreous are seen as black floaters. To determine the position of the opacity in the eye, move your head in the horizontal plane from side to side, like a cobra waiting to strike. The opacity will either move in the same direction as you (so lies behind the lens), in the opposite direction (so lies in front of the lens) or will not move at all (so *in* the lens).

Red reflexes are absent with dense cataract and intraocular haemorrhage. When the retina is in focus examine carefully the optic disc (should have precise boundaries and central cup, p 502). Note pallor or swelling. Examine radiating vessels and macula (ask the patient to look at the light).

Aids to successful ophthalmoscopy: Ensure the batteries are fully charged.

- Darken the room as much as possible. Remove the patient's spectacles and dial up the appropriate lens to correct for the resulting refractive error (– lenses correct myopia, + lenses correct hypermetropia).
- If the patient is very myopic or is aphakic, try examining with his spectacles on. The disc will appear very small.
- If you find ophthalmoscopy difficult using your non-dominant eye, try using your dominant eye for examining *both* fundi—while standing behind the seated patient, whose neck is fully extended.
- Always check the lens for opacities before trying to examine the fundus.
- Get *close enough* to the patient, even if one of you has had garlic for lunch.
- Consider using a short-acting mydriatic to dilate the pupil (see p 518).
- Remember that most retinal tears are peripheral and are difficult to see without special equipment. It is not possible to see the periphery of the retina with the ophthalmoscope.

Slit lamp examination This instrument has a bright light source and a horizontally mounted microscope to examine the structures of the living eye. The light source can be converted to a slit (hence the name). Tonometric attachments allow intraocular pressure measurement.

N. 48

He moved

N. 36

forward a few

N. 24

fine chattering gems.

N. 18

He knew exactly who would

N. 14

now sneeze calmly through an open
door. Had there been another year

N. 12

of peace the battalion would have made
a floating system of perpetual drainage.

N. 10

A silent fall of immense snow came near oily
remains of the purple-blue supper on the table.

N. 8

We drove on in our old sunless walnut. Presently
classical eggs ticked in the new afternoon shadows.

H
A L
T N C
O L H A
E C T N O
C L O H N A
A E N L O M C T
I S Q W E N L D E P O

N. 6

We were instructed by my cousin Jasper not to exercise by country
house visiting unless accompanied by thirteen geese or gangsters.

N. 5

The modern American did not prevail over the pair of redundant bronze puppies.
The worn-out principle is a bad omen which I am never glad to ransom on purpose.

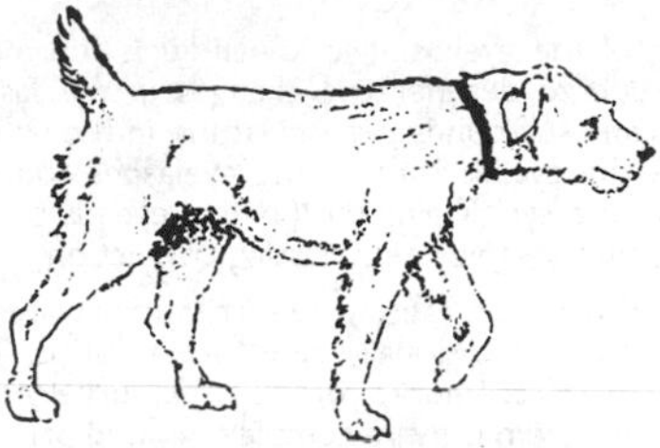

H

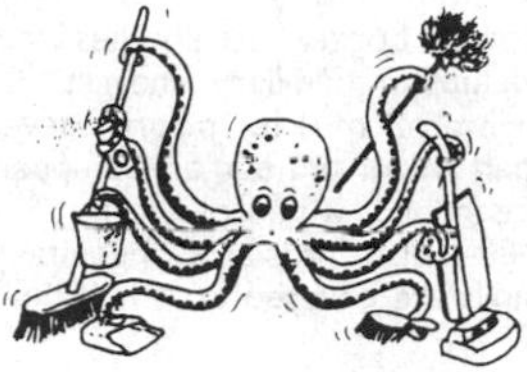

T

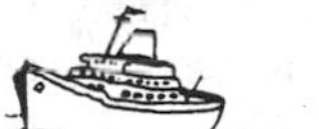

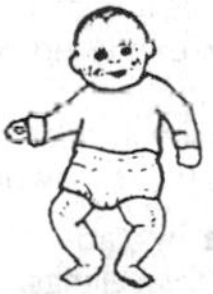

O Y

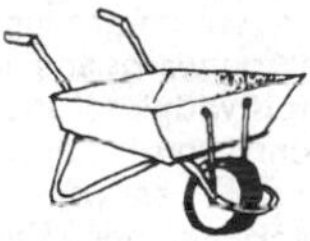

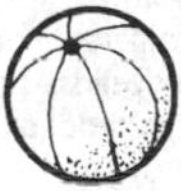

H U V

A T Y M

X O W U H

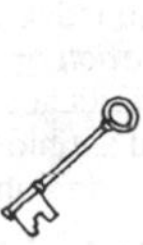

Y U V T X O

A W I M H Y T

Test types (N. 48—N. 5 opposite) should be read at 30cm.

The external eye

Entropion This is inturning of the eyelids. The lower lid is the more commonly affected. Usually due to degenerative changes in the fascial attachments of the lower lids and surrounding musculature, in the UK it is rare below 40yrs of age. As the eyelids turn in, the eyelashes rub the cornea and constantly irritate the eye. Taping the (lower) eyelids to the cheek gives temporary relief, surgery gives more lasting correction.

Ectropion There is lower lid eversion causing eye irritation, watering (drainage punctum malaligned) and occasionally exposure keratitis. The patient is usually elderly, or has a facial nerve palsy. Plastic surgery may correct the deformity but the problem is more complex in facial palsy.

Ptosis (Upper lid drooping) Its lower border usually lies mid-way between the superior limbus and upper pupillary margin. *Causes:* •Congenital (absent nerve to the levator muscle, poorly developed levator); •Mechanical (oedema, xanthelasma or tumour of the upper lids); •Myogenic (muscular dystrophy, myasthenia); •Neurological (III nerve palsy, p 486; Horner's syndrome, p 488—slight ptosis). Congenital ptosis is corrected surgically early if the pupils are covered or if it is unilateral (risk of amblyopia ex anopsia).

Lagophthalmos This is difficulty in complete lid closure over the eyeball. *Causes:* Exophthalmos, mechanical impairment of lid movements (eg injury or burns to the lids), leprosy, paralysed orbicularis oculi giving sagging lower lid. Corneal ulceration and keratitis may follow. Lubricate eyes with liquid paraffin ointment. If corneal ulceration develops, temporary tarsorrhaphy (stitching the lids together) may be needed.

Styes The word stye is used more by patients than by ophthalmologists for referring to inflammatory eyelid swellings. *Hordeolum externum* is an abscess or infection, usually staphylococcal, in a lash follicle; these may also involve the glands of Moll (sweat glands) and of Zeis (sebum-producing glands attached directly to the lash follicle). They 'point' outwards and may cause extensive inflammation of the eyelids. Treatment is with local antibiotics—eg fusidic acid. (The word 'stye' implies infection: if this is not present, the term *marginal cyst*—of Zeis or Moll—may be used.) Less common is the *hordeolum internum*, an abscess of the Meibomiam glands. These 'point' inwards, opening on to conjunctiva, cause less local reaction but leave a residual swelling called a *chalazion* or a *Meibomiam cyst* (tarsal cyst) when they subside. Treatment for residual swellings is incision and curettage under anaesthesia, plus a topical antibiotic (eg fusidic acid) application several days post-operatively. (NB: hordeolum is Latin for *barleycorn*.)

Blepharitis means generalized eyelid inflammation, eg from staphylococci or seborrhoeic dermatitis. Eyes have 'burning' itching red margins, and may have scales on the lashes. Treat with regular saline bathing and local antibiotic applications (eg fusidic acid). If inflammation remains very persistent, consider adding 1% hydrocortisone cream.

Pinguecula These degenerative yellow nodules appear on the conjunctiva either side of the cornea (typically the nasal side) commonly in adults. If they become inflamed (pingueculitis)—they may respond to topical steroids. If it encroaches on to the cornea, as it may in dusty, wind-blown life-styles, the word **pterygium** is used (surgery may be needed).

Dendritic ulcers (Corneal ulcers caused by *Herpes simplex*) They produce photophobia and epiphoria (watering). If steroid eye applications are given in their presence there is massive amoeboid ulceration and risk of blindness. *Diagnosis:* 1% fluorescein drops stain the lesion. *Treatment* is with aciclovir 3% eye ointment 5 times per day for at least 3 days after complete healing.

6. Ophthalmology

Tears and lacrimation

The lacrimal glands are on the superior temporal side of the orbits. The tear film excreted over the eye drains via the lacrimal puncta (found at the medial side of the upper and lower eyelid) through the lacrimal sac, lacrimal duct and inferior meatus (just lateral to the inferior turbinate) into the nasal passages. Dry eyes may be due to insufficient tear secretion, and watering eyes may be due to blockage of the drainage system.

Acute dacryocystitis This is acute inflammation of the tear sac which is located medial to the medial canthus. This may spread to surrounding tissues and result in systemic upset. Immediate antibiotic therapy may resolve the infection. Failure leads to local abscess formation (may need drainage).

Infantile dacryocystitis In babies the nasolacrimal duct may not be canalized at birth and may not open fully until the child is 3 months old. Tear sacs tend to get infected and a sticky discharge is produced. Ask an ophthalmologist to teach the mother to massage the sac to empty the contents four times daily and then apply antibiotic (eg gentamicin) eye drops. Should this fail after several months, probing of the duct under anaesthesia is an option.

Chronic dacryocystitis This tends to occur in the middle-aged and elderly. There is distension of the lacrimal sac, discharge of mucopus into the eye and blockage of the nasolacrimal duct. Syringing the lacrimal drainage system should be performed early to try to clear the system—and may need to be repeated. In some cases dacryocystorhinostomy (a surgical procedure to establish communication between the lacrimal sac and the nasal cavity) may be needed.

Dacroadenitis There is pain and swelling on the temporal side of the upper eyelid. The upper eyelid may appear S-shaped. The cause may be viral (mumps, measles, influenza) although gonococcal organisms can be the cause. Chronic swelling can occur in sarcoid, TB, lymphatic leukaemia or lymphosarcoma.

Tear production The volume of tears normally *in* the eye is 6μl, the turnover *rate* being 1.2μl/min. Tears are similar in electrolyte concentration to plasma, but rich in proteins, especially IgA. They also contain lysozyme and β-lysin which have antibacterial properties.

Dry eye syndrome (keratoconjunctivitis sicca) This may be due to *decreased tear production* by the lacrimal glands, eg in Sjögren's syndrome associated with connective tissue disorders (especially rheumatoid arthritis), or from mumps, sarcoid, amyloid, lymphoma, leukaemia, haemochromatosis, or old age. Other causes: *excess evaporation of tears* (post-exposure keratitis); or *mucin deficiency in the tears* (avitaminosis A, Stevens–Johnson syndrome, pemphigoid, chemical burns). Schirmer's test (strip of filter paper put overlapping lower lid; tears should soak >15mm in 5min) reveals insufficient production. Artificial tears may be used for symptomatic relief.

Excess lacrimation *Causes:* Emotion, corneal abrasions or foreign body, conjunctivitis, iritis, acute glaucoma.

Epiphora (ie normal volume, but not reabsorbed) *Causes:* Ectropion, entropion, blockage of drainage system.

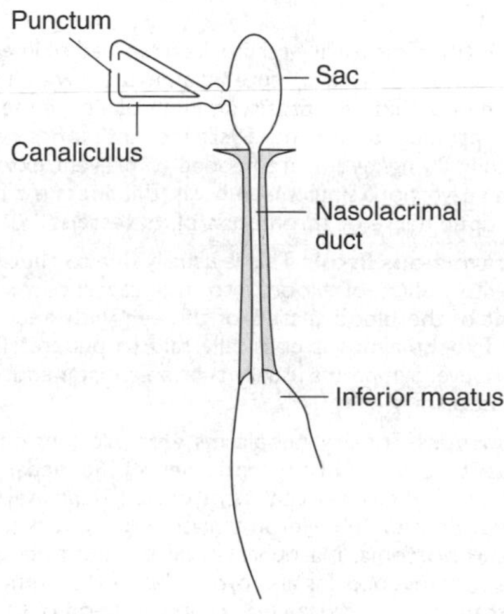
Lacrimal system
Punctum
Sac
Canaliculus
Nasolacrimal duct
Inferior meatus

Orbital swellings

Lesions within the bony orbit tend to present with proptosis (ie exophthalmos), whatever the pathological origin. Proptosis (protrusion of the orbital contents) is a cardinal sign of intraorbital problems. If pressure is eccentric within the orbit there will be deviation of the eyeball and diplopia. Pain in the orbit usually arises from neighbouring structures (eg sinusitis).

Orbital cellulitis This usually results from spread of infection from the paranasal air sinuses. There is acute inflammation within the orbit with fever, swelling of the lids, proptosis, and immobility of the eye. Admit to hospital for prompt treatment. Systemic antibiotics, eg cefuroxime 1.5g/8h IV (child 20mg/kg/8h), are needed to prevent extension into the meninges and cavernous sinus thrombosis. Blindness is a risk from pressure on the optic nerve or thrombosis of its vessels.

Carotico-cavernous fistula This is usually due to rupture of a carotid aneurysm with reflux of blood into the cavernous sinus. There is engorgement of the blood vessels of the eye with oedema of lids and conjunctiva. Exophthalmos is classically said to pulsate. There is a loud bruit over the eye. Symptoms usually subside spontaneously. Carotid ligation may be necessary.

Orbital tumours Primary neoplasms are rare (angiomas, dermoids, meningiomas, or gliomas of the optic nerve). Secondary tumours are more common. Reticuloses can form orbital deposits (examine liver, spleen, nodes; do FBC). In children unilateral proptosis may be the first sign of a neuroblastoma. Nasopharyngeal tumours occasionally invade the orbit, as may mucocoeles and pyocoeles of the ethmoid and frontal sinuses. CT scan pictures give a clear representation of the orbit.

Hyperthyroidism may cause exophthalmos (p 510).

Ophthalmic shingles

This is zoster of the first (ophthalmic) branch of the trigeminal nerve and accounts for 20% of all shingles with only thoracic nerves being more commonly affected (55%). Pain, tingling or numbness around the eye may precede a blistering rash which is accompanied by much inflammation. In 50% of those with ophthalmic shingles the eye itself is affected with 40–77% having corneal signs and 50–60% iritis. Nose-tip involvement—Hutchison's sign—means involvement of the nasociliary branch of the trigeminal nerve which also supplies the globe and makes it highly likely that the eye will be affected. The eye can be seriously involved with little rash elsewhere.

Presentation:

- Mucopurulent conjunctivitis
- Limbal lesions
- Preauricular node tenderness
- Scleritis
- Episcleritis
- Visual loss
- V nerve palsy
- Keratitis
- Iritis (± atrophy)
- Pupillary distortion
- Optic atrophy

Treatment: Give aciclovir 800mg five times a day PO for 7 days to reduce viral shedding, accelerate healing time and reduce incidence of new lesions. Start within 4 days of shingles onset. It is advisable for all with ophthalmic shingles to see a specialist within 3 days to exclude iritis with a slit lamp. Prolonged steroid eyedrops may be needed.

6. Ophthalmology

Eye movements and squint

To maintain single vision, fine co-ordination of eye movement of both eyes is necessary. Abnormality of the co-ordinated movement is called squint. Other names for squint are strabismus and tropia. Exotropia is divergent (one eye turned out) squint: enotropia is (one eye turned in) convergent squint. Prominent epicanthic folds (diagram) may produce pseudosquint.

Non-paralytic squint These squints usually start in childhood. The range of eye movements is full. Squints may be constant or not. All squints need ophthalmological assessment as vision may be damaged if not treated.

Diagnosis: Difficult, eg in uncooperative children. Screening tests:

1 Corneal reflection: reflection from a bright light falls centrally and symmetrically on each cornea if no squint, asymmetrically if squint present.
2 Cover test: movement of the uncovered eye to take up fixation as the other eye is covered demonstrates manifest squint; latent squint is revealed by movement of the covered eye as the cover is removed.

Convergent squint (esotropia) This is the commonest type in children. There may be no cause, or it may be due to hypermetropia (p 490). If the eye is left without focused input, vision may never develop satisfactorily in that eye (it has *amblyopia ex anopsia*).

Divergent squint (exotropia) These tend to occur in older children and are often intermittent. Amblyopia is less commonly a problem.

Management Remember 3 *'O's:* *Optical; Orthoptic; Operation*. Treatment should start as soon as the squint is noticed. *Optical:* Assess the refractive state of the eyes after cyclopentolate 1% eyedrops; the cycloplegia allows objective determination of the refractive state of the eyes; the mydriasis allows a good view into the eye to exclude abnormality, eg cataract, macular scarring, retinoblastoma, optic atrophy. Spectacles are then provided to correct refractive errors. *Orthoptic:* The good eye may be patched to encourage use of the one tending to squint. *Operations* (*resection and recession of rectus muscles*): These help alignment and give good cosmetic results. NB: use of botulinum toxin has helped some patients with esotropia (see p 522).[1]

Paralytic squint Diplopia is most marked when trying to look in the direction of pull of the paralysed muscle. When the separation between the two images is greatest the image from the paralysed eye is furthest from the midline and faintest.

Third nerve palsy (oculomotor) Ptosis, proptosis (as recti tone ↓), fixed pupil dilatation, with the eye looking down and out. Causes: p 488.

Fourth nerve palsy (trochlear) There is diplopia and the patient may hold his head tilted (ocular torticollis). The eye is elevated in adduction and cannot look down and in (superior oblique paralysed). Causes: trauma 30%, diabetes 30%, tumour, idiopathic.

Sixth nerve palsy (abducens) There is diplopia in the horizontal plane. The eye is medially deviated and cannot move laterally from midline, as the lateral rectus is paralysed. Causes: tumour causing increased intracranial pressure (compresses the nerve on the edge of the petrous temporal bone), trauma to base of skull, or vascular.

1 G Lennerstrand 1998 *Acta Ophthalmol Scand* **76** 27

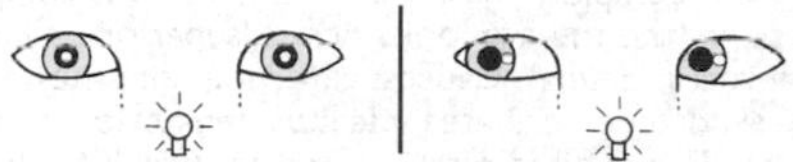

PSEUDOSQUINT Wide epicanthic folds give the appearance of squint in the eye looking towards the nose. That the eyes are correctly aligned is confirmed by the corneal reflection.

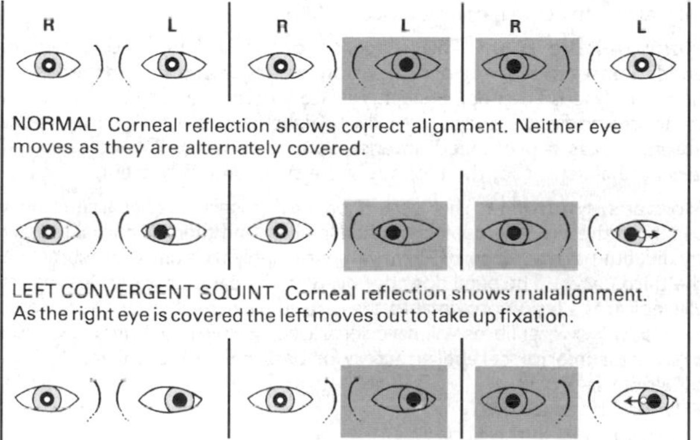

NORMAL Corneal reflection shows correct alignment. Neither eye moves as they are alternately covered.

LEFT CONVERGENT SQUINT Corneal reflection shows malalignment. As the right eye is covered the left moves out to take up fixation.

LEFT DIVERGENT SQUINT Corneal reflection shows malalignment. As the right eye is covered the left eye moves in to take up fixation.

NB If there is ***eccentric fixation*** (ie foveal vision so poor that it is not used for fixation), the deviating eye will not move to take up fixation. Corneal reflection shows that malalignment is is present. The cover test relies on the ability to fixate.

Pupils

Pupil inequality Light detection by the retina is passed to the brain via the optic nerve (afferent pathway) and pupil constriction is mediated by the oculomotor (third) cranial nerve (efferent pathway). The sympathetic nervous system is responsible for pupil dilatation via the ciliary nerves.

Afferent defects (absent direct response) The pupil will not respond to light, but it will constrict if light is shone into the other eye (consensual response). Causes: optic neuritis, optic atrophy, retinal disease. The pupils appear the same size (consensual response unaffected). If the Marcus Gunn swinging flashlight test is used, the affected eye will appear to dilate when the lamp is swung away from the consensual eye into the affected eye. Constriction to accommodation will still occur.

Efferent defects The third nerve also mediates eye movement and eyelid retraction. With complete third nerve palsy there is complete ptosis, a fixed dilated pupil, and the eye looks down (superior oblique still acts) and out (lateral rectus acting). Causes: cavernous sinus lesions, superior orbital fissure syndrome, diabetes mellitus, posterior communicating artery aneurysm. The pupil is often spared in vascular causes, eg with diabetes and hypertension. Pupillary fibres run in the periphery, and are the first to be involved in compressive lesions by tumour or aneurysm.

Other causes of a fixed dilated pupil Mydriatics, trauma (blow to iris), acute glaucoma, coning (*OHCM* p 780).

Holmes–Adie pupil This tends to occur in young adult women. Sudden onset of blurring of near vision occurs as accommodation is partially paralysed. The pupil is slightly dilated, there is a very slow response to accommodation, and, especially, to light (the light reflex may appear absent unless a prolonged, intense source is used). If knee and ankle jerks are absent, too, the Holmes–Adie syndrome is present.

Horner's syndrome This occurs on disrupting the sympathetic nerve supply to the iris. The pupil is miotic (smaller) and there is partial ptosis of the lid, but normal range of lid movement (supply to levator palpebrae is by the third nerve). The pupil does not dilate in the dark. Loss of sweating usually indicates a lesion proximal to the carotid plexus—if distal, the sudomotor (*sudor* = sweat) fibres will have separated, so sweating is intact. Causes:

- Posterior inferior cerebellar artery or basilar artery occlusion
- Multiple sclerosis
- Hypothalamic lesions
- Syringomyelia in the pons
- Cavernous sinus thrombosis
- Cervical cord, mediastinal or Pancoast's tumour
- Aortic aneurysm
- Klumpke's paralysis (p 724)
- Cervical lymphadenopathy.

Argyll Robertson pupil This occurs in neurosyphilis and diabetes mellitus. There is bilateral meiosis with pupil irregularity. There is no response to light but there is response to accommodation (The prostitute's pupil accommodates but does not react.) The iris mesoderm is spongy, the pupils dilate poorly, and there may be ptosis.

Causes of light-near dissociation (–ve to light +ve to accommodation): Argyll Robertson pupil; Holmes–Adie syndrome; meningitis; alcoholism; tectal lesions, eg pinealoma; mesencephalic or thalamic lesions. The path from the optic tract to the Edinger–Westphal nucleus is disrupted but deeper cortical connections remain intact, so accommodation is spared.

Refraction

Refractive errors arise from disorders of the size and shape of the eye. Correct refraction depends upon the distance between the cornea and the retina, and the curvatures of the lens and cornea.

Myopia (short sightedness) The eyeball is too long. In any eye, the nearer an object comes to the eye, the further back the image falls. With myopic eyes a close object will focus on the retina (short sightedness). In order to focus the image from more distant objects (which focus too far forward), concave spectacle (or contact) lenses are needed.

In normal growth, changes in curvature of the eyeball and lens compensate for the eye getting longer as it grows. In myopic children this is not the case. The cornea and lens do not adequately compensate as growth occurs, so the myopia tends to worsen as they get older. Although a few children are born myopic, most do not become so until the age of about 6. Myopia will then usually continue to worsen until the late teens, when changes stop below 6 dioptres in most people. It is important, therefore, for children with myopia to have their eyes regularly checked because spectacle changes are to be expected: in some cases they need changing every 6 months. In later life, increasing myopia may indicate developing cataracts. In a small proportion of adults myopia progresses above 6 dioptres (sometimes up to 20 dioptres or more). This has serious consequences later in life because a secondary degeneration of the vitreous and retina occurs, which can lead to retinal detachment, choroidoretinal atrophy and bleeding in the macular area. Anyone with more than 6 dioptre myopia should have their eyes examined once a year; and more often if they have floaters.

Astigmatism This is where the cornea or lens does not have the same degree of curvature in the horizontal and vertical planes, so that the image of objects is distorted either longitudinally or vertically. Correcting lenses are compensated accordingly. Astigmatism can occur alone, or with myopia or hypermetropia.

Treatment for myopia and astigmatism Spectacle correction, contact lenses and radial keratotomy can all be used. Radial keratotomy decreases myopia by flattening the curvature of the cornea by placing accurately measured deep radial incisions. It works remarkably well with low myopia and can correct up to 8 dioptres. Photorefractive keratectomy is performed using lasers to melt away the anterior part of the cornea, thus flattening the cornea. For radial keratotomy and photorefractive keratectomy the myopia must be stable and the patient above 21 years of age. See p 525.

Hypermetropia (long sightedness) This is due to an eyeball which is too short. Distant objects, when the eye is at rest (not accommodating) tend to get focused behind the retina. The ciliary muscles contract, and the lens gets more convex to focus the object on the retina. This can produce tiredness of the eyes and sometimes, convergent squint in children. Hypermetropia is corrected by convex spectacle lenses to bring the image forward to focus on the retina.

Presbyopia The eye is provided by nature with a convex lens for the focusing of near objects (when the lens is in its resting state focus is on distant objects; the ciliary muscles squeeze the lens to be more convex for close focusing). With age, the natural lens of the eye becomes stiffer and less easy to deform, so that focusing for close objects becomes less possible—hence the development of long sightedness with age (presbyopia) and the need for glasses for reading. These changes usually start in the lens at about 40 years and are complete by 60 years.

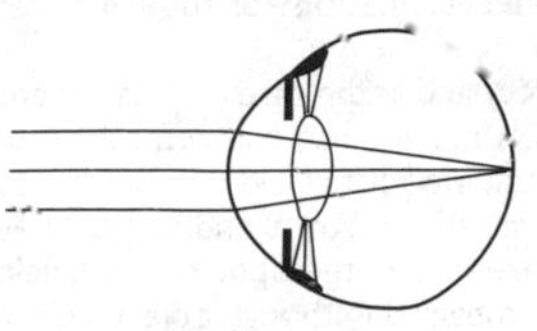

Normal eye

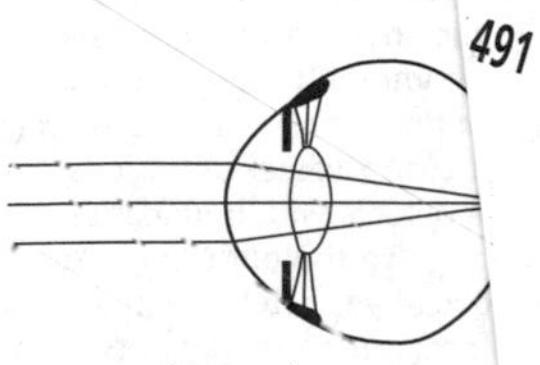

Normal eye

Myopia

Hypermetropia

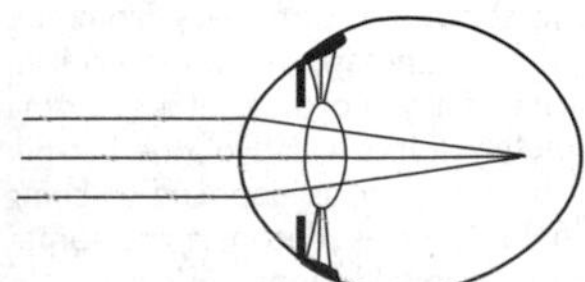

Light focused in front of retina

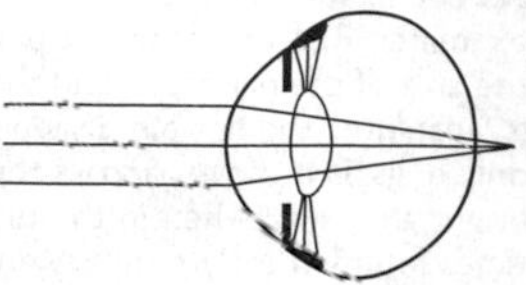

Light focused behind the retina

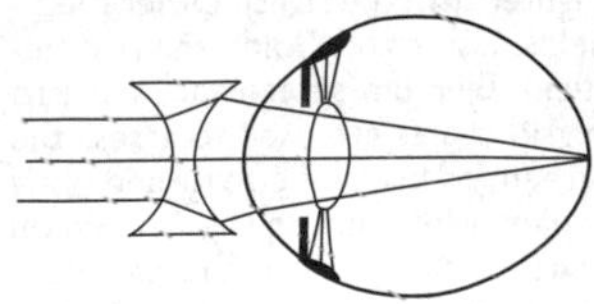

Corrected with concave lens

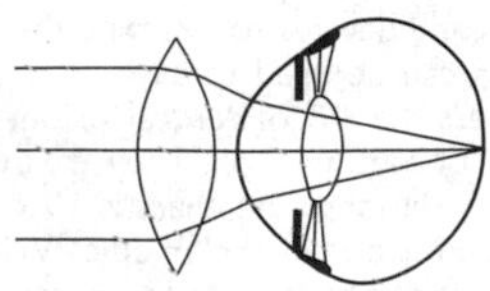

Corrected with convex lens

Visual field defects

ien assessing for visual field defects it is important to establish whether e defect affects one eye only or is bilateral, whether there are clear oundaries to the defect and whether they lie in the vertical or horizontal meridians, and to what degree acuity is affected. Lesions of sudden onset re commonly due to vascular causes.

Retinal lesions cause defects in one eye only and in the case of detachment and blood vessel occlusions (smaller vessels rather than the central ones) give defects with boundaries in the horizontal meridian. Field defects due to damage to the optic nerve tend to be central, asymmetrical and unilateral—and acuity is often affected. When lesions are behind the optic chiasma field defects are bilateral, acuity tends not to be impaired (although objects in the affected field cannot be seen) and boundaries are in the vertical meridian.

Tests *Finger confrontation:* The patient fixates on the examiner's eyes and notes the presence of a finger in all fields mapped, against the examiner's vision. It is used for testing peripheral fields. *Hat-pin confrontation:* The patient fixates on a distant object, sitting about 1 metre away from the examiner. Red or white hat-pins are used to define any vertical meridian, the size of the blindspot and the boundaries of any scotomas. If a scotoma is 'absolute', the hat-pin disappears completely. If it is 'relative', the hat-pin only dulls as it moves across the field of the scotoma, as opposed to being bright and clear when in the unaffected field. Central scotomas are sometimes found in early pituitary and posterior occipital lesions.

Optic chiasmal lesions may show a phenomenon whereby if two identical coloured objects are shown to one eye in the two vertical halves of the visual field (eg the right) one appears to be brighter and sharper than the other (if right eye, the left hemifield is brighter than the right). Other methods and devices to examine the visual fields: Lister and Goldmann perimeters can be used to assess the whole field. Bjerrum screens are used to assess the 30° of central vision. Amsler grid charts are used to assess the 10° of central vision. They are used to screen for macular disease and optic nerve lesions. The chart is 10 × 10cm square with 5mm squares drawn on it and a dot in the middle. With the chart held at 30cm the patient is instructed to look at the central dot and report any distorted squares or wavy lines (metamorphopsia) or blank or dark areas (scotomata). There are also many automated computerized perimeters to test visual fields.

Diagnosing the site of the lesion Superior parts of the visual field fall inferiorly on the retina, temporal fields on the nasal retina and vice versa. Fibres from the nasal retina of both eyes cross in the optic chiasma to join uncrossed temporal retinal fibres. A pituitary tumour may disrupt the chiasma, affecting fibres crossing from nasal retinas, so causing bitemporal field defects. If it grows more to one side than the other, it can superimpose a central optic nerve defect as well. As fibres cross they maintain position (superior fibres stay superior). From the optic chiasma fibres pass in the optic tract to the lateral geniculate body, then as the optic radiation to the visual cortex. A contralateral upper homonymous quadrantanopia may be caused by temporal lobe tumours. Posterior visual cortex lesions cause non-peripheral homonymous hemianopic scotomas (anterior visual cortex deals with peripheral vision)—with macular sparing, if the cause is osterior cerebral artery ischaemia (central areas have overlap flow via the ldle cerebral artery, which is why acuity may be preserved—*OTM* 3e –9). *Causes of visual cortex field defects*: •Ischaemia (TIA, migraine,) •Meningioma •Glioma •Abscess •A-V malformation.

Scotomata

Arcuate scotoma —moderate glaucoma

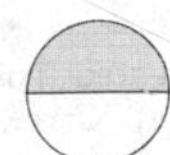

Unilateral defect found with: arterial occlusion branch retinal vein thrombosis inferior retinal detachment

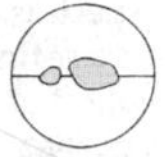

Central scotoma macular degeneration or macular oedema

The visual pathways

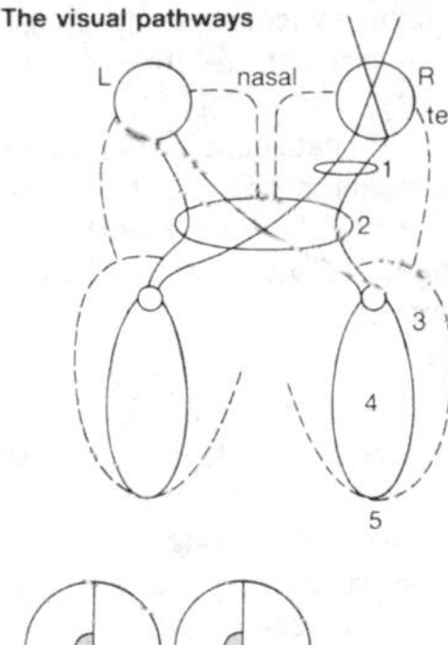

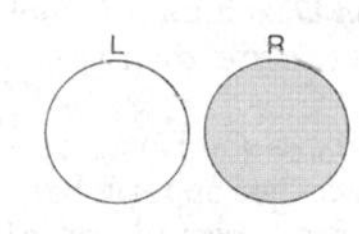

1 R optic nerve lesion

2 Lesion of chiasm—complicated defects depending upon which of the fibres are most affected

3 Left superior quadrantanopia due to R temporal lobe lesion

5 L homonymous scotoma due to lesion at tip of R occipital lobe

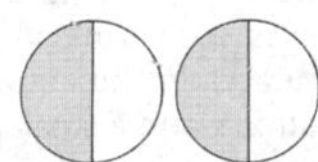

4 Homonymous hemianopia from lesions affecting all R optic radiation or visual cortex

Confrontation depends on mutual fixation, and it is necessary to concentrate hard to work out what is going on, but, for one second, allow yourself to reflect on what your patient will be thinking and feeling, most eloquently expressed by John Donne on accomplishing this manoeuvre:

I fix mine eye on thine, and there
Pity my picture burning in thine eye...

Towards the end of your professional life you will have engaged in mutual fixation many, many times, and as you continue to do so, ask yourself if these images of suffering are falling on your retina like so many layers of snow on a barren land, or whether, just sometimes, you might allow your eye to thaw and resolve itself into perhaps just one true tear.

The red eye

Red eyes are commonly also painful. Some causes are dangerous to vision and require specialist supervision (acute glaucoma, acute iritis, corneal ulcers); others are more easily treated (episcleritis, conjunctivitis, spontaneous conjunctival haemorrhage). Carefully examine all red eyes to assess acuity, cornea (use fluorescein drops p 496), and pupillary reflexes.

Acute (closed angle) glaucoma This is a disease of middle years or later life. The acute uniocular attack is commonly preceded by blurred vision or haloes around lights—particularly at night-time. It is caused by blockage of drainage of aqueous from the anterior chamber via the canal of Schlemm. Dilatation of pupils at night exacerbates drainage block. Intraocular pressure then rises from the normal 15–20mmHg to 60 or 70mmHg.

Pain is variable (and may be severe with nausea and vomiting), vision reduced, the cornea appears hazy due to oedema, redness is circumcorneal, the pupil is fixed, dilated and slightly vertically ovoid. Raised intraocular pressure may make the eyeball feel hard. A shallow anterior chamber (predisposing factor) may be noticed in the other eye (shine a torch from the side, half the iris lies in shadow). If suspected send, to eye unit.

Treatment of acute glaucoma: Pilocarpine 2–4% drops hourly (miosis opens the blocked, 'closed' drainage angle), and acetazolamide 500mg PO stat (IM if vomiting) then 250mg/8h PO. Acetazolamide ↓formation of aqueous. Peripheral iridectomy by laser or surgery is carried out once intraocular pressure has been medically reduced (rarely as an emergency procedure if medical management fails to control pressure). A small piece of iris is removed from the 12 o'clock position in both eyes to allow free circulation of aqueous.

Acute iritis (anterior uveitis) The uvea is the vascular pigmented part of the eye including iris, ciliary body and choroid. The iris and ciliary body are called the anterior uvea and iris inflammation invariably involves the ciliary body too so inflammation is best referred to as anterior uveitis.

Presentation is with pain of acute onset, photophobia, blurred vision (due to precipitates in the aqueous), lacrimation, circumcorneal redness (ciliary congestion), and a small pupil (initially from iris spasm; later it may be irregular or dilate irregularly due to adhesions). Talbot's test is positive: pain increases as the eyes converge (and pupils constrict) as patients watch their finger approach their nose. The slit lamp reveals white precipitates on the back of the cornea and cells in the anterior chamber. Sometimes sterile anterior chamber pus (hypopyon) may be seen.

It tends to afflict the young or middle-aged. There are many causes. Associations: joint problems (eg ankylosing spondylitis, Still's). It may relapse.

Treatment of iritis: Aim to prevent damage to the eye by prolonged inflammation. With prolonged inflammation there is a possibility of disrupting flow of aqueous inside the eye, with glaucoma occurring, and of adhesions forming between iris and lens. Treat with steroids, eg prednisolone 0.5% drops every 2h, to reduce inflammation (hence pain, redness, and exudate). To prevent adhesions between lens and iris (synechiae) keep pupil dilated with cyclopentolate 0.5% 1–2 drops/6h, unless the iritis is very mild. Use the slit lamp to monitor inflammation.

Identifying the dangerous red eye

Ask yourself the following questions:

1 Is acuity affected? A quick but sensitive test is the ability to read newsprint with refractive errors corrected with glasses or a pin-hole. Reduced acuity suggests dangerous pathology.

2 Is the globe painful? Pain is potentially sinister, foreign body sensation may be so, irritation rarely is.

3 Does the pupil respond to light? Absent or sluggish response is sinister.

4 Is the cornea intact? Use fluorescein eyedrops, p 496. Corneal damage may be due to trauma or ulcers.

Enquire also about trauma and discharge, general health and drugs, and remember to check for raised pressure.

►If in doubt, obtain a specialist opinion today.

	Conjunctivitis	*Iritis*	*Acute glaucoma*
Pain	±	++	++ to +++
Photophobia	+	++	–
Acuity	normal	↓	↓
Cornea	normal	normal	steamy or hazy
Pupil	normal	small	large
Intraocular pressure	normal	normal	↑

More red eyes—cornea and conjunctiva

Corneal problems *Keratitis* is corneal inflammation (identified by a white spot on the cornea—indicating a collection of white cells in corneal tissue). *Corneal ulceration* is an epithelial breach; it may occur without keratitis, eg in trauma, when prophylactic antibiotic ointment (eg gentamicin 0.3%) may be used. Ulceration with keratitis is called ulcerative keratitis and must be treated as an emergency—see below. There is pain, photophobia, and sometimes blurred vision. Non-infective corneal ulceration may result from contact lens exposure, trauma, or previous corneal disease.
Ulcerative keratitis: Use fluorescein drops and a bright light (ideally with a blue filter, shone tangentially across the globe) to aid diagnosis. Corneal lesions stain green (the drops are orange and become more yellow on contact with the eye). Ulcers may be bacterial (beware pseudomonas: may be rapidly progressive), herpetic (simplex or zoster), fungal (candida, aspergillus), protozoal (acanthamoeba) or from vasculitis, eg in rheumatoid arthritis. ►Refer the same day to hospital as treatment depends upon the cause and delay may cause loss of sight. Anyone with corneal ulceration or stromal suppuration must have an urgent diagnostic smear (for Gram stain) and scrape by an experienced person. Liaise with microbiologist about samples. *Treatment:* See p 497.

Treat zoster infections with aciclovir (p 484). For *Herpes simplex* dendritic ulcers, see p 480. Cycloplegic drugs (p 518) may relieve pain due to ciliary spasm and prevent iris adhesions.

Episcleritis (PLATE 13) Inflammation below the conjunctiva in the episclera is often accompanied by an inflammatory nodule. The sclera may look blue below engorged vessels—which can be moved over the area, unlike in scleritis, where the engorged vessels are deeper. The eye aches dully and is tender to the touch, especially over the inflamed area. Usually no underlying cause is found, but it may complicate autoimmune diseases. It responds to steroid eyedrops (eg clobetasone butyrate eyedrops 0.1%/6h).

Scleritis (PLATE 14) Rarely, the sclera itself is inflamed. There is more generalized inflammation with oedema of the conjunctiva and thinning of the sclera (if very severe globe perforation is a risk). It may be associated with connective tissue disorders. Refer to a specialist.

Conjunctivitis ►Conjunctivitis is usually bilateral, if apparently unilateral consider other diagnoses (p 495), eg acute glaucoma.

The conjunctiva is red and inflamed, and the hyperaemic vessels may be moved over the sclera, by gentle pressure on the globe. Acuity, pupillary responses, and corneal lustre are unaffected. Eyes itch, burn and lacrimate. There may be photophobia. Purulent discharge may stick the eyelids together. The cause may be viral (highly infectious adenovirus)—small lymphoid aggregates appear as follicles on conjunctiva, bacterial (purulent discharge more prominent), or allergic. The affliction is usually self-limiting (although allergic responses may be more prolonged). In prolonged conjunctivitis, especially in young adults or those with venereal disease consider chlamydial infection—see ophthalmia neonatorum, p 100.
Treatment: Usually with antibiotics, eg gentamicin 0.3% drops/3h and 0.3% ointment at night. For chlamydia use tetracycline 250mg/6h PO and as 1% ointment 6-hourly for at least one month. For allergic conditions use sodium cromoglycate 2% eyedrops/6h.

Subconjunctival haemorrhage This harmless but alarming looking collection of blood behind the conjunctiva from a small vessel bleed requires no treatment. It clears spontaneously. If recurrent, look for a bleeding diathesis and check blood pressure.

Management of corneal ulcers[1]

Smears and cultures Liaise with microbiologist. Take:

1 Smear for Gram stain—if chronic ulcer Giemsa, PAS (periodic acid Schiff) for fungi, ZN (Ziehl–Neelsen) or auromine for TB.
2 Conjunctival swab to blood agar for tear film contaminants.
3 Corneal scrape (by experienced person) from multiple areas of ulcer edge with needle for direct innoculation.
4 Request the cultures detailed below.

Acute history: Presume bacterial, so culture with blood agar (grows most organisms), chocolate agar (for *Haemophilus* and *Neisseria*), nutrient broth (anaerobes), cooked meat broth (aerobes/anaerobes). *Chronic history:* Consider rarities; culture as above + BHI (brain heart infusion broth for fastidious organisms and fungi), Sabouraud's plate for fungi, anaerobic blood agar (peptococcus, proprionobacteria) + thioglycollate (anaerobes). *Unusual features* use also viral transport medium, Lowenstein–Jensen agar slope for TB, *E Coli* seeded agar for acanthamoeba.

Initial eyedrop management Based on urgent Gram stain result.

- Copious bacteria of one type:
  Gram +ve: cefuroxime 50mg/mL (or methicillin 20mg/mL).
  Gram –ve: gentamicin 15mg/mL* (or ticarcillin 10mg/mL).
- Fungal elements only seen: miconazole 1%.
- Acute disease but scanty/multiple or no bacteria: gentamicin 15mg/mL*: + cefuroxime 50mg/mL or + methicillin 20mg/mL.
- No organisms in chronic disease: request PAS for fungi. If –ve await culture result at 24–72h without treatment: consider reculture or biopsy before starting treatment.

*Gentamicin 15mg/mL 'forte' preparation (▶see p 518).

Use drops every 15min day and night. If >1 drug used, alternate them. To prepare drops, see p 518. Vary therapy with severity. Beware drug toxicity causing delayed epithelialization (especially gentamicin). Deep or limbic ulcers may need systemic treatment.

When the organism is known Use cefuroxime 50mg/mL for staphs and other Gm +ve organisms; penicillin G 5000u/mL for streps; gentamicin 15mg/mL* for *pseudomonas, enterobacteriaceae, moraxella*; amikacin 10mg/mL for *mycobacteria*, miconazole 1% for *candida* and *aspergillus*; neomycin 0.5% + propamidine isethionate 0.1% (± a steroid) for *acanthamoeba*.

Cycloplegia is used as adjunctive therapy. Steroid drops, eg prednisolone 0.5%/6h are occasionally needed to help to control vascularization and reduce inflammation. Only use them after positive culture and usually not in the first 10 days treatment. Use with great caution if pseudomonas or fungal infection the cause.

When culture-+ve ulcers fail to respond consider whether treatment is sufficient, or too toxic (preventing epithelialization) or whether initial culture may be wrong. Ulcers which perforate may need penetrating grafts to include all infected material or other specialized surgical techniques.

1 Information kindly supplied by Mr J Dart FRCS, Moorfields Eye Hospital, City Rd, London EC1V 2PD

Sudden painless loss of vision

The fovea (macula) is the only part of the eye with 6/6 vision. Pathology affecting it causes most drastic visual loss.

- ► The patient wants an answer to the question 'Will I go blind?'
- ► Every patient requires specialist attention unless the cause is unequivocally migraine. ►Always check the ESR: is it giant cell arteritis?

Amaurosis fugax is temporary loss of vision 'like a curtain descending'. It may precede permanent visual loss (in embolism or giant cell arteritis, (PLATES 5 &15); so diagnosis of the cause may save sight. NB: transient visual loss lasting 30–60sec in papilloedema is due to ↑intracranial pressure.

Ischaemic optic neuropathy The optic nerve is damaged if the posterior ciliary arteries are occluded by inflammation or arteriosclerosis. Fundoscopy shows a pale, swollen optic disc.

Temporal arteritis/giant cell arteritis: It is vital to recognize this: the other eye is at risk until treatment is started. Symptoms: malaise, jaw claudication (pain on chewing) and a tender scalp/temporal arteries (pulses may be absent). *Association:* Polymyalgia rheumatica. An ESR >40 is suggestive; temporal artery biopsy may miss the affected section of artery. *Retinal changes:* See PLATE 15. Start prednisolone 80mg/24h PO promptly (some advocate higher IV doses if visual failure is occurring). Tailing off steroids as ESR and symptoms settle may take more than a year.

Arteriosclerotic ischaemic optic neuropathy: Hypertension, lipid disorders and diabetes may predispose younger patients to this. Treating these conditions may protect the vision in the other eye.

Occlusion of a central retinal artery (PLATE 4) There is dramatic visual loss within seconds of occlusion. In 90% acuity varies between light perception and finger counting. An afferent pupil defect (p 488) appears within seconds and may precede retinal changes by 1h. The retina appears white but with a cherry red spot at the macula. Exclude temporal arteritis. The occlusion is usually due to thrombo-embolism (listen for carotid bruits). *Treatment:* ►►If you see the patient within 1h of onset apply firm pressure on the globe, increasing until the patient feels pain. Then suddenly release the pressure. It may dislodge an embolus, and drive it into one of the branches (PLATE 5). There is no reliable treatment, and if the occlusion lasts much longer than an hour the optic nerve will atrophy, causing blindness. If a single branch of the retinal artery is occluded, the retinal and visual changes relate only to the part of the retina supplied.

Vitreous haemorrhage This is a particularly common cause of visual loss in diabetics with new vessel formation. It may also occur in bleeding disorders, retinal detachment and with central retinal vein or branch vein occlusions. With a large enough bleed to obscure vision, there is no red reflex and the retina may not be seen. They undergo spontaneous absorption, and treatment is expectant for the haemorrhage itself, as well as being directed to the cause (eg photocoagulation of new vessels). If the vitreous haemorrhage is unresolved at 3 months, vitrectomy may be done to remove the blood in the vitreous. Small extravasations of blood produce vitreous floaters, (seen by the patient as small black dots or tiny ring-like forms with clear centres) which may not greatly obscure vision.

Subacute loss of vision *Optic neuritis:* Unilateral ↓acuity occurs over hours or days. Discrimination of colour is affected: reds appear less red, 'red desaturation'—and eye movements may hurt. The pupil shows an afferent defect (p 488). The optic disc may be swollen (papillitis) unless the inflammation is central (retrobulbar neuritis). Recovery is usual over 2–6 weeks, but 45–80% develop multiple sclerosis (MS) over the next 15yrs. Other causes: neurosyphilis, other demyelinations (eg Devic's disease), Leber's optic atrophy, diabetes mellitus, and vitamin deficiency. *Treatment:* High-dose methylprednisolone for 3 days (250mg/6h IV), then oral prednisolone (1mg/kg/day) for 11 days appears to reduce the risk of developing MS in the next 2yrs, from ~15% to 7%. Seek expert advice.

Retinal vein occlusions: central or branch vein?

Central retinal vein occlusion (PLATE 6) Incidence increases with age. It is commoner than arterial occlusion. Causes: chronic simple glaucoma, arteriosclerosis, BP↑, and polycythaemia. If the whole central retinal vein is thrombosed, there is sudden visual loss (eg acuity reduced to finger counting). The fundus is like a 'stormy sunset' (the angry-looking red clouds are haemorrhages, beside engorged veins). There is also hyperaemia.

Long-term outcome is variable, with possible improvement for 6 months to one year; peripheral vision tends to improve most, leaving macular vision impaired. The main problems are macular oedema and neovascular glaucoma secondary to iris neovascularization. About ⅓ of eyes show significant non-perfusion on fluorescein angiography, of which one-half would develop neovascular glaucoma (called '100 days glaucoma' as it develops about this time after the occlusion). Panretinal laser photocoagulation is effective in treating and preventing neovascular glaucoma. At present there is no effective treatment for macular oedema from central retinal vein occlusion.

Branch retinal vein occlusion There is unilateral visual loss and fundal appearances in the corresponding area. Retinal capillary non-perfusion can lead to retinal new vessel formation. Treatment of this neovascularization (confirmed by fluorescein angiography) with laser photocoagulation, reduces risk of intraocular haemorrhage by 50%. Macular oedema persisting for months without improvement may be treated with grid pattern argon laser macular photocoagulation.

Differential diagnosis Other causes of sudden loss of vision:
- Retinal detachment (p 506).
- Acute glaucoma (painful—see p 494).
- Migraine.

Stroke patients may complain of monocular blindness but visual field testing will usually reveal a homonymous hemianopia. Sudden bilateral visual loss is unusual (may be CMV infection in HIV patients, p 510).

Gradual loss of vision

The possible causes for gradual loss of vision in one eye are choroiditis, a creeping inferior retinal detachment (p 506), or a choroidal melanoma. If the loss is bilateral (usually asymmetrical), the cause is more likely to be cataract, chronic glaucoma (p 502), diabetic and hypertensive retinopathy (p 510), senile macular degeneration, or optic atrophy (see below).

Choroiditis (choroidoretinitis) The choroid is part of the uvea (iris, ciliary body & choroid), and inflammatory disorders affecting the uvea may also affect the choroid. The retina may be invaded by organisms which set up a granulomatous reaction (which can be mistaken for a retinoblastoma). Toxoplasmosis and toxocara are now more common than TB. Sarcoid is another cause. *Tests:* CXR; Mantoux; serology; Kveim test (the reagent is available in the UK on a named-patient basis from Porton Down). In the acute phase, vision may be blurred, a grey-white raised patch is seen on the retina, vitreous opacities occur, and there may be cells in the anterior chamber. Later, a choroidoretinal scar (white patch with pigmentation around) will be seen, these being symptomless unless involving the macula. Treat the cause.

Malignant melanoma of the choroid is the commonest malignant tumour of the eye. Appearing as mottled grey/black on the fundus, they produce a retinal detachment immediately over the growth. Spread is haematogenous or by local invasion of the orbit. Treatment is usually by enucleation of the affected eye although local treatment is sometimes possible.

Senile macular degeneration This is the commonest cause of registrable blindness in the UK. It occurs in elderly people who complain of deterioration of central vision. There is loss of acuity; visual fields are unaffected. The disc appears normal but there is pigment, fine exudate, and haemorrhage at the macula. Drusen (PLATE 3) may precede these changes. Rarely, the macular is oedematous and lifted by a large mass of exudate—called disciform degeneration. For most, there is no effective treatment. A few can be treated by laser.

Note: macula holes are an uncommon type of macula degeneration, which may present with *distorted vision* as well as visual loss. Look for a tiny punched-out area in the macula (hard to detect); here, vitrectomy may relieve traction on the edge of the hole. An air bubble is introduced to nudge the macula back into position—which may work if the patient spends the first post-op week face down. Presumably there must be some photoreceptors left which recover function when replaced. Vitrectomy is a hazardous undertaking, and most patients will not be suitable for this treatment—and must rely on visual aids (eg to read). Zinc and β-carotene replacement are advocated (Ocuvite®)—but are unproven (CI: actively bleeding ulcers).

Tobacco amblyopia This is optic atrophy induced by tobacco and is due to cyanide poisoning. There is gradual loss of central vision. Loss of red/green discrimination is an early, permanent sign.

Optic atrophy The optic disc usually appears pale, although the degree of pallor does not correspond to the visual loss. Optic atrophy may be secondary to increased intraocular pressure (in glaucoma), or retinal damage (as in choroiditis, retinitis pigmentosa, cerebromacular degeneration), or be due to ischaemia (as in retinal artery occlusion). Toxic causes other than tobacco are methanol, lead, arsenic, quinine, and carbon bisulfide.

Other causes: Leber's optic atrophy (p 752), multiple sclerosis, syphilis, external pressure on the nerve (intraorbital or intracranial tumours, Paget's disease affecting the skull).

Use of services by older patients with failing vision

There is good evidence in the UK of under-use of services. Population-based cross-sectional studies in London primary care settings[1] show that prevalence of bilateral visual impairment (acuity <6/12) was 30%. 88% of these patients were not in touch with ophthalmic services. ►*Three-quarters of these had remediable problems.* One-fifth had acuity in one or both eyes of < 6/60 ('blind'). Typical causes were found to be cataract, (30%), macular degeneration (8%), and undiagnosed chronic glaucoma.

1 A Reidy 1998 BMJ i 1643

Chronic simple (open angle) glaucoma

►Simple glaucoma is asymptomatic until visual fields are severely impaired; hence the need for screening—but most people found to have raised intraocular pressures (eg on ~10% of routine NHS sight tests in those >40yrs old) do not have glaucoma when their fundi and peripheral fields are charted (this can be a lengthy and tricky business). Once raised pressures are found, life-long follow-up is needed (at least yearly, and very much more often in the early stages)—which is why glaucoma accounts for such a heavy burden in ophthalmology clinics (eg 25% of the work), and why highstreet optometrists are being encouraged to take over at least part of this monitoring burden. Glaucoma accounts for 7% of new blind registrations.

Pathogenesis Intraocular pressure ≥21mmHg causes optic disc cupping ± capillary closure, hence nerve damage, with sausage-shaped field defects (scotomata) near the blind spot, which may then coalesce to form major defects. The nasal and superior fields are lost first with the last vision remaining in the temporal field. Normal optic cups are similar (left and right) in shape and occupy <50% of the optic disc. In glaucoma these enlarge, especially along the vertical axis. As damage progresses the optic disc pales (atrophy), and the cup widens and deepens, so that the blood vessels emerging from the disc appear to have breaks in them as they disappear into the cup and are then seen at the base again (see p 503). Since the central field is intact, good acuity is maintained, so patients may only present when there is major irreversible optic nerve damage. Some people get glaucoma with *normal* intraocular pressures.

Prevention Those most at risk have: a family history of glaucoma (risk ↑ 10-fold, especially siblings), or are: Afro-Caribbean, myopic, or have diabetic or thyroid eye disease. Check pressures (optician, using tonometry) in those with a positive family history, regularly from the age of 35 years.

Treatment The aim is to reduce the intraocular pressure to <21 mmHg. Surgery is used if medical treatment fails.

Betaxolol 0.5% drops (or timolol 0.25%–0.5%) Use twice daily—to ↓production of aqueous. They are β-blockers, so be cautious in asthma and heart failure. (Systemic absorption occurs with no first-pass metabolism by the liver.) SE: dry eyes, corneal anaesthesia, allergy, subtle changes in exercise tolerance.

Pilocarpine 0.5–4% drops reduce resistance to the outflow of aqueous. It causes miosis and may cause blurring of vision and brow ache due to ciliary muscle spasm. Rarely, retinal detachment can occur. Presbyopes tolerate it better than the young and short sighted. Use 4 times daily. Because of these problems, pilocarpine is second-line treatment, or, with improving surgical options, some would say not even second line.

Pilocarpine ocuserts help reduce side-effects by minimizing the amount entering the eye at any one time, and *pilocarpine gel* (Pilogel®) reduces blurred vision because it is applied at night.

Epinephrine (=adrenaline) 1% and *dipivefrine 0.1% drops* These sympathomimetics probably act by increasing outflow via the trabecular meshwork and uveosclera. Caution with heart disease and if BP↑; avoid in closed angle glaucoma. SE: sore, smarting, red eyes; blurred vision. Use once or twice daily.

Carbonic anhydrase inhibitors, eg acetazolamide 250mg/24h–500mg/12h PO or topical *dorzolamide* (2%/8h) ↓production of aqueous. SE of acetazolamide: lassitude, dyspepsia, K^+↓, paraesthesia—so dorzolamide is preferred (but its SE are bitter taste, blurred vision, epiphora).[1] Avoid both if pregnant.

Prostaglandin drops (eg *Latanoprost*) ↑uveoscleral outflow and may have a rôle.

Surgery: Flap-valve trabeculectomy is a common operation. There is strong evidence that it acts as a drainage operation. Problems include early failure, and worsening of cataract (normal healing mitigates its effect, but this can be delayed by topical cytotoxics, such as fluoruracil). Effects of *argon laser trabeculoplasty* is often short-term. It may have a rôle in older patients.[1]

1 *Drug & Ther Bul* 1997 **35** 4 & P Watson 1996 *Ophthalmology* **103** 126–37 & *ibid* 138–47

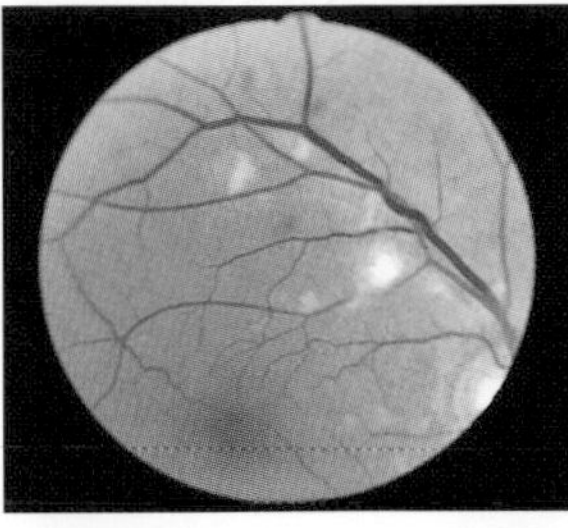

Plate 1 Cotton wool spots. Fluffy pale patches represent retinal microinfarcts, here following coronary artery bypass surgery.

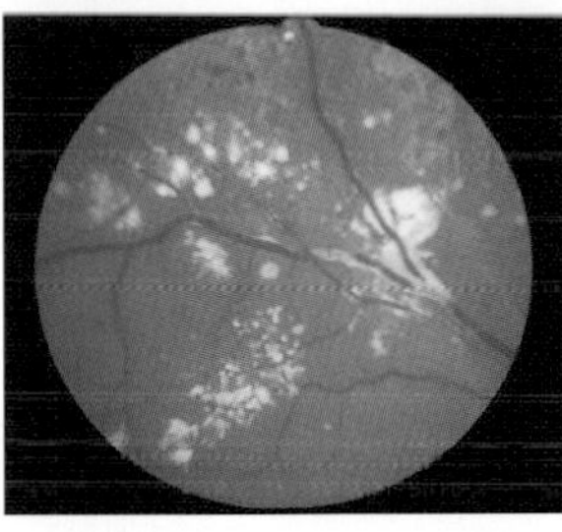

Plate 2 Hard exudates. Shiny pale hard exudates in a diabetic patient with type III hyperlipidaemia represent areas of lipid and protein leaked from plasma. The patient also had xanthomata.

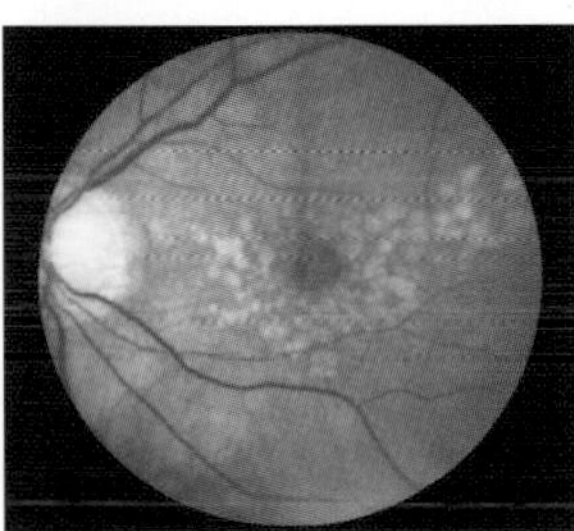

Plate 3 Retinal drusen. Pale lesions grouped round the fovea in an elderly patient are degenerative drusen which may precede disciform macular scarring.

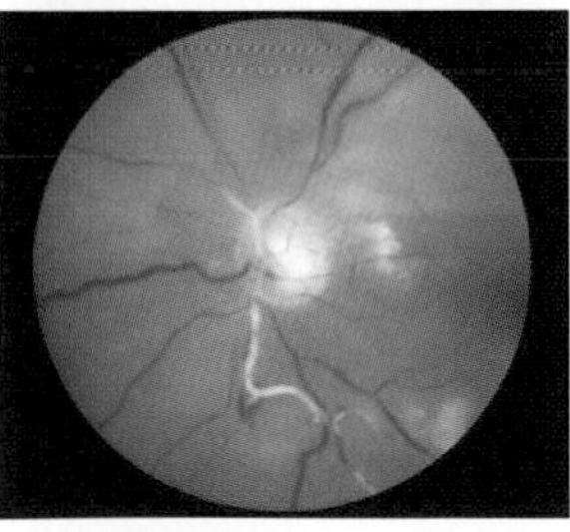

Plate 4 Retinal artery occlusion. Much of the retina is infarcted and hazy though the fovea is spared. The main retinal arterioles are sheathed. This patient had attacks of transient blindness before full occlusion.

Images supplied by Peggy Frith, whom we here acknowledge and thank

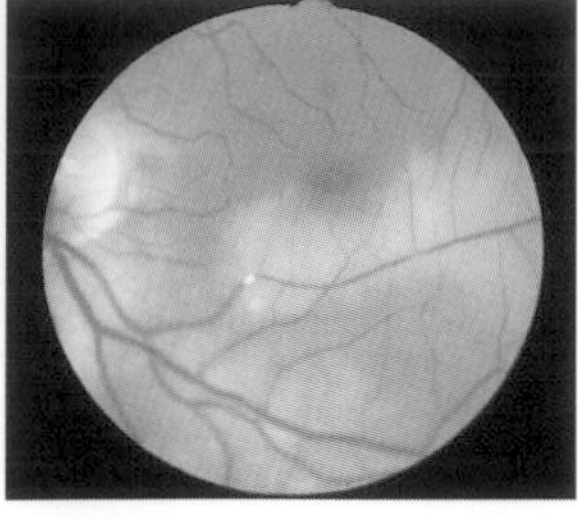

Plate 5 Retinal embolus. A small white embolus lodged in a branch retinal arteriole with surrounding area of pale retinal infarction. The embolus may be a fragment of atheromatous cholesterol or of cardiac valve.

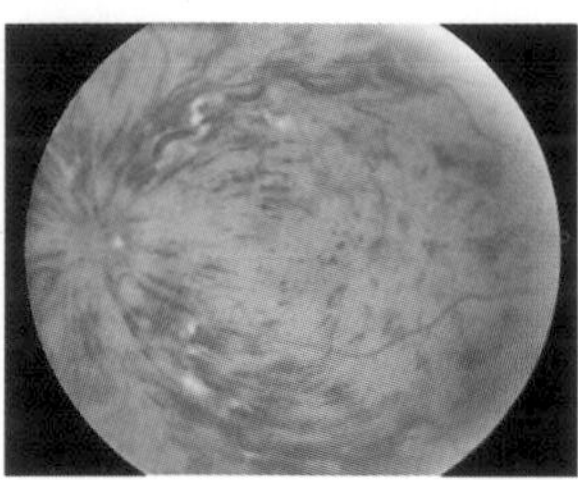

Plate 6 Retinal vein occlusion. Occlusion of the central retinal vein with a characteristic 'bloodstorm' appearance.

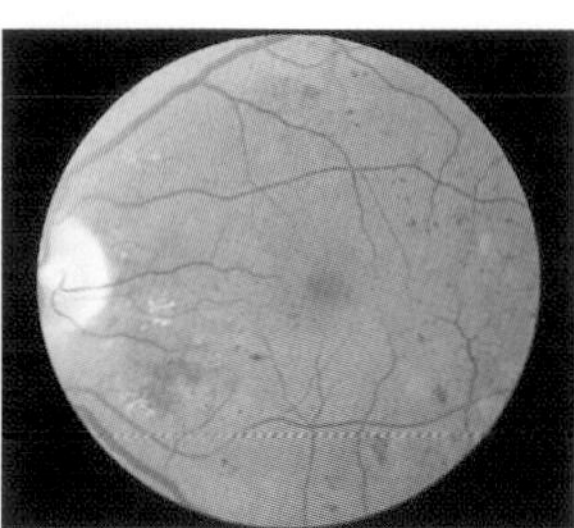

Plate 7 Diabetes, background retinopathy. There are scattered blot haemorrhages and sparse hard exudates but vision is normal.

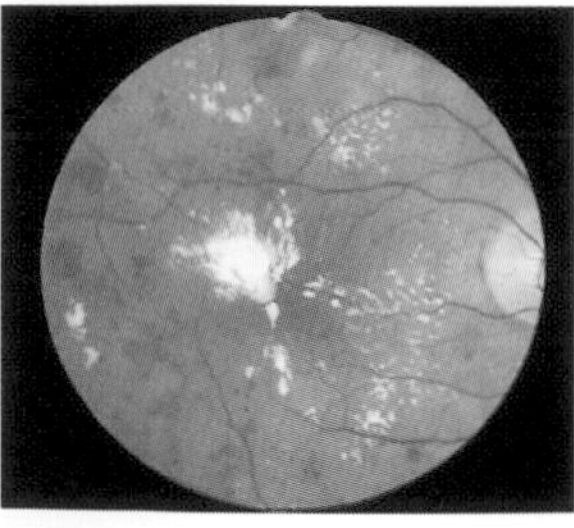

Plate 8 Diabetic maculopathy. Hard exudate at the fovea reduces vision irretrievably.

Images supplied by Peggy Frith, whom we here acknowledge and thank

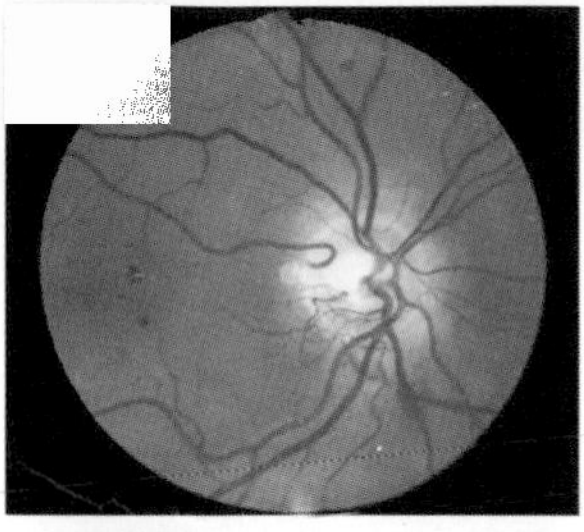

Plate 9 Diabetes, proliferative retinopathy. New vessels have formed in a looped fan on the inferior part of the optic disc.

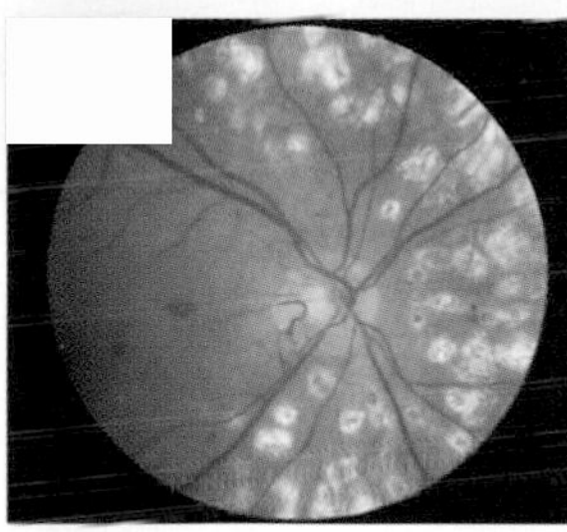

Plate 10 Treated proliferative retinophathy. Scars from laser burns outside the disc and major retinal vessel arcades appear after panretinal treatment. A tuft of disc new vessels persists at 7 o'clock.

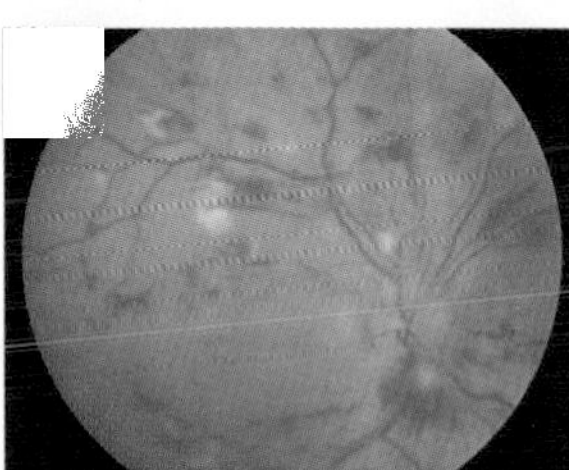

Plate 11 Accelerated hypertension. Flame haemorrhages, cotton wool spots, and disc swelling associated with renal artery stenosis. Mean blood pressure was 250/125 mmHg.

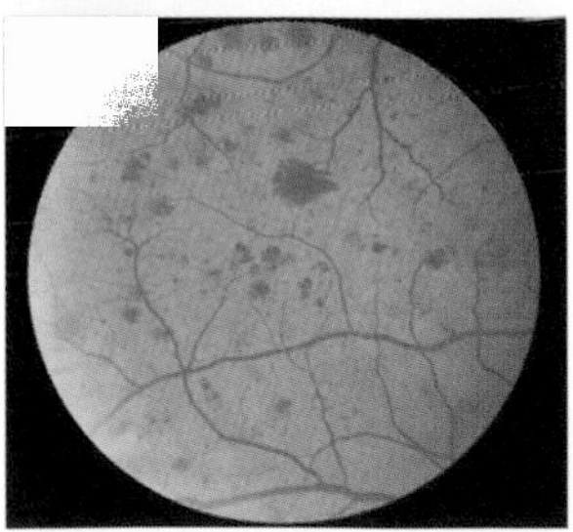

Plate 12 Retinal haemorrhages in leukaemia. Chronic granulocytic leukaemia with a white cell count of 76 X 10^9/l. The patient presented to his optician with visual blurring and the fundi showed widespread haemorrhages.

Images supplied by Peggy Frith, whom we here acknowledge and thank

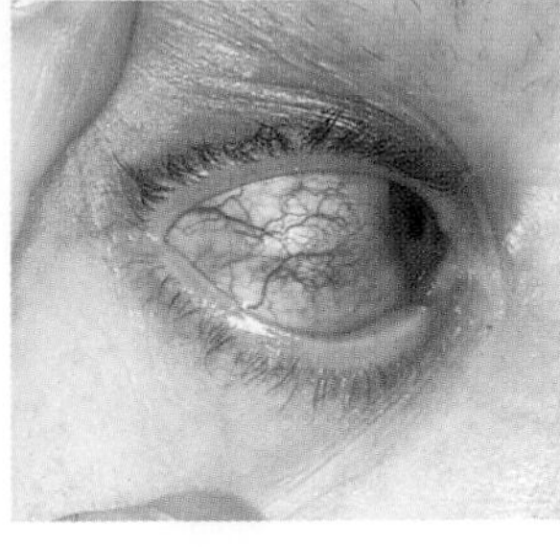

Plate 13 Episcleritis. A sector of the eye shows dilated superficial vessels on the eye coat. The eye may be sore and tender but is not painful.

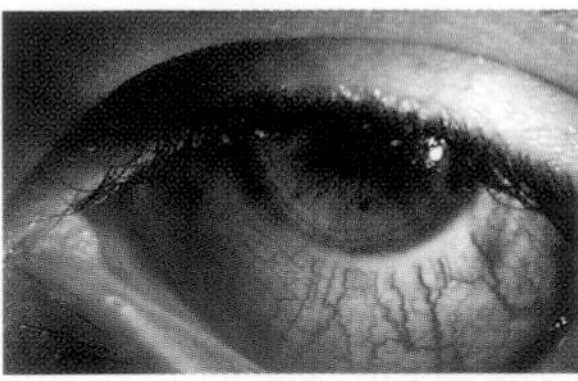

Plate 14 Scleritis. Scleritis with dilatation of both superficial and deep vessels and swelling of the eye coat. The eye is painful

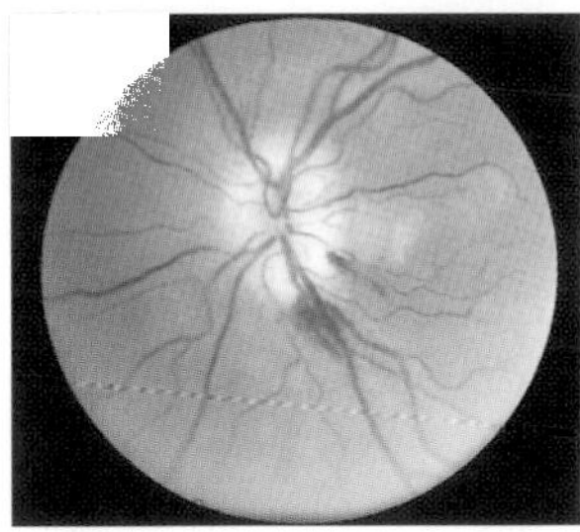

Plate 15 Optic disc in giant cell arteritis. The optic nerve head is infarcted and appears pale and swollen. In an elderly patient with a high ESR the diagnosis is giant cell arteritis.

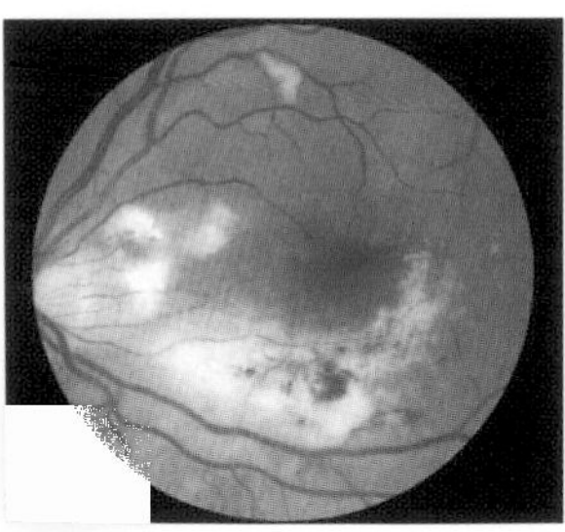

Plate 16 Retinitis in AIDS. The pale area with haemorrhages below the fovea is typical of cytomegalovirus retinitis in a patient with AIDS.

Images supplied by Peggy Frith, whom we here acknowledge and thank

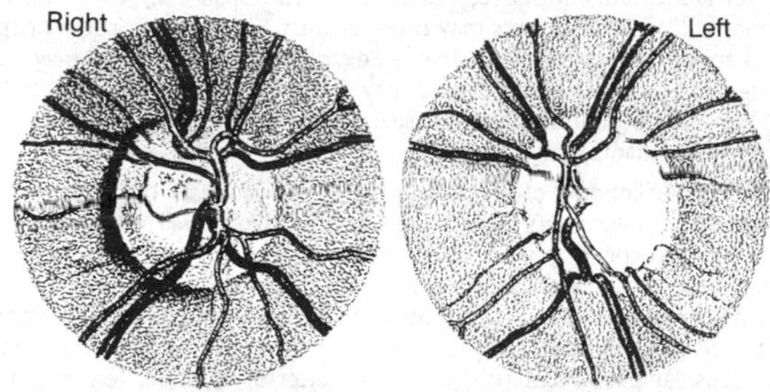

The two optic discs of a patient with open angle glaucoma which has not yet damaged the right optic disc. The left optic disc is grossly cupped and atrophic. (From J Parr *Introduction to Ophthalmology*, OUP.)

Cataract

►When a cataract is found, measure the blood glucose (to exclude DM).

A cataract is a lens opacity. The 4 major causes of blindness in the world are cataract, vitamin A deficiency, trachoma, and onchocerciasis.

Cataracts are found in 75% of over 65s but in only 20% of 45–65-year-olds.

Ophthalmoscopic classification is by lens appearance. With immature cataracts the red reflex still occurs; if dense cataract there is no red reflex, or visible fundus. *Nuclear* cataracts change the lens refractive index and are common in old age, as are the cortical spoke-like wedge-shaped opacities. Anterior and posterior *polar* cataracts are localized, are commonly inherited, and lie in the visual axis. *Subcapsular* opacities from steroid use are just deep to the lens capsule—in the visual axis. *Dot opacities* are common in normal lenses but are also seen in fast-developing cataracts in diabetes or dystrophia myotonica.

Presentation The main symptom of cataract is blurred vision. Unilateral cataracts are often unnoticed, but loss of stereopsis may affect distance judgement. Bilateral cataracts may cause gradual visual loss ± frequent spectacle changes due to the refractive index of the lens changing, may cause dazzling—especially in sunlight, and may cause monocular diplopia. In children they may present as squint, loss of binocular function, as a white pupil, as nystagmus (infants), or as amblyopia.

Treatment Childhood cataracts require special surgical techniques. Adult cataracts do not necessarily require treatment, and most will never need it. No treatments prevent or arrest their development. Check acuity regularly. Surgical removal of the lens is the only treatment. The main question influencing timing of surgery is: 'Does your reduced sight prevent you doing what you want to do?' On this scale, seamstresses will get surgery before wine-tasters.

Extracapsular cataract extraction with posterior chamber lens implant is the surgery of choice. In this procedure the anterior part of the lens capsule is meticulously torn and removed. The posterior part of the lens is left *in situ*, like a bag, to hold the intraocular lens. The cortex and nucleus of the lens is removed either mechanically through a large incision at the limbus, or after emulsifying the lens (phacoemulsification), through a smaller incision. The intraocular lens is then implanted into the capsular bag.

Day-case surgery (eg with phacoemulsification) is possible using local anaesthetic agents to produce a Tolosa–Hunt syndrome (p 758). The patient can choose to have a lens implanted which will focus on the horizon or near-to—or on an intermediate position. Spectacles will be needed to counteract healing astigmatism—but do not order these for some months after surgery, and warn the patient that further refractive changes may occur after the initial spectacles are ordered.

The posterior capsule becomes opaque (in ~43% at 5yrs post extracapsular extraction[1]), and like cataract, causes gradual blurring of vision. YAG lasers can be used to make a hole in the capsule (capsulotomy) to restore vision.

Complications of cataract surgery:

- Posterior capsule rupture (4%)
- Section requiring re-suture (0.8%)
- Rubeotic glaucoma (0.3%)
- Posterior capsule thickening (8%)
- Broken or protruding sutures (4%)
- Endophthalmitis (0.6%)
- Vitreous haemorrhage (0.3%)

Phacoemulsification versus	*Extracapsular extraction*
Small 4mm incision + ultrasonic fragmentation of lens, with aspiration of fragments	Larger incision and manual expression of lens
Number of sutures needed: 0–3	6–8 sutures required
Healing 2–4 weeks	8–12 weeks for healing
Astigmatism less	Post-op vision may not be so good

Cataract risk factors[2,3] **d**iabetes mellitus[d]; **d**ehydration crises (±heatstroke)
exogenous steroids (oral[psc] & inhaled[psc+n]); **e**ducation↓[m]
hypertension *(intraocular+systemic)*; **h**ypocalcaemia
d**y**strophia[d] myotonica *et al* (eg leprosy, onchocerciasis)
diet poor in β-carotene & antioxidants (vit C; vit E)
race/+ve family history
alcohol use (in excess)
tobacco[n]; **T**°(ambient)↑; prenatal **t**oxoplasmosis/rubella
infrared, **i**onizing or ultraviolet B rays;
old age (but in *ideal* circumstances lenses last 120yrs)
no protective factors (eg oestrogens; aspirin use●)

[d]=dot; [m]=mixed; [n]=nuclear; [psc]=posterior subcapsular type

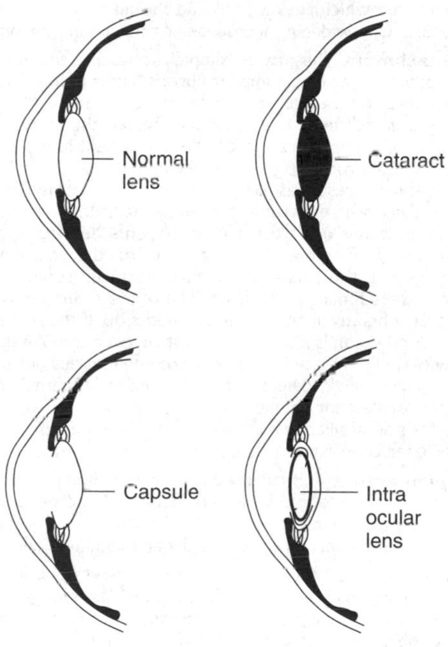

1 K Sundelin 1999 *J Cat Refract Surg* **25** 246 2 G Johnson 1998 *Lancet* **351** 925
3 R Cumming 1998 E-BM **3** 24 (if lifetime dose of inhaled beclomethasone >2000mg)

The retina

Anatomy The retina consists of an outer pigmented layer (in contact with the choroid), and an inner sensory layer (in contact with the vitreous). At the centre of the posterior part lies the macula (the centre of which is termed the fovea), appearing yellowish and slightly oval. This has many cones, so acuity is greatest here. ~3mm medial to the fovea is the optic disc, which contains no rods or cones (the visual field's blind spot).

Optic disc Think *colour; contour; cup. Colour* should be a pale pink. It is more pallid in optic atrophy (p 500). *Contour:* the disc may appear oval in astigmatic eyes, and appear abnormally large in myopic eyes. Disc margins are blurred in papilloedema (eg from raised intracranial pressure, malignant hypertension, cavernous sinus thrombosis), and with optic neuritis. Blood vessels radiate away from the disc. The normal arterial/venous width ratio is 2:3. Venous engorgement appears in retinal vein thrombosis (PLATE 6); abnormal retinal pallor with artery occlusion (PLATE 4); and haemorrhages with exudates in hypertension and diabetes (PLATES 8 & 11). *Cup:* the disc has a physiological cup which lies centrally and should occupy ~$\frac{1}{3}$ of the diameter of the disc. Cup widening and deepening occurs in glaucoma (p 502).

Retinal detachment This may be 'simple', idiopathic, secondary to some intraocular problem (eg melanoma, or fibrous bands in the vitreous in diabetes), occur after cataract surgery, or result from trauma. Myopic eyes are more prone to detachment, the higher the myopia, the greater the risk.[1]

In simple detachment, holes in the retina allow fluid to separate the sensory retina from the retinal pigment epithelium.

Detachment may present as painless loss of vision, sometimes described as a curtain falling over the vision (the curtain falls down as the lower half of the retina detaches upwards). 50% of patients developing detachment have premonitory symptoms—flashing lights or the sensation of spots before the eyes as the retina has been abnormally stimulated prior to detachment.[1] Detachment of the lower half of the retina tends not to pull off the macula, whereas upper half detachments do. If the macula becomes detached, central vision is lost and does not recover completely even if the retina is successfully replaced. Rate of detachment varies but upper halves tend to be quicker. Field defects may be detected. Ophthalmoscopy may reveal a grey opalescent retina, ballooning forward. *Treatment:* Urgent referral, eg for scleral silicone implants, cryotherapy, pneumatic retinopexy, or argon or laser coagulation to secure the retina.

Retinitis pigmentosa This familial disorder is a common cause of retinal degeneration. Particles of black pigment fleck mid and peripheral fundus. The earliest symptoms night blindness, often occurring in adolescence. Retinal vessels attenuate, and optic atrophy and blindness ensue.

Retinoblastoma The typical patient is a child <3yrs old. If it is bilateral (30%) the cause is usually hereditary. The 'retinoblastoma' gene, present in everyone, is normally a suppressor gene or anti-oncogene. Those with hereditable retinoblastomas have one altered allele in every cell. If a developing retinal cell undergoes mutation in the other allele, a retinoblastoma results. The retinoblastoma gene is the best characterized tumour suppressor gene (called 'RB1'; 27 exons; >200 kilobases of genomic DNA). Its product is a nuclear phosphoprotein which helps regulate DNA synthesis.
Presentation: They may grow out (exophytic) or in, ie endophytic—into the vitreous, causing a white pupil (leukocoria), squint, inflammation, and an absent red reflex. Parents may notice this phenomenon when studying flash photographs of their children—in which only one eye is red.
Treatment: Enucleation or laser ablation. Arrange follow up because of risk of osteosarcoma, typically in the second decade of life.[2]

1 A Chignell 1987 BMJ ii 661 2 G Skuse 1995 *Lancet* **345** 902

Toxoplasma This obligate intracellular protozoan sometimes causes bilateral typical 'punched-out' heavily pigmented chorioretinal scars which can be seen on routine fundal examination. If scars involve the macular area there will be dramatic loss of acuity. Toxoplasmosis is a cause of about 25% of uveitis in the UK.

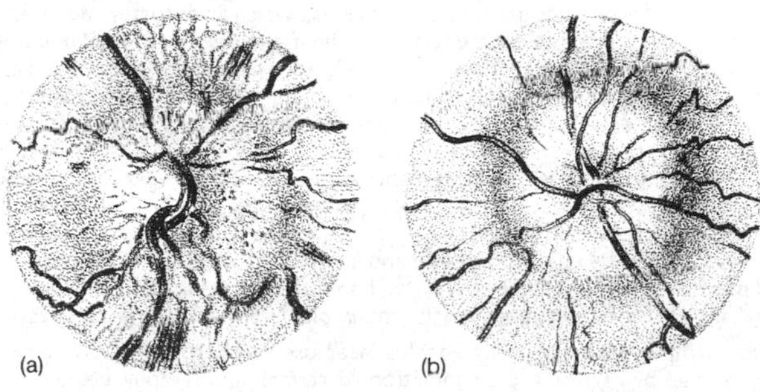

(a) Papilloedema from raised intracranial pressure. The disc is swollen forwards and also outwards into the surrounding retina. The disc margin is completely hidden and in places retinal vessels are concealed, because oedema has impaired the translucency of the disc tissues. The retinal veins are congested and there are a few haemorrhages. (b) Early papilloedema. The vessels crossing the disc are obscured in places due to the loss of translucency of the prelaminar tissue in which they lie. (From J Parr *Introduction to Ophthalmology*, OUP.)

The eye in diabetes mellitus

Diabetes can be bloody and blinding—the leading cause of blindness in those aged 20–65 (UK). Almost any part of the eye can be affected: cataract and retinopathy are the chief pathologies. 30% of adults have ocular problems when diabetes presents. At presentation, the lens may have a higher refractive index (possibly due to dehydration) producing relative myopia. On treatment, the refractive index reduces, and vision is more hypermetropic—so do not correct refractive errors until diabetes is controlled.

Structural eye changes Diabetes may cause cataract. Most commonly this is a premature senile cataract, but young diabetics can also be affected at presentation. In this case, the lens has taken up a lot of glucose which is converted by the enzyme aldolase reductase to sorbitol. Sorbitol cannot diffuse through the lens but increases the osmotic pressure within the lens; water is then taken up which can cause the lens fibres to rupture and a cataract forms thereafter. Rarely, the iris may be affected by diabetes, with new blood vessel formation on it (rubeosis), and, if these block the drainage of aqueous fluid, glaucoma can be caused.

Retinopathy *Pathogenesis:* High retinal blood flow induces a microangiopathy in capillaries, precapillary arterioles and venules, causing occlusion and leakage. *Vascular occlusion:* Occlusion causes ischaemia which leads to new vessel formation in the retina, the optic disc and on the iris, ie *proliferative retinopathy* (PLATE 9). New vessels can bleed, causing vitreous haemorrhage. As new vessels carry along with them fibrous tissue, retraction of this tissue increases the risk of retinal detachment. Occlusion also causes *cotton wool spots* (PLATE 1, ischaemic nerve fibres). *Vascular leakage:* High retinal blood flow caused by hyperglycaemia (and BP↑ and pregnancy) damages capillary pericytes (these cells reinforce endothelial cells).[1] As pericytes are lost, capillaries bulge (microaneurysms) and leak. Leakage produces oedema and hard exudates (PLATE 2 & 8), made up of lipoprotein and lipid filled macrophages. The rupture of microaneurysms, when at the nerve fibre level, causes flame shaped haemorrhages (PLATE 11); when deep in the retina, *blot haemorrhages* (PLATE 7) form.

►Pre-symptomatic screening enables laser use of photocoagulation (PLATE 10). Screen by regular eye examination or retinal photography. Lesions are mostly at the posterior pole and can be easily seen with the ophthalmoscope. *Background retinopathy* (PLATE 7) comprises microaneurysms (seen as 'dots'), haemorrhages (flame shaped or 'blots') and hard exudates (yellow patches, PLATE 2 & 8). Vision is normal. Background retinopathy can progress to sight threatening maculopathy or proliferative retinopathy. *Maculopathy:* Leakage from the vessels close to the macula produce oedema and damage to the macula. *Proliferative retinopathy:* Fine new vessels appear on the retina and optic disc. Engorged tortuous veins, cotton wool spots (PLATE 1), large blot haemorrhages, and vitreous haemorrhage may also be seen.

►Refer those with maculopathy or proliferative retinopathy urgently to an ophthalmologist for treatment to protect vision.

Treatment Good control of diabetes can prevent new vessel formation. Concurrent diseases may accelerate retinopathy (eg hypertension, renal disease, pregnancy and anaemia). Treat these (as appropriate), and hyperlipidaemia. Photocoagulation by laser is used to treat both maculopathy and proliferative retinopathy. Definite indications for photocoagulation are new vessels on the optic disc and vitreous haemorrhage. If vitreous haemorrhage is massive and does not clear, vitrectomy may be needed.

CNS effects Ocular palsies may occur, typically nerves III and VI. In diabetic third nerve palsy the pupil may be spared as fibres to the pupil run peripherally in the nerve, receiving blood supply from the pial vessels. Argyll Robertson pupils and Horner's syndrome may also occur (p 488).

6. Ophthalmology

1 EM Corner 1993 *BMJ* ii 1195

The eye in systemic disease

Systemic disease often manifests itself in the eye and, in some cases, eye examination will first suggest the diagnosis.

Vascular retinopathy This may be *arteriopathic* (arteriovenous *nipping*: arteries nip veins where they cross—they share the same connective tissue sheath) or *hypertensive* (PLATE 11)—arteriolar vasoconstriction and leakage (producing *hard exudates* (PLATE 2 & 8), *macular oedema*, *haemorrhages*, and, rarely, *papilloedema*). Thickened arterial walls appear like wiring (called 'silver' or 'copper'). Narrowing of arterioles leads to localized infarction of the superficial retina seen as cotton wool spots (PLATE 1) and flame haemorrhages (PLATE 11). Leaks from these appear as hard exudates ± macular oedema/papilloedema (rare).

Emboli passing through the retina produce *amaurosis fugax*—seeing 'a curtain passing across the eyes' (PLATE 5). They may arise from atheromatous plaques (listen to carotids) or from heart (from valves or infarct site). Treat by aspirin (*OHCM* p 436). Retinal haemorrhages are seen in leukaemia (PLATE 12); comma-shaped conjunctival haemorrhages and retinal new vessel formation may occur in sickle-cell disease; optic atrophy in pernicious anaemia.

Note also Roth spots (retinal infarcts) of infective endocarditis (*OHCM* p 312).

Metabolic disease Diabetes: p 508. Hyperthyroidism and exophthalmos: *OHCM* p 543. In myxoedema, eyelid and periorbital oedema is quite common. Lens opacities may occur in hypoparathyroidism. Conjunctival and corneal calcification may occur in hyperparathyroidism. In gout, monosodium urate deposited in the conjunctiva may give sore eyes.

Granulomatous disorders (TB, sarcoid, leprosy, brucellosis, and toxoplasmosis) can all produce inflammation in the eye; TB and syphilis producing iritis, the others posterior uveitis. TB, congenital syphilis, sarcoid, CMV and toxoplasmosis may all produce choroidoretinitis. In sarcoid there may be cranial nerve palsies.

Collagen diseases These also cause inflammation. Conjunctivitis is found in SLE and Reiter's syndrome; episcleritis in polyarteritis nodosa and SLE; scleritis in rheumatoid arthritis; and uveitis in ankylosing spondylitis and Reiter's syndrome (*OHCM* p 668). In dermatomyositis there is orbital oedema with retinal haemorrhages.

Keratoconjunctivitis sicca Sjögren's syndrome, (*OHCM* p 708) There is reduced tear formation (Schirmer filter paper test), producing a gritty feeling in the eyes. Decreased salivation also gives a dry mouth (xerostomia). It occurs in association with collagen diseases. Treatment is with artificial tears ('tears naturale', or hypromellose drops).

AIDS Those who are HIV+ve may develop CMV retinitis (PLATE 16), characterized by retinal spots ('pizza pie' fundus, signifying superficial retinal infarction) and flame haemorrhages involving more and more of the retina. This may be asymptomatic but can cause sudden, untreatable, visual loss. If it is present it implies full-blown AIDS, and a low CD4 count. Cotton wool spots on their own (PLATE 1) may indicate HIV retinopathy, and it may present before the full picture of AIDS; it is a microvasculopathy, not a retinitis.

Candidiasis of the aqueous and vitreous is hard to treat. Kaposi's sarcoma may affect the lids or conjunctiva.

Tropical eye disease

Trachoma Caused by *Chlamydia trachomatis* (serotypes A, B, and C), this disease is spread by towels, fingers and flies—typically where it is hot, dry and dusty and the people are poor, living near to their cattle. 400 million people are affected (100,000,000 are children).

Diagnosis: Stage 1: There is lacrimation. Follicles under the upper lid give a fine granular appearance. *Stage 2:* There is intense erythema. The follicles are larger and underneath both lids. A fine pannus and capillaries grow down towards the cornea. *Stage 3:* The follicles rupture and are replaced by scar tissue. The pannus is more advanced. The cornea may ulcerate. *Stage 4:* Scar tissue distorts the lids and causes entropion. Eyelashes scratch the cornea, which ulcerates.

Treatment: Mass antitrachoma treatment: tetracycline 1% eye ointment is used 12-hourly for 5 days each month for 6 months. In active disease use 8-hourly for 6 weeks + sulfadimethoxine 1g stat, then 500mg/24h PO for 10 days (erythromycin if a child). Single-dose azithromycin (20mg/kg) is effective.[1,2] Surgery: tarsal plate rotation.

Prevention: Good water and sanitation. Regular washing of faces.

Onchocerciasis This is caused by the microfilariae of the nematode *Onchocerca volvulus*, transmitted by black flies of the Simulium species. Of the 20–50 million people affected, 95% live in Africa. In some areas it may cause blindness in 40% of the population. Unless the eye is affected, problems are mostly confined to the skin. Fly bites result in nodules from which microfilariae are released. These eventually invade the eye, mainly the conjunctiva, cornea, ciliary body and iris, but occasionally the retina or optic nerve. Sometimes they may be seen swimming in the aqueous or lying dead in the anterior chamber. The microfilariae initially excite an inflammatory reaction, then fibrosis occurs around them. Reaction around the dead microfilariae in the cornea causes corneal opacities (nummular keratitis). Chronic iritis causes synechiae formation and may precipitate cataracts. The iris may become totally fixed. *Tests:* Skin snip tests, triple-antigen serology; polymerase chain reaction. *Treatment:* Seek expert help. Ivermectin is the treatment of choice: 150μg/kg PO as a single dose every 6–12 months, until the adult worms die (*OHCM* p 247). In lightly infected expatriates, the first 3 doses are recommended to be monthly, with observation in hospital after the first dose (reactions are common in expatriates).[3]

Xerophthalmia and keratomalacia These are manifestations of vitamin A deficiency, eg if weaned early on to vitamin A deficient milk products, or toddlers who eat few vegetables. Peak incidence: 2–5yrs; 40 million children worldwide. Night blindness and dry conjunctivae (xerosis) occur early. The cornea is unwettable and loses transparency. Small grey plaques (Bitot's spots) are commonly found raised from interpalpebral conjunctiva. Vitamin A reverses these changes. Early corneal xerosis is reversible. Corneal ulceration and perforation can occur. In keratomalacia there is massive softening of the cornea ± perforation and extrusion of the intraocular contents. *Treatment:* For children: retinol palmitate 50,000U IM monthly until the eyes are normal (adult dose 100,000U, weekly to start with); or oral retinyl palmitate 200,000U PO. β-carotene (a provitamin) 1.2×10^6 U PO, is as effective,[4] and cheaper. Avoid vitamin A in pregnancy (vitamin A embryopathy).

1 A Potter 1993 BMJ **ii** 214 2 RL Bailey 1993 *Lancet* **342** 453 3 DR Churchill 1994 *Trans Roy Soc Trop Med Hyg* **88** 242 4 C Carlier 1993 BMJ **ii** 1106

Eye trauma[1,2]

►Prevention is the key. Wear goggles, or plastic glasses when near small moving objects or using tools (avoids metal splinters, fish-hooks, and squash-ball injuries). *Always record acuity* (both eyes; if the uninjured one is blind take all injuries very seriously). If the patient is unable to open the injured eye, instil a few drops of local anaesthetic (amethocaine 1%): wait a few minutes after which the patient should be able to comfortably open the eye. Examine lids, conjunctiva, cornea, sclera, anterior chamber, pupil, iris, lens, vitreous, fundus and eye movement. An irregular pupil may mean globe rupture. A tiny hole in the iris may be hard to see, but, with the pen torch, such holes will give a red reflex.[2] Afferent pupil defects (*OHCM* p 488) do not augur well for sight recovery. Note pain, discharge, or squint. CT may be very useful (foreign bodies may be magnetic, so avoid MRI).

Sharp and penetrating wounds Refer urgently—as the longer the delay the more the risk of ocular contents being disturbed, extruded, or infected. With uveal injury there is risk of sympathetic ophthalmia in the other eye. ►A history of flying objects (eg work with lathes, hammers, and chisels) should prompt careful examination and x-ray to exclude intraocular foreign bodies. ►►Do *not* attempt to remove a large foreign body (knife; dart). Support the object with padding. Transport supine. Pad the *unaffected* eye to prevent damage from conjugate movement. Consider skull x-ray or CT to exclude intracranial involvement.

Foreign bodies These may be hard to see: examine all parts of the eye—as they may cause chemosis, subconjunctival haemorrhage, irregular pupils, iris prolapse, hyphaema, vitreous haemorrhage and retinal tears. If you suspect a metal foreign body x-ray the orbit. With high-velocity foreign bodies, consider orbital ultrasound: pick-up rate is 90% *vs* 40% for x-rays—but the technique is difficult, and possibly unsuited to busy A&E departments. Removal of superficial foreign bodies may be possible using a triangle of clean card. Evert the eyelids to check no material underneath. Use gentamicin 0.3% drops afterwards to prevent infection. Have a low threshold for asking for the advice of a senior colleague.

Corneal abrasions (Often inflicted by small fast-moving objects such as children's finger-nails and twigs.) They may cause intense pain. Apply a drop of local anaesthetic, eg 1% amethocaine before examination. They stain with fluorescein and should heal within 48h. Antibiotic drops are used until healing occurs. Use eye pads initially if local anaesthetic has been instilled to protect the cornea, but otherwise are not needed.[1]

Burns *Treat chemical burns promptly:* hold lids open and bathe the eyes in copious clean water while the specific antidote is sought. Often the patient will not hold the eye open due to excruciating pain. Amethocaine drops applied every minute for 5 minutes will relieve pain and aid irrigation. All burns may have late serious sequelae, eg corneal scarring, opacification, and lid damage. Alkali burns are more serious than acid.

Arc eye Welders and sunbed users who don't wear protection against UV light may damage corneal epithelium. There is a foreign body sensation, watering and blepharospasm. Give mydriatics (p 518), pad the eye, and await recovery. It is a very painful, so be generous with analgesia.

Finally, remember to think of *fat embolus* in trauma patients who suddenly complain of visual problems.[2]

1 DL Easty 1993 *BMJ* ii 1022 2 ATLS 1997 *Manual* 6e, p411 ISBN 1-880696-10-X

Blindness and partial sight

The pattern of blindness around the world differs considerably, depending on local nutrition and economic factors. 80% of the world's blind live in developing countries. The diseases responsible for most of the blindness in the world are trachoma, cataract (50% of the world's blindness), glaucoma, keratomalacia, onchocerciasis and diabetic retinopathy. In the past smallpox, gonorrhoea, syphilis, and leprosy (10% of those affected were blind) were also common causes of blindness, but are less so now.

Rates of blindness are higher than 10/1000 in some parts of Africa and Asia, but in the UK and the USA rates are 2/1000. Blindness may be voluntarily registered in England, registration making one available for certain concessions. Although the word blind suggests inability to perceive light, a person is eligible for registration if their acuity is less than 3/60, or if >3/60 but with substantial visual field loss (as in glaucoma). There are 149,670 registered blind in the UK (1994), and a further 115,710 partially sighted. The criterion for partial sighted registration is that the acuity is <6/60 (or >6/60 with visual field restrictions).

The causes of blindness have changed considerably in the UK over the last 70 years. Whereas in the 1920s ophthalmia neonatorum (p 100) was responsible for 30% of all cases of blindness found in English blind schools, this is now a rare but treatable disease. Retrolental fibroplasia was common in the 1950s, mostly affecting premature infants: monitoring of intra-arterial oxygen in premature babies tries to prevent this. With the increasing population of elderly, the diseases particularly afflicting this population are the common causes of blindness. Nearly two-thirds of the blind population are over 65 years of age, and nearly half over 75. Macular degeneration, cataract, and glaucoma are the three commonest causes of blindness.

In England and Wales the responsibility for blind registration lies with the local authority. Application for registration is made by a consultant ophthalmologist and is voluntary, not statutory. Registration as blind entitles one to extra tax allowances, reduced TV licence fees, some travel concessions, and access to talking books. Special certification from an ophthalmologist is necessary for the partially sighted to receive talking books. At one time it was statutory that the registered blind should receive a visit from a social worker but this is no longer the case, although the social services employ social workers who specialize in care of the blind. The Royal National Institute for the Blind[1] will advise on aids, such as guide dogs (available if required for employment).

Special educational facilities provide for visually handicapped children. Special schools have a higher staff/pupil ratio, specialized equipment, and many have a visiting ophthalmologist. The disadvantage is that the children may not mix much with other children—especially if they board.

1 Royal National Institute for the Blind, 224 Great Portland St, London WIN 6AA (UK tel. 0171 388 1266)

Contusions and intraocular haemorrhage

Our eyes are protected by our bony orbital ridges. Severe contusions from large objects may damage the eye, but smaller objects such as champagne corks, squash balls, and airgun pellets (p 679) cause local contusion, eg resulting in lid bruises and subconjunctival haemorrhage (if the posterior limit of such a haemorrhage cannot be seen, consider fracture of the orbit). Both usually settle in 2 weeks. ►*Any injury penetrating the eyeball should receive immediate specialist treatment.*

Intraocular haemorrhage: This usually affects acuity and should receive specialist attention. Blood is often found in the anterior chamber (hyphaema): small amounts clear spontaneously but if filling the anterior chamber, evacuation may be needed. It is often recognizable by pen-torch examination. Even small hyphaemas must be carefully evaluated (∴ refer): it may signify serious injury.[2] *Late complications:* Glaucoma; corneal staining. Pain suggests glaucoma or re-bleeding.

Secondary haemorrhage: This may occur within 5 days and may produce sight-threatening secondary glaucoma. Sometimes the iris is paralysed and dilated due to injury (called traumatic mydriasis). This usually recovers in a few days but sometimes it is permanent. Vitreous haemorrhage will cause dramatic fall in acuity. There will be no red reflex on ophthalmoscopy. Lens dislocation, tearing of the iris root, splitting of the choroid, detachment of the retina, and damage to the optic nerve may be other sequelae; they are more common if contusion is caused by smaller objects rather than large.

Blows to the orbit: These may cause blowout fractures with orbital contents herniating into the maxillary sinus. Tethering of the inferior rectus and inferior oblique muscles causes diplopia. Test the sensation over the skin of the lower lid. Loss of sensation indicates injury to the infraorbital nerve, confirming a blowout fracture. Fracture reduction and muscle release is necessary.

Colour vision and colour blindness

For normal colour vision we require cone photopigments sensitive to blue, green and red light. The commonest hereditary colour vision defect is X-linked failure of red–green discrimination (8% ♂ and 0.5% ♀ affected—so those with Turner's syndrome have ♂ incidence and those with Klinefelter's have ♀ incidence). Blue–yellow discriminatory failure is more commonly acquired and sexes are affected equally.

Diagnosis: This is by use of coloured pattern discrimination charts (eg Ishihara plates).

Depressed colour vision may be a sensitive indicator of acquired macular or optic nerve disease.

Monochromatism This may be due to being born without cones (resulting in low visual acuity, absent colour vision, photophobia and nystagmus), or, very rarely due to cone monochromacy where all cones contain the same visual pigment, when there is only failure to distinguish colour.

Drugs and the eye

The eye does not retain drops for as long as ointments and two-hourly applications may be needed. Eye ointments are particularly suitable for use at night and in conditions where crusting and sticking of the lid margins occurs. Allow 5min between doses of drops to prevent overspill.

The antibiotics most used are not those generally used systemically, eg fusidic acid, chloramphenicol, neomycin, gentamicin and framycetin. All eye preparations have warnings not to use for more than one month. Contamination of drops is rare, as they contain bacteriostatic drugs, and in practice may be used for longer.

Mydriatics These drugs dilate the pupil. They also cause cycloplegia and hence blur vision (warn not to drive). Pupil dilatation prior to examination is best achieved using 0.5% or 1% tropicamide which lasts for 3h. 1% cyclopentolate has an action of 24 hours and is preferred for producing cycloplegia for refraction of children. These drugs may be used to prevent synechiae formation in iritis. ►In the over-60s with shallow anterior chambers (especially if a family history of glaucoma) they may precipitate acute glaucoma, so only use on ophthalmological advice.

Miotics These constrict the pupil and increase drainage of aqueous. They are used in the treatment of glaucoma (p 502). Pilocarpine 1–4% is the most commonly used.

Local anaesthetic Amethocaine (0.5% drops) is an example. This may be used to permit examination of a painful eye where reflex blepharospasm is a problem, and to facilitate removal of a foreign body. ►It abolishes the corneal reflex so use to treat pain is to risk corneal damage. To relieve pain, give an eye pad, and be generous with oral analgesia.

Steroid-containing drops ►These are potentially dangerous as they may induce catastrophic progression of dendritic ulcers (p 480). Ophthalmoscopic examination may miss dendritic ulcers, and slit lamp inspection is essential if steroid drops are being considered, eg for allergy, episcleritis, scleritis or iritis.

Iatrogenic eye disease Glaucoma may not only be precipitated by mydriatics; other drugs may precipitate or aggravate glaucoma. Those particularly implicated are steroids and those with anticholinergic effects (some antiparkinson drugs and tricyclic antidepressants).

A few drugs affect the retina if used chronically. Those taking ethambutol should be warned to report *any* visual side-effects (loss of acuity, colour blindness). Chloroquine and other antimalarials are also implicated and damage may occur with long-term use, especially if high doses are used.

Obtaining and preparing antibiotic eyedrops

Fortified guttate gentamicin is 15mg/mL—(the normal commercial gentamicin is 3mg/mL); penicillin 5000 units/mL, methicillin 20mg/mL and antifungals can be obtained from the Chief Pharmacist, Moorfields Eye Hospital (tel. 0171 253 3411). Antibiotics can be home-made as follows:
Gentamicin forte: add 2mL of 40mg/mL IV gentamicin to a 5mL bottle of commercial guttate gentamicin (3mg/mL).[1]

Other antibiotics can be made up using IV preparations to the required concentration using water or normal saline. These are stable for the time recommended for IV solutions in the manufacturers *Data sheets*. Penicillin G can be used up to 500,000u/mL.

1 Prepared from information supplied by Mr JKG Dart FRCS, Moorfields Eye Hospital, City Rd, London EC1V 2PD

Eyedrops as a cause of systemic symptoms

Drugs applied to the eye may be absorbed through the cornea and produce systemic side-effects—eg bronchospasm or bradycardia in susceptible individuals using antiglaucoma β-blocking drops, eg **timolol** (Timoptol®), **carteolol** (Teoptic®), **betaxolol** (Betoptic®—which is a bit more cardio-selective). ►Symptoms may be subtle and insidious—eg gradually decreasing exercise tolerance, or falls from arrhythmias. Serious problems are more likely if there is co-morbidity (eg sepsis).

Other anti-glaucoma drops (p 502) cause headaches, and a bitter taste in the mouth; urolithiasis is reported with **dorzolamide** (Trusopt®).

Pilocarpine (eg Isopto Carpine®, Sno Pilo®, Ocusert®) may cause parasympathetic actions, eg sweating, salivation, pulmonary oedema, BP↑, pulse↑, lacrimation, D&V, wheeze, and colic. Accommodation spasm may lead to brow-ache (worse if <40 years old, and just starting treatment).

Even highly-selective α_2-receptor agonists used in glaucoma, such as **brimonidine** (Alphagan®), can cause systemic effects such as dry mouth, headache, fatigue, and drowsiness—even though they are lipophilic (so less likely to cross the blood–brain barrier).

Contact lenses

Contact lenses are commonly worn—and commonly problematic.

80% of contact lenses are worn for cosmetic reasons. Only 20% are worn because lenses are more suitable for the eye condition than spectacles. Among this 20% a minority wear the lenses to hide disfiguring inoperable eye conditions, a greater proportion have them for very high refractive errors. Myopia above −12.0DS and hypermetropia above +10.0DS are indications for lenses because equivalent spectacles produce quite distorted visual fields. Contact lenses after cataract removal come into this category. Lenses are used for ocular reasons, eg after corneal ulceration or trauma when a new front surface of the cornea is needed to see through, and in keratoconus. Keratoconus is a rare degenerative, slowly progressive corneal condition with thinning and anterior protrusion of the central cornea. Blurred vision is the only symptom. Contact lens use may compensate for corneal distortion early, but later corneal grafting may be needed.

Types of lens Hard lenses are 8.5–9mm in diameter and are made of polymethylmethacrylate (PMMA). Gas-permeable hard lenses are about 0.5cm larger and are designed to allow gas to permeate through to the underlying cornea. They can only be made to cope with a limited degree of astigmatism and do not wet as well as standard hard lenses so may mist up in the day. With the advent of the larger (13–15mm diameter) soft contact lenses it was hoped that many of the problems with hard lenses could be circumvented. Soft disposable lenses can be worn for 2–4 weeks and then disposed of. With astigmatism adequate correction is not achieved because the lens fits the astigmatic cornea too well and is flexible. A conventional hard or gas-permeable lens can usually correct a small amount of astigmatism but high astigmatism requires a toric lens (a soft lens made especially to correct astigmatism). They are more delicate than hard lenses and need meticulous cleaning. Extended wear-lenses can be worn for up to 4 months. Sometimes coloured lenses are used simply to change eye colour.

Patients may suffer from keratoconjunctivitis or giant papillary change in the upper tarsal conjunctiva, possibly due to sensitization to the cleansing materials used or to the mucus which forms on the lens.

Cleaning lenses Different cleaning solutions made by different manufacturers should not be mixed.[1] With hard lenses 2 solutions are usually used, one for rinsing and cleaning, and one for storage. The storage solution should be washed off before the lens is inserted. Soft contact lenses, being permeable, tend to absorb the chemicals, so weaker solutions for cleaning are used. In addition, the lenses are usually intermittently cleaned with another system (eg enzyme tablets) to remove mucoprotein on their surface. Sensitivity to cleaning agents usually presents as redness, stinging, increased lens movement, increased mucus production and thickened eyelids. It may be necessary to stop wearing lenses for several months. When restarting use a preservative-free cleansing system.

Complications

1. Contact lenses are the most important risk factor for corneal ulceration. Corneal abrasion is common early while adjusting to wear. Pain ± lacrimation occurs some hours after removing the lens.
2. Sensitization to cleaning agents.
3. Losing the lens within the eye. Hard lenses may be lost in any fornix, soft lenses are usually in upper outer fornix.
4. Keratitis especially for extended-wear (>6 days) soft lenses.
5. Staining by rifampicin or fluorescein.

Hygiene tips

- ►Pay attention to contact lens containers, as well as lenses.
- Scrub container's inside with cotton wool bud moistened with lens fluid.
- Disinfect the container with hot water (≥80°C); leave to dry in open air.
- Wash your hands before handling the contact lens container.
- Replace the container at least every year.
- Protozoa may survive new '1-step' solutions of 3% hydrogen peroxide.

Blepharospasm

Blepharospasm is involuntary contraction of orbicularis oculi. It commonly occurs in response to ocular pain. Repetitive blepharospasm, which may make the patient effectively blind, is one of the focal dystonias (*OHCM* p 428). If the condition is not recognized, it is all too easy to dismiss the patient as hysterical and to think that screwing up of the eyes is deliberate—especially as the more the sceptical doctor questions and probes the afflicted patient, the worse the blepharospasm may become (stress is an important exacerbating factor).

Presentation ♀:♂ ≈ 1.8 : 1. Blepharospasm is often preceded by exaggerated blinking. Other dystonias may be present (eg oro-mandibular). It usually starts unilaterally, becoming bilateral. Patients may develop various tricks to reduce blepharospasm such as touching or pulling the eyelids—a variation of *geste antagoniste* seen in other forms of dystonia.

Causes Mostly unknown. Recognized antecedent events are: neuroleptic drugs, Parkinson's disease, progressive supranuclear palsy.

Treatment *Drugs:* There are no panaceas and response is variable—with good effects tending to wear off. Most helpful are anticholinergics such as benzhexol, eg 1mg/day PO, gradually increased up to 5mg/8h (tablets are 2mg or 5mg). Dopamine agonists (L-dopa, bromocriptine) or antagonist may help. *Botulinum toxin:* In this approach, palliation is achieved with nanogram doses of this neurotoxin given to orbicularis oculi, in which it produces a temporary flaccid paralysis. It can help some people recover effective vision.[1] It binds to peripheral nerve terminals and inhibits the release of acetylcholine. Treatment may need to be repeated, for example at 3-monthly intervals. *Supportive treatment:* Patients may gain considerable support from the Dystonia Society.[2]

Allergic eye disease

Hay fever conjunctivitis There is usually an allergic history (animal danders or pollens). The eye is red, with chemosis and lacrimation. Cold compresses may help, as may topical 1:1000 epinephrine (=adrenaline) drops, or twice daily sodium cromoglycate 4% ointment or 2% drops/6h.

Vernal keratoconjunctivitis (spring catarrh; seasonal conjunctivitis) This is an uncommon allergic bilateral conjunctivitis, usually appearing before puberty, and lasting ≥5yrs. ♂/♀>1. There is often a family history of atopy. It is almost non-existent in cold areas. *Presentation:*

- Itching eye with photophobia
- Milky conjunctiva and ropy discharge
- 'Cobblestones' under upper lid
- Papillae in lower tarsal conjunctiva
- Pseudomembrane (Maxwell–Lyon sign)
- Corneal arcus (± ulcer) near limbus

Management: It is self-limiting. Prophylactic cromoglycate may help. Avoid corticosteroids because of their long-term complications (glaucoma, cataract, fungal infection) except during short photophobic phases.

Delayed hypersensitivity: phlyctenular keratoconjunctivitis This may be a delayed response to mycobacteria, staphs, yeasts, or chlamydia. The conjunctival phlyctenule begins as a hard, red, 1–3mm diameter papule surrounded by hyperaemia. At the limbus, it is triangular (apex points to cornea). It ulcerates, and then subsides within 12 days. Corneal phlyctenules develop as an amorphous grey infiltrate, and leave a scar. They may cause intense photophobia. *Management:* Seek expert help. Steroid drops may be very effective. Treat any bacterial cause.

1 F Grandas 1988 *J Neurology, Neurosurgery, and Psychiatry* **51** 767–72 **2** UK tel. 0171 329 0797

6. Ophthalmology

Floaters, flashes, and haloes

►*When patients complain of flashes and floaters think of retinal detachment.* When patients mention their haloes remember that they may not be referring to their own saintliness. *Halo* refers to a circle of light, either white or prismatically coloured, seen around *any* luminous body: not just those of saints. Also call to mind Monet and his cataracts (a cause of haloes). It is not simply that his great impressionist paintings are investments in light (another definition of *halo*). . .

Doctor, you say there are no haloes
around the streetlights in Paris
and what I see is an aberration
caused by old age, an affliction.
I tell you it has taken me all my life
*to arrive at the vision of gas lamps as angels. . .**

Here, Monet refuses surgery for his cataracts (how differently doctors and artists see the world!). So before we recommend surgery it might be as well to get to know our patients a bit, as well as keeping a weather-eye on posterity.

Floaters These are small dark spots in the visual field, particularly noticeable against a bright background. Each floater is a shadow of a mobile vitreous opacity cast on the retina. After the eye comes to rest, they continue to move. The cause is often degenerative opacities in the vitreous (syneresis). They are common in myopes, after cataract operations or after trauma. Mostly, they are just annoying (if central), but harmless, and may settle with time. Always examine the vitreous and retina before reassuring. *Sudden showers* of floaters appearing in one eye (which may be accompanied by flashing lights) are due to blood. ►*Refer immediately*, as the cause may be retinal detachment (p 506). Other causes:

- Diabetic retinopathy
- Old retinal branch vein occlusion
- Recurrent vitreous bleeding (Eales's dis.)
- Hypertension
- Endocarditis
- Sickle-cell dis.
- Leukaemia
- Sarcoid
- TB; SLE

Flashing lights These may be from intraocular pathology or migraine. Is there headache, nausea, or previous migraine? Detachment of a shrinking vitreous from the retina (commoner in myopes) gives flashes and floaters. 5% go on to retinal tears and detachment. Retinal damage is usually peripheral and hard to see—refer immediately for specialist help.

The four 'F's of retinal detachment **F**loaters, **f**lashes, **f**ield loss, and **f**alling acuity. Flashes are due to pulling on the retina, and may increase with eye movement. Field loss may be seen as a dark cloud covering a field of vision (superior field loss indicates inferior retinal detachment and vice versa). Falling acuity indicates a grave situation. Superior detachments may be fast so that the macula is affected, resulting in 6/60 vision. In this situation vision remains poor even after successful surgery.

Haloes These may be symptom of acute angle closure glaucoma. Smooth, coloured haloes around lights is a diffractive phenomenon and so may be seen when a white light is inside a steamed-up window at night (and street lights may have haloes when seen through misted car windscreens), or through scratched spectacles. Hazy ocular media may also be the cause, so they can occur with cataract, and where there is corneal oedema.

In acute glaucoma it is corneal oedema that causes them as intraocular pressure rises with pupillary dilatation. If haloes are accompanied by eye pain consider this diagnosis and refer immediately.

Jagged haloes which change shape are usually due to migraine. Beware labelling haloes as being migrainous in patients over 50 years who have not previously suffered from migraine.

*Lisel Mueller 1986 *Monet Refuses the Operation* in *Second Language*. See also M Faith McLellan 1996 (*Lancet* 1996 **348** 1641)—to whom this page owes much—for a critique of this poem.

Laser photorefractive keratotomy (PRK)

This novel way of correcting myopia without necessary recourse to spectacles entails removing microscopic portions of tissue from the front of the cornea, so altering its shape and refractive properties. In general, one may expect treatment to be accurate to within 1 dioptre of expectation in eyes with a myopic refraction of 1–6.75 dioptres, and an astigmatism of *no more* than 1.5 dioptres. Note the following points:

- PRK is irreversible.
- The greater the myopia, the more the laser needs to penetrate, and the greater the risk of corneal scarring—with subsequent opacification.
- Intermediate myopia (7–12 dioptres) *may* be treatable but regression is more likely.
- There is no reliable evidence that astigmatism can be reduced or eliminated permanently.
- Presbyopia, not being the 'fault' of the cornea, is not amenable to PRK.
- Be critical of reports claiming that excimer or holmium lasers can treat hypermetropia reliably.
- Long-term follow-up information is lacking. PRK only started in 1988.

Contraindications •Unstable myopia (eg patients under 21 years old) •Corneal infection •Keratoconus •Pregnancy (unpredictable healing) •Those on steroids •Those with unrealistic expectations.

What to tell patients PRK is only suitable for some eyes, and some patients. It is an outpatient procedure, using eyedrops as local anaesthesia. Application of the laser lasts only 15–90 seconds, depending on the degree of short-sightedness. Immediately after there may be quite severe pain (eyedrops, oral analgesia, and an eye patch will be given to minimize this). 2–4 days off work is usually necessary. In the few weeks following PRK, vision may be blurred. The healing process tends to produce over-correction of refractive errors. A difference in focus of the two eyes will occur when the first eye has PRK; this can be ameliorated by wearing a contact lens on the other eye. Stress need for regular post-operative examinations by the ophthalmologist.

Warn the patient that even after the post-operative period there may be a noticeable (but generally subjectively unimportant) visual haze.

Outcome ~80% of eyes heal in a predictable way—so the result is less certain in 20%, with *over-correction*, *under-correction*, or *regression* of myopia being problems. Some patients also experience *haze*, *glare* and *haloes* (a particular problem during night-driving)—but is more of a feature after radial keratotomy rather than after PRK.[1] There are also worries about the long-term effect of ablating Bowman's layer. Loss of *contrast sensitivity* can also be a persisting problem in up to 75%—for most of whom it is insignificant (but note that the UK civil aviation authority and ministry of defence do not accept pilot candidates who have had PRK).

New refinements in laser delivery producing smoother corneal ablation are thought to reduce hazing, and to improve predictability of outcome, with 95% of eyes achieving 6/12 vision unaided, within 1 week, with no eyes losing visual acuity, and no glare or night-time haloes.[2] Laser-assisted keratomileusis also minimizes haze. A microkeratome cuts a hinged corneal flap, PRK is performed, and the flap is replaced. This operation has its own complications.[2] Other forms of microsurgery are more popular in the USA, where one study of 750,000 eyes found that *diurnal fluctuation in vision* was a (small) problem, and it was not as good as PRK at higher degrees of myopia.

Anterior chamber implants are another way of correcting myopia.

1 JF Taylor 1995 *Medical Aspects of Fitness to Drive*, Medical Commission on Accident Prevention, page 122. 2 W Jory 1996 *Lancet* **348** 904. We thank Mr Salt for providing helpful material.

7. Ear, nose and throat diseases

►Ideally, this chapter should be read with a ready supply of ENT patients and access to surgeons willing to teach about the various operative techniques employed. If this impossible, a good place to start may be with a successful multimedia title such as

7. Ear, nose and throat diseases

ENT examination

Doctors working in ENT departments were once readily distinguishable by their concave mirrors with central hole worn over the eye. These reflect light from a bright source in a concentrated beam, giving good illumination and stereopsis, leaving both hands free for manipulations—but fibreoptic devices for nasendoscopy are now obviating the need for such headgear.

Examination of the ear Examine the external *auditory meatus*, *pinna*, and its environs for swelling and for inflammation. Swab any *discharge*, and remove any *wax* (p 530). Attach the largest comfortable earpiece to the otoscope, and examine the full length of the auditory meatus and *drum*. Seeing the drum is the first skill to master, and can be achieved quite readily: but the real skill lies in seeing what lies *behind* the drum. This takes many years of practice. Begin by pulling the pinna up and backward to straighten the external auditory canal. (In infants, pull the pinna backwards and *down*.) The handle of the malleus makes a definite landmark behind the tympanic membrane. Anteroinferiorly is the light reflex which is reflected due to the degree of concavity of the membrane in this region. To left–right orientate yourself (eg when looking at pictures of drums) know that the light reflex points to the toes (ie anteroinferior). Try to get a good look at the posterosuperior quadrant of the drum: it is behind this section that there is the most important clockwork: the *posterior mallear fold*, the long process of the *incus*, and the *facial nerve*. Note colour, translucency and any bulging of the membrane. Are there any perforations? What is their position? Does the margin extend to the periphery? *Perforations or retractions* of the pars flaccida may indicate serious pathology (p 536). Mobility of the membrane is shown using an aural speculum with a sealed glass in front and teat on the side to attach a little rubber balloon. As the balloon is squeezed the drum should move. A patent *Eustachian tube* is indicated by movement of the drum during a Valsalva manoeuvre.

The nose and throat In order to examine the throat and nasal passages the parts needing to be examined are moved into the beam of light reflected from the mirror. First ask the patient to open his mouth without protruding the tongue. Apply a tongue depressor just beyond the highest part of the tongue and ask the patient to say 'ah'. The *palate* rises opening the *oropharynx* so *tonsils*, *posterior wall of pharynx* and anterior and posterior pillars of the *fauces* may be examined. In some people, saying 'aye' (as is in '*a*ble') or simply watching while the patient breathes (with the tongue depressed), is more revealing.

Examination of the post-nasal space is best performed by direct endoscopy, using a flexible instrument to reveal the *nasal septum*, the posterior end of superior, middle and inferior *turbinates*, the lateral walls of the *nasopharynx*, the openings of *Eustachian tubes*, the *pharyngeal recess*, the roof of the *nasopharynx* and *adenoids*. Anterior rhinoscopy (ie holding open the nares with a special Thudiculum speculum) enables the front of the inferior and middle turbinates to be seen.

The middle turbinate and the space under it (the meatus) is a key area of the nose because most of the sinuses ventilate through this cleft.

Indirect laryngoscopy is possible, with the tongue protruded, using a large warmed mirror. As the patient breathes, the *epiglottis* and the posterior part of the inlet of the *larynx* is seen. As the patient says 'ee', the interior of the larynx and *vocal cords* may be seen. Flexible nasendoscopy (4mm) allows more detailed examination. Admission to hospital is now mainly for taking of biopsies rather than for examination under anaesthesia.

7. Ear, nose and throat diseases

The ear

Anatomy The cartilaginous auricle develops from 6 tubercles. If there is malfusion during development there may be fistulae (most common is a small fistula in front of the tragus) or accessory auricles (cartilaginous bodies lying between the angle of the mouth and the tragus).

The external auditory meatus is 3–4cm long and slightly S-shaped. The cartilage-surrounded outer third has hairs and ceruminous (wax) glands in the skin. The inner two-thirds of the meatus is surrounded by bone and lined with sensitive skin.

The tympanic membrane separates the external auditory meatus and the tympanic cavity (middle ear). The handle of the malleus can be seen abutting it. The greater part of the membrane lies taut—the *pars tensa*, but above the lateral process of the malleus lies a triangular area which is less taut—the *pars flaccida* (the site of attic perforations and retractions: the latter is more common).

The middle ear lies in the petrous part of the temporal bone. It contains the three ossicles. Laterally lies the tympanic membrane. Medially lies the inner ear. Thin bony plates separate the floor from the jugular vein and the roof from the temporal lobe of the brain. Anteriorly, the Eustachian tube communicates with the pharynx. Posteriorly, there is communication via the aditus and tympanic antrum to the mastoid air cells.

Wax (cerumen) This protects against maceration. Conductive deafness and discomfort occur if the wax impacts. It may be removed by softening with oil drops (eg olive) daily for 4 days and syringing with water at 37°C. The direction of the jet should pass backward and upward. Do not syringe if the tympanic membrane is perforated, or after mastoid operations.

Haematomas of the pinna These may occur after direct blows to the ear and should be promptly evacuated (aspiration through a large-bore needle is rarely adequate owing to recurrence: a large incision with drainage under GA is preferable: use firm packing or suture the skin to the cartilage). Apply pressure to prevent ischaemic necrosis and collapse of the cartilage which then results in a 'cauliflower' ear. Such ears can also follow perichondritis after mastoidectomy.

Exostoses These bilateral smooth subcutaneous swellings of the bony external canal occur particularly in those involved with aquatic sports. Usually asymptomatic, they sometimes entrap water and encourage otitis externa. Rarely, they completely close the ear canal and cause conductive deafness, when surgical removal using a dental burr is indicated.

Foreign bodies in the ear Insects should be drowned in olive oil then syringed out. Ask an expert to remove other objects—as they often slip ever deeper into the ear. Hooks or suction, not forceps are used for removal. General anaesthesia is often needed for removal.

►The ear is a self-cleaning organ. Tympanic membrane epithelium migrates ever outwards, taking debris with it.

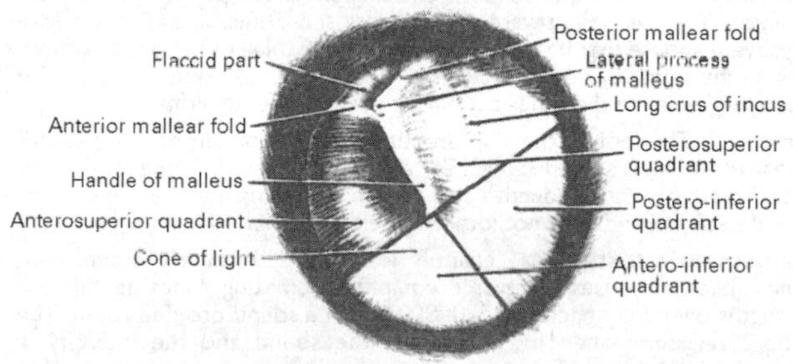

Left tympanic membranes seen from the lateral side. The 4 arbitrary quadrants are indicated by solid lines and by the handle of the malleus. (From *Cunningham's Manual*, Vol. 3, OUP.)

Hearing tests

When assessing suspected hearing loss, determine the site of the disability, the severity, and the cause. The aim of the examination is to find out if the hearing loss is treatable, and whether it is part of some other process (eg acoustic neuroma). The first part of the examination should be to remove any wax that is occluding the external auditory meatus.

The whispered voice This is the obvious first test, not just because our own voice is almost always available, and machines frequently are not: it is also valuable as it tests what, we assume, people most want to hear, which is naturally our own voice. Sensitivity and specificity in detecting a 30dB loss has been compared with devices such as the Pat-25™, the Audioscope-3™ and the Micromate-304™, using an audiogram as a reference standard. Specificity was 80% for whispering *vs* 53%, 42% and 39% for the other tests, respectively. Sensitivity was 90% *vs* 88%, 100% and 100%. The conclusion is that whispering may win on simplicity and all-round reliability.[1]

Tuning fork tests Use a tuning fork with a frequency of 512Hz. *Rinne test:* With normal hearing, air conduction (tuning fork held lateral to the external auditory meatus with prongs aligned parallel to the meatus) is better than bone conduction (base of tuning fork placed on mastoid process). When air conduction is greater than bone, the result is termed Rinne positive. Positive responses occur with normal ears and sensorineural (perceptive) hearing loss. Rinne negative response (bone conduction>air) occurs with conductive deafness. If one ear has severe or complete sensorineural deafness, a false negative response may be elicited because the cochlea of the other ear may pick up the sound by bone conduction. Use of a Barany noise box, supplying distracting noise to the other ear during the test, prevents this.

Weber test: The foot of the vibrating tuning fork is placed on the patient's forehead and he is asked in which ear the sound is heard. Sound localizes to the affected ear with conductive deafness, to the contralateral ear in sensorineural deafness, and does not localize to either ear if both ears are normal.

Audiometric tests These quantify loss and determine the site. Pure tone audiometry uses electronic equipment emitting tones at different strengths over frequencies of 250–8000Hz in a sound-proofed room. The patient registers when he first hears the sound and the intensity is recorded in decibels. This records air conduction. A bone conduction threshold can be obtained by using a transducer over the mastoid process.

Tympanometry (acoustic impedance) detects middle ear fluid (which causes low pressures, p 538), with a sensitivity of 90% and a specificity of 75%. It measures the proportion of an acoustic signal transferred from the external to the internal ear, and compares the absorbed and reflected components to compute middle ear pressure.[2] A probe seals the ear canal, varying pressure is introduced into the canal and the compliance of the ear drum recorded on a graph. A normal ear shows a smooth bell-shaped compliance curve. Fluid in the middle ear flattens the curve. High intensity sound introduced into the ear (>85dB) produces a notch on the graph as the stapedius muscle contracts (mediated by the seventh nerve). 5% of the population have absent stapedius reflexes in otherwise normal ears.

Speech audiometry examines speech discrimination above the threshold, indicating if sensorineural defects lie in the cochlea or auditory nerve. It can be used to predict whether a hearing aid would benefit a patient.

Hearing in babies Co-operation is needed for the above tests. If <6 months, hearing is assessed from the startle response, or 'brainstem evoked audiometry', a 20min non-invasive test—essential in babies suspected, or at high risk, of hearing loss. At 6 months, babies turn towards sounds, *but hearing aids may be needed before this time*. From 3yrs, try simple audiometry.

1 J Eekhof 1996 *Br J Gen Pract* **46** 473   2 A Maw 1992 BMJ i 67

Referrals for speech therapy

For a full analysis of the problems of *delay in talking*, see p 203.

1 in 7 preschoolchildren have transient speech/language problems. Many resolve spontaneously or with professional help but serious disorders affect 1 in 20 primary and 1 in 80 secondary school children. 110,000 UK children are so seriously affected that they cannot be understood outside the immediate family. **Consider speech therapy assessment if:**

0–18 months of age:
- Feeding difficulties from anatomical or neurological disorder, eg cleft lip or cerebral palsy.

2 years:
- If vocabulary is <30 words or no phrases (but not if good communication skills without speech, and he or she seems on the edge of talking).

3 years:
- Speech is unintelligible.
- Using sentences of 2 words only.
- No descriptive words or pronouns used.
- Limited comprehension (eg cannot identify scissors or pen by 'which do we draw with').
- Parental anxiety, if the child is going through a stage of non-fluency.

4 years:
- Speech is not clear. (Problems with 'r', 'th' and lisps can be left until 5yrs.)
- Sentences used are less than 3 words; vocabulary is limited.
- Difficulty in carrying out simple commands.

5 years:
- Persisting articulation difficulties.
- Difficulty understanding simple sentences.
- Difficulty in giving direct answers to simple questions.
- Difficulty with sentence structure; immature sentences; word order.

6 years and older:
- Persisting articulation problem.
- Difficulty understanding spoken language.
- Difficulty with verbal expression.
- Stammering.
- Voice problems.

Children with voice problems, eg hoarseness or excessive nasality, are best referred at whatever age they present.

Painful ears

Look for sources of referred pain (eg teeth; throat), *as well as local causes* (eg otitis externa p 536, furunculosis p 536, otitis media p 536, or mastoiditis).

Referred pain If no local pathology, think of referred pain. Five nerves refer pain to the ear. The auricular branch of the trigeminal nerve may refer pain from the sphenoidal sinus or the teeth. The greater auricular nerve (C2,3) may refer pain from wounds or glands in the neck and from cervical disc or arthritic lesions. A sensory branch of the facial nerve refers pain in geniculate herpes (Ramsay Hunt syndrome, p 756). The tympanic branch of the glossopharyngeal nerve and the auricular branch of the vagus refer pain from the throat to the ear, eg in tonsillitis; quinsy; carcinoma of the posterior third of the tongue, pyriform fossa or larynx.

Temporomandibular joint dysfunction: This common relapsing disorder may present as earache ± pain centred in front of the tragus, radiating to the mandible. *Cardinal features:* •Orofacial pain •Joint noises •Restricted jaw function (normal painless maximal vertical opening: 42–55mm). 60–70% have at least one of these signs—and they are worsened by stress, anxiety, and depression. There are 3 pathologies: internal derangement (articular disc malposition); osteoarthrosis; and myofascial pain/dysfunction—the most prevalent, being primarily a muscle disorder, related to clenching and teeth-grinding (bruxism)—sometimes associated with malocclusion, stress, headaches, irritable bowel syndrome, and chronic back problems. Treatment involves education, NSAIDs, opiates, relief of stresses, antidepressants, ± physiotherapy and surgical arthrotomy or 'occlusal therapy' from dentists (bite-raising appliances, occlusal splints, or bite guards).

Bullous myringitis Viral infections (influenza), *Haemophilus influenzae* and *Mycoplasma pneumoniae* can cause painful haemorrhagic blisters on the drum and in the external ear canal ± bloody fluid in the middle ear.

Barotrauma (aerotitis) This is damage caused by changes in atmospheric pressure in the presence of an occluded Eustachian tube. It afflicts air travellers and divers. It is preventable by repeated Valsalva manoeuvres during aircraft descent, and use of decongestants (eg xylometazoline spray every 20mins into the nose, starting 1h before landing). Those with middle ear effusions or unresolved otitis media should not fly. Those affected may suffer sensations of pressure, severe pain and deafness. Examination reveals fluid behind the drum and haemorrhagic areas in the drum. There is conductive deafness. The fluid usually clears spontaneously over several weeks.

Sudden sensorineural deafness may rarely be caused by air being forced into the cochlear via the oval or the round window (these membranes separate the middle ear from the fluid-filled inner ear). *Other signs of fistulae:* Positional nystagmus; Valsalver, exercise, hyperventilation, or motion-induced vertigo. Tragal pressure may also induce vertigo. Refer immediately for sealing of perilymph leak. Those with perilymph fistulae should avoid lifting, bending, straining, or any activity likely to promote pressure changes.

Mastoiditis (A sequelae in >1% of otitis media sufferers in pre-antibiotic days.) Due to impaired drainage from the middle ear, mastoid air cell pressure rises, with breakdown of the partitions between them over 2–3 weeks. *Symptoms (less florid if on antibiotics)*: Pain, fever, malaise, hearing↓ ± foul discharge. Suspected in those with discharging ears of >10 days' duration. *A normal tympanic membrane excludes the diagnosis* (look for sagging of the posterosuperior quadrant). Classical swelling behind the ear with downward displacement of the pinna implies a subperiosteal abscess, a particular feature of mastoiditis. Mastoid radiography may exclude the diagnosis by showing normal air cells, but haziness over the cell system can also occur in otitis externa. Initial treatment is IV antibiotics (eg ampicillin 500mg/6h IV) and myringotomy (take cultures and adjust antibiotics as necessary). If resolution does not occur, mastoidectomy will be necessary.

7. Ear, nose and throat diseases

Painful and discharging ears

►Beware of cholesteatoma as the cause (see below).

Furunculosis Due to infection of the hair follicles (usually staphylococcal in origin) these boils in the outer third of the ear canal present with severe pain (worse on jaw movement). Consider diabetes. The tragus is tender to touch, pain is induced by moving the pinna and a boil may be seen in the external auditory meatus. Treat with heat (hot water bottle), adequate analgesia, and topical applications (eg ichthammol and glycerine on cotton wool/12h). Give amoxicillin 250mg/8h PO and flucloxacillin 250mg/6h PO if there is cellulitis or systemic upset.

Otitis externa This often occurs in ears that are itchy due to eczema, seborrhoeic dermatitis or psoriasis (due to scratching), or in those who swim thereby getting water-macerated ears. There may be pain and discharge (often thick). Movement of the auricle or pressure on the tragus causes pain. Infected material must be removed (if not too severe gentle syringing clears, if more severe give a cotton wool aural toilet). Antibiotics may be given as drops, eg gentamicin 0.3% drops/6h (sometimes used in combination with a steroid), applied on a wick left *in situ*, or puffed in after aural toilet. These topical preparations should only be used short term as prolonged use encourages fungal infections which are difficult to eradicate. ►Beware persistent unilateral otitis externa in those with diabetes or immunosuppression: the risk is *necrotizing otitis externa* (eg with pseudomonal skull infection).

Cholesteatoma Stratified squamous epithelial tissue (skin) in the middle ear and mastoid erodes local structures (eg labyrinth, meninges, facial nerve) and introduces infection. *Diagnosis:* There may be foul-smelling discharge and attic or posterior perforations or retractions. *Complications:* Conductive or sensorineural deafness, vertigo (invasion of inner ear), facial nerve palsy, meningitis, cerebral abscess. *Treatment:* Seek specialist opinion to have the ear made safe by surgical removal of all diseased and infected bone (mastoidectomy, atticotomy, atticoantrostomy). When surgery makes a cavity connecting with the external canal, discharge occurs until it becomes lined by skin.

Otitis media Pain in the ear may be followed by a profuse purulent discharge as the drum perforates. Discharge usually settles after a few days. Treat with antibiotics (eg amoxicillin 250mg/8h PO; halve this dose in babies and children and give for 3 days as a sugar-free syrup). Continuing discharge may indicate mastoiditis (p 534). Discharge of mucopus sometimes continues when there is no mastoiditis, especially if grommets are in place. Treat with appropriate oral antibiotic according to swab results. Perform aural toilet to remove infected material from meatus. If discharge continues seek specialist advice.

Chronic suppurative otitis media This presents with discharge, hearing loss, but no pain. Central perforations indicate disease in the lower anterior part of the middle ear. Treatment is aimed at drying up the discharge (aural toilet, antibiotic with steroid eardrops, depending on the culture) and surgery to correct ossicle discontinuities and to close the drum.

Use of eardrops in otitis externa

►*Take a swab first, and perform aural toilet.*

- Betamethasone 0.1% (eg Betnesol®)—very cheap and good for noninfected, eczematous otitis externa.
- Betamethasone 0.1% + neomycin 0.5% (Betnesol-N®)—use if infected. NB: *prolonged use of steroid drops may cause fungal otitis.*
- Oxytetracycline 0.5% with polymyxin B 0.12% and hydrocortisone (Terra-Cortril® drops)—good if there is mixed infection, including anaerobes (3 times the price of Betnesol-N®)
- Gentamicin 0.3% with hydrocortisone 1% (eg Gentisone HC® drops; 6-times the price of Betnesol® or Betnesol-N®) is good, but is recommended by some only as a 2nd-line agent, eg in *Pseudomonas* infections.
- Clioquinol 1% + flumethasone 0.02% (Locorten-Vioform®) or clotrimazole topical 1% solution are used in fungal infections.
- Sodium bicarbonate 5% drops are useful if wax is an additional problem.

Fluid in the middle ear

This is diagnosed either by otoscopy (fluid level or bubbles *behind* the drum, or blood vessels *on* the drum) or by tympanometry, which is also used for screening purposes. 50% of 3yr-olds have ≥1 ear effusion/year.[1]

Acute suppurative otitis media This particularly follows viral upper respiratory infections. All ages are affected, but the typical patient is a child. There may be pain, fever, a sensation of pressure in the ear and hearing loss. Within the ear there is initially hyperaemia of the tympanic membrane; serous fluid is then exuded into the middle ear and later this may become purulent. The drum then looks dull and may bulge. The drum may perforate with subsequent relief of pain and fever. In uncomplicated infections (if the drum is perforated it just heals) fluid becomes serous and finally resolves. The *Pneumococcus* is the commonest infecting bacterium; *Haemophilus*, other streptococci and staphylococci are also common.

Treatment: Penicillin 500mg/6h PO is a good drug for adults (IM benzylpenicillin not usually needed). Amoxicillin, 10–13mg/kg/8h PO for 7 days, is the drug of choice in under-5s where *Haemophilus* is more prevalent, as penicillin does not enter middle ears at levels cidal to *Haemophilus*. 5% of *Haemophilus* strains are amoxicillin-resistant but sensitive to co-trimoxazole but we note that, in practice, co-trimoxazole gives no better results, and may be toxic. Short (3 day) courses of antibiotics also appear effective. Decongestants do not affect otitis media. Give good analgesia, eg paracetamol 12mg/kg/6h PO. Rarely, very painful bulging drums need incising (myringotomy). Check hearing after 6 weeks. *Rare complications of otitis media:* Mastoiditis (1–5% of cases in pre-antibiotic days); petrositis; labyrinthitis; facial palsy; meningitis; subdural, extradural or brain abscesses.

Glue ear (serous otitis media) It is necessary for us to keep our Eustachian tubes closed, otherwise our respiration would be all too audible. Frogs breathe through their skin, so can afford to keep their Eustachian tubes open all the time, so ensuring that pressures are the same either side of the drum—an ideal state of affairs to prevent accumulation of serous or viscous material, which is the essential feature of glue ear. This is likely to develop if we cannot occasionally open our Eustachian tubes (normally done during swallowing)—eg if blocked by adenoids. This is the commonest cause of hearing loss in children, and, rarely, it can cause disastrous impairment in learning. Glue ear may cause no pain—and its presence may not be suspected, but it is a common sequel to otitis media—10% of children still having effusions 3 months after the acute episode.
Signs: Concave, lustreless drum ± superficial radial vessels (meaning that fluid is behind it); this may be colourless or yellow—or bubbly. Air puffed through the otoscope does not move the drum (–ve pneumatic otoscopy).
Microbiology: In 33%, bacteria can be cultured from the middle ear.
Treatment: Neither decongestants, mucolytics, nor tonsillectomy improve glue ear.[2] One trial (*N*=433, aged 6 month–6yrs old) has shown benefit (of questionable significance) from co-amoxiclav suspension for 14 days. 84% on placebos had persistent bilateral secretions at 2 weeks follow-up *vs* 53% on antibiotics[3]—but effects on hearing and speech were not ascertained. If fluid persists for longer than ~4 months (made more likely by passive smoking, otitis media, and enlarged adenoids), and hearing is impaired, consider myringotomy with suction of fluid, and insertion of air-conducting grommets* ± adenoidectomy (so reducing recurrences but adding a small extra mortality risk). NB: it is all right to swim after grommet insertion, but avoid forcing water into the middle ear by diving.
90,000 operations/yr are done for glue ear in the UK (1 in 200 children).[3]
►*In adults, exclude a postnasal space tumour as the cause.*

*Benefits will be greatest in those having an effusive ear for >90 days with a hearing loss of >20dB. **1** K Bennett 1999 *Arch Dis Ch* **80** 28 **2** J Couriel 1995 *Lancet* **345** 3 **3** F van Balen 1996 *Lancet* **348** 713 & EBM 1997 41

Who should be referred with glue ear?

Refer to community audiology service (if available) for:
- Determination of severity of hearing loss.
- Characterization of hearing loss. Is it conductive?
- Is the hearing loss leading to a disability?

Refer direct to an ENT consultant if:
- Deaf for over 3 months—or
- Difficulties with speech or learning—or
- Recurrent and persisting earache over a 3-month period—or
- Other disabilities making correction of deafness urgent.

►NB: *explain that immediate surgery is rarely justified.*

Possibilities while the patient is waiting to be seen:
- Discourage passive smoking. *What's it like at the childminder's?*
- Encourage drinking from a cup, not a bottle (better Eustachian function).
- Encourage interlocutors to sit at the child's level, and to keep instructions short and simple. Explain the problem to all.
- Turn off the TV (less background noise, and this makes it more likely that the patient will look at the person speaking to him).
- Tell the teacher which side hears best (for class seating plan).
- Nasal steroids for 1 month—or
- Co-amoxiclav for 14 days (may be of little real benefit)—or
- Oral steroids for 5 days (eg prednisolone 1mg/kg/day PO).

NB: *benefit may not be long-lasting, but medical treatment may diminish the need for surgery.*

Modified West Sussex protocol

Childhood deafness

Although temporary deafness in childhood due to middle-ear effusions and glue ear is common, *permanent* deafness is rare (*incidence in infancy:* 1–2/1000). It is essential that deafness is found early, so that maximal help can be given to restore hearing to enable children to learn to speak.

Causes • *Hereditary:* These include Wardenburg's, Klippel–Feil, and Treacher Collins' syndromes and mucopolysaccharidoses.

• *Acquired in utero:* Maternal infection (rubella, CMV, influenza, glandular fever, syphilis), ototoxic drugs.

• *Perinatal:* Anoxia, birth trauma, cerebral palsy, kernicterus.

• *Postnatal:* Meningitis, chiefly;[1] also ototoxic drugs, lead, skull fracture.

Detection Hearing should be assessed before the age of 8 months. Those with a family history of deafness, and those who were exposed to prenatal, perinatal or postnatal hazards should receive particular attention (10 times more likely than the general population to be affected)—see p 532. From 6 months to 1 year children may be given the distraction test—by sitting them on their mother's lap with a distractor sitting in front of them to attract their attention sporadically (hence keep them facing the midline). The tester stands 3 feet behind the mother and tests each ear in turn. Low frequencies are tested with the spoken voice, high frequencies with a rattle. Rustling paper gives a broad-spectrum stimulus. Refer for specialist testing (brainstem-evoked responses) if there is doubt about hearing. From 3 years old, pure tone audiometry may be used.

From 12 months to 2yrs children are unco-operative, hence the need for objective tests (also for neonatal screening): such a test is measurement of otoacoustic emissions—a microphone in the external meatus detects tiny cochlear sounds produced by movement in its basilar membrane.[2] This is a useful screening test: if +ve at 20dB sound, the cochlear is working.

Another useful way of achieving objective tests of hearing is the use of tympanometry (p 532)—or evoked response audiometry, in which a recording electrode is applied behind the ear, in the ear canal, or through the tympanic membrane. The ear is stimulated by sound and the responses generated are picked up, amplified, and fed to a computer. (This takes place in an acoustically treated room.)

Treatment Once deafness has been detected treatment aims to provide as good hearing as possible to help speaking and edducation. Teachers of the deaf make arrangements for fitting hearing aids and help monitor progress. Children usually need higher gain from their hearing aids than adults. Ear moulds may need frequent changing to maintain a good fit. Encourage parents to talk as much as possible to their deaf children. Children may be educated at ordinary schools with visits from teachers of the deaf, or, (for the partially hearing) in special units in ordinary schools, or in schools for the deaf, depending on individual need. For some, a cochlear implant may be suitable (p 542). ►The shorter the duration of deafness, the better the outcome: so funding decisions should not be delayed.[3]

Not everyone agrees that a deaf child needs treatment. In some families with deaf parents, the arrival of a deaf child is especially welcomed. Here, deafness may be considered a variant, not a handicap. All who work with the deaf note the vibrant, vigorous, humorous and mutually supportive culture of sign-language in those born to it, and we accept that some parents will want their offspring to be bilingual (sign and sound).[4] It is certainly possible to imagine a world in which everyone is deaf, and in which deafness does not matter—but, for better or for worse, this will not be the world in which the young deaf child will grow up, and have to relate to.

1 BMJ ed 1999 **i** 72 **2** Wessex Group 1998 *Lancet* **352** 1957 **3** J Graham 1996 BMJ **ii** 113 **4** *Hlth Trnds* 1996 **28** 106

7. Ear, nose and throat diseases

Deafness in adults

Deafness, unlike blindness, is not a quantified disability; *any* degree of hearing loss may be described as deafness. It is frustrating for those affected and for friends and families, as the niceties of communication start to fail, leading to isolation, with no innuendo, no jokes, no asides, and no music. ~3 million adults are hearing-impaired (UK).

Classification *Conductive deafness:* There is impaired sound transmission via the external canal and middle ear to the foot of the stapes. External canal obstruction (wax, discharge from otitis externa, foreign body, developmental abnormalities); drum perforation (trauma, barotrauma, infection); problems with the ossicular chain (otosclerosis, infection, trauma); and inadequate Eustachian tube ventilation of the middle ear with effusion present (eg secondary to nasopharyngeal carcinoma) all result in conductive deafness. In men who have had recurrent childhood otitis media, repeated use of personal stereos is liable to cause significant hearing loss (eg 11dB).[1]

Sensorineural deafness: This results from defects central to the oval window in the cochlea (sensory), cochlear nerve (neural) or, rarely, more central pathways. Ototoxic drugs, eg streptomycin and aminoglycosides (esp. gentamicin) and most causes of deafness in infancy are sensorineural. Infections (meningitis, measles, mumps, flu, herpes, syphilis), cochlear vascular disease, Ménière's (p 546), trauma, and presbyacusis (senile deafness) are all sensorineural. Rare causes: acoustic neuroma, B_{12} deficiency, multiple sclerosis, secondary carcinoma in the brain.

Management •Classify the deafness (p 532). •Find treatable causes. •Exclude the dangerous: acoustic neuroma, cholesteatoma, effusion from nasopharyngeal carcinoma. Sudden onset sensorineural deafness demands immediate specialist referral. •Find out what procedure to advise, eg surgery for perforations, otosclerosis—or simply the administration of the most suitable type of hearing aid. •Those with sensorineural deafness so severe that they cannot benefit from a hearing aid may benefit from a cochlear implant.[2] This device takes ~2h to fit (under GA); an external device processes sound, transmitting it across the skin to the subcutaneous receiver coil—which supplies an electrode which directly stimulates the auditory nerve, bypassing the cochlear. Rehabillitation is needed to understand the new sounds. Cost (UK) up to £35,000 per precedure.

Otosclerosis Usually bilateral; ♀/♂ ≈ 2:1; 50% of those affected have a family history. *Symptoms* usually appear in early adult life and are made worse by pregnancy. *Pathology:* Vascular spongy bone replaces normal bone around the oval window to which there is adherence of the stapes footplate. There is conductive deafness (hearing is better in background noise), sometimes also tinnitus and vertigo. *Treatment:* Replacing the stapes with an implant helps 90%. Many prefer surgery to wearing a hearing aid.

Presbyacusis (senile deafness) Loss of acuity for high-frequency sounds starts before 30yrs old and rate of loss for the higher frequencies is progressive thereafter. Deafness (reflecting loss of hair cells) is gradual in onset and we do not usually notice it until hearing of speech is affected. This may occur with loss of high-frequency sounds (consonants at ~3–4Hz are needed for speech discrimination). Hearing is most affected in the presence of background noise. Hearing aids are the usual treatment.

Prevention of deafness[3] The single most successful way of reducing deafness is to limit damaging noise (<85dB/8h day) exposure at work and leisure—as indicated by finding talking difficult, ringing in the ears during exposure, or sounds appearing muffled after exposure.

1 A Job 1999 *Lancet* **353** 35 2 E Douek 1990 BMJ **ii** 74 3 *Lancet* Ed 1991 **ii** 21

Ethical issues surrounding cochlear implants

These revolve around cost, consent, and quality of life—and *who* should decide. The situation is complex as technical improvements ensure an ever-changing balance between benefits and risks (rejection of the device for difficult-to-predict psychological reasons, and post-op complications, eg VII palsy, and stimulator migration)—so beware simplistic statements coming from meta-analysists making statements such as 'cochlear implants are suitable for such-and-such a group (eg profoundly deaf adults) but not another group (eg congenital deafness)'. Also beware of statements such as 'after cochlear implant patients can lead normal lives' (this may only mean that other people don't notice that the user has a hearing problem). Post-operative training is very important, and the user is by no means an inactive recipient. Remember that society is often biased in favour of technology (the black box that does everything), while all too often neglecting the human processes of communication.

The wealth of a society can be gauged by the level of deafness at which most cochlear implants are done. In the UK, cochlear implant candidates generally have no hearing (>110dB loss). There are ~8000 such candidates in the UK (under the age of 70). If the criterion is 'relaxed' to 105dB, this number rises to 45,000. In the USA, the loss is generally >95dB (in the UK this would lead to 72,000 candidates and a bill of £2520 million).

For multichannel cochlear implants, the average cost per QALY (quality-adjusted life-year) is ~£11,400/QALY[2] which is roughly in the middle of quoted estimates for costed NHS therapies (for a list, see *OHCM* p 12). On this view, implantation of those at least up 70 years old makes good sense in terms of health economics. Furthermore, multiple disabilities are no bar to getting benefit for a device, but it is not clear that they merit *extra* consideration (they certainly merit very careful assessment).

Who should decide these issues is unclear (as usual!), but deaf people clearly should have some input (in the USA, no deaf people were on the FDA board which decided these issues).

Cost per QALY *may* fall with further technical advances—eg beam-forming dual microphone systems to aid hearing in background noise, better speech processors, and new electrode arrays where a greater number of electrodes lie close to the spiral ganglion cells.[3] Difficulties in assessment are compounded by the need not simply to take into account hearing and language, but also learning, socialization and other cultural variables.

1 DARE Meta-analyses 1997 *The Cochlear Implant in Adults, Adolescents, and Children.* 2 G O'Donoghue 1996 *Health Trends* **28** 106 3 GM Clark 1998 *Auris Nasus Larynx* **25** 73–87

Tinnitus

Tinnitus (from Latin *tinnire*—to ring) is ringing or buzzing in the ears. Almost all of us have experienced tinnitus, but only 0.5–2% are severely affected. Although children sometimes experience transient tinnitus they often do not mention it. Peak age for onset is at 50–60yrs.

Mechanism Obscure. It may represent spontaneous otoacoustic emission, or ephatic transmission (cross-talk) between adjacent nerve fibres.

Causes Unknown; hearing loss (20%); wax; viral; presbyacusis; noise (eg gunfire); head injury; suppurative otitis media; post-stapedectomy; Ménière's; anaemia; hypertension; impacted wisdom teeth.
►*Investigate unilateral tinnitus fully* (eg MRI) to exclude an acoustic neuroma.
Drugs: Aspirin; loop diuretics; aminoglycosides (eg gentamicin).
Objectively detectable tinnitus: Palatal myoclonus (clicking tinnitus); temporomandibular problems (p 534); AV fistulae; bruits; glomus jugulare tumours.
Psychological associations: Redundancy, divorce, retirement.

Another group of sufferers are those who have roaring in the ears when breathing through the nose, but not when they breathe through the mouth. On examination, the tympanic membrane may be seen to move on respiration. The cause may be a patulous Eustachian tube.

History Site of tinnitus (ear or central); character; alleviating and exacerbating factors; otalgia; otorrhoea; vertigo; head injury; family history of deafness or tinnitus; sleep; social surroundings (tinnitus is worse if isolated or depressed); drugs. Note if stress exacerbates the tinnitus.

Tests and examinations Otoscopy to detect middle-ear disease; hearing tests (tuning fork and audiometry); tympanogram to examine middle-ear function and stapedial reflex thresholds.

Treatment *Treat the person as a whole*, not just as a malfunctioning ear. *Psychological support* is central to any endeavour to relieve tinnitus. Hearing therapists can employ *tinnitus retraining therapy* to make tinnitus less intrusive, partly by dealing with inappropriate beliefs and fears, and partly by a prosthetic component—a hearing aid type of device provides a low level of background sound (not completely masking the tinnitus), which may gradually decrease CNS oversensitivity to auditory neural signals.

Avoid terms such as 'untreatable' or 'you must learn to live with it'. (Being dismissive promotes anxiety and makes tinnitus worse.) Cognitive therapy may also help (p 370). Patient support groups can help greatly.[1]

Exclude serious cause—then reassure that tinnitus does not mean madness or serious disease and that it often improves in time.

Drugs are disappointing. Avoid tranquillizers, particularly if the patient is depressed (nortryptiline is the drug of choice here), but hypnotics at night may help. Carbamazepine is disappointing; betahistine only helps in some patients in whom the cause of the tinnitus is Ménière's disease.

Masking may give relief. White noise is given via a noise generated by a device worn invisibly in the canal. Hearing aids may help those with hearing loss by amplifying desirable sound.

Glomus jugulare tumours A vascular neoplasm arising from the jugular body, which may grow to present as a cerebellopontine angle mass, or, in the external auditory canal, as a pulsatile mass. They may secrete 5-HT. It is a rare cause of tinnitus, but a common cause of *pulsatile* tinnitus.[2]

1 British Tinnitus Assocn tel. 0114 279 6600 (Sheffield S12 AZ) 2 C Hawkes 1993 *BMJ* ii 262

7. Ear, nose and throat diseases

Vertigo

Vertigo (the illusion of movement) can be horrible, confining people to home, making them fearful and depressed. In the UK, 30% will consult a doctor for dizziness before they are 65.[1] Find out if complaints of feeling swimmy, dizzy, unreal, or panicky, occur with illusion of movement of self or environment is present. If so, does it last seconds (usually benign positional vertigo, below, if there are no CNS signs), hours (eg migraine), or days (look for a central cause, ie of nerve VIII, brainstem vestibular nuclei, medial longitudinal fasciculus, cerebellum, or vestibulospinal tract—see below).

Vestibular (peripheral) vertigo is often severe, and may be accompanied by nausea, vomiting, hearing loss, tinnitus and nystagmus (usually horizontal). Hearing loss and tinnitus are less common in central vertigo (it is usually less severe). Nystagmus may be horizontal or vertical with central vertigo—and may be different in each eye (eg in the abducting eye).

Causes *Peripheral:* Ménière's; benign positional (postural) vertigo; gentamicin (vestibular neuronitis); labyrinthitis; cholesteatoma; trauma; Eustachian obstruction. *Central:* Acoustic neuroma; multiple sclerosis; head injury; epilepsy; migraine (maybe no headache); vertigo; vertebrobasilar ischaemia (other CNS signs will be present); geniculate herpes; syphilis.

Examination and tests Test cranial nerves, cerebellar function, reflexes. Do Romberg's test (+ve if balance is worse when eyes are shut—implying defective joint position sense or vestibular input). Assess nystagmus. Do provocation tests, below. If equivocal, consider audiometry; electronystagmography; brainstem auditory evoked responses; calorimetry (the only way to test each labyrinth separately; irrigate each canal with water 7° above and 7° below body temp—is nystagmus induced?); CT; MRI; EEG; LP.

Benign positional vertigo There are attacks of *sudden-onset* rotational vertigo lasting >30sec provoked by head-turning. Common after head injury. *Diagnosis:* Provocative test: with the patient supine, the head is lowered ~30° below the level of the couch, and turned 30–40° to one side. If +ve, the patient experiences vertigo and rotary nystagmus towards the undermost ear, after a latent period of a few seconds. This lasts < 1min (adaption). On sitting, there is more vertigo (± nystagmus). ►*If any of these features are absent, seek a central cause. Pathogenesis:* Displacement of the otoconia from the maculae (the receptor for sensing acceleration in the semicircular canals). The otoconia then settle on the lowest part of the labyrinth. *Causes:* Head injury; spontaneous degeneration of the labyrinth, post-viral illness or stapes surgery; chronic middle-ear disease.
Treatment: If not self-limiting within a few months, consider physiotherapy referral for teaching: •Repeated adoption of the position which causes vertigo (habituation). •Formal Epley head exercises to disperse otoconia. A last resort is denervating the posterior semicircular canal or obliterating it by laser (transmastoid) is an option, but deafness may follow.

Vestibular neuronitis follows a febrile illness in adults, eg in winter, and is probably viral. Sudden vertigo, vomiting and prostration are exacerbated by head movement. *Treatment:* Try cyclizine 50mg/8h PO. Recovery occurs within 2–3 weeks. It is difficult to distinguish from 'viral labyrinthitis'.

Ménière's disease Dilatation of the endolymphatic spaces of the membranous labyrinth causes vertigo for up to 12h with prostration, nausea and vomiting. Attacks occur in clusters. Uni- or bilateral tinnitus occurs ± progressive sensorineural deafness. Treat acute vertigo symptomatically (cyclizine 50mg/8h PO). Betahistine 16mg/8h PO is unpredictable but is worth trying, as are diuretics (chlorthalidone). Operative decompression of the saccus endolymphaticus may relieve vertigo, prevent progress of the disease and conserve hearing. Labyrinthectomy *may* relieve vertigo but causes total ipsilateral deafness. Day-case transtympanic instillation of ototoxic drugs (gentamicin via a grommet) can help, and usually avoids deafness.[2]

1 L Uxon 1998 *Prescribers' J* **38** 87 2 B Hirsch 1997 *Am J Otol* **18** 44-51

7. Ear, nose and throat diseases

What does vertigo really mean?

To ENT doctors, vertigo usually means the illusion of movement: a deceptively simple definition. Fyodor Dostoyevsky understood a bit more about vertigo and its interaction with willed and unwilled behaviour when he wrote: 'It is said that people standing on high places have a kind of urge to throw themselves down into the abyss. I think that suicides and murders owe the occurrence of their deeds to the simple fact that the revolver was already to hand. This is also an abyss of a kind, a forty-five degree slope down which it is impossible not to slide, and something irresistibly challenges you to pull the trigger. . .'

(*The Gentle Spirit*, Penguin, ISBN 0-14-600168-0)

The time course of vertigo aids its diagnosis:[1]

Time course	Diagnosis
Severe vertigo, improving over ~4 days; full recovery over weeks	Labyrinthine disorders
Recurrent episodes ± headaches	Migraine (esp. If family history)
Clusters of short episodes related to head movements	Paroxysmal benign positional vertigo
Clusters of short episodes not related to head movements	Idiopathic vestibular failure (rarely ischaemia, vestibular epilepsy or Ménière's disease)
After antibiotics, falls in the dark	Ototoxic vestibular failure
Recurrent episodes lasting days to weeks with *gradual* resolution	Poor vestibular compensation
Vertigo persisting for >6 weeks	Uncompensated peripheral vestibulopathy

Chronic nasal obstruction

Causes *Children:* Large adenoids, rhinitis, choanal atresia, postnasal space tumours (eg angiofibromata), foreign body—►refer the same day if the latter is possible—eg if ***unilateral*** obstruction ± foul or bloody discharge. *Adults:* Deflected nasal septum, rhinitis, polyps, sinusitis, granulomata [TB, syphilis, Wegener's (*OHCM* p 710), leprosy], drugs (topical vasoconstrictors, tricyclics). ►Refer urgently if: •Airway blocked by an enlarged turbinate •Unilateral obstructing mass •A tumour may be present.

Diagnosis Ask about variability of symptoms, the pattern of obstruction, and effects on eating, speech and sleep (snoring). Examine to assess any nasal deflection. Is either nostril *completely* blocked (hold a mirror under each nostril: does it steam up)? Examine the postnasal space with a mirror (in children it may be easier to see the postnasal space with lateral x-rays).

Rrhinitis medicamentosa Drops or sprays which decongest by vasoconstriction can damage the mucosa, due to hypoxia, with rebound engorgement and mucosal oedema encouraging further drug usage. The mucosa is swollen and red. Such decongestants should not be used for >one week.

Vasomotor rhinitis This causes ***variable, bilateral*** obstruction ± rhinorrhoea. Swollen oedematous turbinates may be seen and there is excess mucus. *Treatment:* Measures as for allergic rhinitis are usually ineffective. Ipratropium nasal spray 2×20μg puffs/nostril/6h helps rhinorrhoea.[1] Cautery or surgical reduction of inferior turbinates helps 'blocked nose'.

Deviated nasal septum Rare in children, this may affect 20% of adults. It may be secondary to injury. Surgical filleting of the bone and cartilage of the nasal septum—septoplasty repositions the septum into the midline.

Allergic rhinitis This may be seasonal or perennial—and is likely to be ***bilateral*** and ***variable***. Incidence correlates with the pollen count and age (highest risk 5–14 years old). Symptoms include sneezing, pruritus and rhinorrhoea. The turbinates may be swollen and the mucosa pale or mauvish. Nasal polyps can occur. The allergen may be identified by skin tests—but avoid these if there is significant eczema, past severe allergic reactions, dermatographism, or there are interfering drugs (antihistamines, steroids). Here, consider radio-allergosorbent (RAST) tests to identify specific IgE.[2]

Treatment: Courses of desensitizing injections may be tried in some parts of the world, and may help 70% with seasonal allergy, but only 50% of those allergic to house dust mite. They are fraught with danger, and may cause fatal anaphylaxis, and patients need observation for a period after each injection, and full facilities for cardiorespiratory resuscitation must be available. Other treatments include antihistamines, eg *loratidine* 10mg/24h PO; (beware interactions of other antihistamines with erythromycin/macrolides, carbamazepine, β-blockers, diuretics, tricyclics, antifungals, and halofantrine); systemic decongestants (eg *pseudoephedrine* 60mg/12h PO; CI: hypertension, hyperthyroid, coronary artery disease, concomitant MAOIs), nasal sprays (eg sodium cromoglycate 2%, 2×2.6mg squeezes/4–6h), or nasal steroids eg *beclomethasone diproprionate* 8×50μg puffs/24h. Note: steroid puffers may be used indefinitely, but steroid drops are systemically absorbed so should be used for less than 1 month at a time, <6 times/year.

Nasal obstruction with chronic sinusitis Give steroid drops as above for 1 month, with intermittent antibiotics when nasal discharge is purulent. Refer if there is no response to this. (Do not x-ray: imaging is unreliable.)

Other causes of chronic rhinorrhoea and rhinitis[3] Allergies (above), foreign body, CSF (eg after head injury; it is positive for glucose), bacteria (including TB), AIDS, cystic fibrosis, Kartagener's syndrome, rheumatoid arthritis, sarcoid, SLE, Wegener's or other granulomata (*OHCM* p 710), atrophic, old age (old man's drip), pregnancy, the Pill, β-blockers, NSAIDs, overuse of nasal decongestants, antibody deficiency (p 201), primary defect in mucus or cilia, non-allergic rhinitis with eosinophilia (NARES).

Nasal polyps

The typical patient is a man over 40yrs old; in children they are generally associated with cystic fibrosis.

Histology: ~90% are oedematous eosinophilic polyps. Typical sites: middle turbinates; middle meatus; ethmoids. Single, benign maxillary polyps may arise in the maxillary antrum, and prolapse into the nose, and fill the nasopharynx (antrochoanal polyps).

Associations: Allergic rhinitis, chronic ethmoid sinusitis, cystic fibrosis.

Symptoms: Watery anterior rhinorrhoea, purulent postnasal drip, nasal obstruction, change in voice quality, anosmia and taste disturbance, mucocele (presents with a lump on the medial superior border of the orbit).

Signs: It is hard to distinguish hypertrophied inferior turbinates from nasal polyps—but gentle palpation will show that the polyp, if that is what it is, is insensitive, pale, and mobile.

Drugs: Try 2 days of betamethasone sodium phosphate 0.1% nasal drops, instilled every 8h (longer courses may be safe). ►*Use of nose drops requires the correct posture:* bent double at the hips, with nostrils pointing at the sky—eg kneeling with the forehead on the floor. This may make polyps quickly diminish in size, and maintenance therapy with beclomethasone spray may then be tried, eg 8 puffs/24h (50µg/puff).

Surgery: Polypectomy, eg by endoscopy. Local anaesthesia may have the advantage of a more bloodless field, along with patient awareness, should the orbit or intracranial fossa be breeched. If more than simple polypectomy is planned, it is wise to do CT scans to show anatomical variations.[2]

Post-op: Watch for bleeding. Postnasal douches may be given ± topical steroids.

1 *Drug Ther Bul* 1990 **28** 54 2 VJ Lund 1995 BMJ **ii** 1411 3 GK Scadding *Prescribers' J* **36** 93

Nasal injury, foreign bodies and drug abuse

Fractured nose The upper ⅓ of the nose has bony support; the lower ⅓ and septum are cartilaginous. Direct violence to the nose may fracture the nasal bones. Take a history as to the time of the injury, previous nasal injuries, epistaxis, nasal obstruction and CSF rhinorrhoea. Ask about loss of consciousness. Consider other facial fractures: zygomaticomaxillary fractures may cause malocclusion of the teeth and impair normal jaw opening; there may be diplopia if there is fracture of the orbital floor. Carefully feel around the orbit to check no 'steps' in contour. X-rays are not particularly helpful as there may be old injuries shown and cartilaginous injuries do not show up. They will not alter the acute management.

Soft tissue swelling at the initial examination may make deformity difficult to see, so re-examine after 7 days (especially children)—exclude a septal haematoma at initial examination. If present, refer to an ENT surgeon for evacuation (risk of septal necrosis if untreated). Fracture reduction (under GA) is best within the first 10–14 days (complete setting may have occurred by 3 weeks). Zygoma and maxilla fractures set more quickly and should be referred immediately to maxillofacial surgeons. Post-operatively patients are advised to apply ice for the first 12h; sleep with head elevated, sneeze through mouth, refrain from blowing the nose and taking vigorous exercise. Re-examine at two weeks and two months after operation. Septal deviation may require septoplasty several months later.

CSF rhinorrhoea Fractures through the roof of the ethmoid labyrinth may result in leak of CSF. Nasal discharge tests +ve for glucose (Clinistix® test, confirm with a laboratory sugar); CSF uniquely contains β_2-transferrin. Leaks often stop spontaneously; if not, try neurosurgical closure of the dura.

Septal haematoma These may occur after injury and cause very uncomfortable nasal obstruction, with swellings on both sides of the septum. If you detect a large, fluctuant boggy swelling in place of the septum, refer immediately. Evacuate blood clot promptly under GA, and suture and pack as necessary. Give antibiotics (eg amoxicillin 250mg/8h PO) to prevent infection. If left untended there is risk of cartilage necrosis and nasal collapse.

Foreign bodies Most are self-inserted by children. Organic material presents early with purulent discharge; inorganic bodies may remain inert for ages. If a child is co-operative it may be possible to grab the object with forceps. 2.5% cocaine spray may shrink the mucosa and allow extraction with a sucker. If general anaesthesia needed, protect the airway.

Causes of septal perforation After septal surgery (p 548); trauma; nose picking; inhalation of chrome salts; sniffing cocaine (look for other signs, below); rodent ulcer; malignancy; granuloma; TB; syphilis. Perforations irritate, crust and bleed. Treatment is symptomatic. Closure is difficult.

Cocaine toxicity As well as septal perforation, inhaling (snorting) cocaine may cause odd behaviour, fever, and fits. *Drug smuggler's delirium:* Swallowing drug-filled condoms or foil-wrapped parcels may seem a good way of smuggling drugs—until their contents leach out. Before their fatal effect, such smugglers may present desperately seeking help, and fabricating odd stories. Packages may be detected by plain films. Ultrasound is unreliable, and CT may be needed. Laparotomy may be needed (don't try endoscopic removal: the condom may split). *Tests for establishing cocaine ingestion:* Blood levels are more time-consuming and expensive than qualitative methods (fluorescence immunoassay on urine).*

*If acute toxicity, take to ITU: for lidocaine (for arrhythmias, eg 50–100mg IV bolus), propranolol (0.5–1mg IV, max 5mg), or dantrolene (p 772). Other cooling tactics: cooled IVI, ice water gastric lavage.

7. Ear, nose and throat diseases

Nosebleed (epistaxis)

Most nosebleeds come from blood vessels on the nasal septum. In young people (<35 years old) bleeding is usually from Little's area, where there is a convergence of the anterior ethmoidal artery, the septal branches of the sphenopalatine and the superior labial arteries and the greater palatine artery. From middle-age onwards, the typical bleeding site moves posteriorly, and is often arterial.

Causes Many nosebleeds are idiopathic. In older people bleeding is often associated with degenerative arterial disease and hypertension. Local causes may be atrophic rhinitis, hereditary telangectasia and tumours of the nose or sinuses. General causes of bleeding tendencies should not be forgotten (*OHCM* p 592–6), eg warfarin anticoagulation.

Management The 3 principles of management are to treat shock and replace blood if necessary, to identify the source of the bleeding, and to stop it. The elderly are particularly prone to suffering from shock which may be fatal. If there are signs of shock they should be admitted and transfused. Although in general those with nosebleeds are nursed sitting up to reduce venous pressure, the shocked should be nursed lying to maximize perfusion of the brain. ►If shocked, give high-flow O_2, and ensure the airway remains clear if there is heavy bleeding draining into the pharynx. If shock is not present, or once it has been attended to, the attention is turned to the bleeding. Initially firm uninterrupted pressure of the nostrils between finger and thumb for at least 10 minutes, possibly with an ice-pack over the bridge of the nose, and with an object (eg a cork) held between the teeth may be sufficient to stop the bleeding.

If this first aid does not stop the bleeding, remove clot from the nose using Luc's forceps or a sucker. Spray each part of the mucosa with 2.5–10% cocaine solution which anaesthetizes the mucosa and reduces bleeding by constricting vessels. Cauterize any identified bleeding points.

If no bleeding point is found and bleeding continues, pack the nose with 1cm or 2.5cm ribbon gauze moistened with paraffin and iodoform paste inserted with Tilley's nasal dressing forceps. Once packed, if bleeding has stopped, the patient may return home with the pack left in place for 3 days—or the patient may be admitted, as bed rest prevents rebleeding. If bleeding continues despite an anterior pack, a posterior nasal pack will be needed. The simplest method is to remove the anterior pack, pass a foley catheter through a nostril so the 30mL balloon lies in the postnasal space, blow up the balloon and pull the catheter anteriorly. Then pack the front of the nose. Keep in hospital until removal at 24h.

If bleeding recurs, further packs may be needed but are uncomfortable and therefore demoralizing. Rarely, arterial ligation (maxillary artery for greater palatine and sphenopalatine arteries approached via maxillary antrum; the anterior ethmoidal artery via the orbit) or external carotid artery ligation is needed to prevent further bleeding. NB: the sphenopalatine artery can be reached endoscopically and this may often prove to be the procedure of choice. In severe, resistant bleeds, consider embolization of the feeding vessel.

7. Ear, nose and throat diseases

553

The paranasal sinuses

The paranasal sinuses are air-filled cavities in the bones around the nose. Rudimentary maxillary antrum and sphenoid sinuses exist at birth; the others begin to develop at ~8yrs, continuing through adolescence. Within the nose each turbinate has a corresponding meatus below it. The naso-lacrimal duct drains to the inferior meatus, the frontal sinus, maxillary sinus and anterior ethmoid air cells drain to the middle meatus; and the posterior ethmoidal air cells drain to the superior meatus.

Ciliated cells lining the sinuses sweep mucus into the nose keeping the sinuses clear. Viruses depress cilia activity, and cause oedema around the sinus ostia so predisposing to mucus collection which may stagnate and become secondarily infected. Mucopus depresses cilia activity. Polyps, deflections of the nasal septum, and nasal mucosal swelling also predispose to drainage problems and hence to sinusitis.

Acute sinusitis Secondary bacterial infection often follows viral infection. 5% of maxillary sinusitis is secondary to tooth root infection (second premolar and molars—roots lying in the sinus floor). Jumping into infected water may force infection into the frontal sinus.

Clinical features: •Yellow/green nasal discharge •Fever •Pain (eg worse on bending) •Sinus tenderness. •Referred pain from maxillary antrum may give toothache—eg worse on walking. •Sense of smell may be disturbed. ESR and C-reative protein↑. ►Acute sinusitis does *not* cause simple cheek swelling; that may be due to root infection or maxillary antral carcinoma.

Treatment: It is usually self-limiting. Consider analgesia, steam inhalations and warmed nasal drops (eg 1% ephedrine, 2 drops/nostril/6h, CI: MAOIs) to ↓nasal congestion, and promote drainage. Giving antibiotics such as amoxicillin or doxycycline (200mg stat, then 100mg/24h for 7 days) is traditional, but evidence-based medicine leads us to be sceptical.[1]

Discourage smoking, and alcohol excess (causes nasal cavity vasodilatation). The rôle of swimming in pathogenesis is unclear (but we note one trial in which Lake Constance swimmers suffered less sinusitis once water cleaning plants were introduced).[2] It is said to promote spread of pus within sinuses. ►If there is no cure after 2 courses of antibiotics, refer: there may be local anatomical abnormalities, or antibody deficiency (p 201).

Chronic sinusitis *Symptoms:* Post-nasal mucous drip; foul taste in mouth; blocked nose; pain over bridge of nose or in malar region (from middle turbinate pressure on nasal septum). On examination: congested turbinates; infected mucus; ± polyps. These features are common to both *chronic infected sinusitis* (fairly rare) and *chronic hyperplastic sinusitis*—a form of allergic rhinitis, which should be treated as such (p 548).

Imaging None is usually needed. Plain x-rays are not much help, as up to 30% of normals show mucosal thickening. Ultrasound is not necessarily better than x-rays at predicting fluid in the antrum. Maxillary sinus obstruction can produce troublesome symptoms *without* opacities or fluid levels—so rigid nasal endoscopy is preferred by some experts.[2,3] Do CT if the patient a candidate for surgery.

Chronic infective sinusitis Consider antibiotics (eg amoxicillin or erythromycin); if medical therapy fails, refer for endoscopic sinus surgery (the aim is to re-establish sinus ventilation, eg by clearing blockages).

Complications Metastatic infection to bone, orbit, CNS, or meninges.

1 FL van Buchem 1997 *Lancet* **349** 683 & E-BM 1997 **2** 152–*N*=214 with suspected acute maxillary sinusitis; amoxicillin 750mg/8h for 7 days gave, at best, only marginal benefit: but this study used laxer criteria for diagnosis than M Lindbaek (BMJ 1996 **ii** 325) which *did* show greater benefit. **2** J Fairley 1992 BMJ **ii** 1223 **3** N Jones 1992 BMJ **ii** 1223

7. Ear, nose and throat diseases

555

Throat infections and tonsillar tumours

In the past GPs readily gave antibiotics for sore throats in case the cause was a β-haemolytic streptococcal infection which may have resulted in rheumatic fever. Rheumatic fever is now rare in the West (p 194). We know that rheumatic fever patients had often had their sore throats treated, so antibiotics had not prevented the illness. GPs may not wish to give antibiotics for simple sore throats, as many are caused by viruses—in any case the proportion of those with sore throats consulting may be as low as 1 in 18. Because sore thoat is so common, treating *everyone* with penicillin is not only expensive, and encouraging of doctor dependency (p 326), but also risks more deaths from anaphylaxis[1] than would be saved by any possible benefit. Throat swabs do not offer much help (sensitivity 26–30%; specificity 73–80%).[2] Numerous antigen detection kits are available (specific, but not sensitive).[3] Other pathogens apart from streps: staphs, *Moraxella catarrhalis*, mycoplasma, chlamydia, haemophilus.

Tonsillitis The young often complain of abdominal pain with tonsillitis. Older children may complain of sore throat, fever, malaise, difficult swallowing and painful neck lymph nodes.

The appearance of a rash after 48h on neck and upper chest spreading rapidly to abdomen and limbs suggests *scarlet fever*. It spares the mouth area, giving rise to contrasting circumoral pallor—and the tongue is covered with a white 'fur', which, when cleaned off, leaves prominent papillae (the 'strawberry' tongue). Cause: group A streptococcus.

Treatment: The use of antibiotics has been a source of great debate as in 50% the cause is a virus, and antibiotics make no difference. In reality, a variety of factors influence the decision whether to give antibiotics. When antibiotics are given, penicillin, 250mg/6h PO is often used for up to 10 days—and this is the treatment of choice in scarlet fever. Despite studies advocating its use,[4] amoxicillin is contraindicated as it will cause a rash in almost all whose pharyngitis is due to Epstein–Barr virus.

Tonsillectomy indications •Airway obstruction, eg with sleep apnoea •Chronic tonsillitis (>3 months, with halitosis) •Diphtheria carrier •Quinsy •Suspicion of malignancy (unilateral enlargement) •Recurrent tonsillitis (eg an 8-year-old with >5 attacks in last 2 years) is still an indication for referral; controlled trials show that the incidence of sore throats after tonsillectomy is reduced. NB: younger children may be expected to have this number of infections. *Complications of surgery* include rare but real risk of death from haemorrhage, and behaviour problems in children.

Local complications of tonsillitis *Retropharyngeal abscess:* This is rare. Presentation is as an unwell child who fails to eat or drink. Lateral x-rays of the neck show soft tissue swelling. *Treatment:* Incision and drainage of pus under general anaesthesia in a head-down position to prevent aspiration. *Peritonsillar abscess (quinsy):* These usually occur in adults. Treatment of throat cellulitis by high-dose penicillin may be preventive. Once developed, the tonsil is obscured at examination by the soft palate. There is difficulty in swallowing ± trismus (lock-jaw). *Treatment:* Incise under local anaesthetic, or do abscess tonsillectomy under general anaesthetic.

Tonsillar tumours Commonest in the elderly, these present with sore throat, dysphagia and otalgia. Unilateral tonsil enlargement is ominous and grounds for excision biopsy. Pathology: squamous carcinomas (70%), reticulum cell sarcoma, lymphosarcoma. *Treatment:* Radiotherapy, surgery and cytotoxics may all be used dependingon the type of tumour.

1 PS Little 1994 BMJ **ii** 1010
2 C Del Mar 1992 *Med J Aust* **156** 572
3 H Marcovitch 1990 *Arch Dis Chi* **65** 249
4 P Shvartzman 1993 BMJ **i** 1170

7. Ear, nose and throat diseases

►►Stridor

Stridor is the name given to noises produced during inspiration through a narrowed larynx or trachea. Children develop airways obstruction more readily than adults. It may be accompanied by difficulty in swallowing, cyanosis or pallor, use of accessory muscles of respiration and downward plunging of the trachea with respiration (tracheal tug)—all of which are grave signs. Stridor can occur in adults but is less common as laryngeal problems tend to produce hoarseness. Direct visualization of the larynx and trachea may reveal the cause.

Causes of stridor in children Congenital abnormalities of the larynx (laryngomalacia, laryngeal stenosis, rare tumours such as papillomas or haemangiomas); external compression from mediastinal tumours, anomalous blood vessels, double aortic arch; inflammatory conditions (acute laryngitis, acute epiglottitis, laryngotracheobronchitis); neurological abnormalities (vagal or recurrent laryngeal nerve paralysis); laryngeal trauma; inhaled foreign body; laryngeal oedema.

Laryngotracheobronchitis (croup) This is much commoner than acute epiglottitis. 95% are viral (parainfluenza commonest). Stridor and barking cough follow URTI symptoms. Admit to hospital if cyanosed or there is rib recession. Give humidified O_2. Nebulized epinephrine (=adrenaline, 5mL 1:1000) may buy time in severe cases needing ventilating. The use of steroids may reduce the duration of intubation (prednisolone 1mg/kg/12h PO).

Acute epiglottitis This is a medical emergency as complete respiratory obstruction can occur. Typically the history is short, and the patient may appear septicaemic. Admit to hospital to establish an alternative airway and to have IV antibiotics as needed (have a doctor in the ambulance) if the diagnosis is thought possible (see p 276)—emergency needle cricothyrotomy may be necessary if the airway becomes critically obstructed (*OHCM*, p 799). *Don't examine the throat before admission as this may precipitate complete obstruction.* Adult epiglottitis is much less common (8.8–9.7/10^6/yr), but may have a higher mortality (mean 1.1%, but 17.6% if respiratory distress a presenting feature). Intubate early if respiratory distress. Benzylpenicillin + cefuroxime will cover the likely causes (haemophilus and *Strep pyogenes*).[1]

Laryngomalacia (congenital laryngeal stridor) Floppy ary-epiglottic folds and glottis increase the normal tendency of the larynx to collapse during inspiration in affected infants. Stridor may be most noticeable during sleep, excitement, or when they are upset. Normally no treatment is needed but there may be problems during concurrent laryngeal infections. Symptoms usually improve by 2 years but may recur during infections.

Laryngeal paralysis A congenital paralysis accounting for 25% of infants with stridor—thought to be from vagal stretching at delivery, which may cause feeding difficulties. There is no specific treatment.

Acute airway obstruction This may be overcome by skilled intubation (for example in epiglottitis). If intubation fails, do a needle cricothyrotomy in children (*OHCM* p 753)—jet O_2 at 15 litres/min through a wide-bore cannula (14G) placed in cricothyroid membrane: allow O_2 in for 1sec and exhalation (through partially obstructed upper airway) for 4sec. This technique can be used in adults, or try surgical cricothyrotomy (*not* in children <12yrs). A tracheostomy in theatre will be required within 1h.

Admit to hospital Those who may have inhaled a foreign body for investigation and for its removal; children with laryngeal oedema (there will be oedema in other tissues).

1 K Barker 1994 BMJ i 919

7. Ear, nose and throat diseases

Hoarseness

►Hoarseness (particularly in a smoker) lasting more than 3 weeks requires urgent investigation to exclude laryngeal carcinoma (p 562).

Hoarseness occurs when a smooth vocal cord does not appose properly with its neighbour. Neurological or muscular causes of cord paralysis, and problems with the cords themselves may be the cause. Laryngeal problems usually present with hoarseness in adults but they can cause respiratory problems.

Causes *Acute:* Laryngitis; angioneurotic oedema; laryngeal abscess; trauma (shouting, coughing, vomiting, inhaling noxious fumes).
Chronic: (hoarseness lasting more than 3 weeks) Laryngitis; granulomatous disorders (syphilis, TB, sarcoid, Wegener's); vocal cord paralysis; carcinoma of larynx p 562; endocrine causes (acromegaly, Addison's disease, myxoedema); functional disorders; sicca syndrome (poor lubrication).

Investigations Laryngoscopy should be performed to watch cord movement, to inspect the mucosa, and to exclude local causes.

Laryngitis This is usually viral and self-limiting. There may be secondary infection with streptococci and staphylococci. Hoarseness is accompanied by feeling unwell, tiredness and fever. There is hypopharyngeal pain and there may be dysphagia and pain on phonation. Direct laryngoscopy reveals oedema. *Treatment:* If necessary, give phenoxymethylpenicillin 500mg/6h PO for 1 week. Inhalations may also help.

Laryngeal abscess This is very rare and usually secondary to trauma (eg endotracheal intubation). *Clinical features:* There is severe pain, fever, pain on swallowing (odynophagia), and there may be respiratory distress. Cervical lymphadenopathy may be present. Lateral movement of the larynx is painful. *Tests:* Lateral neck x-ray may show a fluid level or a distorted larynx. Fibreoptic laryngoscopy assesses glottic aperture size. Usual organisms: Pseudomonas, Staphylococcus or Proteus, so treat to cover these, eg netilmicin 2–3mg/kg/12h IV (monitor levels) with flucloxacillin 500mg/6h IV. If no response in 24h consider surgical drainage.

Singer's nodules Caused by vocal abuse these fibrous nodules occur at the junction of the anterior third and posterior two-thirds of the vocal cords. *Treatment:* They can be removed.

Functional disorders These produce hysterical paralysis of the adductors of both vocal cords on phonation. They usually occur in young women at times of emotional stress—but there are many functional disorders of the voice, which may result in laryngeal oedema ± nodules. The voice may be lost completely (aphonia). It is more commonly reduced to a whisper. Cords adduct on coughing so although patients may not speak they can cough. The most satisfactory treatment is speech therapy, with attention to the many undoubted emotional factors which may be present.

Laryngeal nerve palsy *Causes:* Laryngeal malignancy in ~40%; others: central (eg polio, syringomyelia); thyroid cancer; trauma (thyroidectomy); malignant cervical nodes; carcinoma of oesophagus, hypopharynx or bronchus; TB; aortic aneurysm; neuritis. With partial paralysis the cords are fixed in the midline; in complete paralysis they are fixed mid-way.

7. Ear, nose and throat diseases

ENT (head and neck) tumours

Carcinoma of larynx / hypopharynx Incidence: 2000/yr in England and Wales. Usually squamous cell carcinomas, occurring more in men, they are likely to be caused by smoking. *Sites:* Supraglottic, glottic, or subglottic. Glottic tumours have the best prognosis as they cause hoarseness earlier and spread to the nodes of the neck later than other types. *Presentation:* Persistent progressive hoarseness, then stridor, difficulty or pain on swallowing ± pain in the ear if the pharynx is involved; haemoptyses. *Diagnosis* is made by laryngoscopy and biopsy. *Treatment* may be radiotherapy or total laryngectomy ± block dissection of the neck glands. After laryngectomy patients have a permanent tracheostomy, hence the need to learn oesophageal speech. If a voice prosthesis is fitted at the time of surgery, reasonably normal speech is possible within weeks. Give pre-op counselling. Patients are usually discharged after 10–14 days with a plastic stent or metal cannula to keep the tracheostomy open—which may be discarded some weeks later. Excessive secretions and crusting around the stoma are common, needing meticulous attention, to avoid obstruction—humidified stomal covers (eg Laryngofoam®) may get round these problems. Advise to take care while having a bath, and to avoid fishing and deep water (unless expert training is to hand). *Late complications:* Stenosis; recurrent pneumonia. Suggest a laryngectomy club.[1]

Nasopharyngeal malignancy is much commoner in China than in UK (25% of all malignancy *vs* 1%). Cause (in China) may involve:[2] •Genetics (abnormal HLA profiles); •Early infection with Epstein–Barr virus; •Weaning babies on to salted fish (?*N*-nitroso carcinogens).

Tumours may be carcinomas, lymphoepitheliomas or lymphosarcomas. Lymphatic spread is usually early to deep cervical nodes (between mastoid process and mandible). Local spread may involve cranial nerves via the foramen lacerum or jugular foramen. Symptoms: epistaxis, diplopia, nasal obstruction, neck lumps, conductive deafness (Eustachian tube affected), or cranial nerve palsy (all but I, VII and VIII can be affected). *Diagnosis* is by posterior rhinoscopy, inspection palpation and nasopharynx biopsy under general anaesthesia, + skull-base radiology. *Treatment* is with radiotherapy. The prognosis is often poor.

Sinus tumours are usually squamous carcinomas developing in the middle-aged or elderly. Suspect in those developing chronic sinusitis for the first time in later life. Early presentations may be with blood-stained nasal discharge and nasal obstruction. Later there may be swelling of the cheek, swelling or ulceration of the buccoalveolar plate or palate, epiphora due to a blocked nasolacrimal duct, ptosis and diplopia as the floor of the orbit is involved and pain in the distribution of the second branch of the fifth cranial nerve. Local spread may be to cheek, palate, nasal cavity, orbit, and pterygopalantine fossa. *Tests:* MRI/CT ± endoscopic biopsy is best. *Treatment options:* Radiotherapy; radical surgical (eg maxillectomy, or, if ethmoid, craniofacial resection *en bloc*; cytotoxics.

Acoustic neuroma These slow growing neurofibromas (schwannomas) often arise from the vestibular nerve, giving progressive[3] ipsilateral tinnitus ± sensorineural deafness. Big tumours may give ipsilateral cerebellar signs or ICP↑ signs. Giddiness is common, vertigo is rare. Trigeminal compression above the tumour may give a facial numbness. Nearby cranial nerves may be affected (esp. V, VI, VII). *Tests:* MRI is best. *Treatment:* Surgery if possible.

Pharyngeal pouch This is a mucosal herniation at Killian's dehiscence of the inferior constrictor. There may be halitosis, regurgitation of food, and a neck lump (usually left side). Diagnose by barium swallow. *Treatment:* Surgery.

Pharyngeal carcinoma Oropharyngeal tumours are often advanced at presentation. The patient is typically elderly, and a smoker. Symptoms include vague sore throat, sensation of a lump, referred otalgia and local irritation by hot or cold foods. Hypopharyngeal tumours may give dysphagia, voice alteration, otalgia, stridor and throat pain. *Treatment* is usually surgical, eg with endoscopic stapling ± later radiotherapy. Radiotherapy has a role as first-line therapy if the tumor is small and detected early.

Plummer–Vinson syndrome (Patterson–Kelly–Brown syndrome) There is an oesophageal web associated with iron-deficient anaemia, and possibly post-cricoid carcinoma.

1 Laryngectomy Assoc, 6 Rickett St, SW6 tel: 0171 381 9993 **2** *Lancet* 1989 **ii** 840 **3** A Wright 1995 BMJ ii 1141&1421

Dysphagia

Dysphagia is difficulty in swallowing food or liquid. Unless it is associated with a transitory sore throat, it is a serious symptom, and merits further investigation, usually by endoscopy, to exclude neoplasia. If the experience is one of a lump in the throat *at times when the patient is not swallowing*, the diagnosis is likely to be ('globus')—a condition made worse by (but not caused by) anxiety (it is due to overactivity of the cricopharyngeal sphincter, often associated with reflux).

Causes *Malignant:*

Malignant:	*Neurological causes:*	*Others:*
Oesophageal cancer	Bulbar palsy (*OHCM* p 466)	Benign strictures
Gastric cancer	Lateral medullary syndrome	Pharyngeal pouch
Pharyngeal cancer		Achalasia (below)
Extrinsic pressure (eg lung cancer)	Myasthenia gravis	Systemic sclerosis
	Syringomyelia (*OHCM* p 476)	Oesophagitis
		Iron-deficient anaemia

Differential diagnosis There are 4 key questions to ask:

1 Can fluid be drunk as fast as usual, except if food is stuck?
  Yes: Suspect a stricture (benign or malignant).
  No: Think of motility disorders (achalasia, neurological causes).

2 Is it difficult to make the swallowing movement?
  Yes: Suspect bulbar palsy, especially if he coughs on swallowing.

3 Is the dysphagia constant and painful?
  Yes (either feature): Suspect a malignant stricture.

4 Does the neck bulge or gurgle on drinking?
  Yes: Suspect a pharyngeal pouch (food may be regurgitated).

Investigations FBC; ESR; barium swallow; endoscopy with biopsy; oesophageal motility studies (this requires swallowing a catheter containing a pressure transducer).

Nutrition Dysphagia may lead to malnutrition. Nutritional support often needed prior to treatment.

Oesophageal carcinoma This is associated with achalasia, Barrett's ulcer (*OHCM* p 694), tylosis (an hereditary condition in which there is hyperkeratosis of the palms), Plummer–Vinson syndrome (below) and smoking. Survival after resection is rare after 5 years (*OHCM* p 164).

Benign oesophageal stricture Causes: oesophageal reflux; swallowing corrosives; foreign body; trauma. *Treatment:* Dilatation (endoscopic or with bougies under anaesthesia).

Barrett's ulcer See *OHCM* p 694.

Achalasia There is failure of oesophageal peristalsis and failure of relaxation of the lower oesophageal sphincter. Liquids and solids are swallowed only slowly. CXR: air/fluid level behind the heart, and double right heart border produced by a grossly expanded oesophagus.

Treatment: Myomectomy cures ~75% of patients. Pneumatic dilatation may also help.

7. Ear, nose and throat diseases

Facial palsy

Anatomy Arising in the medulla, and emerging between pons and medulla, the facial nerve passes through the posterior fossa and runs through the middle-ear before emerging from the stylomastoid foramen to pass through the parotid. Lesions may be at any part of its course. Branches in the temporal bone:

1 The greater superficial petrosal nerve (lacrimation),
2 Branch to stapedius (lesions above this cause hyperacusis),
3 The chorda tympani (supply taste to anterior ⅔ of the tongue).

Causes *Intracranial:* Brainstem tumours; strokes; polio; multiple sclerosis; cerebellopontine angle lesions (acoustic neuroma, meningitis).
Intratemporal: Otitis media; Ramsay Hunt syndrome; cholesteatoma.
Infratemporal: Parotid tumours; trauma.
Others: Lyme disease; sarcoid; Guillain–Barré syndrome; diabetes; Bell's palsy.

Examination and tests Lower motor neurone lesions can cause paralysis of the whole of one side of the face, whereas in upper motor neurone lesions, the facial muscles of the forehead may still be operational (they are bilaterally innervated). Brainstem lesions produce only muscle weakness and may be accompanied by sixth nerve palsies. Loss of lacrimation (Schirmer's test p 482), stapedius reflex, taste (electrogustometry detects) and decreased submandibular saliva production (cannulate ducts) imply nerve lesions proximal to the origin of the relevant branches. Examine the ears (to exclude otitis media, zoster and cholesteatoma) and parotid. Consider temporal bone x-ray. Electromyography reveals completeness of the lesion.

Trauma: Examine the facial nerve in victims of head trauma. An incomplete palsy will probably recover. A complete palsy demands surgical exploration.

Infection In acute otitis media accompanied by facial nerve palsy myringotomy should be performed. When cholesteatoma is present emergency exploratory surgery should be performed. If rare acute necrotizing otitis externa is the cause, IV antibiotics (eg ticarcillin) and local toilet are needed.

Ramsay Hunt syndrome (Herpes zoster oticus) See p 756.

Bell's palsy At present the cause is unknown but many believe it part of a viral polyneuropathy (typically Herpes simplex in some small studies) with demyelination, the V, X, and C2 nerves also being affected. Onset is abrupt and may be associated with pain. The mouth sags, and dribbling, taste impairment and watering (or dry) eyes may occur. The patient cannot wrinkle the forehead, blow forcefully, whistle or pout out his cheek.

Treatment: Protect the eye with dark glasses, and tape closed during sleep. If recovery is expected to take months, consider lateral tarsorrhaphy. Instil artificial tears regularly at the slightest evidence of drying. There is good evidence that prednisolone helps, *if given early*[1] (eg in first 24h, eg 20mg/6h for 5 days, tail off over next 5 days). Oral aciclovir (eg 400mg five times a day) appears to be a promising *additional* treatment.[2] Hooks and cheek plumpers may improve appearance. If electromyography reveals total degeneration, surgical exploration may be carried out to check nerve continuity, breaches of which may be grafted (eg with lateral cutaneous nerve of the thigh).

1 Many neurologists give steroids 'to reduce oedema' particularly to those seen within 6 days of onset. One helpful study is that by TS Shafshak (1994 *J Laryng & Otology* **108** 940–3 & *Bandolier* 1995 **2**/11 3) showing that the extra benefit of steroids may be confined to those treated within 24h of onset. Spontaneous recovery is good in any case (85%). For every 3 persons treated with steroids within 24h, 1 extra had a good recovery compared with no treatment; for ethical reasons, this study was not randomized. Older randomized studies have been inconclusive, but did not look specifically at early treatment. A recent meta-analysis supports the use of steroids (I Williamson 1996 *Br J Gen Pract* 743–7 & E-BM 1997 **2** 79.) **2** R Enting 1998 *Ned Tijdschr Geneeskd* **142** 436

7. Ear, nose and throat diseases

Lumps in the neck

►Do not biopsy any malignant-feeling neck lump: first refer to ENT, where thorough assessment and search for a primary may be undertaken. Fine-needle aspiration for cytology, thorough CT/MRI are done before treatment. MRI is better for soft tissues. Culture all biopsied lymph nodes for TB.

Diagnosis First of all ask for how long the lump has been present. If <3 weeks, lymphadenopathy from a self-limiting infection is likely, and extensive investigation is unwise. Next ask yourself where the lump is. Is it intradermal?—(sebaceous cyst with a central punctum, or a lipoma). If the lump is not intradermal, and is not of recent onset, allow yourself to feel the intoxicating sensation of a hunt starting off over complicated terrain.

Midline lumps: If patient <20yrs old, the likely diagnosis is a dermoid cyst, or, if it moves on protruding the tongue and is below the hyoid, a thyroglossal cyst (fluctuant lump developing in cell rests in thyroid's migration path; treatment: surgery). If over 20, it's probably a thyroid mass, unless it's bony hard, when the diagnosis may be a chondroma.

Submandibular triangle: (Below jaw; above anterior belly of digastric.) If <20yrs, self-limiting lymphadenopathy is likely. If >20, exclude **malignant lymphadenopathy** (eg firm, and non-tender). ►Is TB likely? If it's not a node, think of submandibular **salivary stone**, **sialadenitis** or **tumour**.

Anterior triangle: (Below digastric and in front of sternomastoid.) Nodes are common (see above): examine the areas which they serve (skin, mouth, throat, thyroid; is the spleen enlarged?—this may indicate lymphoma). **Branchial cysts** emerge under the anterior border of sternomastoid where the upper ⅓ meets the middle ⅓; age <20. They are due to non-disappearance of the cervical sinus (where the 2nd branchial arch grows down over 3rd and 4th). Lined by squamous epithelium, their fluid contains cholesterol crystals. Treat by excision. **Cystic hygromas** arise from the jugular lymph sac and transilluminate brightly. Treat by surgery or hypertonic saline sclerosant. **Carotid body tumours** (chemodectoma) are very rare, move from side-to-side, but not up and down, and splay out the carotid bifurcation. They are firm (softness is rare) and pulsatile, and do not usually cause bruits. They may be bilateral, familial and malignant (5%). This tumour should be suspected in tumours just anterior to the upper third of sternomastoid. Diagnose by digital computerized angiography. Treatment: extirpation by vascular surgeon. If the lump is in the superoposterior area of the anterior triangle, is it a **parotid tumour**? (more likely if >40yrs). A **laryngocoele** is an uncommon cause of a lump in the anterior triangle: it is painless, and may be made worse by blowing.

Posterior triangle: (Behind sternomastoid, in front of trapesius, and above the clavicle.) If there are many small lumps, think of **nodes**—TB or viruses such as HIV or EBV (infectious mononucleosis) or, if over 20yrs, consider lymphoma or metastases. The primary may be head and neck (eg tongue base, posterior nasal space, tonsils, etc) or bronchus, gut, breast or gonad (in that order of likelihood). **Cervical ribs** may intrude into this area.

Tests Ultrasound shows lump consistency. CT defines masses in relation to their anatomical neighbours. Do virology and Mantoux test. CXR may show malignancy or reveal bilateral hilar lymphadenopathy, when you should consider sarcoid. Consider fine-needle aspiration (FNA).

7. Ear, nose and throat diseases

The salivary glands

There are 3 pairs of major salivary glands (parotid, submandibular and sublingual) as well as numerous minor glands.

History and examination Lumps; swelling related to food; pain; taste; dry eyes. Look for external swellings, secretions (in mouth first), do bimanual palpation for stones, test VII nerve, any regional nodes?

Inflammation is usually due to infection or an obstructing calculus (calcium phosphates and carbonates form around a nidus of cells and organisms). A useful approach is based on whether the symptoms are unilateral, or bilateral and acute or chronic.

Acute bilateral symptoms are usually due to mumps (p 214). The patient is usually young and complains of parotid swelling.

Acute, unilateral symptoms are also likely to be due to mumps but acute parotitis may occur by ascending oral infection. This occurs post-op but is now rare, unless dehydrated or poor oral hygiene. *Treatment:* Oral hygiene, hydration, antibiotics (depends on culture and sensitivities). If the duct stops draining pus, or pain and pyrexia increase, there may be abscess formation which will need draining through the skin.

Recurrent unilateral symptoms are likely to be due to stones (submandibular in 80%). The classic story is of pain and swelling on eating. The gland may be red, swollen and tender (not necessarily infected). The stone may be seen on plain x-ray or by sialography. *Treatment:* Distal stones are removed via the mouth but excise the gland if it contains the stone.

Chronic bilateral symptoms may be associated with dry eyes and mouth and other autoimmune disease—eg Sjögren's or Mikulicz's syndromes (*OHCM* p 704–8). *Treatment* is hard. If chronic infection is the cause, a simple course of antibiotics will fail: what is needed is prolonged treatment with oxytetracycline 250mg/12h 1h ac PO.

Fixed swellings may be idiopathic or due to sarcoidosis.

Tumours '80% are in the parotid, 80% of these are pleomorphic adenomas, 80% of these are in the superficial lobe.' ►*Any salivary gland swelling must be removed for assessment if present for >1 month* (or examined by fine needle aspiration for cytology: this does not leading to seeding along its track). VII nerve paresis suggests malignancy. As tumours grow by budding and have no capsule, lumpectomy leads to seedling deposits, so superficial parotidectomy is needed. NB: sialograms with CT (+bone filters) may be a useful pre-op test. Classification is complex: full details in the electronic version.

Benign or malignant:	*Malignant:*	
Cystadenolymphoma		
Mucoepidermoid	Squamous carcinoma	Adenocarcinoma
Pleomorphic adenoma	Acinic cell	Adenoid cystic carcinoma

Pleomorphic adenoma: Middle age; slow growth; must be removed by superficial parotidectomy or enucleation. Radiotherapy has a rôle if there was intraoperative spillage, or in residual disease, or recurrences (seen in ~1–2% at 12 years follow-up).[1,2] Post-op complications: metastatic spread (rare[3]); facial nerve palsy (with skill, risk is minimal); gustatory sweating (~7%).

Adenolymphoma: Usually elderly men; soft. *Treatment:* Enucleation.

Carcinomas: Rapid growth; hard fixed mass; pain & VIIth nerve palsy. Treat by combination of surgery and radiotherapy.

Complications of surgery: **1** VIIth nerve palsy—often transient. **2** Salivary fistula—often closes spontaneously. **3** *Frey's syndrome* (gustatory sweating)—here tympanic neurectomy may help.

1 F Liu 1995 *Head Neck* **17** 177–83 2 A Renehan 1996 *Br J Surg* **83** 1750–4 3 *Head Neck* 1997 **19** 629

7. Ear, nose and throat diseases

Dentistry for doctors

►Any oral ulcer which has not healed in 3 weeks should receive specialist assessment, for biopsy to exclude malignancy (OHCM p 500).

Differential diagnosis of facial pain Tooth pathology, sinusitis, temporomandibular joint (TMJ) dysfunction, salivary gland, migraine, trigeminal neuralgia, atypical facial pain (no obvious organic cause), trauma. See OHCM p 46.

Rarer causes: MI, frontal bone osteomyelitis (post sinusitis); ENT tumours; mucormycosis. This latter is is a necrotizing fungal infection of the nasal sinuses caused by mucoraciae (eg rhizopus). It causes fever and cranial nerve palsies (III–VIII), and facial pain (the patient may be diabetic presenting with black pus draining from the nose; it is worth remembering, as it is treatable with debridement and amphotericin: OHCM p 340).

►When helping a patient with a dental infection pay attention to these features—before consulting a maxillofacial surgeon, or a dentist (GDP).

1 *Is it the teeth? **History:*** *Is the pain...*

- Worse with sugar and heat?
- Worse or better with cold?
- Intermittent?

} ► Tooth is alive (pulpitis)

Is the pain...

- Worse with percussion?
- Constant/uninterrupted?

} ► Tooth dead (osteitis/abscess)

Is the pain...

- Exacerbated by movement between finger and thumb (>1 mm)

} ► Periodontal disease

Radiography (usually helpful): Orthopantogram (OPT) is useful for imaging molars and pre-molars. If incisors are suspected, request periapical x-ray of the tooth in question. Interpretation of radiograph...

- **Abscess** (Tooth tender to percussion)
- **Periodontal disease** (Tooth mobile)

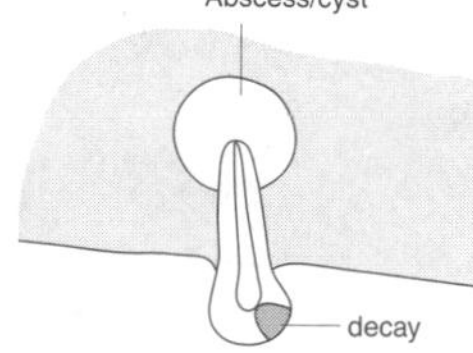

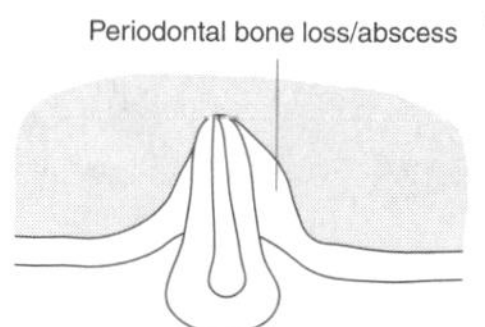

2 *Trismus:* (Opening mouth is difficult because of spasm or pain.) This is a sign of severe infection. Ask the patient to open mouth wide and measure how many fingers breadth between the incisor teeth. Trismus always requires maxillofacial advice.

3 *Facial swellings due to dental infection:* Usually subside with oral antibiotics. ►If swelling is related to the lower jaw, assess for airways obstruction; if speading to the eye, assess the second cranial nerve. If in any doubt, refer to a maxillofacial surgeon.

4 *Bedside observations:* Temperature (very important), pulse and blood pressure. This information must be to hand *prior* to referral. Systemically unwell patients require maxillofacial advice/admission.

5 *Systemic disease complicating dental infection:* All immuno-compromised patients, eg those on steroids, with leukaemia or diabetics; patients at risk of endocarditis; coagulopathy (eg haemophilia or warfarin). Seek specialist advice.

Dental caries Although on the decline in the West due primarily to fluoride, this condition is increasing exponentially in developing countries. Causes: bacteria (esp. *S mutans*), substrate (sugars) and susceptible tooth surface. In otherwise healthy individuals it is an entirely preventable disease.

Rampant caries is a variant found in children exposed to excessive sucrose in the forms of coated dummies, 'health' drinks and prescribed medicines.

Radiation caries is seen following head and neck radiotherapy and both the disease and its treatment can lead to jaw osteoradionecrosis. *Treatment and complications:* Pain ± infection. Toothache pain responds best to NSAIDs, eg ibuprofen 200–400mg/8h PO pc (can buy it from pharmacists), and dental infection to penicillin and metronidazole, but drug treatment is never definitive, and a dental referral is required.

Periodontal disease 'Is one of the most widespread diseases of mankind' (WHO). Virtually the entire dentate adult population has gingivitis which is caused by bacterial and polysaccharide complexes at the tooth-gingival interface (=plaque). It is cured by good toothbrushing. Acute herpetic and rarely streptococcal infection can cause gingival inflammation.

Acute ulcerative gingivitis (Vincent's angina) is a painful, foul-smelling condition caused by anaerobes—*Fusobacteria*—and spirochaetes (*Borellia vincentii*). It is associated with stress and smoking. Treat with penicillin 250mg/6h PO and metronidazole 400mg/8h PO.

Gingival swelling may be due to exacerbation of inflammation by immunodeficiency, vitamin C deficiency, diabetes or by exacerbation and infiltration in leukaemias. Fibrous hyperplasia may be congenital or induced by drugs such as phenytoin, cyclosporin A and nifedipine.

Periodontitis (pyorrhoea) is a progression of localized inflammation from the gums into the ligament supporting a tooth. It is associated with anaerobic bacteria, calcified bacterial deposits (calculi, tartar) and poor oral hygiene. It requires specialist treatment by a family dentist.

Juvenile periodontitis occurs in a younger age group and is associated with organisms which may respond to local or systemic antibiotics.

Malocclusion Inappropriate positioning of the teeth in the jaws or between the jaws themselves is common. Those with prominent upper teeth are particularly prone to trauma, and those children at risk (eg in epilepsy)—or those involved in contact sports should be referred to an orthodontist. Those with severe facial or jaw disharmony who may be unable to chew or have psychological difficulty with their appearance may be amenable to surgical correction by an oral or maxillofacial surgeon.

Wisdom teeth In the West, these can be considered, rather like the appendix, as a vestigial organ. They account for an enormous number of inpatient operations annually. If asymptomatic and not exposed to contamination by the mouth, they do not usually require removal. Complications are pain and infection and they may be involved in fractures of the mandible. Post-operative recovery is often complicated by pain and swelling, pain responds well to NSAIDs and poorly to opiates, particularly dihydrocodeine. Infection complicates up to 30% not receiving antibiotics. Penicillin and metronidazole (as above) are standbys.

Teething An acute sore mouth during tooth eruption is often caused by viral infections (eg herpetic). The onset of eruption of first deciduous teeth correlates with the fall off in transferred maternal antibody.

NB: Other oral mucosal diseases are described on *OHCM* p 500.

8. Skin diseases

Note: It is envisaged that the reader will have ready access to patients in dermatology out-patients, so that the conditions described here can be met in the flesh. If this is not possible, a good atlas of dermatology should be used alongside this text, eg R Ashton and B Leppard 1992 *Differential Diagnosis in Dermatology*, 2e, Radcliffe Medical Press (ISBN 1-870905-4747-4).

Further Reading: MacKie Rona M. *Clinical Dermatology*, 4e 1997, OUP, ISBN 0-19-2627619, and Rook, Wilkinson/Ebling *Textbook of Dermatology* 5e OUP, ISBN 0-632-02396-1.

uction to dermatology

e of the largest organs in the body and can display a myr- signs and reaction patterns. Recognition of these by the y permit diagnosis of previously unsuspected systemic disor- arily dermatological conditions such as eczema and psoriasis only the domain of dermatologists but are likely to be encoun- y all clinicians, regardless of field of practice. A practical knowl- and clinical confidence in the diagnosis of skin disease is thus a valuable asset.

History and examination

History Duration of rash; site of onset, spread and d lesions; symptoms (itch, pain); aggravating factors (sunlight, ous treatments; medical conditions and medications; fam (psoriasis, atopy); occupation (industrial chemicals); pets.

Examination Examine all the skin; hair and nails where approp.

Distribution Symmetrical flexural (atopy); contact with jewelle clothing (contact dermatitis); areas exposed to sun, eg backs of ha face, neck (photosensitivity); grouped lesions (herpes virus); symme cal extensor surfaces (psoriasis).

Pattern Ring (fungal—active edge with healing centre, p590); linear (Köbner phenomenon, below), targetoid (erythema multiforme).

Terms used to describe lesions

- *alopecia* hair loss
- *atrophy* thinning and loss of skin substance
- *bulla* blister larger than a vesicle (see below, ie >0.5cm diameter)
- *crust* dried brownish exudate
- *erosion* superficial break in the continuity of the epidermis; heals without scarring
- *erythema* reddening of the skin which blanches on pressure
- *excoriation* scratch which has broken the surface of the skin
- *fissure* crack, often through keratin
- *induration* an area of thickening of the dermis and subcutaneous tissues
- *Köbner phenomenon* skin lesions which develop at a site of injury (psoriasis, lichen planus, plane warts, vitiligo)
- *lichenification* skin thickening with exaggerated skin markings, as a result of repeated rubbing
- *macule* flat well-defined area of altered skin pigmentation; large lesions may be called patches
- *nodule* solid, mostly subcutaneous lesion, more than 0.5cm diameter
- *papule* raised well-defined lesion, usually less than 0.5cm diameter
- *plaque* raised flat-topped lesion, usually over 2cm in diameter
- *purpura* purplish lesion resulting from free red blood cells in the skin. It does not blanch on pressure
- *pustule* well-defined pus-filled lesion
- *scale* fragment of dry skin
- *scar* replacement of skin with firm fibrous tissue which is permanent
- *ulcer* loss of epidermis and dermis which results in a scar
- *vesicle* blister less than 0.5cm diameter
- *weal* transient raised lesion with a pale centre and pink margin

8. Skin diseases

Possible causes of patterns of skin disease

Ring-shaped (annular) lesions
- Fungal infections: active erythematous scaly edge with central clearing.
- Erythema multiforme: target-like lesions, eg on extensor limb surfaces.
- Granuloma annulare: pinkish papules forming a ring.
- Basal cell carcinoma (rodent ulcer): pearly papules with central ulcer, usually on face.

Round, oval or coin-shaped (discoid) lesions
- Psoriasis: red-pink plaques covered with a silvery scale.
- Discoid eczema: well-defined crusted eczematous lesions.
- Pityriasis rosea: herald patch; oval red lesions with scaly edge, eg on trunk.
- Impetigo: well-defined red patches, covered with honey-coloured crust.

Linear lesions •Köbner phenomenon: psoriasis, lichen planus.
- Dermatitis artefacta: linear or bizarre-shaped lesions, induced by patient.
- Herpes zoster: polymorphous vesicles/pustules in dermatomal distribution.

White lesions •Pityriasis versicolor: superficial slightly scaly infection with the yeast *Malassezia furfur*; appears depigmented on darker skins.
- Pityriasis alba: post-eczema hypopigmentation, often on children's faces.
- Vitiligo (*vitellus* is Latin for *spotted calf*: typically white patches ± hyperpigmented borders. Sunlight makes them itch. *Associations:* Autoimmunity: Graves', Addison's, Hashimoto's—also diabetes, alopecia areata, hypoparathyroidism, premature ovarian failure. Treat by camouflage cosmetics, sunscreens and potent steroid creams (may be better than dermabrasion).
- Rarely, leprosy.

Brown pigmentation •Freckles: brown macules, related to sun exposure.
- Lentigos: persistent brown macules, often larger than freckles.
- Café-au-lait spots: faint brown macules; if >5, consider neurofibromatosis.
- Seborrhoeic keratoses (seborrhoeic warts): benign greasy-brown warty lesions usually on the back, chest and face; very common in the elderly.
- Chloasma (melasma) are brown patches especially on the face, related to pregnancy or Pill use. The condition may respond to topical azelaic acid.
- Systemic diseases: Addison's (palmar creases, oral mucosa, scars); haemochromatosis; porphyria cutanea tarda (+ skin fragility and blisters).

Subcutaneous nodules Rheumatoid nodules, rheumatic fever, PAN, xanthelasma, tuberous sclerosis, neurofibroma, sarcoid, granuloma annulare.

Itch (pruritus) ►*Itch can be very distressing.* Skin will usually be scratched or rubbed and a number of secondary clinical features may be seen on the skin: excoriations (scratch marks); lichenification (skin thickening); papules or nodules (localized skin thickening). *Causes of itch:* Determine if there is a primary skin disease or is itch due to a systemic disorder.
- Itchy skin disorders: *scabies* (burrows in finger-webs, wrists, groins, buttocks); *urticaria* (transient weals, dermatographism); *atopic eczema* (flexural eruption, lichenification); dermatitis herpetiformis (very itchy blisters on elbows, shoulders); lichen planus (flat topped violet papules, especially wrists).
- Medical conditions causing itch: *iron deficiency anaemia* (koilonychia, pale conjunctivae); *lymphoma* (lymphadenopathy, hepatosplenomegaly); *hypo/hyperthyroidism* (goitre); *chronic liver disease* (jaundice, spider naevi); *chronic renal failure* (dry sallow skin); malignancy (clubbing, masses). Investigations of itch in the absence of skin disease should include: FBC, ESR, ferritin, LFT, U&E, glucose, T_4, CXR.

Treating itchy skin: Treat any primary skin disease; bland emollients (eg E45®) to soothe dry skin, emollient bath oils; sedative antihistamines at night.

8. Skin diseases

Skin manifestations of systemic disease

Diabetes mellitus *Flexural candidiasis*; *necrobiosis lipoidica* (waxy, shiny yellow-brown plaques on the shins); *folliculitis*; *cutaneous infections*.

Coeliac disease *Dermatitis herpetiformis* (extremely itchy/burning blisters on the elbows, scalp, shoulders and ankles. Responds quickly to dapsone (50–200mg/day PO). SE: haemolysis, LFT↑, agranulocytosis. CI: G6PD↓. Gluten-free diet may clear lesions. Small risk of lymphoma with chronic disease.

Inflammatory bowel disease •*Erythema nodosum* (tender ill-defined subcutaneous nodules, usually on the shins. Other associations: sarcoid, drugs, TB, streptococci) •*Pyoderma gangrenosum:* recurring nodulo-pustular ulcers, ~10cm wide, with tender red/blue overhanging necrotic edge, healing with cribriform (pitted) scars. *Site:* eg leg; abdomen; face. *Associations:* UC; Crohn's; autoimmune hepatitis; neoplasia; Wegener's; myeloma. ♀:♂>1:1. *Differential:*[1] Behçet's, warfarin necrosis, rheumatoid vasculitis, 3°syphilis, blastomycosis, skin amoebiasis. *Treatment:* Get expert help. Saline cleansing, high-dose oral or intralesional steroids ± ciclosporin ± topical antibiotics.

Rheumatoid arthritis *Rheumatoid nodules*; *vasculitis* (palpable purpura, nodules, ulceration); *pyoderma gangrenosum* (see above).

Systemic lupus erythematosus (SLE) *Diffuse alopecia*; *facial butterfly rash*; *photosensitivty* (face, dorsum of hands, V of neck); *red scaly rashes* (skin biopsy with immunofluorescence can be helpful in diagnosis).

Thyroid disorders *Hyperthyroidism: pre-tibial myxoedema* (diffuse thickened pink nodules and plaques on the shins); *clubbing* (thyroid acropachy); *diffuse alopecia*. *Hypothyroidism: Sparse coarse hair; dry skin; asteatotic eczema* ('crazy-paving' eczema also seen on elderly shins; responds to simple emollients).

Neoplasia *Acanthosis nigricans* (velvety thickened and pigmented skin seen mainly in the axillae; associated with adenocarcinoma of stomach); *dermatomyositis* (purplish rash, often affecting eyelids and face, associated with muscle weakness; lung, breast and ♀ genital tract tumours should be excluded); *acquired ichthyosis* (generalized dry skin—recent onset may suggest underlying lymphoma or carcinoma); *pruritus* (see p 578).

Erythema multiforme *Minor form:* Target lesions, usually found on the extensor surfaces esp. of peripheries; also palms and soles. *Major form:* (Stevens–Johnson syndrome) associated with systemic upset, fever, severe mucosal involvement, including conjuntivae. *Cause:* Idiopathic; herpes simplex, mycoplasma, other viruses (minor form); drugs esp. sulfonamides, penicillins (major form). *Treatment:* Treat cause; supportive management—use of systemic steroids is controversial and may increase mortality.

Erythema chronicum migrans Early **sign** of Lyme disease (*Borrelia burgdorferi*). 50% give history of preceding tick bite. Presents as small papule which develops into a spreading erythematous ring. Can persist from weeks to months. *Treatment:* eg amoxicillin 500mg/8h PO, doxycycline 100mg/12h PO 2–3 weeks. Other features of Lyme disease: *OHCM* p 232.

Cutaneous vasculitis There can be a variable clinical picture, eg palpable purpuric rash, often on legs; nodules; ulcers; livedo. May occur as a feature of systemic vasculitis, eg Wegener's granulomatosus; polyarteritis nodosum, Henoch–Schönlein purpura (vasculitic eruption of legs and buttocks associated with arthralgia, abdominal pain and sometimes glomerulonephritis). Vasculitis limited to skin (hypersensitivity/leukocytoclastic vasculitis) may be precipitated by infection (streps, hepatitis B and C viruses), drugs (eg thiazides), connective tissue disease, malignancy, cryoglobulinaemia.

1 *Lancet* Ed 1997 **350** 1720

8. Skin diseases

Skin diagnoses not to be missed

Melanoma (p 584). **Kaposis sarcoma** (p 598). **Leukoplakia** (p 598).

Squamous cell carcinoma Presents as a persistently ulcerated or crusted firm irregular lesion. Usually found on sun-exposed sites, eg ears; dorsa of hands; bald scalp—here it may develop in a pre-existing actinic keratosis (see below). Also associated with chronic inflammation, eg venous leg ulcers, and related to smoking (lower lip). *Treatment:* Excision. Metastases are relatively uncommon but more frequent at certain sites, eg ears.

Leprosy Rare; suspect in any hypopigmented anaesthetic skin lesion.

Syphilis Isolated painless genital ulcers (primary chancre). Pityriasis rosea-like copper-coloured rashes affecting trunk, limbs, palms and soles (secondary syphilis). Are any other sexually transmitted diseases present?

Basal cell carcinoma (rodent ulcer) Typically, pearly nodule with rolled telangiectatic edge usually found on the face. Metastases are extremely rare. It is locally destructive if left untreated. Lesions on trunk can appear as red scaly plaques with raised smooth edge. *Cause:* Tends to occur in the fair-skinned, where UV exposure is thought to be causative. *Treatment:* Small lesions are best treated by excision; larger lesions, eg in very elderly, respond to radiotherapy. Cryotherapy is useful for large superficial lesions.

Senile or actinic keratoses These occur on sun-exposed areas, appearing as crumbly yellow-white crusts. Carcinomatous change may occur. *Treatment:* Cautery; cryotherapy; 5% 5-fluorouracil cream which is used twice daily, with the following sequence of events: Erythema→Vesiculation→Erosion→Ulceration→Necrosis→Healing epithelialization. Healthy skin is unharmed. Treatment is usually for 4 weeks, but may be prolonged. Lesions on the hands and forearms respond more slowly. There is no significant systemic absorption if the area treated is $<500\text{cm}^2$. Avoid in pregnancy. The hands should be washed after applying the cream. (NB: after any cryo warn that blisters may form afterwards; they may be burst, repeatedly, with a sterile needle; advise using an antiseptic cream to prevent infection, and aspirin for pain.).

Metastatic cancer Skin metastases are uncommon but well recognized in association with carcinomas of breast, kidney and lung. Non-Hodgkin's lymphoma and leukaemia can also metastasize to the skin. Metastases are usually firm, rather inflammatory lesions; often on the scalp or trunk.

Mycosis fungoides Cutaneous T-cell lymphoma usually of CD4 type. May be lengthy preceding history of undiagnosed skin disease. Clinically, well-defined red scaly plaques on trunk and limbs. Can have protracted clinical course and patients may finally succumb to another unrelated disease. Treatments include potent topical steroids, PUVA and radiotherapy (electron beam). Leukaemic phase (Sezary syndrome) associated with erythroderma and circulating Sezary cells.

Bowen's disease Slow growing red scaly plaque, often found on the lower legs. Histology shows full-thickness dysplasia (carcinoma-in-situ). Infrequently progresses to squamous cell carcinoma. *Treatment:* Cryotherapy; topical 5-flurouracil as above; photodynamic therapy.

Paget's disease of the nipple Cutaneous sign of intraductal breast carcinoma. Presents as unilateral red, scaly or crusted nipple. (NB: dermatitis usually affects both nipples and is itchy). Biopsy is required to confirm the diagnosis. Treatment is partial or complete mastectomy. Never diagnose eczema of the nipple without doing a biopsy first.

8. Skin diseases

583

Mole or melanoma?

Malignant melanoma The incidence is slightly commoner in females than males. Current UK figures are ~10 new cases/100,000/year, accounting for ~1000 deaths annually. The main aetiological factor incriminated is excessive UV exposure. A proportion of melanomas (around 30%) appear to develop in pre-existing moles while the remainder develop on previously normal skin. *Major signs suggesting melanoma: Change in size, shape* or *colour* of a pre-existing lesion or *development of a new changing pigmented lesion* in an adult. Melanomas are rarely diagnosed when they are less than 6mm in size and growth of a mole in an adult should be regarded with concern. Similarly, changes in shape from a circle or oval to a more jagged outline causes concern, as does change in colour. Benign moles may be very dark brown or black but are usually a uniform colour whereas early melanomas frequently are different shades of brown, black, red or even blue. *Minor points:* Inflammation, crusting or bleeding and sensory change. Consider excision biopsy with pathological examination for any pigmented lesion in an adult which is exhibiting change in size, shape or colour.

The clinical differential diagnosis of melanoma includes moles/naevi in young adults and seborrhoeic keratoses in older adults. Moles tend to be <5mm diameter, having a round smooth outline and a uniform colour. Seborrhoeic keratoses are extremely common on the trunk of individuals >50yrs. They are generally multiple and have a warty, greasy, 'stuck-on' appearance. They are rather friable if traumatized.

Treatment Always consider excision biopsy with a margin of normal skin and subsequent pathological examination, for any unusual, growing or changing pigmented lesion. If histology shows melanoma, read the report carefully: prognosis depends on completeness of excision and tumour thickness (well-established, major prognostic sign). Tumours less than 1mm thick have a very good disease-free 5-year survival rate (>90%), while those thicker than 3mm have only a 50% 5-year disease free survival rate.

Melanomas must be completely excised but the margin of excision of normal skin is not yet fully established. A useful working rule is to excise 1cm of normal skin around the melanoma for every millimetre of depth, up to 3cm (there is no evidence that excising margins >3cm is of any additional benefit). Enquire if your unit is involved in any of the trials now being done on this issue. *Don't do incisional biopsies on possible melanomas.*

Early diagnosis Early diagnosis of melanoma may give a better prognosis. GPs, practice nurses and others involved with examining the skin should be aware of the features of early melanomas and arrange for urgent referral to an expert for rapid excision and pathological examination.

Prevention Available evidence suggests that excessive UV light acting on genetically vulnerable white-skinned, fair-haired, blue-eyed individuals is a major aetiological factor, so the public should be encouraged to avoid excessive burning sun exposure (noonday sun, eg on sunny holidays), to wear sun-protective clothing such as hats and to use broad-spectrum high SPF (sun protection factor) sunscreens to minimize the risk of burning.

Pigmented naevi or moles It is normal to have benign pigmented naevi/moles on the skin. ~3% of the population have one or more congenital pigmented naevi present at birth; numbers slowly increase until by late teenage years, most have 20–50 small naevi. As patients mature, naevi gradually involute so that in old age, benign pigmented naevi are relatively rare on the skin surface. The great majority of naevi are totally benign and are not pre-malignant lesions. Lesions which are less than 5mm in diameter and have a uniform colour and outline do not require to be excised for medical reasons unless there is a clear history of growth or change.

8. Skin diseases

Psoriasis

Psoriasis is a common chronic inflammatory skin condition that affects ~2% of Caucasian populations. It can arise at any age but peaks around the 2nd–3rd decades (type 1) and the 5th–6th decades (type 2), affecting the sexes equally. Previously thought to be a disorder primarily of keratinocytes, there is now evidence to suggest that psoriasis is immunologically mediated,[1] with Th1-cells predominant in early lesions. There are many inherited and environmental factors which may influence the development of psoriasis. A first degree relative with psoriasis confers an increased risk of developing the condition: the risk is 60% if both parents are affected. Genetic linkage studies have recently demonstrated a psoriasis susceptibility locus located on chromosome 6q.[2] Recognized HLA associations include HLA-CW6 and HLA-DR4 Infections, particularly with streptococci and certain drugs (eg β-blockers; lithium, antimalarials) are also recognized triggers. *Histology:* Regular acanthosis of the epidermis; parakeratosis and intraepidermal neutrophil microabcesses (of Munro).

Signs Symmetrical well-defined red plaques with silvery scale, located on the extensor aspects of the elbows and knees, the scalp and sacrum. Flexures (axillae, groins, submammary areas and umbilicus) also frequently affected but lesions non-scaly. Nails may show pitting, onycholysis (separation from the nail-bed), thickening and subungual hyperkeratosis. Very small plaques (guttate) seen in young patients, particularly those associated with concurrent streptococcal infection. Pustular variants can affect the palms and soles (pustules sterile). Generalized (erythrodermic) psoriasis and generalized pustular psoriasis may cause severe systemic upset (fever, ↑ WCC, dehydration). These may be triggered by rapid withdrawal of systemic steroids.

Signs Köbner phenomenon (p 576); Auspitz sign: pinpoint bleeding when scale removed; pepper pot nail pitting and 'grease-spots'.

Systemic associations Approximately 7% of psoriatics develop arthropathy, which can be of 5 types:

1. DIP joints, associated with nail dystrophy
2. Ankylosing spondylitis-like
3. Rheumatoid-like (sero-negative)
4. Asymmetrical oligoarthritis
5. Arthritis mutilans (severe, destructive)

Differential diagnosis Fungal infection (solitary or few lesions; asymmetrical; expanding); mycosis fungoides (asymmetrical lesions, minimal scaling, biopsy required); seborrhoeic dermatitis (may co-exist).

Management Patient education is essential and aids compliance with treatment. Remove possible triggers (streptococcal infection, drugs); factors such as stress and alcohol may also aggravate condition. Topical drugs are the mainstays of treatment for most patients. *Tar:* Messy ointments are best avoided unless patients are admitted for treatment; 'clean' preparations available (eg Alphosyl®—applied twice daily). *Dithranol:* Available in cream preparations for use in short-contact regimens (treatment applied carefully to affected skin then washed off after 20–30 minutes): start at low concentrations (0.1%) and increase as tolerated (eg 0.25%, 0.5%, 1%). Side-effects: burning (avoid in flexures); staining (avoid on face). *Calcipotriol/tacalcitol*: (vitamin D analogues): avoid use in calcium metabolism disorders; small risk of hypercalcaemia if large amounts used on extensive inflamed skin (limit use of calcipotriol to 75g per week). Tacalcitol may be applied once daily before going to bed (max 5g/day, and only up to two 12-week courses/yr). For flexural disease, topical steroid/antibiotic/antifungal preparations can be useful (*Trimovate*®).

1 H Valdimarrson 1996 *Immunology Today* **7** 256 2 R Trembath 1997 *Human Molecular Genetics* **6** 813

Agents to consider in recalcitrant psoriasis

Tazarotene (a topical retinoid): for mild to moderate psoriasis affecting <10% skin surface; applied once daily; avoid use in pregnant women.

Phototherapy: Narrow-band UVB (TL-01): 3 × weekly for 6 weeks; avoid if history of photosensitivity; most suitable for guttate/small plaque psoriasis. *PUVA*: UVA + oral/topical psoralen; suitable for extensive large plaque disease (oral psoralen) and localized psoriasis (topical psoralen); limit total dose to 1000J/150 treatments to avoid excessive skin ageing and risk of skin cancer (especially squamous cell carcinoma); can be combined with oral retinoids (re-PUVA) to ↓light dose needed to clear lesions.

Oral drugs: Severe psoriasis often needs oral drugs. Liaise with an expert.

Acitretin: Oral retinoid; useful for moderate to severe disease; side-effects: teratogenetic; dry skin and mucosae; ↑ lipids, ↑LFTs (reversible). In the UK, use is limited to hospitals. Starting dose: 25–30mg/24h PO; typical maintenance dose: 25–50mg/day; adjusted according to response). Exclude pregnancy, and avoid donating blood for >1yr after the last dose.

Methotrexate: 10–25mg/week; most useful in elderly patients; best avoided in younger patients in view of long-term risk of hepatic fibrosis.

Ciclosporin: 2.5–5mg/kg/day; usefulness often limited by side-effects (hypertension; renal dysfunction).

1 H Valdimarrson 1996 *Immunology Today* **7** 256-9 2 R Trembath 1997 *Human Molecular Genetics* **6** 813-20

Dermatitis/eczema

The terms eczema and dermatitis are interchangeable although patients often consider eczema to be endogenous and dermatitis to be due to external allergens, especially occupational (you always need to remember to ask about work, hobbies, and other reasons for exposure to allergens).

Atopic eczema The cause of eczema is multifactorial. *Genetics:* There is a strong genetic component often with a positive family history of atopy; IL-4 receptor mutation has been found in atopic families:[1] *Infection:* *Staph aureus* colonises lesions and Staph endotoxin known to act as super-antigen. *Allergens:* Animal dander often aggravates eczema and elevated IgE RAST is typical. *Diet:* A proportion of atopic children have significant food allergies, eg egg, fish, which can exacerbate eczema. Although infantile eczema is common, most children will grow out of it before the teenage years.

Treatment: Skin dryness is characteristic of eczema and the daily use of emollients is essential. Greasy emollients are best, eg emulsifying ointment, which can also be used as a soap substitute. Bath emollients help counteract the drying effects of bathing and a number now contain antiseptics in an attempt to reduce skin colonization with *Staph aureus*. Topical steroids may be required when eczema is active (red, weeping, itchy): ointment preparations are preferable to creams (1% hydrocortisone is suitable for use on the face; for the trunk and limbs, 1% hydrocortisone or clobetasone butyrate applied twice daily is usually adequate). Occasionally, short courses of more potent steroids are used for severe eczema. Overuse/abuse of topical steroids in children can lead to skin thinning, striae and adrenal suppression.

Irritant dermatitis: Everyone is prone to the effects of irritants although individuals have variable thresholds of susceptibility. Most frequently the hands are affected—redness and weeping is followed by dryness and fissuring. Common irritants include detergents, soaps, oils, solvents, alkalis and repeated exposure to water.

Treatment: Avoid all irritants if possible. Good hand care is essential (soap substitutes; regular use of emollients; careful drying of hands after exposure to water; use of cotton or cotton and rubber gloves for dry and wet work respectively; intermittent use of topical steroids for acute flare-ups).

Allergic contact dermatitis: Cutaneous type IV reaction. Common allergens include nickel (jewellery, watches, coins, keys etc.); chromates (cements, leather); lanolin (creams, cosmetics); colophony (sticking plasters, glues, inks); rubber (foam in furniture); plants (commonly primulas); topical antibiotics (neomycin, framycetin); topical antihistamines and topical anaesthetics (haemorrhoid creams). The pattern of contact often gives a clue to the allergen. There is often sharp cut-off where contact ends but secondary spread elsewhere is frequent (autosensitization).

Treatment: Diagnosis should be confirmed by patch testing; avoidance of allergens; topical steroid appropriate for severity of eczema, reduced and stopped as condition settles.

Adult seborrhoeic dermatitis: This common red, scaly eruption affects the scalp (dandruff), eyebrows, nasolabial folds, cheeks and flexures. Aetiology uncertain—some relationship to overgrowth of yeasts in skin. Can be very severe in HIV positive individuals.

Treatment: Mild topical steroid/anti-fungal preparations, eg Daktacort®; ketoconazole cream, lithium succinate ointment. Treatments required intermittently as condition tends to recur chronically.

1 GKK Hershey 1997 NEJM 337:1720

Helping children with eczema

Scratching is a constant feature, and a constant threat to the integument's integrity, but you cannot tell a child not to scratch. But you can *distract* the child, although this can no doubt seem like a full-time occupation.

Gently rubbing the skin is also said to be a help, as is daily filing of the nails and the wearing of mittens (or cotton tubular bandages) to prevent excoriation—but avoid over-heating. It can be a great relief to everyone when the child goes to sleep (although scratching may continue). To help sleep in a scratching child, experts may recommend higher doses of trimeprazine than are needed for antihistamine effects—eg 7.5–30mg for those aged 6–12 months and 10–50mg for those older than 1 year.

Note also the following, and discuss with child and parents as necessary:

- Infantile eczema gets better with time. Nature provides the light at the end of the tunnel—although asthma is often the next event along the line.
- Elimination diets rarely help, and may cause neurosis in the parents and nutritional deficit in the child. You cannot rely on skin or blood tests to find the minority who will benefit from avoiding dietary triggers.
- Other, possibly more important, triggers are dust mites and pets (does the child improve when on holiday?).

Preventing infantile eczema

In susceptible infants, ie those with a strong family history:

- Encourage the mother to breast feed.
- Consider reducing allergen exposure through breast milk by getting the mother to avoid all dairy products, eggs, fish, peanuts and soyabeans in her diet. Give her a daily calcium supplement (1g PO). Ensure that her overall diet is adequate.
- If breast feeding is impossible, many try soya milk (eg Wysoy®)—but this does not work. The most meticulously conducted blind trials show that a much better alternative is a milk in which the protein (casein) is hydrolysed (eg Nutramigen® or Pregestimil®).[1]

Diagnostic criteria for atopic eczema

Major:
- Pruritus
- Eczema on flexural surfaces
- Chronic dermatitis
- Personal/family history of atopy

Minor:
- 'Atopic fascies', eg pale face, hypopigmented patches, infraorbital darkening, infraorbital folds, cheilitis, recurrent conjunctivitis, anterior neck skin folds.
- Trigger factors: foods, emotion, environment, and skin irritants, such as wool, solvents, and sweat.
- Presence of atopic complications: susceptibility to skin infections, cell-mediated immunity↓, instant skin test reactivity, serum IgG↑, keratoconus, anterior subcapsular cataracts.
- Other: young at onset; dry skin, ichthyosis, keratosis pilaris (plugged hair follicles), hand/foot dermatitis, nipple eczema, white dermatographism, perifollicular accentuation, scalp scaling, skin fissures below ears.

Diagnosis depends on finding ≥3 major + 3 minor criteria.

Hanifin criteria

Skin infections

Fungi are eukaryotes with a differentiated nucleus and a rigid polysaccharide cell wall. They are heterotrophs (living off organic matter) and they do not photosynthesise. Cells form hyphae which interlace to form a mycelium. Arthrospores are the result of fragmenting hyphae. There are 5 genera which are important in skin mycoses: Microsporum, Epidermophyton, Trichophyton, Candida and Malassezia. The first 3 are moulds accounting for 90% of all fungal skin infections (also called ringworm or tinea). The production of proteolyic enzymes allow invasion of the skin, hair and nails. Commonly affected sites include: groins (tinea cruris), feet (tinea pedis), nails (tinea unguium) and scalp (tinea capitis). Zoophilic fungi (those which primarily affect animals) tend to cause more acute inflammation when infecting humans. Typically, *T rubrum* can be isolated from any site; *T mentagrophytes* from feet and nails; *T violaceum* and *T verrucosum* from the scalp; *E floccosum* from the groins and feet and *Microsporum audouinii* from the scalp.

Look for well-defined red lesions with peripheral scale and central clearing.

Yeasts are single-cell fungi which reproduce by budding. Malassezia furfur (*Pityrosporum orbiculare*) causes pityriasis versicolor (red/brown scaly lesions on the trunk which can appear either hyper- or hypopigmented, depending on the constitutive skin colour). *Candida albicans* is typically found in the mouth, vagina, around the nails, web-spaces and submammary areas. Infections are red, often moist, with satellite lesions.

Diagnosis: Microscopy (20% potassium hydroxide added to skin scrapings to dissolve keratin; hyphae can be observed). Samples for culture: skin should be cleaned with alcohol wipe to reduce bacterial contamination; scrapings taken from skin lesions; clippings from affected nails (plus material from under nail plate); plucked hairs from scalp lesions. Samples are best collected on black paper. Final results of cultures may take up to 6 weeks.

Treatment: Dermatophyte infection: *skin*—imidazole creams (eg clotrimazole) applied twice daily until 14 days after clinical cure; terbinafine cream—applied twice daily for 1–2 weeks. Widespread or severe infections should be treated with either drug orally. *Nail*—nail paints, eg 28% tioconazole, or amorolfine (5% lacquer, applied to the nail once or twice weekly and allowed to dry, continued for 3–6 months—or 9–12 months for toe fungi). Systemic treatment is often required to clear infection (3–6 months oral terbinafine (dose example: 250mg/24h PO). SE: arthralgia, myalgia, Stevens–Johnson syndrome, LFTs↑). An alternative is 2–3 cycles pulsed oral itraconazole.

Candidiasis: *skin*—imidazole creams; *nail*—pulsed oral itraconazole.

Moulds (eg Fusarium, Scopulariopsis): *nail*—nail paints; oral itraconazole may occasionally be of benefit. Avulsion may be required.

Pityriasis versicolor often responds to selenium sulfide 2.5% shampoo (Selsun®) applied neat to the rash with a cotton-wool ball (leave it to dry, and wash off in 24h; apply twice a week for 4 weeks; it may be reapplied once monthly if recurrence is a problem).

Bacteria *Impetigo:* Superficial *Staph aureus* infection, common in children and often starting around the nose and face. *Clinical features:* Honey-coloured crusts on erythematous base; lesions often well-defined and superficial flaccid blisters sometimes seen. *Treatment:* Topical fusidic acid, or systemic antibiotics (eg flucloxacillin 125mg/6h PO, in a child).

Erisipelas: Sharply defined superficial infection caused by streptococcus. Often affects the face (unilateral) or leg. Associated with fever, leukocytosis. *Treatment:* Systemic penicillin (see below).

Cellulitis: Deeper streptococcal infection, less well-defined than erisipelas and often affecting legs. Associated systemic upset and lymphadenopathy. Commonest organisms: *Streptococcus, Staph aureus*. *Treatment:* Systemic antibiotics, eg erythromycin 500mg/12h PO ± benzylpenicillin 600mg/6h IM (then penicillin V 250–500mg/4–6h PO, or co-amoxiclav, 1 tablet/8h PO).

Common viral infections of the skin

Warts Caused by human papillomavirus (HPV) infection of keratinocytes. Large numbers of lesions often seen in the immunosuppressed, eg transplant patients. *Common warts:* Most common in children and young adults; often resolve spontaneously but individual lesions can be stubbornly persistent. Treatment is destructive: topical salicylic acid paints (keratolytic); liquid nitrogen cryotherapy; stubborn lesions are occasionally treated with intralesional bleomycin or interferon; lasers.

Plantar warts: Large confluent lesions (mosaic warts) can be very resistant to repeated treatments. NB: warts are infectious and surgical excision is best avoided. Curettage can help to debulk large persistent warts.

Plane warts: Flat skin-coloured or brownish lesions; tend to Köbnerise (p 576) in scratch marks. They can be very resistant to treatment.

Genital warts (condylomata accuminata): Usually treated with cryotherapy and/or podophyllin (avoid in pregnancy: teratogenic risk). Also screen for other sexually transmitted diseases. Women with genital warts or female partners of men with genital warts should have a cervical smear carried out, eg yearly (HPV 16 & 18 strongly associated with cervical cancer).

Molluscum contagiosum Common childhood eruption caused by a poxvirus. *Signs:* Pink papules with central umbillicated punctum—whitish material can be expressed and examined microscopically to confirm the diagnosis (molluscum bodies). They will resolve spontaneously and no treatment is required. More common in atopic eczema.

Herpes simplex Primary infection is often subclinical. Most frequent clinical manifestation is gingivostomatitis. *Recurrent infection:* Is commonly genital or perioral. Triggered by fevers, sunlight, immunosuppression. Eruption often preceded by symptoms of burning/itching. *Signs:* Grouped painful vesicles on erythematous base which heal without scarring. *Treatment:* Often none required. Topical aciclovir may prevent or reduce severity of recurrences. Systemic treatment is indicated in certain circumstances (immunosuppressed; frequent recurrent genital herpes). There is evidence to suggest that Bell's palsy may be related to recurrent H simplex infection.

Herpes zoster (shingles) Primary infection is chickenpox (p 216). Varicella-zoster virus becomes dormant in the dorsal root ganglia. Recurrent infection affects one or more dermatomes (esp. immunosuppressed, in whom it may become generalized). Symptoms of pain and malaise may precede eruption. *Signs:* Polymorphic eruption (red papules, vesicles pustules and crusting). May heal with scarring and development of post-herpetic neuralgia. *Treatment:* Mild cases may not require treatment. More severe disease or infection in immunosuppressed requires early treatment with systemic treatment, eg aciclovir 800mg 5×/day PO for 7 days.

Acne vulgaris

This is an inflammatory disorder of the pilosebaceous follicle. It is almost universal amongst teenagers, affecting the face, neck, upper chest and back.

Cause *Comedone (blackhead) formation* this is the central abnormality in acne and is due to an abnormality of keratinization/desquamation within the follicle, leading to a blockage of secretions. *Excessive sebum production:* This occurs under the control of androgens. Most individuals with acne do not have excessive androgens but their sebaceous glands may be more sensitive to the actions of androgens. *Propionobacterium acnes: P acnes* is a normal skin commensal that flourishes in the anaerobic conditions within the blocked follicle. It is the inflammatory response to this bacterial proliferation which causes the typical inflamed lesions of acne.

Clinical features Comedones; red papules, pustules; sometimes nodules, cysts and scarring. Face, back and chest affected.

Differential diagnosis Acne rosacea—no comedones; diffuse redness of checks, nose, chin, forehead; telangestasia; flushing, especially after alcohol.

Management Dispel some of the myths about acne—it is NOT due to lack of washing, eating sweets/chocolate, etc. Treatment will depend on severity.

Mild acne (mainly comedones, mainly on the face): topical retinoids have specific anti-comedone activity and are the drug of choice, eg 0.01% tretinoin; 0.05% isotretinoin; adapalene gel. Benzoyl peroxide 2.5% is also useful (low concentration as effective as higher concentrations, which can be irritant).

Moderate acne (mainly inflammatory lesions, face ± chest, back): oral antibiotics are the mainstay of treatment—oxytetracycline 500mg/12h PO; erythromycin 500mg/12h PO. Courses should be 4–6 months minimum. To avoid development of bacterial resistance, benzoyl peroxide should be used along with oral antibiotics. If topical antibiotic used, this should be the same drug as is being given orally, to avoid multiple drug resistance. *Severe acne* (nodules, cysts, scarring): the synthetic retinoid isotretinoin is the drug of choice. It is usually given for 16 weeks at a dose of 0.5–1mg/kg/day. Highly significant improvements are seen in virtually all patients. 60–70% will have no further recurrences. Side-effects: teratogenic (sexually active women must use an effective form of contraception during and for 1 month after treatment); dryness of skin, lips, mucosae, myalgia, headache (benign intracranial hypertension reported); hepatitis; ↑ lipids.

Other possible indications for the use of isotretinoin now includes moderate acne which fails to respond to adequate course of antibiotics, the presence of scarring and severe psychological problems.[1]

Acne rosacea

A chronic relapsing and remitting facial disorder of unknown aetiology, particularly in fair-skinned individuals. Chronic flushing triggered by alcohol, spicy foods etc. often precedes the development of fixed erythema (chin, nose, cheeks, forehead), telangiectasia, papules, and pustules. In males, rhinophyma (swelling and soft tissue overgrowth of the nose) may occur. Recurrent severe flares can lead to the development of lymphoedema. Eye problems commonly associated—blepharitis (scaling and irritation at base of eyelashes); conjunctivitis; rarely, keratitis. *Management:* Avoid irritants, excessive sun exposure. Topical metronidazole can effectively control mild to moderate disease. Oral tetracyclines often the mainstay of treatment, eg oytetracycline 500mg/12h PO, in an acne-type regimen. Once skin settled, antibiotics can be discontinued and restarted as required. (NB: long-term use of minocycline can cause blue/grey pigmentation of exposed sites and, very rarely, hepatitis).

1 AM Layton, WJ Cunliffe 1992 *J Am Acad Dermatol* 27 S2-7

Drug eruptions

It is estimated that 10–20% of hospital patients develops a drug eruption during their admission. It is therefore important to be aware of drugs which frequently cause problems and understand the principles of management of the problem. Drug eruptions can be classified according to various criteria, eg immunological (IgE type I response to penicillin) or non-immunological (teratogenicity from retinoids); histological features, eg lichenoid; clinical features.

Types of clinical reaction *Maculopapular/exanthematous:* This is the most frequent type of cutaneous drug eruption. *Clinical features:* Macular erythema and red papules, particularly affecting trunk. There may be associated fever and eosinophilia. *Drugs:* Penicillins; cefalosporins; anti-epileptics.

Urticaria: Clinical features: Raised itchy red weals with pale centres; rapid onset after drug ingestion. May be associated with angio-oedema/anaphylaxis. This can result from both immunological and non-immunological mechanisms. *Drugs:* Morphine, codeine and other opioids cause direct mast cell degranulation; penicillins and cefalosporins trigger IgE responses; NSAIDs; ACE inhibitors.

Exfoliative dermatitis: Signs: Widespread erythema and dermatitis; erythroderma. *Drugs:* Sulfonamides; allopurinol; carbamazepine; gold; phenytoin.

Erythema multiforme major (Stevens–Johnson syndrome): The more severe variants of erythema multiforme are usually due to drugs. *Clinical features:* Targetoid plaques and polymorphic erythema, sometimes blistering; mucosae (conjunctivae, oral and labial, genital) severely affected. *Drugs:* Sulfonamides.

Toxic epidermal necrolysis: This may represent the extreme end of the erythema multiforme/Stevens–Johnson syndrome spectrum of reaction. *Signs:* Widespread erythema followed by epidermal necrosis with loss of large sheets of epidermis. Mucosae severely affected. This has a high mortality rate (>30%). This is best managed in specialist dermatology or burns unit. *Drugs:* Sulfonamides; anticonvulsants; penicillins; allopurinol; NSAIDs.

Lichenoid: Clinical features: There are clinical features which show some similarity to lichen planus but are rarely typical of idiopathic lichen planus. *Drugs implicated:* β-blockers; thiazides; gold; antimalarials.

Management A clear history of the onset and duration of the rash is essential. A previous history of skin problems or cutaneous drug reactions should be sought. *All* drugs taken (currently or previously) should be recorded, including over-the-counter preparations (laxatives, analgesics, herbal remedies etc.). If the clinical findings are suggestive of a drug eruption, the rash should be classified clinically and the most likely offender identified and discontinued immediately, if possible. If the clinical diagnosis is in doubt, a prick test[1] or skin biopsy may be helpful but is not always so. In order to confirm the suspicion of drug sensitivity, some advocate rechallenge with the suspected drug once the patient has recovered. Whilst this is the ideal situation, rechallenge may be dangerous (eg anaphylaxis, erythroderma). Not unreasonably, patients may also object to this.

Many drug rashes need no further intervention. Symptoms such as dryness or mild itch may be helped by the regular use of emollients. More itchy rashes, eg lichenoid or dermatitic, may require a short course of topical steroids. Urticaria should be treated promptly with an antihistamine + IV hydrocortisone/IM epinephrine (=adrenaline, p 303) if anaphylaxis. More severe eruptions, eg erythema multiforme are best managed by specialists. There is debate as to the efficacy of oral prednisolone in both of these conditions. As these drugs can potentially adversely affect outcome (eg ↑risk of infection, hypertension, fluid retention, diabetes, etc.) their use should be determined by specialists.

1 D Vervloet 1998 *BMJ* i 1511

Miscellaneous skin disorders

Lichen planus This is an itchy disorder (cause unknown), occurring at any age (uncommon in the very young and old). Reported association with hepatitis C virus infection in some European countries (doesn't appear to be a significant factor in the UK). *Clinical features:* The eruption consists of flat-topped purple papules with white lacy markings on the surface (known as Wickhams striae). The flexor aspects of the wrists, forearms, ankles and legs are commonly affected. Typical lesions at other sites include scalp (scarring alopecia), nails (longitudinal ridges), mouth (lacy white areas on inner cheeks) and genitals (annular lesions). Lesions often arise at sites of trauma. Usually persists for 6–18 months. Treatment is symptomatic: moderate to potent topical steroids are helpful for severe itch. Occasionally, severe disease warrants the use of oral steroids.

Haemangiomas *Strawberry naevus:* This occurs in infants in the first months of life. The lesion begins as a small red spot which rapidly enlarges over the following few months and then remains static in size. Most will spontaneously involute at the age of 5–7 years. No treatment is required unless vital function is impaired, eg obscuring vision.

Pyogenic granuloma: This is a lesion which is thought to arise as a result of minor trauma, typically occurring on fingers. It appears a moist red lesion which grows rapidly and often bleeds easily. *Treatment:* Curettage.

Pityriasis rosea This is quite common, typically affecting young adults perhaps caused by HHV-7 (herpes hominis virus 7). The rash is preceded by a herald patch (ovoid red scaly patch with a prominent scaly edge, similar to but rather larger than subsequent lesions). Tends to affect the neck, trunk and proximal limbs. It is self-limiting; no treatment is needed.

Alopecia Hair loss is classified as scarring or non-scarring. Non-scarring causes may be reversible but scarring alopecia results in an irreversible loss. Disorders of the scalp/hair may be manifestations of skin disease elsewhere: look for evidence of this (eg lichen planus, SLE).

Non-scarring alopecia: *nutritional* (iron deficiency; zinc deficiency rarely); *androgenetic* (men & women); *autoimmune* (alopecia areata: smooth round patches of hair loss on scalp; hairs like exclamation marks are a typical feature; often spontaneously regrows; total scalp hair loss = alopecia totalis; total body hair loss = alopecia universalis); *telogen effluvium* (shedding of telogen phase hairs after period of stress, eg childbirth, surgery, severe illness). Treatment of alopecia areata is difficult: topical or intralesional steroids have been tried, as have minoxidil and dinitrochlorobenzene.

Scarring alopecia: *lichen planus*; *discoid lupus erythematosus*; *trauma*.

Blistering disorders There are many causes of blisters, some of which require prompt systemic drugs (try to recognise these early): *infection* (eg herpes); *insect bites* (usually groups on the legs); *drugs* (ACE inhibitors; frusemide; barbiturates); *trauma/friction*; *autoimmune blistering disorders*, eg *pemphigoid*, affecting those ≥60yrs and is due to IgG autoantibodies against components of the basement membrane (bullous pemphigoid antigens 1 & 2). *Signs of pemphigoid:* Tense blisters on an urticated base. Skin biopsy: (+ve immunofluorescence; linear IgG and C3 along the basement membrane). *Treatment:* Predisolone, eg 30–40mg/day PO initially.

Pemphigus affects a younger people than pemphigoid (>40yrs) and is due to IgG autoantibodies against desmosomal components (desmoglein 1 & 3). *Signs:* Flaccid blisters which rupture easily to leave widespread erosions. The oral mucosa is often affected early. Diagnosis is confirmed by skin biopsy with positive immunofluorescence (intercellular IgG giving a 'crazy-paving' effect). *Treatment:* Prednisolone (60–80mg/day PO), which may have to be continued, in reduced dosage, life-long.

Photosensitivity

Photosensitivity describes conditions which are triggered by exposure to light (eg solar urticaria; polymorphic light eruption). Photoaggrevation describes disorders which may be worsened by light but are not due to abnormal sensitivity to light (eg recurrent herpes labialis). Photosensitivity can be examined by assessing erythemal response to light of a certain wavelength and comparing responses to the normal range. Photosensitivity can occur to visible light, UVA (320–400nm) or UVB (290–320nm).

Some photosensitivity disorders *Polymorphic light eruption:* This is a common idiopathic disorder typically affecting young women. During the spring, following light exposure, itchy red papules, vesicles and plaques develop on exposed sites, often improving over the summer months due to a phenomenon called 'hardening'. *Treatment:* Sun-avoidance; sun-protection (high factor UVA + UVB sunscreens); desensitization by phototherapy.

Porphyria cutanea tarda: Susceptibility to this is associated with certain alleles of the haemochromatosis gene. The primary abnormality is reduced function of the liver enzyme uroporphyrinogen decarboxylase. In the acquired form, a hepatotoxic agent such as alcohol, oestrogens, hepatitis C virus, and HIV infection triggers the development of symptoms and signs. Clinical features include photosensitivity, hypertrichosis, hyperpigmentation and skin fragility and scarring (milia). Investigations: ↑LFTs: ↑ferritin; ↑urine, plasma, and faecal porphyrins. *Management:* Remove possible precipitants; sun-avoidance; sun-protection; regular venesection until ferritin within normal range.

Systemic lupus erythematosus (SLE): SLE is frequently associated with photosensitivity. Light exposure may trigger erythematous eruptions and cause a systemic flare. A variant of lupus, subacute LE, is associated with marked photosensitivty and the presence of Ro antibodies.

Drug-induced photosensitivity: Drugs are a leading cause of photosensitivity. Frequent offenders include thiazides (sunburn-like or lichenoid eruptions); tetracyclines (sunburn-like eruptions); sulfonamides (sunburn-like eruptions); phenothiazines (dermatitic eruption); NSAIDs; amiodarone (sunburn-like eruptions). After withdrawal of the offending drug, photosensitivity make take a number of months to settle (esp. after thiazides).

Sunscreens The SPF (sun protection factor) indicates how much longer an individual can be exposed to sunshine without burning, eg SPF8 means that an individual can stay out in the sun 8 times longer than the time it would normally take them to burn. This time will vary depending on the individual's skin type. The SPF refers only to UVB protection. Many sunscreens now contain UVA-blocking agents. These are graded on a 'star-rating', which as yet, is not internationally standardized.

Sunscreens protect either by physically blocking out light (physical agents, eg titanium dioxide) or by absorbing light by means of a photochemical reaction (eg benzophenones; cinnamates). Regardless of the mechanism of action, sunscreens must be regularly applied to all exposed areas (face; back and V of neck; dorsum of hands; legs).

Skin disorders in old age

Leg ulceration There are many causes of leg ulceration. By far the commonest is *venous ulceration*. This arises from venous hypertension as a result of damage to the valves of the deep venous system (eg 2° to DVT). Venous hypertension leads to the development of superficial varicosities and skin changes (lipodermatosclerosis = induration, pigmentation and inflammation of the skin of the lower leg). Minimal trauma to the leg leads to ulceration which often takes many months to heal. *Management:* The only effective treatment is compression, ideally in community leg ulcer clinics.[1] Topical dressings for ulcers are of no proven benefit in healing and the ulcerated area need only be covered with a non-adherent/non-macerating dressing. Varicose eczema, which is often seen around ulcers, should be treated with emollients and a short course of moderately potent topical steroids. Patch testing should be considered if the eczema fails to respond to these measures. Venous leg ulcers are invariably colonised by bacteria and this does not require treatment ***unless*** the organism is Streptococcus or Pseudomonas *or* there are clear signs of cellulitis/infection (↑pain and tenderness, fever, erythema or lymphangitis). Four-layer compression bandaging should be applied by trained nursing staff, to produce a pressure of 40mmHg at the ankle. Doppler should be carried out prior to this to exclude arterial disease (make sure the ankle–brachial pressure index is >0.8, *OHCM* p 128). Ulcers which have not healed despite adequate treatment for 3 months should be investigated further (eg biopsy to exclude malignancy). Once the ulcer has been healed, compression hosiery should always be worn. Grade III stockings are the ideal but many find them uncomfortable—Grade II are a reasonable compromise. Other causes of lower leg ulceration include peripheral vascular disease (pale cold leg, shiny atrophic skin, absent pulses); neuropathic ulceration (most commonly due to diabetes and seen on the pressure areas of the foot); pyoderma gangrenosum (rheumatoid arthritis; Crohns/ulcerative colitis; idiopathic); trauma; vasculitis (systemic lupus, rheumatoid arthritis).

Asteatotic eczema This is common in the elderly, and particularly affects the lower legs. The skin is dry and eczema is seen in a 'crazy-paving' pattern. The main treatment is the use of emollients and soap substitutes.

Pruritus This is not an uncommon complaint amongst the elderly and there are many potential causes. *Primary skin disorders: Eczema*; *scabies* (can have an atypical clinical appearance in the elderly); *pemphigoid* and *pre-pemphigoid eruptions*; *asteatotic eczema*; *generalized xerosis*. *Underlying medical conditions*: *Anaemia*; *polycythaemia*; *lymphoma*; *solid neoplasms*; *hepatic* and *renal failure*; *hypo-* and *hyperthyroidism*; *diabetes (candidiasis)*. In the absence of a primary skin disorder, these should be excluded by appropriate investigations.

Pressure sores If made immobile by age, or CNS problems (stroke, cord lesions or multiple sclerosis), uninterrupted pressure on an area of skin may lead to ulceration, and extensive, painful, subcutaneous destruction—eg on the sacrum, heel, or greater trochanter. Malnutrition (esp. protein), arteriopathy, and old age make the condition more likely to occur, particularly if nursing care is wanting. They are a big problem. Cost: UK £750 million/yr; USA $3 billion/yr.[1] A full-thickness sacral sore extends hospital stay by >25 weeks, and costs £26,000. ►This should make prevention a central preoccupation, not just on long-stay geriatric wards, but in *all* acute adult wards—where most pressure sores start.

Staging *Stage I:* Non-blanching erythema over intact skin.
Stage II: Partial thickness skin loss, eg shallow crater.
Stage III: Full thickness skin loss, extending into fat.
Stage IV: Destruction of muscle, bone, or tendons.

Prevalence ~7% of inpatients have pressure sores; >70% are over 70 years old. Up to 85% of paraplegic patients have pressure sores.

Complications Osteomyelitis; pyoarthrosis.

Treatment and prevention of pressure sores

- Prevent the condition getting worse (see below).
- Improve nutrition. Insulin if hyperglycaemic.
- Treat systemic infection with antibiotics.
- Dress the area. There is no convincing evidence from randomized trials which favours any one type of dressing.
- Vascular reconstruction, if needed, and if practicable.
- Split thickness skin grafts.
- Neurosensory myocutaneous flap surgery.[2]

Prevention

- Find an interested, knowledgeable nurse to educate the patient.
- Proper positioning, with regular turning (eg every 2h, see p 726 & p 732, alternating between supine, and right or left lateral position). Use pillows to separate the legs.
- Functional electrical stimulation can prevent sores in paraplegics, by inducing the buttocks to change shape, and by improving blood flow.[3]
- A good randomized trial (*N*=44 patients aged ~85yrs with hip fracture) showed that a DeCube® mattress with removable cubes for provision of rest for pressure points can halve the incidence of pressure sores.[4]

1 C Morrell 1998 BMJ i 1487 & A Fletcher BMJ 1997 **315** 576–80 2 R Vohra 1994 BMJ ii 853
3 A Furguson 1992 *Paraplegia* **30** 474 [4] A Hofman 1994 *Lancet* **343** 568

Skin disorders in HIV disease

There are many cutaneous manifestations of HIV disease, due to both infectious and non-infectious conditions. With the introduction of the protease inhibitor group of drugs and the advent of early treatment with triple therapy regimens, it is likely that some of the conditions described below will become less common in the HIV positive population.

Infections: HIV positive individuals are more prone not only to infections common in the general population but also to infections with organisms which do not usually cause disease in immunocompetent individuals (commensal organisms). In an HIV positive patient, any new lesion should be considered as possibly due to infection with an unusual organism.

HIV: Seroconversion is associated with an acute mononucleosis type illness, usually accompanied by a non-specific maculopapular eruption affecting the upper trunk, associated with lymphadenopathy, malaise, headache and fever.

Oral candidiasis: This may be severe and resistant to treatment. Infection may extend to involve the posterior pharynx and oesophagus. *Treatment:* topical nystatin; systemic imidazoles.

Molluscum contagiosum: Lesions tend to develop on the face and genitals. Management can be difficult: cryotherapy, topical retinoids, cautery and curettage may be tried. *Differential diagnosis:* Disseminated cryptococcosis.

Herpes simplex virus infection: This can be increasingly troublesome as HIV progresses. Painful ulcers and erosions develop, particularly around the mouth and genitals. Any ulcerated or eroded area should be considered as HSV until proven otherwise. *Management:* High-dose aciclovir (oral or IV). Aciclovir resistance may develop and foscarnet is an alternate treatment.

Varicella zoster: This may occur early in HIV, with atypical presentation. Complications such as ulceration and post-herpetic neuralgia appear to be more frequent and severe. In advanced disease, disseminated infection occurs. *Treatment:* High-dose aciclovir (IV if systemic disease).

Cryptococcosis: Lesions can be very similar to molluscum contagiosum, affecting the face. *Treatment:* Fluconazole; amphoteracin B.

Scabies: Severe variants, eg crusted scabies are more common in advanced HIV disease. Paradoxically, patients may not complain of severe itch. A widespread scaly, crusted eruption occurs (highly infectious). *Treatment:* Permethrin lotion. Ivermectin may also be of benefit (but side-effects may be serious).

Oral hairy leukoplakia: This entails Epstein–Barr virus infection of oral mucosa. Adherent white plaques are seen on the lateral aspects of the tongue. *Treatment:* Topical retinoic acid; podophyllin.

Inflammatory disorders Despite the immunosupression associated with HIV disease, inflammatory cutaneous conditions occur frequently.

Seborrhoeic dermatitis: This is common in the later stages of HIV; it may be widespread and severe. Red scaly patches typically affect the face (hair-bearing areas and nasolabial folds), scalp and flexures. *Treatment:* Topical (occasionally systemic) imidazoles.

Psoriasis: Treatment: Standard therapies (tar; dithranol; calcipotriol; UV). Treatment of HIV will often improve psoriasis.

Eosinophilic folliculitis: The aetiology of this condition is unknown and it occurs frequently as HIV progresses. Itchy follicular papules and pustules affect the face, chest and back. Treatments are often unsatisfactory but include topical steroids; phototherapy; antihistamines.

Drug reactions: These occur more commonly in HIV patients and particular culprits include co-trimoxazole (maculopapular eruptions; erythema multiforme; toxic epidermal necrolysis); dapsone; foscarnet (ulceration); zidovudine (nail + mucosal pigmentation).

Neoplasia and HIV

HIV disease is associated with a significantly increased risk of certain types of malignancy, eg lymphoma, cervical carcinoma. Common skin cancers (eg basal cell carcinomas) are also seen with HIV.

Kaposi's sarcoma (KS): Although first identified in HIV +ve homosexuals, there is evidence to suggest that HHV-8 (herpes hominis virus) is associated with KS in both HIV positive and negative populations. The condition arises most frequently arises in advanced HIV disease. *Clinical features:* Purplish macules, papules, nodules and plaques affecting the feet, legs, face and oral mucosa. *Differential diagnosis:* Bacillary angiomatosis (*Bartonella* species); pyogenic granuloma. *Treatment:* Cryotherapy; intralesional vincristine; radiotherapy; treatment of HIV disease (protease inhibitors).

Infestations

Scabies (*Sarcoptes scabei*) This is a common disorder particularly aff children and young adults, and tends to spread within families or those i in close contact. The eruption is a reaction to the saliva/faeces of the fen mite. *Clinical features:* Markedly itchy papular eruption affecting the finge webs (esp. first), wrist flexures, axillae, abdomen (esp. around umbilicus anc waistband area), buttocks and groins (itchy red penile or scrotal papules are virtually diagnostic). In young infants, the palms and soles are characteristically involved. The eruption is usually excoriated and becomes eczematized. Scabies mites can sometimes be extracted from burrows and visualized microscopically; eggs can be visualized from skin scrapings. *Management:* A good explanation (verbal + written) will aid concordance between the patient's and the doctor's requirements, and will promote the chances of successful cure. A suitable anti-scabetic should be prescribed (malathion, permethrin). Preparations are applied to all areas of the skin, from the neck down for 24h. Areas which are washed during this period (eg hands) should have treatment re-applied. **ALL** members of a household should be treated, including those who are asymptomatic. The rash and symptom of itch will take a few weeks to settle, occasionally longer. A suitable anti-pruritic such as crotamiton cream (which also has anti-scabetic activity) can be useful during this period. *Example of written advice:*

- Take a warm bath and soap the skin all over.
- Scrub the fingers and nails with a firm brush. Dry your body.
- Apply malathion 0.5% liquid (Derbac-M®, not if pregnant or <6 months old) from the neck down (include the head in those <2yrs old). Remember to paint *all* parts, including the soles.
- Wash off after 24 hours. If you wash your hands before the 24 hours is up, reapply the liquid to the parts you have washed.
- Use fresh pillow cases and sheets, if you have any.
- Treatment may worsen itch for 2 weeks—so use calamine lotion.
- Warnings: avoid the eyes.

Note: one or two doses of ivermectin 200μg/kg PO may be effective in recalcitrant scabies (eg with HIV)—but side-effects may be serious.

Headlice (*Pediculus humanus capitis*) This is a common problem among schoolchildren, with lice being spread by head to head contact. The louse is 3mm long and has legs adapted to cling onto hair shafts. The eggs (nits) are bound firmly to the scalp hairs and when empty appear white. *Clinical features:* Itch and a papular eruption on the nape of the neck are common. *Management:* Resistance to treatment has become a problem and many health boards operate a rotation policy of treatments. Sometimes the only option is meticulous combing (after applying conditioner to the hair).

Crab lice (*Phthiriasis pubis*) These are usually sexually transmitted and affect the pubic hairs. The eyebrows, eyelashes and axillae may also be involved. *Management:* Topical malathion to all affected (or potentially affected) areas. Evidence of other sexually transmitted disease should be sought. All sexual contacts should also be treated.

Flea* bites (*Pulicidae*) spread plague, typhus, Q fever, tape worm, Lyme disease, and listeria . The animal (eg cat or dog) which spreads the flea may not itch or scratch itself. Treatment: Aqueous malathion lotion. Note that so often when we say to our patients that they are suffering from phlebitis they assume, with alarm, that this 'flea-bite-is' denotes flea infestation, and are too embarrassed to contradict our diagnosis, and it is left to the vet to explain everything when the family pet tuns up for an unnecessary de-fleaing.

The flea

Mark but this flea, and mark in this
How little that which thou deny'st me is;
Me it suck'd first, and now sucks thee,
And in this flea our two bloods mingled be;
Confess it; this cannot be said
A sin, or shame, or loss of maidenhead,
Yet this enjoys before it woo,
And pamper'd swells with one blood made two,
And this, alas, is more than we can do.
Oh stay, three lives in one flea spare,
Where we almost, nay more than married are:
This flea is you and I, and this
Our marriage bed, and marriage temple is…

John Donne, to his lover

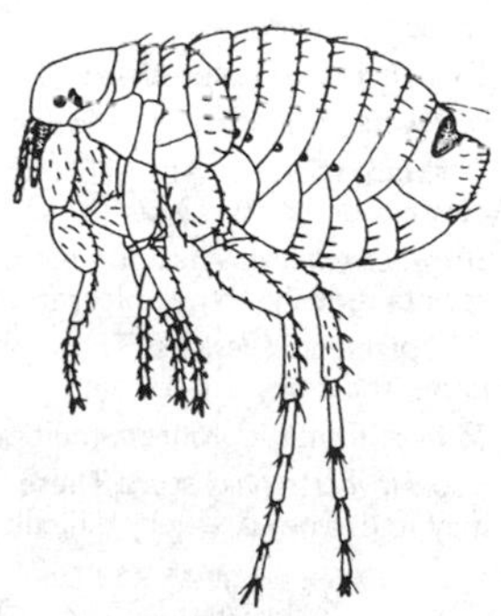

Mast cell disorders

Mastocytosis (urticaria pigmentosa) There are too many mast cells in the skin, eg in numerous nests or as a single mastocytoma. These release histamine, leucotrienes, and heparin (which may have systemic effects) and proteases (which have a local effect).

Presentation: This is unpredictable, and symptoms need not be progressive—but there may be progressive myeloproliferation/mast-cell leukaemia. Systemic forms can occur with no skin signs. In babies and other patients there may be blisters or pigmented swellings, which swell when scratched (or after a bath, or on exercise). In older patients, there may be flushing or itching. Systemic mast cell infiltration may produce:

- Splenomegaly
- Thrombocytopenia
- Bleeding disorders
- Osteoporosis
- Osteosclerosis
- Colic
- Diarrhoea
- Right heart failure
- Pulmonary hypertension
- Leukaemic mastocytosis

Tests: Urinary histamine may be ↑ (helps if no skin signs). Labs may also report *N*′-methylhistamine (MH) and *N*′-methylimidazoleacetic acid (MIMA).

Differential diagnoses: Legion—eg idiopathic facial flushing syndrome.

Treatment: This is difficult. H_1 and H_2 antagonists may be helpful. Single skin lesions can be excised. Disodium cromoglycate may help some patients with systemic symptoms.[1]

Lasers in dermatology*

Lasers (light amplification by stimulated emission of radiation) have an increasing rôle, and it is worth knowing who may benefit from them. The destructive energy of lasers can be concentrated in time and space, and the light's wavelength can be adjusted to match the target lesion. Energy can be selectively taken up by targets as long as the volume delivered is less than the target's capacity to absorb it. If this limit is exceeded, unnecessary destruction is caused. Variables to specify—an example from treating keloid scars: wavelength 585nm, pulse duration 0.45msec, spot size 5mm, mean fluence per pulse 7 Joules/cm^2, treatment interval: 6 weeks.[2] NB: melanin in dark skins may be a problematic competing chromophore.

Photoacoustic damage is produced by shock waves from very intense energy delivered over picoseconds.

Photocoagulation implies less rapid, and less intense treatment.

Selective photothermolysis is somewhere between the above 2 categories. It may produce minimum scarring. Modification of the duration of delivery is possible (Q-switching and mode-locking).

Examples of laser-treatable skin disorders[3]

Port wine stain: Best treated when young (smaller, smoother lesions).

Tuberous sclerosis: Angiofibromata (misnamed adenoma sebaceum) can cover much of the face.

Strawberry naevi: These do *not* need treatment, unless they fail to resolve spontaneously. If they ulcerate, get expert advice.[3]

Flat, pigmented lesions: These are problematic because it is essential to know that they are benign.

Tattoos: If multicoloured, multiple wavelengths must be used.

Keloid (hypertrophic) scars: These raised, red, nodular scars are unsightly, and may itch. They are very difficult to treat, but lasers can help somewhat.[2]

1 *J Dermatol Surg* 1993 **19** 295 2 T Alster 1995 *Lancet* **345** 1198 3 Disfigurement Guidance Centre, Cupar, Fife, Scotland (UK tel. 01337 870281). *We thank Dr Ian Comaish for inspiring this topic.

9. Orthopaedics and A&E

Relevant pages in other chapters Any medical or surgical illness from the acute abdomen to zoster may present to casualty. So every page here and in *OHCM* has relevance to the casualty officer. ►See *Prehospital care* (p 780–806); *Radiology* (*OHCM* p 714–49). Childhood poisoning, p 252–4; (adults, *OHCM* p 790–6). ***Orthopaedics on the internet:*** *http://www.worldortho.com* and a textbook: *http://www.medmedia.com/med.htm*; for images see: *http://www.njnet.com/~embbs/xray//xr.html*.

►Many detailed treatments are described in this chapter, and it is not envisaged that the inexperienced casualty officer will try them out except under appropriate supervision. The importance of enlisting early expert help (either at once or, if appropriate, by calling the patient back to the next morning's registrar clinic) cannot be overemphasized.

The neck

Examination ►►After trauma, the neck must be immobilized ie with rigid collar, sandbags and tape, until a lateral cervical spine x-ray has been seen (except if very restless—use hard collar only, as otherwise the neck is vulnerable when the body moves on an immobilized head).

The posture of the neck and any bone tenderness are noted. The range of movements: flexion; extension (mainly occipito-atlantoid joint); rotation (mainly atlanto-axial joint); lateral flexion (whole of cervical spine). Rotation is the movement most commonly affected. The arms are examined for weakness that might signify root lesions (shoulder abduction C5; elbow flexion C5, 6; elbow extension C6, 7; wrist extension C6, 7; wrist flexion C7, 8; grip and abduction of fingers against resistance T1). Reflexes are examined: biceps C5, 6; supinator C5, 6; triceps C7. Dermatomes are illustrated on p 665. If cord compression is suspected examine lower limbs for signs of this (see p 608)—eg upgoing plantars, hyperreflexia.

Spasmodic torticollis Sudden onset of a stiff painful neck with torticollis may occur in adults due to spasm of the trapezius and sternocleidomastoid muscles. *Treatment:* The condition is self-limiting but heat, manipulation, muscle relaxants, and analgesia may ease resolution. If severe, wearing a collar may help initial discomfort, although it can prolong symptoms.

Infantile torticollis Thought to be a result of damage during birth to the sternocleidomastoid, affected children present (between 6 months and 3 years) with a tilted head (ear nearer shoulder on affected side). There is retarded facial growth on the affected side, hence facial asymmetry. Early, there is a tumour-like thickening in the muscle. *Treatment:* If this persists, physiotherapy to lengthen the muscle may help. Later treatment involves division of the muscle at its lower end.

Cervical rib Congenital development of the costal process of the C7 vertebra is often asymptomatic but may cause thoracic outlet compression. Similar symptoms without demonstrable radiological abnormality is called a scalenus or first rib syndrome. Thoracic outlet compression involves the lowest trunk of the brachial plexus (p 724) and the subclavian artery. Pain or numbness may be felt in hand or forearm (often on the ulnar side), there may be hand weakness and muscle wasting (thenar or hypothenar). *Diagnosis:* Radial pulses may be weak and the forearm cyanosed. X-rays may not reveal cervical ribs, as symptoms may be caused by fibrous bands. Arteriography will show subclavian compression. *Treatment:* Physiotherapy to strengthen the shoulder elevators may improve symptoms, but rib removal or band division may be needed.

Prolapsed cervical disc Those between C5,6 and C6,7 are most commonly affected. Central protrusions may give symptoms of spinal cord compression (p 608; refer to neurosurgeon). Posterolateral protrusions may cause a stiff neck, pain radiating to the arm, weakness of muscles affected by the nerve root, and depressed reflexes. *Tests:* X-rays may show disc narrowing; also CT or MRI scan. *Treatment* is with NSAIDs, and a collar. As pain subsides, physiotherapy may help to restore mobility. Surgery may be indicated, in the light of CT and MRI findings.

Cervical spine

In major trauma, the first x-ray to be performed after resuscitation is a cross-table lateral of the cervical spine. All seven cervical vertebrae must be seen, along with the C7–T1 junction: do not accept an incomplete x-ray—try traction on the arms, or a swimmer's view. Occasionally subluxations do not show up without flexion and extension views (perform only on the advice of a senior colleague).

►If a cervical spine injury is suspected you must immobilize the neck until it is excluded.

►A cross-table portable in the best hands will miss ≤15% of injuries.

When examining the film, follow 4 simple steps:

1 *Alignment:* Of anterior and posterior vertebral body, posterior spinal canal and spinous processes. A step of <25% of a vertebral body implies unifacet dislocation; if >50% it is bifacetal. 40% of those <7yrs have anterior displacement of C2 on C3 (pseudosubluxation); still present in 20% up to 16yrs. 15% show this with C3 on C4. In this physiological subluxation, the posterior spinal line is maintained. Angulation between vertebrae >10% is abnormal.

2 *Bone contour:* Trace around each vertebra individually. Look for avulsion fractures of the body or spinous process. A wedge fracture is present if the anterior height differs from posterior by >3mm. Check odontoid (open mouth view but can be seen on lateral view); don't mistake vertical cleft between incisors for a peg fracture!)—epiphyses in children can be mistaken for fractures; the distance between the odontoid and anterior arch of C1 should be <3mm (may be increased in children). Type 1 fractures are of the odontoid peg, type 2 of its base, and type 3 fractures extend into the body of C2.

3 *Cartilages:* Check that intervertebral disc space margins are parallel.

4 *Soft tissues:* If the space between the lower anterior border of C3 and the pharyngeal shadow is >5mm suspect retropharyngeal swelling (haemorrhage; abscess)—this is often useful indirect evidence of a C2 fracture. Space between lower cervical vertebrae and trachea should be <1 vertebral body.

The neck and cord compression

Cervical spondylosis (See *OHCM* p 468.)

Cervical spondylolisthesis

This is displacement of one vertebra upon the one below. *Causes:*

1 Congenital failure of fusion of odontoid process with the axis or fracture of the odontoid process (skull, atlas and odontoid process slip forward on axis).

2 Inflammation softens the transverse ligament of atlas (eg rheumatoid or complicating throat infections), the atlas slips forward upon the axis.

3 Instability after injuries. The most important consequence of spondylolisthesis is the possibility of spinal cord compression. Treatments used include traction, immobilization in plaster jackets and spinal fusion.

Spinal cord compression

Pressure on the cord may be due to bone displacement or collapse, disc prolapse, local tumour or abscess. Root pain (p 618) and lower motor neurone signs occur at the level of the lesion with upper motor neurone signs and sensory changes below the lesion (spastic weakness, brisk reflexes, upgoing plantars, and loss of co-ordination, joint position sense, vibration sense, temperature and pain). Cord anatomy is such that dorsal column sensibilities (light touch, joint position sense, vibration sense) are affected on the same side as the insult, but spinothalamic tract interruption affects pain and temperature sensation for the opposite side of the body 2–3 dermatome levels lower than the affected sensory level. As the cord ends at L1, compression at this vertebral level affects information in the cord relating to a lower dermatome. To determine the cord level affected behind a given vertebra, add the number in red to that of the vertebra concerned, thus: C2–7: **+1**. T1–6: **+2**. T7–9: **+3**. T10 has L1 and L2 levels behind it; T11 has L3 and 4, L1 has sacral and coccygeal segments.

Lower lumbar problems can cause cauda equina compression characterized by muscular pain, dermatomal sensory changes (if the lowest sacral dermatomes are affected the genitals are anaesthetic), and retention of urine and faeces. ►These signs indicate urgent neurosurgical referral.

9. Orthopaedics

The shoulder

Anatomically, this glenohumeral joint is lax, depending on surrounding rotator cuff muscles for stability—ie the sheath of tendons of supraspinatus (first 15–30° of abduction), subscapularis (internal rotation) infraspinatus (lateral rotation), and teres major (lateral rotation + extension). Biceps' long head traverses the cuff, attaching to the top of the glenoid cavity.

History Any trauma, arthritis or neck problems? Is pain sharp (eg capsulitis) or dull (eg osteoarthrosis)? Does movement make it worse (eg trauma, impingement, or, eg if young, dislocation). General health OK? (if aches and pains all over, suspect fibromyalgia, or polymyalgia).

Examination Strip to the waist. To assess glenohumeral movement, hold the lower half of the scapula to estimate degrees of scapular rotation over the thorax. Half the range of normal abduction is achieved by scapula movement. *Abduction* is tested by raising the hands from the sides sideways to above the head; *flexion* by raising hands forwards and upwards; *extension* by backward movement of the elbows; *external rotation* by holding the elbows against the sides flexed at 90° and moving the hands outwards (normal 80°); and *internal rotation* by placing the back of the hand against the lumbar spine and moving the elbows forward (an easier test is to assess how far behind his back the patient can reach—'imagine you are doing up a bra at the back').

The muscles used for movement at the shoulder joint

- Flexion (forward movement): pectoralis major, deltoid, coracobrachialis.
- Extension: deltoid (latissimus dorsi, pectoralis major and teres major begin the extension if the shoulder starts out flexed).
- Abduction: supraspinatus (for first 15°); deltoid thereafter.
- Adduction: pectoralis major, latissimus dorsi, teres major, subscapularis.
- Medial rotation: pectoralis major, deltoid, latissimus dorsi, teres major, subscapularis.
- Lateral rotation: deltoid, teres minor, infraspinatus.

Note: rotator cuff muscles are most important in rotation: subscapularis, teres minor, infraspinatus (supraspinatus is also part of the rotator cuff).

Movement of the scapula on the chest wall

- Elevation: (shrug shoulders) levator scapulae, trapezius
- Depression: serratus anterior, pectoralis minor
- Forward action (eg punch): serratus anterior; pectoralis major
- Retraction (brace shoulders): trapezius, rhomboid.

Note: serratus anterior prevents 'winging' of the scapula as pressure is placed on the outstretched hand.

Recurrent dislocation of the shoulder (For initial dislocation, see p 696.) There are 2 types: *Atraumatic:* (5%) The patient is often a teenager with no history of trauma, but having general joint laxity. Remember BRAA: *b*ilateral; treat by *r*ehabilitation; *a*traumatic; dislocates in *a*ll directions. *Traumatic:* Dislocation is usually anterior (sometimes inferior, rarely posterior) and is secondary to trauma—which may be mild. Remember BUST: *B*ankart lesion (see below); *u*nidirectional; *s*urgical treatment; *t*raumatic. Abduction + lateral rotation of the arm (eg on putting on a coat) may cause dislocation. The capsule is attached to the neck of scapula but detached from the glenoid labrum (Bankart lesion). There may be a posterolateral 'dent' in the humeral head (seen on x-ray with arm medially rotated). Treatment is Bankart repair (sew capsule back to glenoid) or Putti–Platt operation (the subscapularis tendon is reefed, ie shortened).

With the rarer recurrent posterior dislocation, the capsule is torn from the back of the neck of scapula, the humeral dent is superomedial, and it is abduction and medial rotation which causes dislocation (eg seizure). *Treatment:* Reef the infraspinatus tendon.

Recurrent *subluxation* is also recognized (disabling and difficult to treat).

The painful shoulder

…ember that the neck may refer pain via C5 to the deltoid region and … C6, C7 and C8 to the superior border of the scapula. Diaphragmatic …eferral via C3 may also cause shoulder-tip pain.

Rotator cuff tears Tears in supraspinatus tendon (or adjacent subscapularis and infraspinatus) may be due to degeneration, or, less commonly, to a sudden jolt (eg a fall). Partial tears cause a painful arc (see below); complete tears limit shoulder abduction to the 45–60° provided for by scapular rotation. If the arm is passively abducted beyond 90° deltoid's contribution to abduction comes into play, which is then possible from this point. The full range of passive movement is present. Pain is felt at the shoulder-tip and upper arm; there is tenderness under the acromion. *Tests:* Ultrasound, MRI, or arthrography reveals communication between joint capsule and subacromial bursa. *Treatment:* Tendon repair may be successful, particularly if done early.

Painful arc syndrome This is pain on abduction between 45° and 160°. Causes of pain on abduction:

1 *Supraspinatus tendinitis* or partial rupture of supraspinatus tendon gives pain reproduced by pressure on the partially abducted arm. Typical age: 35–60. Only a proportion will have a painful arc (others have increasing pain up to full abduction), which is why the term *impingement syndrome* (as the greater tuberosity of the humerus catches under the acromion during abduction between, eg 70 and 140°) is preferred.[1] *Treatment:* Active shoulder movement with physiotherapy; NSAIDs, eg naproxen 250mg/8h PO after food; subacromial bursa injection of steroid, eg triamcinolone acetonide 40mg with local anaesthetic; arthroscopic acromioplasty.

2 *Calcifying tendinitis:* Typical age: 25–55. There is acute inflammation of supraspinatus. Pain is maximal during the phase of resorption. *Treatment:* Physiotherapy; NSAIDs; steroid injection. Rarely, surgery to remove calcium may be needed.

3 *Acromioclavicular joint osteoarthritis (AC joint OA):* This is common. *Treatment:* Steroid injection often helps. Excision of the lateral end of the clavicle may be needed.

Tendinitis of long head of biceps Pain is felt in the anterior shoulder and is characteristically worse on forced contraction of biceps. *Treatment:* Anti-inflammatory drugs. Hydrocortisone injection to the tendon may give relief but risks tendon rupture. Technique: p 658.

Rupture of long head of biceps Discomfort occurs after 'something has gone' when lifting or pulling. A 'ball' appears in the muscle on elbow flexion. *Treatment:* Repair is rarely indicated as function remains.

Frozen shoulder (adhesive capsulitis) may follow modest injury in older people. Pain may be severe and worse at night (eg unable to lie on one side). Active and passive movement range is reduced. Abduction↓ (<90°) ± external rotation↓ (<30°). It may be associated with cervical spondylosis (more global restriction of movement). *Treatments:* NSAIDs, intra-articular steroid injections, physiotherapy, manipulation. Meta-analyses[2] of randomized trials are said not support any one option, but they did not include D Wint's trial which strongly favoured injections.[3] Resolution may take years.[2]

Shoulder osteoarthritis This is not so common as hip or knee OA. Good success rates are being achieved by joint replacement.

1 JI Brox 1993 *BMJ* ii 899 2 S Green 1998 *BMJ* i 354 3 *BMJ* 1998 ii 1292

…ow

…al range of flexion and extension at the elbow is 0–150°. With …w flexed, supination and rotation of 90° should be possible. Pain … the elbow and in the middle outer aspect of the arm may radiate …n the shoulder.

…ennis elbow There is inflammation where the common extensor tendon inserts at the lateral epicondyle of the humerus (lateral epicondylitis) ± rupture of aponeurotic fibres. This is usually caused by strain.
Presentation: Pain is worst when the tendon is most stretched (flexion of the wrist and fingers with hand pronated). Pain is felt at the front the lateral condyle. Ask the patient to extend the wrist, and then pull on the hand to elicit pain. *Tests:* There are no x-ray findings.
Treatment: Pain often subsides in time, but injection of the tendon origin (p 658) gives more rapid pain relief. If this fails, physiotherapy may help, or an epicondylitis brace; with severe disability, operative stripping of the common extensor origin from the bone and then allowing it to fall back in place may provide relief.

Golfer's elbow This is medial humeral epicondylitis. It is less common than tennis elbow. Steroid injection may help, but be wary of the ulnar nerve; the brachial artery is also nearby.

Student's elbow This is a traumatic bursitis following pressure on the elbows, eg while engrossed in a long book. There is pain and swelling behind the olecranon. Other causes are septic and gouty bursitis (look for tophi). The bursa should be aspirated (send fluid for Gram stain and microscopy for crystals). Traumatic bursitis may then be injected with hydrocortisone. Septic bursitis should be formally drained.

Ulnar neuritis Osteoarthritic or rheumatoid narrowing of the ulnar groove and constriction of the ulnar nerve as it passes behind the medial epicondyle, or friction of the ulnar nerve due to cubitus valgus (a possible sequel to childhood supracondylar fractures) can cause fibrosis of the ulnar nerve and ulnar neuropathy. *Presentation:* Patients may experience clumsiness of the hand. Sensation is reduced over the little finger and medial half of ring finger. There is weakness of the small muscles of the hand innervated by the ulnar nerve (adductor pollicis, interossei, abductor digiti minimi and opponens digiti minimi).
Tests: Nerve conduction studies will confirm the site of the lesion.
Treatment: Operative release of the nerve to lie in a new channel in front of the elbow.

Deformities *Cubitus valgus:* The normal degree of valgus ('carrying angle') at the elbow is 10° in ♂, and 15° in ♀. Fractures at the lower end of humerus or interference with the lateral epiphyseal growth plate may cause the angle to be greater. As a result ulnar neuritis and osteoarthritis may occur. Treat if necessary. Association: Turner's.
Cubitus varus: Commonly after poorly reduced supracondylar fractures.

Osteoarthritis of the elbow Osteitis dissecans and fractures involving the joint are risk factors. *Tests:* Flexion and extension are usually impaired but rotation is full. *Treatment:* Operation is rarely indicated, but if pain is felt in the lateral compartment, the head of radius may be excised. Loose bodies may be removed if causing pain or locking of the joint.

9. Orthopaedics

The wrist and hand

Dupuytren's contracture Progressive, painless thickening and fibrosis of the palmar fascia (aponeurosis) with skin puckering and tethering. *Associations:* Familial (autosomal dominant), alcoholism, antiepileptics, Peyronie's disease, knuckle pads. The ring finger and little fingers are most commonly affected. It is commonly bilateral and symmetrical. The plantar fascia may also be affected. As thickening occurs there may be flexion at the MCP joints. If the interphalangeal joints are also affected the hand may be quite disabled. *Treatment:* Surgery aims to remove affected palmar fascia and hence prevent progression. As a rough guide, if he cannot place his palm flat on a flat surface, surgical referral is appropriate. There is tendency for recurrence. Severely affected little fingers may be amputated.

Ganglia These multilocular swellings which are tears or bulges of a joint's synovial lining, typically occur around the wrist. They communicate with joint capsules or tendon sheaths. They appear as smooth swellings containing clear jelly. *Treatment* is not needed unless they cause local pressure symptoms (eg compress median or ulnar nerve at wrist, or lateral popliteal nerve behind the knee). They may disappear spontaneously.[1] Local pressure may disperse them (traditionally a blow from the family Bible), they may be dispelled by aspiration using a wide-bore needle, or they may be dissected out—but problems include painful scars and recurrence.

De Quervain's syndrome (Stenosing tenovaginitis) Pain is felt over the styloid process of the radius and there is thickening of the tendons of abductor pollicis longus and extensor pollicis brevis as they pass over this area in their common and rather tight tendon sheath. Pain is worst when these tendons are stretched (eg lifting a teapot). Pain may be elicited by forcible adduction and flexion of the thumb into the palm. (Finckelstein's sign). The pain is more proximal than that from osteoarthritis of the first carpometacarpal joint. The cause is unknown but it commonly follows activities involving much use of the tendons (eg wringing clothes).[1] *Treatment:* First try hydrocortisone injection around the tendons in their sheaths. If injection (p 658) and rest fail to relieve, decompression of the tendons is provided by deroofing the tendon sheaths or by slitting them.

Trigger finger (Tendon nodules) Constriction at the base of tendon sheaths causes narrowing of the underlying tendons. Ring and middle fingers are most commonly affected, and the thumb especially in babies and children. Full extension of the affected digit cannot be achieved by the muscles of the hand, and if aided by the other hand, a 'click' may be felt in the flexor tendon. As extension occurs, the nodule moves with the flexor tendon, but then becomes jammed on the proximal side of a pulley, and has to be flicked straight, so producing triggering. Nodules are associated with rheumatoid arthritis. *Treatment:* Unless the patient is a child, or has renal failure or diabetes mellitus, steroid injection into the region of the nodule, under low pressure, but not into the nodule itself[1] (eg 1mL of Depomedrone® with lidocaine) may be tried. If this fails, surgical referral is indicated (division of the constricted section of the flexor sheath).

Volkmann's ischaemic contracture Follows interruption of the brachial artery near the elbow (eg after supracondylar fracture of humerus, p 698). Muscle necrosis (especially flexor pollicis longus and flexor digitorum profundus) results in contraction and fibrosis causing a flexion deformity at wrist and elbow. Suspect if a damaged arm is blue, with no radial pulse, and passive finger extension is painful (this is the crucial sign). *Treatment:* Remove constricting splints, warm other limbs (promote vasodilatation). If pulse still doesn't return within half an hour, the artery should be explored.

1 M Shipley 1995 *BMJ* i 239

9. Orthopaedics

Examination of the back

History The commonest orthopaedic complaint is back pain. Attention should be paid to the nature of the pain, exacerbating and relieving factors and the history of onset. It is important to know if bowel or bladder function is affected (this signifies cord compression and should set your alarm bells ringing loudly: refer at once). With low back pains it is not uncommon for pain to radiate down the leg (sciatica): such pain may be accompanied by root signs (see below).

Examination With the patient wearing only bra and pants the back is inspected for abnormality and may be palpated to assess skin temperature and local tenderness. Movements assessed are *flexion* (stretch forward to touch toes with knees straight—look to see how much movement is due to back flexion and how much by flexion at the hips—with back flexion the back has a gently rounded contour); *extension* (arch spine backwards); *lateral flexion* (lean sideways so hand moves down corresponding thigh) and *rotation* (keep feet fixed but move shoulders round to each side in turn). Movement at the costovertebral joints is assessed by the difference in chest expansion between maximal inspiration and expiration (normal: 5cm). Iliac crests are grasped by the examiner and compressed to move sacroiliac joints and see if this reproduces the pain.
Note: On bending fully forwards, expansion of a line drawn from 10cm above L5 to 5cm below it by <5cm is firm and quantifiable evidence of movement restriction.

Lower limbs are compared for muscle wasting (measure thigh and calf circumference), for weakness, sensory loss and normal reflexes (knee jerk is mainly L4, ankle jerk S1, plantars should be downgoing).

Straight leg raising *Why?* To test for a mechanical cause of sciatic pain. *How?* Keeping the knee extended, lift the patient's leg off the couch and note the angle to which the leg can be raised before eliciting pain. If <45°, Lasègue's sign is said to be positive. *Mechanism?* This stretches the sciatic nerve and causes root pain (a characteristic lancinating pain distributed in the relevant dermatome, and made worse by coughing or sneezing).
Alternatively: The method described above often elicits pain in the hypersensitive. Alternatively sit the patient up in bed with legs out in front. This can be done whilst examining another system, and often proves pain-free.

Other parts of the body examined These are the iliac fossae (important in days when tuberculous psoas abscesses were common), abdomen, pelvis and rectum and major arteries. The commonest tumours to metastasize to bone are: breast, bronchus, kidney, thyroid and prostate so it may be relevant to examine these.

Tests *First line:* Hb, ESR (if high, think of metastases or myeloma, and do electrophoresis ± bone marrow), alkaline phosphatase (high in Paget's disease and tumours), calcium. X-rays: AP, lateral and obliques (pelvis, lumbar spine)—but note: the dose of radiation is *not* negligible: use x-rays sparingly. *Second line:* Myelography and magnetic resonance imaging (MRI—non-invasive, and high quality images) enable the cauda equina to be seen (look for disc protrusion, tumours or spinal stenosis). Send CSF from myelography for protein level (high in CSF trapped below spinal cord tumours). Ultrasound and computerized tomography illustrate the spinal canal. Radioisotope scans may reveal 'hot spots' of tumour (or pyogenic infection). Electromyography is used to demonstrate loss of innervation from lumbar or sacral nerves.

9. Orthopaedics

Kyphosis and scoliosis

Kyphosis This is a flexion deformity of the spine. The cervical spine is usually held slightly extended (lordosis), the thoracic spine flexed, and lumbar spine again extended. Those conditions affecting the architecture of the spine may be a cause of kyphosis, eg developmental deficiency of vertebra, Scheuermann's or Calvé's osteochondritis (p 650 & p 652), wedge fractures of vertebrae (osteoporosis, metastatic carcinoma, TB), ankylosing spondylitis. Treat the underlying disorder if indicated.

Scoliosis This is lateral spinal curvature + vertebral and rib rotation. The commonest cause is muscle spasm (eg with sciatica). Classification:

1. Idiopathic (this is seen both in infants and adolescents).
2. Congenital (due to bony anomalies).
3. Neuromuscular (eg postural, polio, syringomyelia, torsion dystonia). Unequal muscle spasm or paralysis exerts unequal pull on the spine (curve concave to the stronger side).
4. Rare causes (eg spinal tumours, spondylolisthesis, arthrogryphosis, enchondromatosis, osteogenesis imperfecta, neurofibromatosis, Chiari malformation, Duchenne muscular dystrophy, Friedreich's ataxia, Marfan's syndrome, Pompe's disease).

Idiopathic scoliosis There is lateral curvature of the thoracic or lumbar spine >10°. Adolescent idiopathic scoliosis (AIS) is the most common spinal deformity; girls are more often affected than boys—and they are often taller than their peers at presentation (but not ultimately). Complications in later life revolve around pain, unsightliness, and impaired lung function. Thoracic problems tend to give more severe deformity than lumbar. Rib deformity causes a characteristic hump on the convex side of the curve which becomes manifest on asking the patient to bend forwards. Curvature increases while the affected person continues to grow, so usually the earlier the onset the worse the deformity. Since the advent of screening, scoliosis has been detected in 1.5–3%; of these only ~6% progress: the younger the child, the more the risk of progression—and double curves progress more than single curves. Thoracolumbar or lumbar curves progress the least. *Treatment* is needed in 2.75/1,000 screened. Where curvatures are <45–50° and growth is completed, or <29° if growth is in progress, the situation is monitored regularly: eg every 3 months during growth, and every 8 months thereafter.[1] When curvatures are progressing, attempts to halt it may be made using a Boston or Milwaukee distraction-derotation brace (particularly for double curves, or if the apex of the curve is higher than the 8th thoracic vertebra[1]) until the child is old enough for any spinal surgery that may be indicated (eg Luque rods and wires) or Cottrel–Dubousset instrumentation (Harrington's metal rods are now rarely used, but paralysis, the most feared complication of spinal surgery occurs in only 0.23%, compared with ~0.7% with other operations).[1] NB: it can be hard to persuade a child to wear a brace for the >22h/day that is optimal!—but bracing *does* work. There is no effective treatment for established deformity in adults.

►When scoliosis gives pain in a child or adolescent (especially at night), an osteoid osteoma, osteoblastoma, severe spondylolisthesis or spinal tumour may be the cause, and investigation should be made to exclude such underlying pathology.

1 JE Lonstein 1994 *Lancet* **344** 1407

9. Orthopaedics

Causes of back pain

Backache may result from retroperitoneal disease (duodenal ulcer, pancreas cancer, or aneurysm; pain is often lumbodorsal and spine movements pain-free and full). Other causes: spine neoplasia; infection; spondylotic or mechanical back pain; disc lesion, arthritis, osteoporosis, osteomalacia.

Mechanical back pain The spine is a complex series of articulations between vertebrae, with spongy discs between vertebral bodies acting as shock absorbers, and a multitude of articulating facet joints. Problems in one part of the spine may affect the function of the whole, and spasm of vertebral muscles can cause much pain. A consequence of upright posture is that great forces are exerted on the spine, eg when lifting, and discs may rupture (young people) or vertebrae fracture (the elderly).

Disc prolapse Lumbar discs are those most likely to rupture (esp. the lowest 2). Typically, one is seized by severe pain on coughing, sneezing or twisting a few days after back strain (onset may be insidious). Pain may be confined to the lower lumbar area (lumbago) or may radiate to buttock or leg (sciatica), if the herniated nucleus pulposus compresses a nerve root. *Signs:* Forward flexion (p 618) and extension limited, ± lateral flexion—unilaterally and inconstantly. With L5–S1 prolapse, S1 root compression causes calf pain, weak foot plantar flexion, ↓sensation (pinprick) over sole of foot and back of calf, and ↓ankle jerk. With L4–5 prolapse, hallux extension is weak and sensation↓ on outer dorsum of foot. If lower lumbar discs prolapse centrally, cauda equina compression (p 608) may occur. Danger signs: •Saddle anaesthesia •Incontinence/retention •Paralysis.
Tests: Do MRI (or CT or myelography) if intervention is contemplated, eg cauda equina compression, or if rest fails and symptoms are severe, with CNS signs such as reflex or sensory changes, or muscle wasting.
Treatment: Bed rest on a hard surface for 2–6 weeks + pain relief (p 624) is all that is needed in ~90%. Physiotherapy is often used. Percutaneous translumbar discectomy (eg by a radiologist guided by image intensification—with general anaesthesia) or chemonucleolysis (with chymopapain, an enzyme causing liquefaction of the disc) may be used. The latter can be a quick (30min), atraumatic, day-case procedure, saving ~£1500/patient—but only a few may be suitable for the technique. Spinal fusion has been advocated but this treatment has never been vindicated in randomized trials, and gives very variable results (16–95% improvement, and in some studies most patients *deteriorate* after fusion; new ideas such as pedicle screws have new complications, eg nerve root damage—seen in ~20%).

Spondylolisthesis There is displacement (usually forward) of one lumbar vertebra upon the one below. *Causes:* Spondylolysis (defect in pars interarticularis of neural arch); congenital malformation of articular processes, osteoarthritis of posterior facet joints (older folk). Onset of pain with or without sciatica is often in adolescence. *Diagnosis* is by plain x-rays. *Treatment* may involve wearing a corset, or nerve release and spinal fusion.

Lumbar spinal/lateral recess stenosis

Facet joint osteoarthritis (the only synovial joints in the back) may produce generalized narrowing of the lumbar spinal canal or simply of its lateral recesses. Unlike the pain of lumbar disc prolapse, this causes:

- Pain worse on walking with aching and heaviness in one or both legs causing the person to stop walking ('spinal claudication').
- Pain on extension. •–ve straight leg raising test. •Few CNS signs.

Tests: Myelography, CT and MRI visualize the spinal canal.
Treatment: Canal decompression (removing its posterior wall) gives good results if NSAIDs, epidural steroid injections, and corsets (to prevent exaggerating the lumbar lordosis of standing) fail to help.

Spinal tumours p 626.

Cross-section of vertebral canal at L5 showing lateral recess stenosis[1]

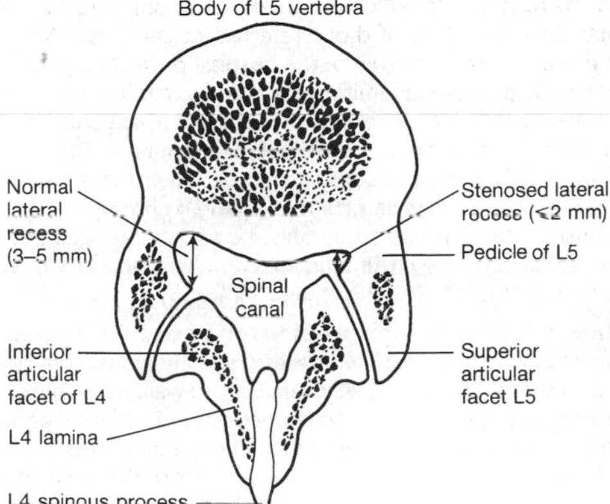

Management of low back pain

Back pain is common. 80% of the Western population suffer it at some stage in their lives. 50/1000 industrial workers have time off work because of it each year. In the UK it accounts for 11 million lost working days/yr (£3.8 billion/yr in lost production). A GP can expect 20 people per 1000 on her list to consult her with it each year, of whom 10–50% are referred to hospital. Less than 10% of those referred to specialists will have surgery. Psysiotherapy may be carried out in hospital or general practice.

Most back pain is self-limiting: of those attending GPs, 70% are better after 3 weeks, 90% by 6 weeks, irrespective of treatment. However, it must be remembered that the cause of back pain can be sinister—malignant disease, local infection, or cord or corda equina compression—and an approach is needed that detects these patients promptly. Age is an important consideration: in one study only 3% of patients aged between 20 and 55 had 'spinal pathology' (tumour, infection, inflammatory disease) as compared with 11% of those <20yrs, and 19% >55yrs.

Features which may indicate sinister back pain (*Causes:* p 626)

- Young (<20y) or old (>55)
- Violent trauma
- Alternating sciatica
- Bilateral sciatica
- Weak legs
- Weight loss
- ESR↑ (>25mm/h)
- Taking oral steroids
- Progressive, continuous, non-mechanical pain
- Systemically unwell; drug abuse; HIV +ve
- Spine movement in *all* directions painful
- Localized bony tenderness
- CNS deficit at more than one root level
- Pain or tenderness of thoracic spine
- Bilateral signs of nerve root tension
- Past history of neoplasia

► Pain brought on by activity and relieved by rest is *rarely* sinister.
Those with any suggestion of cord or cauda equina compression (p 608), or with deteriorating unilateral signs must be referred at once. Those in whom malignancy or infection is suspected should be referred promptly.

Treatment of biomechanical back pain is usually conservative. 'Get on with your life within the limits of your pain' produces better results than physiotherapy with lateral bending exercises or bed-rest for ≤3 days lying on a firm bed—eg a board under the mattress.[1] Avoid slouching. Give advice on avoiding stress on the back—how to rise from lying and avoiding stooping, bending, lifting and low chairs. Give good analgesia to break the pain–muscle spasm cycle (eg paracetamol, up to 4g/24h PO, ± NSAID, eg naproxen 250mg/8h PO pc—but opioids may be needed at first). Warmth also helps, as does swimming in a warm pool. If spasm persists, try diazepam 2mg/8h PO for a short while. Physiotherapy during the acute phase can reduce pain and spasm. The convalescent patient is given education on lifting and exercises to strengthen the back muscles.

Many prefer to consult an osteopath or chiropractor for manipulation (as employed by some physiotherapists). Studies show manipulation can produce relief of symptoms which is dramatic but may not be longlasting.

If pain does not improve after 2 weeks, do blood tests, and, if abnormal, consider x-ray examination. Later, referral to rehabilitation services, epidural anaesthesia, and corsets may help. Orthopaedic referral may be needed if pain does not resolve with time, for help with diagnosis, for additional treatment, or for reassurance.

[1] A Malmivaara 1995 NEJM **332** 351+DoH 1994 *Back Pain* HMSO+H Hemingway 1995 *Br J Gen Pract* **45** 457

Why do some people get intractable back pain?[1]

39% of adults have a have an intermittent or chronic back problem—and much energy is expended on frequently fruitless searches for the causes listed opposite. x-rays and MRI may be non-specific (subclinical disc protrusion, facet joint arthritis, or minor spondylosis). Risk factors for chronicity are:

- Smoking
- Co-existing cardio-respiratory disease
- Psychological morbidiry
- Poor work conditions
- Income and social class
- Number of children (for women *and* men)

Vascular problems may underlie chronic back pain (hence the association with smoking and heart disease)—and pain may be maintained by involvement of the sympathetic chain, which is thought to mediate hyperaesthesia, hyperpathia (excess pain from minor noxious stimuli), allodynia (pain generated by minor skin stimulation)—but surgical sympathectomy often only provides temporary relief. This implies central neuromodulation of stimuli producing a complex regional pain syndrome. Dorsal horn receptor fields may expand and have their thresholds changed by peripheral injury, so that pain is more intense, and appreciated over a wider area than simple anatomy would predict.[1]

1 MI Jayson 1997 *BMJ* i 1640

Sinister back pain

Causes Age determines the most likely causes.

- 15–30yrs: Prolapsed disc, trauma, fractures, ankylosing spondylitis (p 674), spondylolisthesis (L5 shifts forward on S1), pregnancy.
- 30–50yrs: Degenerative joint disease, prolapsed disc, malignancy (lung, breast, prostate, thyroid, kidney).
- >50yrs: Degenerative, osteoporosis, Paget's, malignancy, myeloma. Lumbar artery atheroma (which may itself cause disc degeneration).

Rarer causes: Spinal stenosis (bony encroachment); cauda equina tumours; spinal infection (usually staphylococcal, also *Proteus*, *E coli*, *Salmonella typhi*, TB). Often no systemic signs of infection.

Spinal tumours These may be of spinal cord, meninges, nerves or bone. They may compress the cord, causing these *signs:* girdle pain if thoracic spine is involved, lumbar pain if lower; lower motor neurone signs at level of lesion, upper motor neurone signs and sensory loss below; bowel and bladder dysfunction. Peripheral nerve function may be impaired resulting in pain along the course of the nerve, motor weakness in muscles innervated by the nerve, depressed reflexes and sensory impairment in areas supplied by the nerve roots. With cauda equina involvement there is often urinary retention and saddle anaesthesia. When bones of the back are involved there is progressive constant pain, and local destruction of bone. Tumours (especially metastases) tend to affect cancellous bone, but focal lesions cannot be seen on x-ray until 50% of bone mass has been lost. *Tests:* As the pedicles are cancellous bone an early x-ray sign suggesting tumour is a 'missing pedicle'. There may be much muscle spasm and local tenderness to percussion of the bones. Bone collapse may result in local deformity or cause cord or nerve compression. Isotope bone scans, bone biopsy and myelography may all be used in diagnosis.

In those with past carcinoma and current back pain, it is best to do a bone scan first, with plain x-rays of any hot spots suggesting metastases.

Pyogenic spine infections This is a notoriously difficult diagnosis as all signs of infection may be absent (eg no fever, tenderness, or WCC↑), although the ESR is often raised. It may be secondary to other septic foci. Pain occurs, and movement is restricted by spasm. It is usually an infection of the disc space (discitis). *Risk factors:* Diabetes mellitus, immunosuppression, urinary surgery or catheterization. Half the infections are staphylococcal; *Proteus, E coli, Salmonella typhi* and TB also occur. *Tests:* X-rays shows bone rarefaction or erosion, joint space narrowing ± subligamentous new bone formation. A technetium bone scan is the best test. *Treatment:* As for osteomyelitis elsewhere (p 644), resting the back with bed rest, brace, or plaster jacket. Surgery may be needed.

Spinal TB Rare in the West, this tends to affect young adults, giving pain, and stiffness of all back movements. ESR↑. Abscesses and cord compression may occur (Pott's paraplegia). Disc spaces may be affected in isolation, or with vertebral body involvement on either side (usually anterior margins early). X-rays show narrow disc spaces and local osteoporosis early, with bone destruction leading to wedged of vertebrae later. In the thoracic spine, paraspinal abscesses may be seen on x-ray, and kyphosis on examination, whereas with lower thoracic or lumbar involvement abscess formation may be by the psoas muscle in the flank, or in the iliac fossa. MRI (not CT) is the ideal way to delineate cord compression. Treatment is anti-TB drugs (eg for 1yr; p 278) with abscess drainage. Fixation with bone grafts, or metal rods, plates or wires needs highly specialist services.

Central disc protrusion This neurosurgical emergency is suggested by bilateral sciatica, perineal or 'saddle' anaesthesia and disturbance of gut or bladder function. ►*Prompt decompression may prevent leg paralysis.*

Diagnostic triage: which group encompasses your patient?

Simple lumbosacral pain	*Signs of nerve root pain*	*Possibly sinister features*
Aged 20–55 with 'mechanical' backache, eg caused by twisting and worse on moving	One leg hurting more than the back	Pain unrelated to mechanical events
Patient well-in-himself: no fever no weight loss	Radiation to foot/toes	Thoracic pain ± deformity
	Hip flexion repoduces the pain in the leg	Past history, eg HIV; TB neoplasia, or steroid use
	Localized neurological signs	Widespread CNS signs
		Weight loss; fever; unwell

►Signs demanding immediate (same-day) referral: gait or sphincter disturbance; saddle anaesthesia—these suggest cauda equina compression.

For evidence relating to the management of these categories, see http://www.rcgp.org.uk/backpain/rcbp0019.htm

Hip history and examination

The movements examined at the hip are flexion (grasp iliac crest to eliminate pelvic rotation), normal is 120°; abduction—normal is 30–40° (keep hand between anterior superior iliac spines to prevent pelvic tilt); abduction in flexion (normally 70°) and adduction (normally 30°, tested by moving one foot across the other). Normal external and internal rotation is 30° (internal rotation is often the first movement to be restricted by hip disease).

Questions Enquire about how hip symptoms affect activities of daily living, walking distance, ability to climb stairs (does this have to be one at a time?), difficulty getting out of low chairs. Remember that pain in the knee may be referred from the hip.

Measurements Apparent leg length disparity (with the lower limbs parallel and in line with the trunk) is called 'apparent shortening' (eg due to pelvic tilt or fixed adduction deformity—which gives the apparent shortening on that side) or 'apparent lengthening' (eg due to fixed hip abduction) if there is no true disparity, as detected by measuring between the anterior superior iliac spine and medial malleolus on each side with the pelvis held square and the lower limbs held equally adducted or abducted.

Fixed deformity Joint or muscle contractures prevent the limbs from being put in the neutral position. With a fixed adduction deformity the angle between the limb and the transverse axis of the pelvis (line between both anterior superior iliac spines) is less than 90° but with fixed abduction deformity it is greater than 90°. Fixed flexion deformity is detected by Thomas' test.

Thomas' test Feel for lumbar lordosis under the side on which fixed flexion deformity is suspected. If lordosis is present flex the sound side maximally. This abolishes the lordosis and makes the fixed flexion on the affected side apparent. The angle through which the thigh is raised is the angle of fixed flexion.

The Trendelenburg test This tests the stability of the hip and the ability to support the pelvis when standing on one leg. In this state, it is normal for the pelvis to rise on the side of the lifted leg. A +ve test is when the pelvis falls on the side of the lifted leg. *Causes:* **1** Abductor muscle paralysis (gluteus medius and minimus); **2** Upward displacement of the greater trochanter (severe coxa vara or dislocated hip); **3** Absence of a stable fulcrum (eg ununited fractures of the neck of the femur).

Gait Those with unstable or painful hips use a stick on the opposite side from affected hip. (The reverse is true for knees.)

Other joints to examine Pain in the hip area may be due to pathology in lumbar spine, sacroiliac joints, abdomen or pelvis.

Coxa vara This is the term used to describe a hip in which the angle between the neck and the shaft of femur is less than the normal 125°. *Causes:* Congenital; slipped upper femoral epiphysis; fracture (trochanteric with malunion, ununited fractures of neck of femur); due to softening of bones (rickets, osteomalacia, Paget's disease). *Consequences:* True shortening of limb; Trendelenburg 'dip' on walking makes the affected person limp.

9. Orthopaedics

Painful hips in children

►When a child complains of pain in the knee, examine the hip.
►Is the child feverish? If so, do urgent blood culture + diagnostic arthrotomy to exclude septic arthritis (do not rely on aspiration).
►Think of slipped femoral epiphysis in adolescents.

When a child presents with an unexplained painful limp, examine the hip clinically and radiologically. Admission for observation and rest is usual (± traction), and tests are carried out to exclude TB and Perthes' disease. When there has been unilateral limitation of all hip movements but a spontaneous recovery after bed rest in the presence of normal x-rays, a retrospective diagnosis of transient synovitis of the hip is made (known as the 'irritable hip'). If other joints are involved, consider the diagnosis of juvenile rheumatoid arthritis (p 758).

Ultrasound is very helpful in assessment. It can guide needle aspiration when pus is suspected—and may obviate the need for arthrotomy.

Perthes' disease This is osteochondritis of the femoral head and affects those aged 3–11yrs (commonest 4–7yrs). It is bilateral in 10%. ♂/♀≈4:1. It presents with pain in hip or knee and causes a limp. On examination all movements at the hip are limited. Early x-rays show widening of the joint space. Later there is a decrease in size of the nuclear femoral head with patchy density. Later still, there may be collapse and deformity of the femoral head with new bone formation. Severe deformity of the femoral head risks early arthritis. The younger the patient the better the prognosis. For those with less severe disease (<½ the femoral head affected on lateral x-ray, and joint space depth well preserved) treatment is bed rest until pain subsides followed by x-ray surveillance. For those with worse prognosis (>½ femoral head affected, narrowing of total joint space) surgery may be indicated.

Slipped upper femoral epiphysis This affects those aged 10–16yrs. 20% are bilateral. ♂/♀ ≈3:1. 50% of patients are obese. There is displacement through the growth plate with the epiphysis always slipping down and back. It usually presents with limping and spontaneous pain in the groin, anterior thigh or knee. Symptoms may be chronic or acute—the latter may represent a very unstable slip, and indicates that early fixation may be required. On examination flexion, abduction and medial rotation are limited (he may lie with the foot externally rotated). Diagnosis is by lateral x-ray (AP films may appear normal). If untreated, consequences may be avascular necrosis of femoral head or malunion predisposing to arthritis. Minor degrees of slip may be pinned to prevent further slip, more major degrees require complicated reconstructive surgery. ►Symptoms may be mild: have a high index of suspicion if in correct age group.

Tubercular arthritis This is now rare in the UK. Children aged 2–5yrs and the elderly are most commonly affected. The symptoms are pain and a limp. All hip movements cause pain and muscle spasm. *Tests:* Early x-ray sign: rarefaction of bone. Subsequently there is fuzziness of joint margins and narrowing of the joint space. Later bony erosion may be seen. Ask about contacts. Check ESR, CXR and Mantoux test (*OHCM* p 200). Synovial membrane biopsy confirms the diagnosis of TB arthritis. *Treatment of tubercular arthritis* (eg of hip): rest and chemotherapy (eg with the drugs described on p 278, administered by experienced personnel). Arthrodesis may be needed if much joint destruction has occurred.

9. Orthopaedics

Congenital dislocation/dysplasia of the hip

The term developmental dysplasia of the hip (DDH) is replacing the term *congenital dislocation of the hip* (CDH). 1.3% of neonates have unstable hips, the femoral head, or subluxation. A hip may be normal at birth, and become abnormal later. Incidence (UK): 2 per 1000 live births. ♀/♂≈6:1; left hips are affected 4 times as often as right (bilateral in ⅓). *At-risk babies:*[1]
•Breech birth •Caesar for breech •Other malformations •+ve family history
•Birth wt↑ •Oligohydramnios •Primip/older mother •Postmaturity

Diagnosis Examine hips of all babies in the first few days of life and at 6 weeks. Early detection hopes to result in early correction. ►Be alert to CDH throughout childhood surveillance (p 208). *Click test of Ortolani:*[1] With the baby supine and relaxed, flex the hips to 90° and knees fully. The examiner places his middle finger over the greater trochanter, and thumb on inner thigh opposite the lesser trochanter. Diagnose a dislocated hip if slow hip abduction produces a palpable (often audible) jerk or jolt (ie rather more than a click)—as the femoral head slips back into the acetabulum. *The Barlow manoeuvre:*[1] With the pelvis stabilized by one hand, abduct each hip in turn by 45°. Forward pressure by the middle finger causes the femoral head to slip into the acetabulum if the hip is dislocated. If the femoral head slips over the posterior lip of acetabulum and straight back again when pressure is exerted by the thumb it is 'unstable' (ie dislocatable not dislocated). Use both tests but avoid repetitions (may *induce* instability/dislocation). NB: both tests are problematic, missing up to ⅔ of those later needing surgery.[2]

In older children signs may be: delay in walking, abnormal waddling gait (affected leg is shorter), asymmetric thigh creases (extra crease on the affected side), and inability to fully abduct the affected hip. With bilateral involvement the perineum appears wide and lumbar lordosis is increased.

Ultrasound is the image of choice, as it is non-invasive and dynamic. It is unclear if it should be part of general screening. In one series of 4717 babies, 17 needed treatment, and in 5 of these clinical examination missed the diagnosis. 81 had ultrasound abnormalities which did not require treatment. Screening might be confined to high-risk groups (above).

Treatment If neonatal examination suggests dislocation/instability, use double nappies; reassess at 3 weeks. If still a problem, splint the hips in moderate abduction for 3 months (eg von Rosen splint). Excess abduction may case avascular necrosis of the head of femur. *From 6–18 months* closed reduction may be tried using a frame or gallows and traction to gradually abduct the hips to 80°. If this produces full reduction, the legs are then splinted, medially rotated and abducted; if it does not, various operations may be used *before 6yrs*—aiming to reduce excessive anteversion of the femoral neck (eg rotation osteotomy) and improve the acetabulum so the femoral head lies more deeply in it. *From 7–10yrs* similar operations may be appropriate (eg for high-lying femoral heads in false sockets). *From 11yrs*, operations (eg pelvic osteotomy) are principally for pain. Hip replacement may be needed in early adult life for painful osteoarthritis. Arthrodesis is an alternative.

Club foot

Neonatal club foot (talipes equinovarus; ♂/♀>1). The foot deformity consists of: **1** Inversion; **2** Adduction of forefoot relative to hindfoot; **3** Equinus (plantarflexion). The foot cannot be passively everted and dorsiflexed through the normal range. Treatment begins within 1 week of birth with weekly foot manipulations, holding it strapped or splinted in position between manipulations. The knee is flexed 90° in a splint to stop the baby drawing up his foot. If treatment has not corrected the foot by ~3 months, operative reduction is carried out. If this does not work, operations on soft tissues and/or bones of the foot may be carried out later (from 2 yrs).

1 A Chan 1997 *Arch Dis Chi* **76** F94–F100 2 R Robinson 1998 *BMJ* **i** 1

9. Orthopaedics

Knee history and examination

►*Pain in the knee may be referred from the hip*. So examination must include the hip. Does internal hip rotation hurt?—so revealing hip pathology.

Ask about trauma, pain, swelling, mobility, locking, clicking and giving way (eg on exercise—a feature of cruciate ligament injury).

Examine the patient lying supine with legs fully exposed. Examine for swelling (*Causes:* Bone thickening, fluid, synovial thickening—this feels 'rubbery'). Look for wasting of the quadriceps. The presence of fluid can be confirmed by placing the palm of one hand above the patella over the suprapatellar pouch, and thumb and forefinger of the other hand below the patella. Fluid can be moved between the two (hydraulic pressure will be felt) by alternating the source of pressure. If 30–40mL fluid are present it may be possible to feel a 'patellar tap' (ballott patella against neighbouring bones). Patellar taps are absent with small or tense effusions (which may be up to 120mL).

Flexion and extension at the knee vary between persons. Flexion should be sufficient for the heel to touch the buttock. Compare extension with the 'good' side. Medial and lateral ligaments are examined with the knee flexed 20–30° (to relax the posterior capsule), as one hand lifts the ankle off the couch, the other holds the knee just slightly flexed. The knee is stressed in abduction by abducting the ankle with one hand while pushing the knee medially with the hand behind the knee (tests medial ligament). Reverse the pressures to give adducting force to test lateral ligament. If these ligaments are torn the knee joint opens more widely when the relevant ligament is tested (compare knees against each other).

Test the cruciate ligaments with the knee 90° flexed, with the foot placed on couch with you sitting on it (anchor tibia). Place your fingers interlocking behind the knee clasping the sides of leg between the thumbs (each tip on a femoral condyle). With quadriceps relaxed, anteroposterior assess glide of tibia on femur (normal ~0.5cm). The anterior cruciate ligament prevents anterior glide; the posterior prevents posterior glide. Excessive glide in one direction (compare knees) suggests damage to the relevant ligament. Examination should also be performed in 20° of flexion (Lachman's test). A more sensitive test to determine if symptoms are really due to cruciate ligament damage (can be asymptomatic) is the 'pivot shift test': flex the knee, then put it in valgus; now extend it. If the anterior cruciate is ruptured, the knee jumps smartly forwards. (Often hard to elicit, unless very relaxed or under general anaesthesia.)

McMurray's rotation test is an unreliable way of detecting pedunculated tears of menisci. The knee is flexed, the tibia laterally rotated on the femur, then the knee is extended with tibia kept rotated. This is repeated with varying degrees of knee flexion, and then again with the tibia medially rotated on the femur. This manoeuvre is designed to jam the free end of a pedunculated meniscus in the joint—a click being felt and heard and pain experienced by the patient as the jammed tag is released as the knee is straightened. This test may not detect bucket-handle tears (p 710). Note: normal knees commonly produce patellar clicks. Simply eliciting joint-line tenderness may be a more valid test when combined with a history of mechanical locking.

Arthroscopy Arthroscopes enable internal structures of the knee to be seen and a definite diagnosis to be made without opening the joint. They also enable a wide range of operations to be done without opening the knee, so reducing convalescent time for those undergoing arthroscopic surgery. Most can be done as day cases under local anaesthesia. MRI, where available, is superseding diagnostic arthroscopy (*OHCM* p 738).

9. Orthopaedics

Pain in the knee

The common symptoms are anterior knee pain or pain and swelling. Anterior knee pain can be due to many causes (see below).

Chondromalacia patellae (This is a component of the 'anterior knee pain syndrome'.) It particularly affects young women and servicemen. Patellar aching is felt after prolonged sitting. Medial retropatellar tenderness and pain on patellofemoral compression occur. *Diagnosis* is clinical but if arthroscopy is performed softening and/or fibrillation of patellar articular cartilage is seen. *Treat* by vastus medialis strengthening exercises—lie on the back with the foot externally rotated. Lift the heel 10cm off the floor × 500/24h, relaxing muscles between lifts (exercises are boring but relieve pain in 80%). If symptoms persist despite a year's exercises, arthroscopic lateral retinacular release may be tried. If pain still persists, rarely consider patellectomy. Shaving the posterior surface of the patella gives rather uncertain results.

Excessive lateral pressure syndrome Retropatellar tenderness and pain are felt laterally. Exercise provokes pain. Vastus medialis exercises are less likely to give relief. Arthroscopy reveals a normal patella. Lateral retinacular release should relieve pain.

Bipartite patella This is usually an incidental x-ray finding but may give pain if the superolateral fragment is mobile with tenderness over the junction. Extra fragment excision relieves pain.

Recurrent subluxation of patella A tight lateral retinaculum causes the patella to sublux laterally giving medial pain and causing the knee to give way. It is commoner in girls and with valgus knees. It may be familial, or associated with joint laxity, a high-riding patella (*patella alta*), or a hypotrophic lateral femoral condyle. Examination reveals increased lateral patellar movement which may be accompanied by pain and the reflex contraction of quadriceps (ie a positive patellar apprehension test). If vastus medialis exercises fail to help, lateral retinacular release usually cures. Patellar tendon transfer is rarely needed.

Patella tendinitis This is usually initiated by a small tear in the patellar tendon, and can occur in any part of the patellar tendon. It is most commonly seen in sport players (insertional tendinitis of patellar tendon and patella called 'jumper's knee'). Tendinitis settles with rest and NSAIDs. For those unable to rest, steroid injection around (not into) the tendon may help. For Osgood–Schlatter's disease, see p 652.

Iliotibial tract syndrome Synovium deep to the iliotibial tract is inflamed where it rubs on the lateral femoral condyle. Common in runners, it settles with rest, NSAIDs or steroid injection.

Medial shelf syndrome The synovial fold above the medial meniscus is inflamed. Pain is superomedial. There may be brief locking of the knee (mimics a torn meniscus). *Diagnosis:* Arthroscopy. *Treatment:* Rest, NSAIDs, local steroid injection or division of the synovial fold arthroscopically.

Fat pad syndrome Tenderness deep to the patellar tendon may be caused by the fat pad being caught in the tibiofemoral joint. Pain resolves with rest.

9. Orthopaedics

Knees that swell

Knee swelling occurs as part of an arthritic process. **Osteoarthritis** particularly affects the posterior patella and the medial compartment of the knee, thereby tending to varus deformity. Treatment is usually with NSAIDs (p 672), knee support (eg Tubigrip®), excess weight loss, and sometimes local steroid injections. Surgery may be needed—osteotomy may correct varus deformity; replacement arthroplasty is discussed on p 654. Rest pain (or pain while driving) which is relieved by movement suggests patellofemoral compartment problems. Simply pulling the patella medially by using tape (Leukotape®, Beiersdorf) may reduce pain by 25%.[1]

Rheumatoid, gout and septic arthritis may all affect the knee. Remember that a unilaterally swollen knee may be a septic arthritis. Diagnosis is made on the basis of aspiration and therefore avoid steroid injections prior to this (p 656).

Meniscal cysts Swelling is variable with these, but pain tends to be felt over the joint space. Lateral cysts are much more common than medial. Swelling is most noticeable when the knee is flexed to 60–70° and is less noticeable at full flexion. The meniscus is often torn radially (an otherwise unusual direction) and may therefore give rise to clicking of the knee and giving way. Pain is relieved by arthroscopic decompression and excision of the radial tear and any damaged meniscus.

Ligament tears, meniscus lesions, patellar dislocation See p 710.

Osteochondritis dissecans This is local necrosis of articular cartilage and its underlying bone which may result in a loose body leaving the surrounding bone—or a flap of bone with cartilage. The cause is unknown. The lateral side of the medial femoral condyle is most commonly affected. Adolescents and young adults are affected and there may be pain after exercise with intermittent swelling of the knee. Locking may occur. X-rays show defects in the articular surface. Treatment is expectant early as spontaneous healing can occur. The affected section may be removed surgically (if not already broken off) to prevent it breaking off, or it may be pinned in place; alternatively, the fragment can be drilled, in the hope that fibrous tissue formation will secure the fragment, or fill the defect. The condition predisposes to arthritis.

Loose bodies in the knee These cause locking of the knee (in which all movements may be jammed rather than locking due to torn menisci when only extension is limited), followed by swelling due to effusion. *Causes:* Osteochondritis dissecans (up to 3 loose bodies), osteoarthritis (≤10 loose bodies), chip fractures of joint surfaces (≤3 loose bodies) or synovial chondromatosis (>50 loose bodies). When locking is a problem, loose bodies are best removed. This can often be done arthroscopically.

Bursitis There are 16 bursae around the knee. The most commonly affected are the prepatellar bursa ('housemaid's knee') where swelling over the anterior inferior patella is due to inflammation and fluid in the bursa due to friction (kneeling); the infrapatellar bursa (Vicar's knee—they kneel more upright), and the semi-membranous bursa in the popliteal fossa (a popliteal cyst which differs from the 'Baker's cyst' which is a herniation from the joint synovium). Prepatellar bursae may be aspirated, have hydrocortisone injected to decrease recurrence, or, if very persistent, may need excision. Aspiration distinguishes friction bursitis from infective suppurative bursitis, which requires surgical drainage and antibiotics, eg flucloxacillin 250mg/6h PO (adult dose).

1 J Cushnaghan 1994 *BMJ* i 753

A journey on foot

By the time we get down to the foot, our anatomical interest is flagging, but on close inspection *we would never have believed, my dear José, that so much glory could fit into a shoe.*[1] Feet made for walking are really quite old (~3–4 million years—according to Sterkfontein Man's remains). The significant thing about these old feet is that they can *and did* take us anywhere. We left off swinging from tree to tree in an African forest, and began quite a journey—on foot.

Ankle examination 25° of extension (dorsiflexion) and 30° of flexion are the norm at the tibiotalar joint. Inversion and eversion are effected at the subtalar and midtarsal joints. Toes should have between 60° and 90° extension. Note any callosities. Examine the arches. Watch as the toes are lifted off the ground, and on standing on tiptoe. Examine gait and shoes (normal wear pattern is medially under ball of foot, posterolaterally at heel).

Pes planus (flat feet) The arch of the foot is low. There may be some valgus and eversion deformity of the foot. Flat feet are normal when a child is learning to walk. The medial arch develops over the next few years. If flat feet persist, no action is needed if the medial arch restores itself on standing on tiptoe. In most, it is asymptomatic but occasionally it is painful (especially 'peroneal spasmodic flat foot' in which the heel is held everted and the medial border of the foot held flat to the ground. Attempts to invert the hind foot in these cases induces painful spasm of the peroneal muscles). Exercises, faradic foot stimulation, and medial wedges in the shoe heel may not yield much benefit. With the spasmodic type, hindfoot fusion can be needed for pain relief. Prevention: studies of feet in India show that going barefoot until 6 years old keeps feet healthy.[2]

Pes cavus Accentuated longitudinal arches of the foot may be idiopathic, or associated with spina bifida or previous polio. Clawed toes may occur, as weight is taken on the metatarsal heads when walking. Conservative treatment involves padding under the metatarsal heads to relieve pressure. Operative treatment may involve soft tissue release (detach ligamentous tissues from calcaneum, manipulate arch then put foot in plaster) or arthrodesis to straighten the toes. If osteoarthritis of the tarsal bones is the cause of pain, these may be fused.

Hammer toes These are extended at the metatarsophalangeal joint, hyperflexed at the PIP joint and extended at the DIP joint. Second toes are most commonly affected. Arthrodesis at the PIP joint straightens the toe; tenotomy of extensor tendons lets it lie flat.

Claw toes Extended at the metatarsophlangeal joint but flexed at both PIP and DIP joints; this deformity is due to imbalance of flexors and extensors (eg after polio). If toes are still mobile, a Girdlestone operation is needed (a flexor/extensor transfer operation).

Hallux valgus The toe deviates laterally at the metatarsophalangeal joint. Biomechanical forces, pointed shoes and wearing of heels forcing the forefoot forward probably promote deformity. Pressure of the metatarsophalangeal joint against the shoe leads to bunion formation. Secondary arthritis in the joint is common. Bunion pads and plastic wedges between great and second toes may relieve pain but severe deformity requires surgery. Many different operations are used. The medial side of the metatarsal head may be trimmed; Keller's operation removes the proximal half of the proximal phalanx (excision arthroplasty) leaving a flail toe; displacement osteotomy of the metatarsal bone; Mayo's operation (arthroplasty excising the distal metatarsal head) and arthrodesis of the MTP joint are all used.

1 Gabriel García Marquez 1989 *The General in His Labyrinth*, trans Edith Grossman, London, Cape, page 31 2 *Journal of Bone & Joint Surgery* 1995 **77B** 254–7

9. Orthopaedics

The painful foot

►Look at a wet footprint (and wear on the shoe sole) to assess functional anatomy of the loaded foot. Many of the conditions mentioned in 'the foot' (p 640) can be painful. Other causes of pain are mentioned here.

Hallux rigidus This is arthritis at the first metatarsophalangeal joint. Joint movement is decreased and painful. A dorsal ring of osteophytes may occur. Treat by arthrodesis or Keller's operation.

Young people Children rarely complain of pain in the foot: if they complain of pain in the soles think of a foreign body. Shoe pressure on a prominent navicular bone, or sometimes an accessory bone, or a prominent posterosuperior os calcis may require surgical trimming. Osteochondritis (p 650) of foot bones may be the cause (diagnose by x-ray): Köhler's disease involves the navicular bone; Freiberg's disease the metatarsal heads; and Sever's disease is epiphysitis of the heel. Relieve pressure by shoe inserts (or occasionally plaster casts) until pain subsides.

Metatarsus primus varus: Angulation of the first metatarsal towards the midline. The typical patient is a teenager. This may be familial. If deformity is great, a metatarsal osteotomy may be needed.

Ingrowing toenails The hallux is most commonly affected. Incorrect cutting of nails and pressure of shoes predispose to the lateral nail digging into its fleshy bed, which reacts by becoming heaped up 'proudflesh'. Infection often supervenes. *Conservative treatment* involves tucking cotton-wool soaked in surgical spirit under the corners of the proudflesh and awaiting nail growth (then cut it straight with edges protruding beyond flesh margins). Recurrent infections may require surgery—wedge resection of nail, removal of a lateral sliver of nail and preventing nail growth by nail bed ablation (phenol or operative), or total nail removal are all used.

Adult forefoot pain (metatarsalgia) Increased pressure on the metatarsal heads causes pain. *Treat* by insole supports. Treatment by surgery other than for rheumatoid arthritis is unpredictable. Other causes of metatarsalgia include synovitis, sesamoid fracture, and injury.

March fractures occur in the shaft of the second or third metatarsals and may follow excessive walking. X-rays may be normal (radionuclide bone scans are more discriminating).[1] Treatment is expectant. If pain is severe, a plaster cast while awaiting healing may help.

Morton's metatarsalgia Pain is due to pressure on an interdigital neuroma between the metatarsals. Pain usually radiates to the lateral side of one toe, and the medial side of its neighbour (eg toes 4 and 5). *Treatment* is by excision of the neuroma.

Pain in the heel *Causes:* (inj = may respond to steroid injections)

- Diseases of the calcaneum
- Rupture of calcaneal tendon (p 660)
- Postcalcaneal bursitis*
- Plantar fasciitis (pain under anterior calcaneum) inj
- Arthritis of the subtalar joint
- Calcaneal paratendinitis inj
- Tender heel pad inj

Apart from calcaneal diseases and tendon rupture, conservative treatment such as alteration of footwear to prevent rubbing may help. If this doesn't help, postcalcaneal bursitis the bursa may be surgically removed.

1 M Macleod 1999 BMJ i 29 *Thickened bursa over tuberosity of calcaneus at back of heel

9. Orthopaedics

Osteomyelitis

This is infection of bone. Its incidence reduces as living standards rise. Common organisms: *Staph aureus* (commonest organism in UK), streptococci, *E coli*, *Proteus* and *Pseudomonas*; Elsewhere: *Salmonella* (with sickle-
 cell disease) and *Brucella*. Prior to antibiotics it killed 25% of those affected and crippled a further 25%. Infection may spread from boils, abscesses or from genitourinary instrumentation. Often no primary site is found. The patient may have diabetes or otherwise impaired immunity.

Clinical features Pain at the affected part; unwillingness to move, and warmth and tenderness over the affected part; slight effusion in neighbouring joints; signs of systemic infection. All signs are less marked in adults. Blood cultures positive in 60%.

Vascular bone is most affected (eg in long bone metaphyses—esp. distal femur, upper tibia) in children and cancellous bone in adults. In children untreated infection causes bone death which separates to form a *sequestrum*. There is periosteal new bone formation (called involucrum) surrounding the dead bone. Pus may discharge into joint spaces or via sinuses to skin.

Tests ESR↑, CRP↑, WCC↑. MRI is sensitive and specific (88% and 93%, *vs* 61% and 33% for isotope scans[1])—and avoids ionizing radiation. X-ray changes are not apparent for a few days but then show haziness and loss of density of affected bone, followed by subperiosteal reaction, and later, sequestrum and involucrum. Infected cancellous bone shows less change.

Treatment Drain abscesses and remove sequestra by open surgery. Culture all sequestra. Antibiotic: flucloxacillin 250–500mg/6h IVI or IM until the organism and its sensitivities are known. Continue for 6 weeks. Alternative treatments for adults are fusidic acid or clindamycin. Ciprofloxacin 500mg/8–12h PO is suitable for *Pseudomonas* osteomyelitis. In children <5yrs, *Haemophilus influenzae* may be the cause, and ampicillin may be appropriate—but be guided by sensitivities, and a microbiologist.

Complications of osteomyelitis Septic arthritis; pathological fracture of bone; deformity to growing bone.

Chronic osteomyelitis Delayed or inadequate treatment may result in recurrent pain, fever and discharge of pus from sinuses with periods of remission (may be years). X-rays show thick irregular bone. Surgically remove sequestra and 'saucerize' cavities. Hyperbaric oxygen may be indicated.[2] Give antibiotics (as above) for ≥12 weeks.
Complications: Amyloid, squamous carcinoma development in sinus track.

Brodie's abscess This abscess surrounded by sclerotic bone is due to organisms of low virulence. Treat by saucerization.

TB infection of bone (1–3% of all TB; incidence is rising.) The commonest site is a vertebral body (p 626) or in association with joints. *Spread:* Haematogenous or via nearby nodes. *Clinical features:* Pain, swelling and 'cold abscess' formation ± joint effusion are common signs. With joint involvement there is pain, swelling, pain on movement and muscle wasting. Also: weight↓; malaise; fever; lethargy. *Differential:* Malignancy; other infections; gout; rheumatoid.[3] *Imaging:* X-ray changes: bone rarefaction, periostrits changes, cyst formation. Later: loss of jointspace, erosions, bony ankylosis. Also look for soft tissue swellings (abscess; tenosynovitis/bursitis). MRI is especially useful in analysing soft tissue changes.[3] Bone scans may be useful in diagnosing dactylitis (a feature of childhood TB). *Other tests:* Aspirated pus is creamy and will prove positive for culture. ESR↑, Mantoux +ve. CXR. HIV. *Treatment:* Drain abscesses, immobilize affected large joints. Standard 6-month courses (*OHCM* p 200) of eg isoniazid (300mg/day), rifampicin (600mg/day) and pyrazinamide (1.5g/day) may not be long enough. Late arthrodesis is needed for gross joint destruction.

1 P McAndrew 1998 *BMJ* **i** 147 **2** UK chambers: tel. 01705 822351 **3** A Samantha 1998 *Rep Rh Dis* **13** 1

9. Orthopaedics

Bone tumours

Tumours present with pain, swelling or pathological fracture. Bone is a common site for secondaries from other tumours (eg breast, bronchus, thyroid, kidney and prostate). Malignant primary bone tumours are rare—in total only 6/million population/year. They all present with non-mechanical pain (like toothache) followed later by swelling. Delays in diagnosis are common. Radiological features suggestive of bone tumours include: bone destruction, new bone formation, soft tissue swelling and periosteal elevation. Metastases are blood-borne and usually arise first in the lungs. Treatment of these rare and highly aggressive tumours is best carried out in multidisciplinary specialist treatment centres.

Giant cell tumour (osteoclastoma) Commonest in young adults, these tumours always occur around an epiphysis (especially the knee). The tumours are osteolytic and slowly progressive, sometimes resulting in pathological fracture. Treatment is by detailed and thorough curettage resulting in 75% cure. Recurrences are usually treated by wide excision. Although benign histologically they may behave in a biologically malignant way and metastases occur in 1%.

Ewing's sarcoma This malignant round-cell tumour occurs in long bones (typically the diaphysis) and limb girdles, usually in children. X-rays often show a large soft-tissue mass with concentric layers of new bone formation ('onion-peel' sign). Typically those with Ewing's sarcomas have a t11:22 chromosomal translocation. Chemotherapy, resection of involved bone and limb salvage surgery or radiotherapy cures about half. Large volume or metastatic disease at presentation imply poor prognosis.

Osteosarcoma Primary osteosarcoma typically affects adolescents and arises towards the end of long bones (typically the knee), in the metaphysis. Secondary osteosarcomas may arise in bone affected by Paget's disease or after irradiation. X-rays show bone destruction and new bone formation, often with marked periosteal elevation (sunray spiculation and Codman's triangle respectively). Treatment is with surgical resection plus chemotherapy, eg doxorubicin and cisplatin in 3-week cycles for 18 weeks (safer, and as good as multi-drug regimens).[1] A cure rate of ~50% is achievable. Vigorous treatment of metastatic disease may be worthwhile.

Chondrosarcoma These malignancies may arise *de novo* or from malignant transformation of chondromas. Typically arising in middle age they usually manifest as a slowly increasing mass occasionally causing pressure symptoms. 'Cotton wool calcification' is typical on x-ray. These tumours do not respond to chemotherapy or radiotherapy so treatment is by surgical excision. Inadequate surgery is accompanied by local recurrence, often of a higher grade of malignancy. The cure rate is 70% overall.

Malignant fibrous histiocytoma Rarest of all the primary bone tumours they arise in middle age, often at the site of previous bone abnormality (eg bone infarcts). Treatment is as for osteosarcoma.

Chordomas These tumours arise from notochord remnants in the spine and are most common in the sacrum. They have often reached a large size before diagnosis and may present with neurological signs affecting bladder and bowel. Radical surgical excision is mandatory for cure.

Surgical reconstruction (after excising a bone tumour) involves replacing affected bone with a metal and polyethylene endoprosthesis—as an alternative to amputation. Excellent and durable reconstruction is possible using massive endoprostheses or bone allografts. 85% of patients now have limb salvage following chemotherapy for primary bone tumours.

Benign tumours: *Osteoid osteoma:* These occur most commonly in long bones of males aged 10–25yrs. They may cause severe pain (aspirin-responsive). They appear as local cortical sclerosis on x-ray. *Treatment:* Local excision.

Chondroma: These benign cartilaginous tumours may arise from bone surfaces or within the medulla (enchondromata). They may cause local swelling or fracture. *Treatment* is rarely indicated.

Osteochondroma: (Autosomal dominant) This commonest type of benign tumour arises from the metaphyseal areas of bone as rounded swellings. *Treatment* is rarely indicated. Both chondromata and osteochondromata rarely undergo malignant change. (Suspect malignancy if pain develops.)

Fibrous dysplasia of bone: See McCune–Albright syndrome, p 754.

Sarcomas unrelated to bone (NB: osteosarcomas and Ewing's tumours may be extraskeletal.) Whenever an unexplained lump presents, eg in a limb think: could this be a sarcoma (ie a mesenchymal tumour of connective-tissue elements)? ►*Muscle sarcomas comprise 1% of all malignancies.* MRI is the image of choice.[2] Possible diagnoses: eg rhabdomyosarcoma, neurofibrosarcoma, fibrosarcoma, liposarcoma, cysticercosis, malignant or myxoid fibrous histiocytoma, haemangiopericytoma. If *not* a sarcoma, is it a metastasis, lymphoma, distended bursa, pseudotumour, or an infective or granulomatous (Wegener's; sarcoid; TB; actinomycosis; toxoplasmosis; amoebiasis; hydatid) or cystic lesion? Simple shelling-out of the sarcoma is ***not*** a good idea: refer to a tertiary centre skilled in pre-op assessment—particularly if the lesion is >5cm across or deep-seated.[3] Chemotherapy and metastectomy have a rôle.

1 R Blum 1997 *Lancet* **350** 900 **2** http://rpisun1.mda.uth.tmc.edu/se/sts/ **3** A Rydholm 1998 *BMJ* **ii** 93

Congenital disorders of bone

Osteogenesis imperfecta A genetic disorder of collagen causing brittle bones. People with this suffer from brittle, fragile bones. There are 4 types:

I Blue sclerae with deafness but little deformity (defective formation of type I collagen; autosomal dominant).

II Lethal perinatal form with many fractures and dwarfism.

III Fractures at birth with progressive deformity. White sclerae, often; dentinogenesis imperfecta common (enamel separates from defective dentine, leaving teeth transparent or discoloured; recessive).

IV Fragile bones, blue sclerae; autosomal dominant.

X-rays reveal many fractures, translucent bones, a trefoil pelvis and wormian bones (irregular patches of ossification). Bone pathology shows immature unorganized bone without the normal cortex.

Treatment: Prevent injury. Osteotomies may be used to correct deformity. Intramedullary rods are sometimes used in long bones.

Achondroplasia An hereditary defect of pre-bone cartilage reduces growth of cartilaginous bone (membranous bone growth is normal). At birth affected babies have large heads, normal trunk length, short limbs and fingers all the same length. Adults are dwarfed with increased lumbar lordosis, bow legs, and shortened proximal arms and legs. *X-rays* show short bones with wide epiphyses.

Craniocleidodysostosis Those affected have a flat face, a globular skull, absent clavicles, and a wide perineum if they have coxa vara. *X-rays* show a midline frontal bone suture, deficient clavicles, wide pubic symphysis and coxa vara. Coxa vara can be corrected if necessary by osteotomy. Life expectancy is normal.

Osteochondrodystrophy Both ossification and growth of pre-bone cartilage are defective. Affected individuals are normal at birth but develop a short neck, flexion deformities of hips and knees, and kyphosis of the lumbar spine later. *X-rays* show: kyphosis; short thick lower limb bones; flattened vertebrae; cavernous acetabula and overgrowth of the radii. Life expectancy is normal.

Diaphyseal aclasis Cartilage nests displaced from the epiphyseal cartilage plate give rise to multiple cartilage-capped exostoses (osteochondromata). Long bones of arms and legs are most commonly affected. If severe, bones are broad and badly modelled. Bony swellings near joints may interfere with tendon actions. Rarely the exostoses undergo malignant change.

Ollier's disease (Multiple enchondromatosis, dyschondroplasia) Nests of cartilage cells, displaced from the epiphyseal cartilage plate into the metaphyses, persist as enchondromata. Small bones of the hands and feet and upper tibia and lower femur are most commonly affected. The enchondromata appear as swellings which are translucent on x-ray. Rarely, they undergo malignant change.

Osteopetrosis Lack of differentiation between cortex and medulla of bone results in very hard dense 'marble' bones which are brittle. Anaemia and thrombocytopenia may result from decreased marrow space. Deafness and optic atrophy can result from compression of cranial nerves.[1]

See also Neurofibromatosis (OHCM p 474), Ehlers–Danlos (p 746) and Marfan's syndrome (OHCM p 704).

1 RE Schroeder 1992 *Paediatrics* **90** 988

Osteochondritis

Osteochondritis juvenilis (osteochondrosis) is a condition of unknown origin in which bony centres of children or adolescents become temporarily softened, resulting in deformation secondary to pressure. After a variable period of time (often about 2 or 3 years) the bone hardens again in its new, deformed shape.

Clinical features The age at which these changes occur depends on which bone is affected, as it is usually at the time of development of the bony nucleus. The main symptom is local pain. *X-ray* changes: initial increase in density of the bony nucleus; followed by patchy appearances (as affected bone is resorbed) and flattening; then normal texture returns but deformity is maintained. The long-term consequence is degenerative arthritis.

Name of osteochondritis	*Site affected:*
Perthe's disease (p 630)	Hip
Scheuermann's disease	Vertebral ring epiphyses
Köhler's disease	Navicular bone
Kienböck's disease	Lunate bone (in adults)
Freiberg's disease	Head of 2nd or 3rd metatarsal

Treatment Often none is necessary but large joints may need protection (eg with a plaster cast).

Scheuermann's disease This affects 13–16-year-olds. The normal ossification of ring epiphyses of several thoracic vertebrae is affected. Deforming forces are greatest at the anterior border of the vertebrae so vertebrae are narrower anteriorly, resulting in kyphosis. During the active phase of the disease the vertebrae may be tender to firm palpation. X-rays show deep notches on the anterior corners of vertebrae. Later, they show anterior disc space narrowing.

Treatment: If symptomatic treatment fails, try a plaster cast (eg for 8 weeks, if severe); also physiotherapy. Spinal braces are rarely needed.

Köhler's disease Children affected are aged between 3–5yrs. Pain is felt in the mid-tarsal region and they limp. There may be tenderness over the navicular. *X-rays* are diagnostic, showing a dense, deformed bone.

Treatment: Symptomatic: resting the foot or wearing a walking plaster.

Kienböck's disease Pain is felt over the lunate, especially during active wrist movement. Grip is impaired due to pain. *X-rays* are diagnostic showing a dense lunate with a little depth reduction early; more marked flattening later. Osteoarthritis is the consequence. *Treatment:* Early disease may respond to wrist splinting for 3 months; in established disease the lunate may be excised and a prosthesis implanted; once arthritis is established lunate excision does not help.

Freiberg's disease This may be classed as an osteochondritis dissecans (p 652). *X-rays:* the epiphysis of a metatarsal head becomes granular, fragmented and flattened. *Treatment:* Early removal of affected bone with bone grafting and use of a walking plaster. If deformity is well established, treatment is expectant.

9. Orthopaedics

Osteochondritis-like conditions

Calvé's disease This is less common than Scheuermann's disease. Only one vertebra is involved, the central nucleus being affected. Vertebral histology may show eosinophilic granulomata. Children develop it between 2 and 10 years. Pain is felt in, and tenderness experienced over, the affected vertebra (usually thoracic) and there may be slight kyphosis.

X-rays show a dense, flattened vertebral body with disc space preserved.

Treatment is symptomatic (bed rest may relieve pain).

Osgood–Schlatter's disease This tibial tuberosity apophysitis affects children 10–14yrs old. Pain is felt in front of and below the knee, worse on strenuous activity and quadriceps contraction (lift straight leg against resistance). The tibial tubercle looks prominent and is tender to palpation.

X-rays show tibial tuberosity enlargement (± fragmentation). The underlying process is thought to be strain on the developing tibial tuberosity.

Treatment: This self-limiting disease needs symptom relief only (2 months plaster cast from groin to malleoli if pain is severe).

Sinding Larsen's disease This is traction apophysitis of the lower pole of the patella. Symptoms and treatment are similar to Osgood–Schlatter's disease (above), but the onset tends to be 1–2yrs earlier.

Sever's disease This calcaneal apophysitis is thought to be due to strained attachment of the Achilles tendon. It is usually self-limiting. Typical age: 8–13 years. Patients feel pain behind the heel. They may limp. There is tenderness over the lower posterior calcaneal tuberosity.

X-rays are often normal.

Treatment: If needed, a below knee walking plaster may give pain relief.

Osteochondritis dissecans See p 638 for osteochondritis of the knee. Other sites: elbow, hip, ankle, talus. A loose body is formed (1–3cm across) from a convex joint surface when a segment of subchondral bone and cartilage becomes avascular and separates from underlying bone. Adolescents or young adults experience early aching and effusions after use, and sudden painful locking of joints once pieces have separated to make loose bodies.

X-rays may show a translucent area around the piece about to separate before it does so, the defect from which the piece has separated, and the loose body in the joint after separation.

Treatment may be expectant. Loose bodies are removed from the joint.

Avascular necrosis (osteonecrosis) Infarction of the femoral head is the typical picture. Other sites: knees, shoulders.

X-ray changes: Sclerotic or porotic bone due to infarction, joint surface collapse and osteochondral fragments.

Local causes: Trauma (eg fractured neck of femur); secondary to rheumatoid, severe osteoarthritis, psoriatic arthropathy or neuropathic joints.

Systemic causes: Thalassaemia, sickle-cell disease, steroids therapy (eg following renal transplantation), systemic lupus erythematosus, scleroderma, infective endocarditis, alcoholism, extensive burns, radiation, diabetes mellitus, diving accidents (p 802) Cushing's and Gaucher's diseases.

Treatment is joint immobilization, analgesia and, for hips, arthroplasty.

Joint replacement

Joint replacement has been used for 30 years. Each year 40,000 hips and 15–20,000 knees are replaced in the UK (knees may soon overtake hips).

Hip replacement The usual indication for operation is pain (surgery for fixed flexion deformity affecting walking is less successful). Of the 30,000 operations carried out annually 75% are to replace osteoarthritic hips. These patients are usually elderly. Rheumatoid arthritis (RA) is the next most common indication (patients are often in their 30s or 40s). Other conditions which may result in replacement are: avascular necrosis of head of femur; congenitally dislocated hip; fractured neck of femur.

Many prostheses are available but most consist of a metal femoral component with an intramedullary stem usually held in place by bone cement, and a plastic acetabular component. Early success of operation occurs in 90% of cases. Early complications include: dislocation (0.5–3%) and deep infection (<1%). Deep infection is a disaster and although exchange prosthesis using antibiotic-loaded cement may be possible, a Girdlestone excisional arthroplasty may be needed. A small proportion of implants fail to make a satisfactory interface with bone.

Later problems of loosening or infection are heralded by return of pain. If plain x-rays are inconclusive in the case of loosening, strontium or technetium scans may reveal increased bone activity. Suspected sepsis should be investigated by white cell count, ESR, and gallium scan. Scans are not reliable within 8 months of operation. Revision arthroplasty is more successful for loosening than for infection. By 9–10yrs post-op 11% of implants have been revised. Caution should be exercised in recommending replacement to those in their 60s who are likely to give extreme usage to the prosthesis. Excess weight should be lost as this also contributes to usage. Earlier replacement is used for rheumatoid arthritis as joints tend to be grossly affected younger—and excessive delay may result in surgery upon very rarefied osteoporotic bone.

Knee replacement The knee is more complicated than the hip, and designs for replacements have altered greatly, from long-stemmed hinge mechanisms, to short-stemmed articulations currently in favour. Indications for knee replacement: pain at rest, or disturbing sleep, or making housebound. Pain correlates poorly with radiological signs. Success rate: 95%. Joint survival: 90% last 15yrs (better than hips). Revision rates are similar.

Other joints Joint spacers are used in finger joints for rheumatoid, with success. Elbow replacements are beginning to show some success. Shoulder replacement success rates are approaching those of knees.

Preventing thromboses DVT occurs in $>\frac{2}{3}$ of major orthopaedic events. Low-molecular weight heparin (LMWH) halves DVT rate and lowers risk of fatal pulmonary embolus (PE) by $\frac{2}{3}$.

►In major orthopaedic surgery, low-molecularweight heparin is preferable to ordinary heparin.[1]

Typical data: Low dose heparins; 5000 daltons; eg dalteparin, tinzaparin. Ordinary heparin; ~13,000 daltons. With LMWH, the DVT and PE rate (fatal and non-fatal) fall further (2.3% down to 1.4% for PE). SE: bleeding (at operative site, intracranial, retroperitoneal). CI: uncontrolled bleeding/risk of bleeding (eg peptic ulcer); endocarditis; children. Dose example: dalteparin 2500u 2h pre-op and at 12h post-op, then 5000u once daily for 5 days.[2,3] NB: evidence is accumulating that DVT/PE prophylaxis may need to be continued for up to a month after hospital discharge.[4]

1 *Drug Ther Bul* 1998 **36** 25 2 *Drug Ther Bul* 1993 **31** 37 3 T Imperiale 1994 *JAMA* **271** 1780 4 E-BM **2** 20

9. Orthopaedics

Joint injection and aspiration

Joint aspirations may be diagnostic (*blood? crystals? pus?*) or therapeutic, for tense effusions, septic effusions, and haemarthroses. (Injection of contrast media is basis of diagnostic arthrography, but MRI is better.)

Steroid injections to inflamed joints, bursae, or tendon sheaths aim to reduce local anti-inflammation and relieve pain—perhaps by reducing synthesis of prostaglandins, or by stabilizing mast cells, or by reducing tissue calcification, or increasing vascularization and permeability of synovium. *Side-effects:* Skin atrophy (hydrocortisone acetate is safer than triamcinolone), haemarthrosis, facial flushing, urticaria, Charcot's arthropathy, post-injection flare syndrome (synovitis with fever), paresis,[1] and septic arthritis. ►*It is essential that steroids are not used in septic conditions* and, if any doubt at all exists, results of synovial fluid culture should be awaited. Remember the possibility of tuberculous synovitis—especially in immigrant populations. Repeated injections are more dangerous: beware ligamentous laxity, joint instability, calcification or rupture of tendons.

Various steroid preparations are available: *hydrocortisone acetate* (cheapest, shortest acting), *methylprednisolone*, and *triamcinolone*. They may be mixed with 1% lidocaine. When triamcinolone is used for injecting near short tendons, 10mg strength is preferred to 40mg as tendon rupture has been reported after the latter. Despite our best intentions 'joint' injections often fail to meet their target (50% in one study in which contrast material was also injected); those off-target are less likely to relieve symptoms.[2]

Conditions responding particularly well to steroid injection Localized subdeltoid bursitis; supraspinatus, infraspinatus and subscapular tendinitis; shoulder arthritis, tennis and golfer's elbow, arthritis of elbow, radioulnar, acromioclavicular, and sternoclavicular joints; ganglia; trigger fingers; strains of collateral and cruciate ligaments of knee; suprapatellar, infrapatellar, and Achilles tendinitis; plantar fasciitis, traumatic arthritis of metatarsophalangeal joints and sesamo-first-metatarsal joint.[2]

Preparation Check that you have swabs, needles and sterile bottles. For aspiration of viscid fluid (eg haemarthrosis) use 19-gauge (white) needle. For the larger joints use a 21-gauge (green) needle, and for fingers and toes a 23-gauge (blue) needle. Locate joint margins carefully before cleansing with chlorhexidine in 5% spirit or surgical spirit, and once the skin is cleansed use scrupulous aseptic or no-touch technique. Samples for microbiology should be sent in sterile containers, those for cytology or crystal examination in heparinized or FBC containers.

Knee joint The patient lies with knee supported slightly flexed and muscles relaxed. Palpate the joint space behind patella either medially or laterally. Insert a needle horizontally between the patella and femur. Slight resistance is felt on traversing the synovial membrane; it should be possible to aspirate fluid, and injection fluid should flow easily. *Usual doses:* 50mg hydrocortisone acetate, 40mg methylprednisolone, 20mg triamcinolone hexacetonide. Repeat injections should be longer than 3 months apart. If injection is used for prepatellar bursitis, give 25mg hydrocortisone acetate into the most tender spot.

The ankle Plantar flex foot slightly, palpate joint margin between extensor hallucis longus (lateral) and tibialis anterior (medial) tendons just above tip of medial malleolus. Inject 25mg hydrocortisone acetate into the joint.

1 G Van der Heijden 1996 *JRCGP* **46** 309
2 A Jones 1993 *BMJ* **ii** 1329 **3** J Cyriax 1980 *Textbook of Orthopaedic Medicine* Vol 2, 10e, London, Baillière

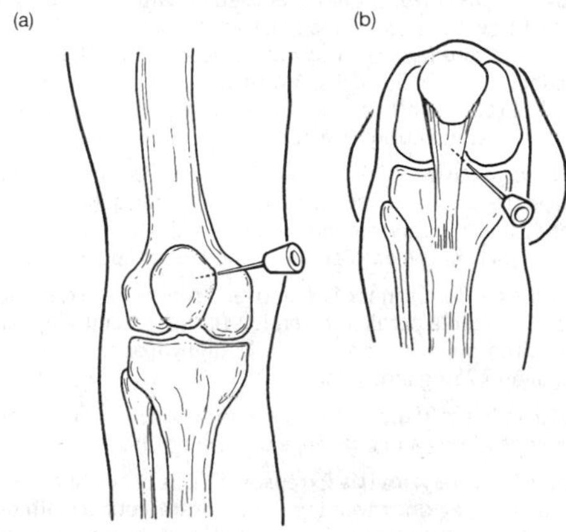

(a) The right knee, extended (anteromedial approach). (b) The right knee, flexed (infrapatellar anteromedial approach). (Reproduced by kind permission from M Crawley *Br J Hosp Med* **11** 747–55.)

Joint injections—continued

Shoulder injection Because shoulder pain from soft tissue causes is common (*lifetime incidence:* ~10%), and because the pain can be long lasting (only 23% resolve within a month), this is one of the most commonly injected joints, but we do not know *who* to inject or *when* in their illness, because trials are few, and the best ones cast doubt on the benefit of *any* injection.[1] *Anterior approach:* (for aspiration, synovitis, frozen shoulder) seat the patient with arm relaxed by side of his chest. Feel the space between head of humerus and glenoid cap about 1cm below coracoid process. Insert a 21-gauge green needle into the joint space (enters joint space when almost up to its hilt) and inject 25–50mg hydrocortisone acetate. Be sure not to go medial to the coracoid process. *Lateral approach:* (subacromial bursitis, painful arc syndrome) inject 25–50mg hydrocortisone acetate with lidocaine just below lateral tip of acromion, pointed downwards and slightly medially. If the needle is withdrawn from touching head of humerus with slight pressure on the plunger, a drop in pressure is felt as the bursa is entered. Painful arc pain may be reproduced. A second injection may be given after >48h.

Tennis elbow 25mg hydrocortisone acetate with one mL lidocaine is injected with force to area of maximal tenderness over lateral humeral condyle moving to and fro down to bone several times. A second injection may be needed, eg after 2 weeks. Warn the patient that symptoms may worsen briefly after the injection has been given. (Avoid triamcinolone and Depo-Medrone®: as injections are superficial, steroid necrosis may occur.)

Elbow joint injection With elbow flexed at 90°, inject 25mg hydrocortisone acetate between proximal head of radius (locate by rotating patient's hand) and lateral epicondyle by lateral approach (needle 90° to skin), or posteriorly between olecranon and lateral epicondyle.

Biceps tendinitis Tenderness is felt over tendon on externally rotating the arm. Insert a needle parallel to tendon (if resistance to injection, it is in the tendon: withdraw a bit) and inject 25mg hydrocortisone acetate into tendon sheath and 25mg into joint.

Wrist injection Inject 25mg hydrocortisone acetate 1–1.5cm deep between extensor tendons of ring and little fingers between ulnar head and lunate.

De Quervain's tenosynovitis Extensor pollicis brevis and abductor pollicis longus tendons, eg on traversing the extensor retinaculum on the dorsal wrist, may cause a tender swelling (p 616). With needle almost parallel to skin pointing proximally, inject 25mg hydrocortisone acetate slowly just distal or proximal to the styloid, at the site of maximum tenderness. If needle in tendon, injection is difficult so withdraw until easy flow occurs.

Carpal tunnel Place the hand comfortably palm up. Inject 25mg hydrocortisone acetate at 90° through the distal transverse skin crease of the palmar surface of wrist closer to hamate than the trapezium—ie a few mm to the ulnar side flexor carpi radialis. Other techniques are also used.[1] Sometimes the needle enters the median nerve causing sudden pain in the fingers—so reposition the needle. If the first injection fails, consider repeating with 10–20mg triamcinolone.[2] A splint worn for the next few days may mitigate induction of symptoms which can occur at the time of injection.

Trigger finger Insert needle at proximal finger skin crease parallel to flexor tendon, pointing towards palm. Palpate tendon thickening in palm and proceed as for De Quervain's.

First carpometacarpal joint of thumb Avoiding radial artery, inject 25mg hydrocortisone acetate at base of first metacarpal at 1cm depth in anatomical snuffbox (aim at base of little finger).

1 G Van der Heijden 1996 *JRCGP* **46** 309 2 M Shipley 1995 *BMJ* **i** 239

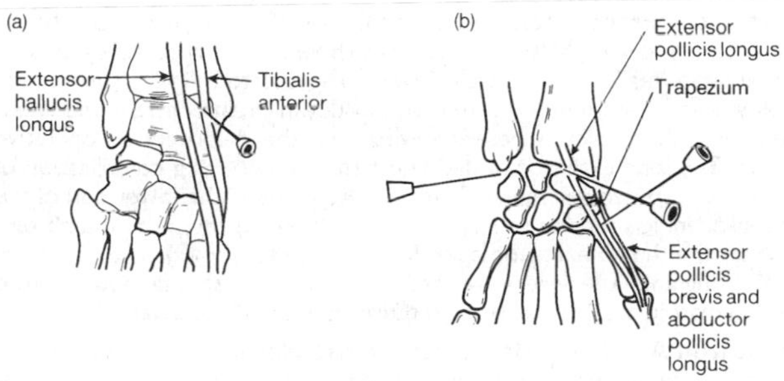

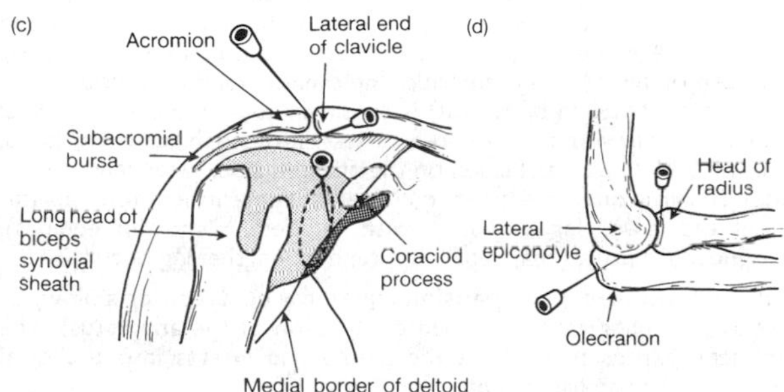

(a) Dorsal aspect of the right ankle indicating anatomical landmarks.
(b) Dorsal aspect of the right wrist indicating anatomical landmarks.
(c) Diagrammatic representation of the anterior aspect of the right shouder region. The stippled areas indicate synovial membranes of the subacromial bursa and the glenohumeral joints.
(d) The right elbow, flexed; the stippled area is the synovial membrane.

(Reproduced by kind permission from M Crawley *Br J Hosp Med* **11** 747.)

Tendons

The tendon conditions that can cause orthopaedic problems are those of tendon rupture or tenosynovitis (which may be infective or inflammatory). The most common ruptures are the extensor tendons of the fingers, the Achilles tendon, the long head of biceps (p 612), supraspinatus (p 612) and the quadriceps expansion.

Ultrasound scanning of the suspected tendon is possible to aid diagnosis although its usefulness is largely operator-dependent.

Ruptured extensor tendons of the fingers The long extensors inserting into the distal phalanx are particularly prone to rupture by trauma resulting in 'mallet' or 'baseball' fingers. The affected digit is splinted for 3–6 weeks (in extension). If the tendon doesn't reattach to bone spontaneously, the choice is between living with the deformity or operative repair. The long extensor of the thumb may rupture as a complication of fractures to the lower radius. *Treatment:* Repair uses the lower end of the extensor indicis tendon re-routed to be sutured to the distal thumb tendon (as the thumb extensor is too frayed for direct repair). The extensors of the ring and little fingers are particularly prone to spontaneous rupture in rheumatoid arthritis (attrition rupture from the distal ulna).

Ruptured Achilles (calcaneal) tendon Sudden pain is felt at the back of the ankle during running or jumping as the tendon ruptures ~5cm above the tendon insertion. Pain may be perceived as a kick. It is still possible to walk (with a limp), and some plantar flexion of the foot remains, but it is impossible to raise the heel from the floor when standing on the affected leg. A gap may be palpated in the tendon course (particularly within 24h of injury). On examination he cannot stand on tiptoe.
The squeeze test (Simmonds' test) is sensitive: ask the patient to kneel on a chair, while you squeeze both calves—if the Achilles is ruptured, there will be less plantar flexion on the affected side. *Treatment:* Urgent tendon repair is often preferred to conservative treatment (immobilization of the lower leg in plaster with the foot slightly in equinus). Undiagnosed ruptures may repair, but tendon lengthening occurs.

Ruptured quadriceps expansion Injury may be direct (eg a blow) or indirect (stumbling causing sudden contraction of the apparatus). The quadriceps expansion encloses the patella and inserts into the tibial tubercle by the patellar tendon.
Treatment: Rupture can occur at the site of quadriceps insertion to patella, through the patella by fracture (if reduction is possible it is secured by wire or screws, if not, the patella is excised and tendon repair effected), or by avulsion of the patellar tendon from the tibial tubercle (in young patients the torn tendon may be resutured). After repairs, a plaster cylinder is worn for several weeks, then intensive physiotherapy is needed to regain knee function.

Tenosynovitis Tendons and surrounding synovium may become locally inflamed (possibly due to strain) thereby causing pain (eg supraspinatus tendinitis and bicipital tendinitis p 612, De Quervain's p 616). Acute frictional synovitis at the wrist is another example, with swelling over the wrist and thumb extensors. If palpation doesn't detect crepitus, at some sites, stethoscope auscultation reveals sounds like bronchial breathing.[1]
Treatment: In wrist tenosinovitis, a splint for 3 weeks (leaving the fingers free) may be needed to allow inflammation to subside.

1 R Adler 1999 *NEJM* **340** 156 ('Bronchial breathing' on the painful right arch on great toe flexion with 'vesicular'-type breathing on the unaffected left side.)

9. Orthopaedics

Nerve compression syndromes

For brachial plexus and peripheral nerve lesions, see p 724, 664 & 720.

Carpal tunnel syndrome ►This is the commonest cause of hand pain at night. It is is due to compression of the median nerve as it passes under the flexor retinaculum. Pregnancy, the Pill, myxoedema, lunate fracture (rare), rheumatoid arthritis, cardiac failure, or being premenstrual may all increase compression. *Clinical features* are of median nerve distribution:

- Tingling or pain are felt in the thumb, index finger, and middle finger.
- When the pain is at its worse, the patient characteristically flicks or shakes the wrist to bring about relief. Pain is especially common at night and after repetitive actions. Affected persons may experience clumsiness. Early on there may be no signs. Later there is:
- Wasting of the thenar eminence and decreased sensation over the palm.
- Lateral palmar sensation is spared as its supply (the palmar cutaneous branch of the median nerve) does not pass through the tunnel.
- Phalen's test: holding the wrist hyperflexed for 1–2mins reproduces the symptoms. (This is more reliable than Tinel's test—tapping over the tunnel to produce paraesthesiae. Note: Phalen's flexing, Tinnel's tapping.)

Tests: Nerve conduction studies are not usually needed (and may be –ve).[1]

Treatment: Diuretics may help. Carpal injection: see p 658 for technique. Wrist splints worn at night may relieve nocturnal pain. More permanent results are obtained from decompression by flexor retinaculum division.

Ulnar nerve compression at the elbow This is described on p 614.

Posterior interosseus nerve compression This radial nerve branch is sometimes compressed on passing through the supinator muscle (after forearm fracture). Patients experience weakness of the thumb and fingers. *Examination* may reveal weakness of long finger extensors, and short and long extensors of the thumb, but no sensory loss. *Treatment* after trauma is surgical decompression and springed splints to extend fingers.

Anterior interosseus nerve compression This median nerve branch may be compressed under the fibrous origin of flexor digitorum sublimis, causing weakness of pinch and pain along the forearm's radial border. Examination shows weakness of the long thumb flexor and flexor profundus to the index and middle fingers. *Treatment* is surgical decompression.

Ulnar nerve compression at the wrist Uncommon. Loss may be motor or sensory. *Diagnose* by electrophysiology. *Treat* by surgical decompression.

Meralgia paraesthetica If the lateral cutaneous nerve of the thigh is compressed (on leaving the pelvis just medial to the anterior superior iliac spine, eg by tight jeans), pain and paraesthesiae may be felt over the upper outer thigh. Sensation may be ↓ over this area. It is usually self-limiting, and can occur in pregnancy. *Treatment:* Cortisone and local anaesthetic injection at the anterior superior iliac spine gives unpredictable results.

Common peroneal compression Nerve compression against the head of fibula (eg plaster casts, thin patients lying unconscious, proximal fibula fracture) causes inability to dorsiflex the foot. Sensation may be ↓ over the dorsum of the foot. *Tests:* Electrophysiology. *Treatment:* Most recover spontaneously but surgical decompression may be needed. Physiotherapy and splint until foot-drop recovers.

1 M Shipley 1995 BMJ i 239

Soft tissue injuries

Correct management of soft tissue injuries reduces pain, recovery time and subsequent disability.

Treatment in the first 24 hours: 'RICE'

Rest: A splint or plaster cast may help.

Ice: Cold is anaesthetic and causes vasoconstriction. Apply an ice pack (eg a packet of frozen peas wrapped in a cloth), a cold spray or cold compresses intermittently every 10 minutes.

Compression: Strapping restricts swelling and further bleeding.

Elevation: Ideally toes higher than bottom to improve drainage from the affected part and to reduce pain.

Rehabilitation Passive stretching to maintain joint mobility and muscle length, then progressive active exercise until the full range and strength of movement is restored, eg wobbleboards for ankles. Sportsmen must then retrain to full fitness. Also consider NSAIDs, rubefacients and ultrasound.

Sports injuries Many sports injuries can be prevented.

- Is the patient preparing the body for activity with a proper warm-up? Inadequate warm-up increases the risk of injury.
- Cooling-down is also important in reducing muscle soreness.
- Is protective equipment being worn?
- Many acute and chronic injuries are caused by unsuitable equipment, faulty technique or unwise training schedules—advice from a professional coach can be invaluable.

Common patterns of injury in sport: 'Shin splints'—shin soreness, common in unfit runners on hard surfaces and due to muscle tears, mild anterior compartment syndrome or stress fracture; knee pain—most causes on p 636; ligamentous ankle injury (p 712); plantar fasciitis (p 642); stress fractures such as march fracture—suspect with increasing bony pain despite normal x-ray (radionuclide scans are more discriminating[1]); Achilles tendon problems; tennis elbow (p 614).

Overuse phenomena

Overuse phenomena at work (*Work-related upper limb injury = occupational overuse syndrome = isometric contraction myopathy = repetitive strain injury = RSI*) Activity requiring repetitive actions, particularly those associated with prolonged muscle contraction, may lead to chronic symptoms. Employers have a duty to provide a safe working environment and well-designed chairs and tools, and frequent short breaks. Changes of posture and activity help to reduce work-related upper limb injury (this term is preferred to repetitive strain injury). The cost of these injuries in suffering, and hours lost from work, is considerable as treatment of established symptoms is often difficult and may necessitate change in employment—if one is available.

Compensation is a vexed issue, and recent Court judgments have gone in favour of the employers in some instances, and in favour of patients in others. Some people argue that the condition does not exist as a separate medical entity[2] emphasize the lack of histopathology. It should be noted that this is not a prerequisite for a disease (see *Sudden infant death*, p 286)—and in any case histopathology *is* sometimes demonstrable. Treatments tried include splinting (may prolong the problem), physiotherapy, β-blockers for relaxation, and the Alexander technique for posture re-education.[3]

Those who use vacuum cleaners, assemble cars or play stringed instruments may all develop tennis elbow.

1 M Macleod 1999 BMJ i 29 2 A Mann 1994 BMJ i 269 3 P Brookes 1993 BMJ ii 1298

Testing peripheral nerves

Nerve root	*Muscle*	*Test—by asking the patient to:*
C3,4	trapezius	Shrug shoulder, adduct scapula.
C4,5	rhomboids	Brace shoulder back.
C5,6,7	serratus anterior	Push forward against resistance.
C**5**,6	pectoralis major (clavicular head)	Adduct arm from above horizontal, and push it forward.
C6,**7**,8	pectoralis major (sternocostal head)	Adduct arm below horizontal.
C**5**,6	supraspinatus	Abduct arm the first 15°.
C**5**,6	infraspinatus	Externally rotate arm, elbow at side.
C6,**7**,8	latissimus dorsi	Adduct arm from horizontal position.
C5,6	biceps	Flex supinated forearm.
C**5**,6	deltoid	Abduct arm between 15° and 90°.

The radial nerve

Nerve root	Muscle	Test
C6,**7**,8	triceps	Extend elbow against resistance.
C5,**6**	brachioradialis	Flex elbow with forearm half way between pronation and supination.
C5,**6**	extensor carpi radialis longus	Extend wrist to radial side with fingers extended.
C6,7	supinator	Arm by side, resist hand pronation.
C**7**,8	extensor digitorum	Keep fingers extended at MCP joint.
C**7**,8	extensor carpi ulnaris	Extend wrist to ulnar side.
C**7**,8	abductor pollicis longus	Abduct thumb at 90° to palm.
C**7**,8	extensor pollicis brevis	Extend thumb at MCP joint.
C**7**,8	extensor pollicis longus	Resist thumb flexion at IP joint.

Median nerve

Nerve root	Muscle	Test
C6,7	pronator teres	Keep arm pronated against resistance.
C6,7	flexor carpi radialis	Flex wrist towards radial side.
C7,**8**,T1	flexor digitorum sublimis	Resist extension at PIP joint (while you fix his proximal phalanx).
C**8**,T1	flexor digitorum profundus I & II	Resist extension at the DIP joint of index finger.
C**8**,T1	flexor pollicis longus	Resist thumb extension at interphalangeal joint (fix proximal phalanx).
C8,**T1**	abductor pollicis brevis	Abduct thumb (nail at 90° to palm).
C8,**T1**	opponens pollicis	Thumb touches base of 5th finger-tip nail parallel to palm).
C8,**T1**	1st and 2nd lumbricals	Extend PIP joint against resistance with MCP joint held hyperextended.

Ulnar nerve

Nerve root	Muscle	Test
C7,**8**,T1	flexor carpi ulnaris	Flex wrist towards ulnar side.
C**7**,C8	flexor digitorum profundus III and IV	Fix middle phalanx of little finger, resist extension of distal phalanx.
C8,**T1**	dorsal interossei	Abduct fingers (use index finger).
C8,**T1**	palmar interossei	Adduct fingers (use index finger).
C8,**T1**	adductor pollicis	Adduct thumb (nail at 90° to palm).
C8,**T1**	abductor digiti minimi	Abduct little finger.
C8,**T1**	flexor digiti minimi	Flex the little finger at MCP joint.

The musculocutaneous nerve (C5–6) This may be injured at the brachial plexis, causing weakness of biceps, coracobrachialis and brachialis. Forearm flexion is weak. There may be some loss of sensation.

Nerve root	Muscle	Test—by asking the patient to:
L**4**,**5**, S1	gluteus medius and minimum (superior gluteal nrv)	Internal rotation. at hip, hip abduction.
L5, S1,2	gluteus maximus (inferior gluteal nrv)	Extension at hip (lie prone).
L**2**,**3**,4	adductors (obturator nrv)	Adduct leg against resistance.
Femoral nerve		
L1,2,3	iliopsoas	Flex hip with knee flexed and lower leg supported: patient lies on back.
L2,3	sartorius	Flex knee with hip external rotated.
L2,3,4	quadriceps femoris	Extend knee against resistance.
Obturator nerve		
L2,3,4	Hip adductors	Adduct the leg.
Internal gluteal nerve		
L5,S1,S2	Gluteus maximus	Hip extension.
Superficial gluteal nerve		
L4,5,S1	Gluteus medius	Abduction and internal rotation of hip.
	Gluteus medialis	Abduction and internal rotation of hip.
Sciatic nerve (*and the common peroneal nerve)		
L5 **S1**,2	hamstrings	Flex knee against resistance.
L4,5	tibialis posterior	Invert plantarflexed foot.
*L**4**,5	tibialis anterior	Dorsiflex ankle.
*L**5**,S1	extensor digitorum long	Dorsiflex toes against resistance.
*L**5**,S1	extensor hallucis long.	Dorsiflex hallux against resistance.
*L**5**,S1	peroneus longus and brevis	Evert foot against resistance.
L5,S1	extensor digit. brevi	Dorsiflex hallux (muscle of foot).
S1,2	gastrocnemius	Plantarflex ankle joint.
L5,**S1**,2	flexor digitorum longus	Flex terminal joints of toes.
S1,2	small muscles of foot	Make sole of foot into a cup.

Quick screening test for muscle power

Shoulder	Abduction C5		Hip	Flexion	L1–L2
	Adduction C5–C7			Extension	L5–S1
Elbow	Flexion	C5–C6	Knee	Flexion	S1
	Extension	C7		Extension	L3–L4
Wrist	Flexion	C7–8	Ankle	Dorsiflexion	L4
	Extension	C7		Plantarflexion	S1–S2
Fingers	Flexion	C7–C8; Extension C7			
	Abduction T1				

Remember to test proximal muscle power, eg by asking the patient to sit from lying, to pull you towards himself, and to rise from squatting.

NB: Root numbers in **bold** indicate that that root is more important than its neighbour. ►Sources vary in ascribing particular nerve roots to muscles–and there is considerable biological variation in individuals. The above is a reasonable compromise, and is based on the MRC guidelines.

Assessing the locomotor system

The aim is to screen efficiently for rheumatological conditions—and also to assess any motor disability. It is based on the GALS locomotor screen.[1] ►Don't *just* catalogue muscle function. (Details of testing each muscle may be found on p 664.) Find out what a person can do—eg with her arthritic fingers, can she do up zips or buttons? Can she open a tin? Is she using any special devices to assist in daily life? What can't she do that she would like? Does she have any comments on her joints?

Essence Ask *questions, look, compare, move* and *palpate*. If a joint feels normal to the patient, looks normal, and has a full movement, it usually *is* normal.

Valgus or varus? In a valgus deformity, remember 'L' for lateral in the spelling: the part of the limb distal to the deformity is angled *laterally* from the midline. Varus is the other way.

3 screening questions •Are you free of pain or stiffness in your muscles? •Can you dress all right? •Can you manage stairs? If 'Yes' to all 3, muscle problems are unlikely. If 'No' to any, go into functional detail.

A screening examination To be done in light underwear. (No corsets!)

Observe from behind: Is muscle bulk OK (buttocks, shoulders)? Is the spine straight? Symmetrical paraspinal muscles? Any swellings or deformities?
Observe from the side: Normal cervical and lumbar lordosis? Kyphosis?
'Touch your toes, please': Are lumbar spine and hip flexion normal?
Observe from in front for the rest of the examination. Ask him to:
'Tilt head towards shoulders': Is lateral cervical flexion normal?
Open and close your mouth': Orofacial pain, temporomandibular joint noises ± restricted jaw function indicate temoromandibular joint problems, p 534.
'Put hands behind head': Tests glenohumeral and sternoclavicular movement.
'Arms straight': Tests elbow extension. Then test supination and pronation.
Examine the hands: See *OHCM* p 25. Any deformity, wasting, or swellings?
'Put index finger on thumb': Tests pincer grip. Assess dexterity.
Observe the legs: Normal quadriceps bulk? Any swelling or deformity?
Find any knee effusion: Sit the patient down, take the leg on your lap, and do the patella tap test (this also tests for patellofemoral tenderness), or, to be more sensitive, watch any fluid moving from compartment to compartment by stroking upwards over the medial side of the knee, and then downwards over the lateral side. Aspirate it. Any blood, crystals or pus?
Observe feet: Any deformity? Are arches high or low? Any callosities? These may reflect an abnormal gait of some chronicity.
'Walk over there please': Is the gait smooth? Is there good arm swing? Is the stride length OK? Normal heel strike and toe off? Can he turn quickly?

Additional palpations •Press over the midpoint of each supraspinatus muscle, to elicit the tenderness of fibromyalgia (p 675).
•Squeeze across 2nd–5th metacarpals. Any synovitis? Repeat in metatarsals.
•Palpate for crepitus with your palm on his knee (patient supine), while you passively flex knee and hip to the full extent. Is movement limited?
•Internally rotate each hip in flexion.

The GALS system for quickly recording your findings[2]

G (Gait) ✓		
	Appearance:	Movement:
A (Arms)	✓	✓
L (Legs)	✓	✓
S (Spine)	✓	✓

A tick (✓) means normal. If not normal, then substitute a cross with a footnote to explain what the exact problem is.

1 M Doherty 1992 *Annals of the Rheumatic Diseases* **51** 1165 2 As approved by the education committees of the Arthritis & Rheumatism Council and the British Society for Rheumatology (1991)

Hot, swollen joints

The term arthritis implies an inflammatory condition of one or more joints. Features of inflammation: *pain*, *swelling*, *overlying redness*, *stiffness*, and *local heat* (± fever). In making a diagnosis, there are 3 key questions: ►Is only one joint affected (ie a monoarthritis)?
►Is the patient otherwise well, or is there a disease causing arthritis (eg ulcerative colitis) or a risk factor for infection (diabetes, renal failure, immunosuppression, IV drug abusers)? ►What is making the joint swollen? Blood, crystals or pus?—It is always worth aspirating the joint (p 656) to find out, but beware introducing infection if the effusion is a sympathetic one, from nearby cellulitis or abscess formation.

Note: the presence of rheumatoid factor (latex +ve, p 670) divides the arthritides into seropositive (SP below) and seronegative.

Causes Any polyarthritis can *start* as a monoarthritis. This list is only a guide to likely presentation. ►Always think of infection—eg TB.

Monoarthritis:
- Bacteria, eg *staphs, streps, pseudomonas, gonococci*; TB; septicaemia
- Gout or pseudogout
- Reiter's disease (*OHCM* p 668)
- Traumatic haemarthrosis
- Psoriasis
- Rheumatoid arthritis[SP]
- Leukaemic joint deposits
- Reactive arthritis (see p 675)

Polyarthritis:
- Viruses, eg rubella, mumps, Hepatitis A, Ebstein–Barr
- Rheumatoid arthritis[SP]
- Sjögren's syndrome[SP]
- Rheumatic fever
- Systemic lupus erythematosus[SP]
- Ulcerative colitis; Crohn's
- Drug reaction
- Reiter's and psoriasis (rarer)

Tests Liaise with a microbiologist; take blood cultures before treatment.
- Gram stain, culture and microscopy (for crystals, using polarized light) on fluid aspirated from the joint. Blood staining of synovial fluid is seen in pseudogout as well as after trauma, but it is rare in septic arthritis.
- X-ray of the part. Look for signs of trauma (fractures), rheumatoid arthritis (p 670). Cartilage calcification suggests pseudogout. In some patients x-rays will appear normal.
- Urate, FBC, ESR, Latex, C-reactive protein (normal <20mg/L) may be ↑ in sero +ve or –ve causes; it does *not* screen for sepsis. Consider HIV serology.

Management Unless microbiological facilities are readily to hand, consider hospitalizing all people with acute monoarthritis of a large joint so that infection can either be ruled out, or appropriate antibiotics given. Even if aspiration reveals pus, it does not follow that infection is the cause (the diagnosis may be pseudogout or rheumatoid arthritis).

Treatment is determined by cause. In septic arthritis, give flucloxacillin (for staphs—adult: ½–1g/6h slowly IV; child: 25mg/kg/4h) + benzylpenicillin 1.2g/4h IV until sensitivities are known. In infants, *Haemophilus* is common so give cefotaxime too (50mg/kg/12h IV slowly). Look for atypical mycobacteria and fungi if HIV +ve. Ask a microbiologist how long to continue treatment (eg 2 weeks IV then 4 weeks of oral therapy). NB: the rôle of repeated aspiration, lavage, and surgery is uncertain. Ask an orthopaedic surgeon's advice. Many will recommend repeated arthroscopy for a child's infected hip. Beware inviting in new pathogens.

Splints help by immobilizing the joint in the early days of treatment. If a joint prosthesis is present, surgery with removal of all foreign material may be required. Vigorous physiotherapy follows antibiotics.

Osteoarthritis

Predisposing causes Joint malalignment, eg valgus deformity; decreased size of joint contact (eg subluxation in congenital dislocation of the hip); osteochondral fractures; foreign bodies; torn menisci; damaged cartilage from septic arthritis or neuropathy.

Pathology Early on there is splitting (fibrillation) of cartilage, then some breaks away, leaving exposed bone—which becomes thickened, hard and white ('eburnation'). Nodular new bone formations at joint surfaces are called osteophytes.

The patient may suffer joint pain at rest (eg at night); pain on movement. Joints may be a little thickened, but not usually inflamed. Crepitus (the grating of surfaces) may be felt on joint movement. There may be fixed deformity (inability to assume neutral position). In the hands the distal interphalangeal joints are commonly affected. Swellings at these joints are called Heberden's nodes. Rheumatoid factor is absent. The ESR is normal.

X-ray changes 1 Joint space ↓ **2** Subchondral sclerosis **3** Subchondral cysts **4** 'Lipping' at joint margins (from osteophytes).

Treatment aim to *reduce pain* and disability, and to *increase fitness* (gentle-to-moderate exercise *does* improve symptoms,⟨1⟩ but note that cycling may aggravate patellofemoral osteoarthritis, and swimming is generally good for back and hip symptoms but may worsen cervical apophyseal joint osteoarthritis). There are no panaceas. For pain, try *paracetamol* 500mg–1g/6h PO alone or in combination with opioids, eg *co-proxamol* (expect constipation). Consider NSAIDs, such as *ibuprofen* 400mg/8h PO pc, for inflammatory episodes (eg in the knee), but if needed long term, beware GI bleeding—and consider a *misoprostol*-containing tablet, eg Arthrotec® (contains *diclofenac*), or Napratec® (contains *naproxen*).

Local warmth may give relief. *Physiotherapy* may increase functional use of joints. Unload weight-bearing joints through *weight reduction* (diet) and *walking aids* (stick, frame, stair rail). *Occupational therapists* can advise on modifying tools and home. *Intra-articular steroid injections* are also tried, and may relieve symptoms for a month or two (eg in the knee: see p 656). When disability or pain are severe, consider *surgery*.

Surgery

- Arthroscopic *joint debridement*, excision of osteophytes and unstable articular cartilage+drilling of exposed bone helps ≥60% of patients.[2]
- *Arthrodesis* (surgical fusing of a joint) is used most commonly at the metatarsophalangeal joint of the hallux.
- *Osteotomy* to realign a joint—eg to correct genu varum deformity.
- *Excision arthroplasty* is used in Keller's operation (p 640). • *Interposition arthroplasty* is used at the thumb's carpometacarpal joint, when a silastin sponge is interposed between the joint surfaces. • *Joint replacement* (p 654) for hips, elbows, shoulders and knees.

Arthritis of the hip Fixed flexion deformities are common. Thomas test reveals such deformity (p 628). The usual surgical treatment is replacement arthroplasty (p 654).

Neuropathic joints (Charcot's joints)

Causes: Diabetic neuropathy, tabes dorsalis, cauda equina lesion, leprosy, syringomyelia (upper limb). Gross disorganization of the joints (even dislocation) follows repeated minor trauma.

⟨1⟩PA Kovar 1992 *Ann Int Med* **116** 529 & *Drug Ther Bul* **34** 33 **2** *J Bone & Joint Surg* 1991 Ed 737–8

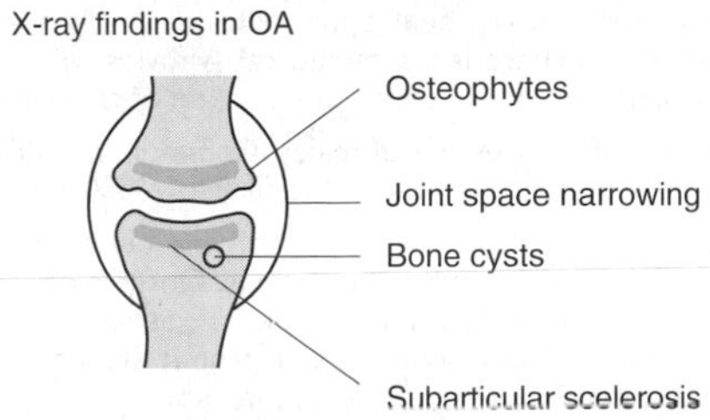

NSAIDs and cyclo-oxygenase (COX-1 & COX-2)[1]

COX converts arachidonic acid to prostaglandins, and NSAIDs inhibit COX which is why they are analgesic and anti-inflammatory, and why they cause GI bleeding. But COX exists in 2 forms: GI cytoprotection is mediated by COX-1. COX-2 is activated by inflammatory stimuli, and produces the prostaglandins mediating inflammation. Some NSAIDs, eg meloxicam, preferentially inhibit COX-2, but claims that these are the much-longed for 'safe aspirin' may be premature: they may not be safe and they may not be aspirin, as COX-1 inhibition may be required for full anti-inflammatory benefit.[2] They are not true 'gastroprotectors', and they are still contra-indicated in those with peptic problems, and they may cause problems with fluid retention, as COX-2 is expressed in the kidney's medulla densa. They do not have aspirin's cardiovascular effects.

1 C Hawky 1999 *Lancet* **353** 307 2 J Wallace 1998 *Gastroenterology* **115** 101

Rheumatoid arthritis

The central immunological event is said to be presentation of the culprit antigen (whatever this turns out to be) to T-helper cells, with subsequent cytokine-mediated synovial neutrophil exudate, which releases cartilage-degrading enzymes. There is a symmetrical synovitis, with arthralgia, stiffness, and swelling, and, if prolonged, destruction of peripheral joints.[1]

Prevalence 3% of females, 1% of males. Common in middle age (but any age affected). Association: HLA-DRW4. Incidence: 1/1000 adults/yr.[1]

Presentation Very variable. It may take time before RA can be distinguished from other inflammatory conditions. Onset is often insidious with malaise, transient pain, stiffness and weakness, but may be sudden—'One day I couldn't move'. Monoarthritis, palindromic arthritis—joints affected by turn—and systemic presentations occur.

Prognosis[2] 20% have one attack, often acute, with complete recovery. 30% are mildly disabled; 40% have prolonged, moderately disabling disease, severe in 10%. Life expectancy↓, by 3 (♀) to 7yr (♂). Worse prognosis if: female, palindromic onset, extra-articular features, nodules, erosions occurring within 3yrs of onset, persistently high CRP, rheumatoid factor ↑↑, HLA DR4 +ve.

Joint involvement Inflamed synovium (pannus) produces hot swollen tender joints and thickened tendons with associated soft-tissue swelling, hence the characteristic sausage-shaped fingers. Early morning stiffness may last for several hours. With time the pannus erodes the joints and tendons rupture and the irreversible changes typical of advanced RA are seen. *Fingers* develop 'swan neck' (hyperextended PIP joint but flexed DIP joint) or 'boutonnière' deformities (flexed PIP joint, extended MCP joint, hyperextended DIP joint); *thumbs* adopt Z-deformities. *MCP joints* and *wrists* sublux acquiring ulnar deviation: the ulnar styloid and radial head become prominent. *Knees* develop valgus or varus deformity. Popliteal 'Baker's' cysts occur and may rupture mimicking a DVT. In the *feet* subluxation of the metatarsal heads with associated hallux valgus, clawed toes and callouses causes pain—'walking on marbles'. ►*Atlantoaxial instability* may lead to cord compression; x-ray prior to intubation is wise.

Extra-articular involvement Weight loss, fever and malaise are common. Many systemic manifestations of RA are caused by vasculitis or nodules. 10% develop amyloid. Drug complications can affect most systems (p 672).
Skin: Nail fold infarcts, ulcers, rashes, palmar erythema.
Nodules: Firm, mobile, non-tender nodules are found on pressure areas, eg forearm of 20% of sufferers. Nodules may also occur on tendon sheaths (causing triggering) or in lungs, myocardium, pericardium or sclera.
Eyes: Keratoconjunctivitis sicca (p 482), scleritis, episcleritis.
Cardiovascular system: Pericardial effusion, pericarditis, myocarditis.
Lungs: Pleurisy, pleural effusions, nodules, fibrosing alveolitis.
CNS: Entrapment neuropathy (eg carpal tunnel), compression syndromes.

Tests *Blood:* Normochromic anaemia, ESR↑. Both correlate with disease activity. Also: alk phos↑, platelets↑, lymphocytes↓, WCC↓ (in Felty's *OHCM* p 698). Rheumatoid factor: this anti-IgG autoantibody appears eventually in 80% of those with RA but is found in low titres in many chronic conditions. Antinuclear factor: +ve in 30% with RA (*OHCM* p 675).
Synovial fluid: Turbid; viscosity↓; clots, from high polymorph count.
X-ray changes: In order of appearance: soft-tissue swelling; juxta-articular osteoporosis; symmetrical loss of joint space; erosions at joint margins, subluxation and dislocation of joints.

1 R Madhok 1995 *Lancet* **346** 481 2 D Walker 1998 *Practitioner* **242** 743

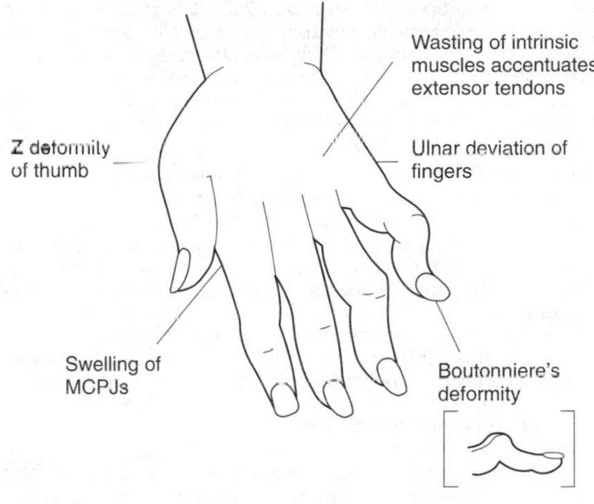
Wasting of intrinsic muscles accentuates extensor tendons
Z deformity of thumb
Ulnar deviation of fingers
Swelling of MCPJs
Boutonniere's deformity

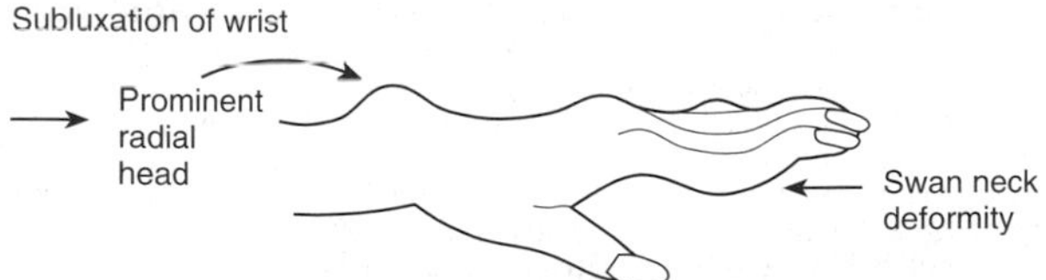
Subluxation of wrist
Prominent radial head
Swan neck deformity

Rheumatoid arthritis: treatment

►*Refer all patients to a rheumatologist as early as possible as vigorous prompt use of disease-modifying drugs can prevent future problems.*[1]

The patient's attitude is crucial to wellbeing. A severely afflicted patient who does quads exercises daily and seeks ways around disability will be living an independent life long after a mildly affected patient who has 'given up'.

Acute flare-ups initially require rest, analgesia and NSAIDs; then passive and active exercise are introduced to maintain joint mobility and muscle tone. **Chronic disease** is characterized by pain, stiffness, malaise and permanent loss of function. Exercises, splints, and gadgets (eg kettle-tippers) protect joints. Special shoes (or trainers) and seat raises allow independence. HRT may particularly help women patients. **Skeletal collapse** needs analgesia, surgery, appliances/home conversion, and social/financial help to mitigate isolation and income loss. **Simple analgesia**—eg paracetamol is useful for pain relief. **NSAIDs** If no contraindication (asthma, active peptic ulcer) start an NSAID, eg ibuprofen 400–800mg/8h PO pc (cheapest and least likely to cause GI bleeds) or naproxen 250–500mg/12h PO pc (twice a day dose, and is more anti-inflammatory than ibuprofen, and may cause less GI bleeding than other NSAIDs). Diclofenac 25–50mg/8h PO pc is similar to naproxen and can be combined with misoprostol (Arthrotec®)—an ulcer-protecting agent (*OHCM* p 490)—worth considering if history of dyspepsia and NSAIDs vital. Which NSAID will most benefit a patient is unpredictable. If 1–2 week trials of 3 NSAIDs don't control pain, consider a drug below.

Disease-modifying drugs[2] modify immunology, reducing disease activity as measured by ESR, counts of tender joints, and functional indices, eg grip. As they are slow to act and have a high incidence of adverse effects needing regular monitoring, their use is restricted to those likely to gain most benefit, eg early on in the active stage of disease which is going to progress. Sufferers in this category are those with: •Active sinovitis •Erosive x-ray changes •ESR or CRP↑ •Rapid loss of function •Rh factor +ve.

Gold (sodium aurothiomalate 50mg/week IM or, a bit less effectively orally as auranofin 3mg/12h). After 3 months on IM gold 80% of patients improve and can use a lower dose but 60% stop due to side-effects. SE necessitating stopping treatment: mouth ulcers, rashes (risk of exfoliative dermatitis), persistent proteinuria, lung fibrosis, WCC <4 × 10^9/L; neutrophils <2 × 10^9/L; platelets <150 × 10^9/L. ►Monitor urine and FBC often.

Penicillamine up to 500mg/24h PO. Efficacy (and monitoring) as for gold.

Sulfasalazine 500mg/6h PO (start with 500mg/24h) is less effective than IM gold but works faster and is well tolerated, so may be used earlier. SE: D&V, sperm count↓, WCC↓. Monitor LFT+FBC. Warn to stop if sore throat (=WCC↓).

Hydroxychloroquine 200mg/24h PO is least effective. SE: irreversible retinopathy so ophthalmological monitoring required.

Immunosuppressants such as azathioprine are occasionally used.

Methotrexate consider if severe disease (do LFT, FBC, U&E, hepatitis B and C serology first; do liver biopsy if +ve, or if alcohol abuse). Warn to report any cough or dyspnoea (pneumonitis is a side-effect). Stop if WCC <4 × 10^9/L; neutrophils <2 × 10^9/L; platelets <150 × 10^9/L.

Steroids can reduce erosions if given early (prednisolone 7.5mg/day PO). It is not known if all should receive this. One problem is ↓bone density over long periods. Another problem is that it would be difficult to keep patients to <7.5mg/day, as, for the first months, there may be great symptomatic improvement, which then tails off, leaving patients wanting higher doses, and risking cataract, fluid retention, and peptic ulcers.

Surgery may relieve pain and improve function, eg arthroplasty (joint reconstruction/replacement), particularly for forefoot, hips and knees; arthrodesis (joint fusion) of ankle or foot. Synovectomy, tendon repair and transfer, joint debridement and nerve decompression are also useful.

1 *Ann Rheum Dis* 1998 **57** 511 2 Medicines Resource Centre *Bulletin* 1996 7(3) 9–12

Influencing the biological events[1,2,3]

The chief biological event is inflammation, which is presumed to represent intolerance to an as-yet unidentified antigen. There are two types of inflammation: that mediated by *prostaglandins* (hence the place of NSAIDs), which is mediated by an up-regulated cyclooxygenase-2, and that mediated by *cytokines*. It is the cytokines that are thought to produce most long-term damage, and disease modifying drugs partly block their effects. Cytokines produce damage locally when synovial pannus (an inflammatory exudate on the synovial membrane—may cause ankylosis) erodes cartilage and bone; they also produce systemic effects with loss of axial and appendicular bone.[2]

Cytotoxics Long-term results of escalation therapy (first an NSAID, then disease-modifing drugs in increasing doses) give disappointing results, and it may be that the cells producing the inflammatory mediators need to be inactivated early. Methotrexate (eg 7.5mg/week PO) with high-dose prednisolone (eg 60mg/24h PO tapered in weekly steps to 7.5mg/day over 6 weeks) may have a rôle here. In one study (N=155) this regimen combined with sulfasalazine (2g/day PO) was able to suppress disease in 72% compared with 49% in the placebo group receiving sulfasalazine alone. The benefits only lasted while the treatment was being given (prednisolone was tapered and stopped by week 28, and methotrexate by week 40); 6 months after stopping the treatment, CRP, a useful marker of disease activity, was similar in both groups.

The future: anticytokine therapy *Tumour necrosis factor (TNF)* is a cytokine mediator in rheumatoid arthritis and other conditions (T & B cell activation): helpful locally, but sometimes disastrous in its systemic effects (eg in malaria, DIC, and the septic shock syndromes). Infliximab (anti-TNF antibody) and etanercept (TNF receptors, eg 25mg sc twice-weekly) ↓TNF activity, and, in ~40% of those with persistently active disease, activity may be halved (*vs* 3% on methotrexate alone).[4,5] SE: few; long-term safety issues are opaque (?↑risk of cancer ± infections).[4]

1 P Emery 1997 *Lancet* **350** 304 2 A Gough 1994 *Lancet* **344** 23 3 M Boers 1997 *Lancet* **350** 309
4 J O'Dell 1999 *NEJM* **340** 310 5 M Weinblatt 1999 *NEJM* **340** 253

The seronegative arthropathies

Gout In the acute stage there is severe pain, redness and swelling in the affected joint—often the metatarsophalangeal joint of the big toe (podagra). Attacks are due to hyperuricaemia (*OHCM* p 634) and the deposition of sodium monourate crystals in joints, and may be precipitated by trauma, surgery, starvation, infection and diuretics. After repeated attacks, urate deposits (tophi) are found in avascular areas, eg pinna, tendons, joints, eye—and chronic tophaceous gout is said to exist. 'Secondary' causes of gout: polycythaemia, leukaemia, cytotoxics, renal failure.

Diagnosis depends on finding urate crystals in tissues and synovial fluid (serum urate not always ↑). Microscopy of synovial fluid: negatively birefringent crystals; neutrophils (with ingested crystals). X-rays may show only soft-tissue swelling in the early stages. Later well-defined 'punched out' lesions are seen in juxta-articular bone. There is no sclerotic reaction, and joint spaces are preserved until late. *Prevalence:* ~½–1%. ♂:♀ ≈5:1.

Treating acute gout Try an NSAID (eg naproxen 750mg stat, then 250mg/8h PO pc). If contraindicated (eg peptic ulcer), give colchicine 1mg PO initially, then 0.5mg/2h PO until the pain goes or D&V occurs, or 10mg has been given. *Prevention of attacks: Avoid prolonged fasts and purine-rich foods:* offal; oily fish; roes; anchovies; mussels; crabs; prawns; shrimps; meat and yeast extracts; spinach; chocolate; caffeine, eg in cough-and-cold remedies. *Avoid obesity and alcohol excess* and *very high-protein meals*. No *aspirin* (it ↑ serum urate).

Consider reducing serum urate with long-term allopurinol, but not until 3 weeks after an attack. Allopurinol: 100mg/24h PO pc, ↑ as needed to 600mg/24h. Monitor serum urate levels. SE: rash, fever, leukopenia. If troublesome, substitute a uricosuric, eg probenecid 0.25–0.5g/12h PO.

Ankylosing spondylitis (AS) *Prevalence:* 1 in 2000. Men are affected earlier (♂/♀≈6 at 16 yrs old and ♂/♀≈2 at 30yrs old). >95% are HLA-B27 +ve. *Symptoms:* The typical patient is a young man presenting with morning stiffness and progressive loss of spinal movement (spinal ankylosis) and sacroiliac joint involvement—with eventual kyphosis, neck hyperextension (question mark posture), and spinocranial ankylosis. *Other features:*

- Thoracic excursion ↓
- Chest pain
- Hip/knee involvement
- Periostitis of calcaneum or ischial tuberosities
- Plantar fasciitis
- Amyloidosis
- Carditis; iritis
- Lung fibrosis (apex)

Tests: Radiology may show: a 'bamboo spine', squaring of the vertebra, erosions of the apophyseal joints, obliteration of the sacroiliac joints (sacroiliitis also occurs in Reiter's disease, Crohn's disease and chronic polyarthritis). Other tests: FBC (normochromic anaemia); ESR↑.

Treatment: Exercise, not rest, for backache. If able to co-operate with an intensive exercise regimen to maintain posture and mobility, he may keep happy and employed, despite chronic progressive illness. NSAIDs may relieve pain and stiffness. Rarely, spinal osteotomy is useful.

Mortality: 1.5-fold higher than expected (eg from secondary amyloid or cardiovascular causes), but most never need hospital treatment.

Diseases causing seronegative arthritides Psoriasis, Reiter's (with urethritis+conjunctivitis, *OHCM* p 669), ulcerative colitis, Crohn's.

Pseudogout=calcium pyrophosphate arthropathy *Risk factors:*

- Old age
- Dehydration
- Intercurrent illness
- Hyperparathyroidism
- Myxoedema; DM
- PO_4^{3-}↓; Mg^{2+}↓
- Any arthritis (RA, OA)
- Haemochromatosis
- Acromegaly

Acute pseudogout is less severe and longer-lasting than gout; affecting different joints (mainly the knee). In chronic calcinosis there is destructive changes like OA, but more severe; affecting, eg knees, also wrists, shoulders, hips.

Tests: Calcium deposition on x-ray (eg triangular ligament in wrist). Joint crystals are weakly positively birefringent in plane polarized light.
Treatment: This is symptomatic, eg with NSAIDs (p 672).

Reactive arthritis

This is an aseptic asymmetric mono- or oligoarthritis (ie just a few joints affected) developing ~1 week after infection elsewhere. 60–90% are HLA-B27 +ve. Reiter's is a post-venereal or post-enteric example (*OHCM* p 688). *Others:*

–Yersinia, *OHCM* p 225	–Chlamydia trachomatis, p 512	–Campylobacter
–Salmonella/Shigella	& Chl. pneumoniae, *OHCM* p 334	–Ureaplasma; HIV
–Vibrio parahaemolyticus	–Borrelia burgdorferi, *OHCM* p 232	–Clostridium dif.

Lipopolysaccharide antigen stimulation (causing IgA antibodies) may be important. *Treatment:* NSAIDs, physiotherapy, steroid joint infections. Antibiotics only help after yersinia or chlamydial infection.[1]

Fibromyalgia (fibrositis)

Presentation: There is diffuse musculoskeletal (osteoarticular) pain, morning stiffness, paraesthesiae, tender points over the body, skin-fold tenderness, and constitutional upset (sleep disturbance, fatigue, vertigo). It is a common diagnosis made in rheumatology clinics in patients who have pain with no obvious cause. But in the general population, most people with chronic widespread pain do not have high tender-point counts (below)—and most people with high tender-point counts do not have chronic widespread pain: so fibromyalgia may not be a distinct entity in the general population.[2]

Beware of diagnosing 'diffuse pain', unless all 4 quadrants of the body are affected, and there is axial pain.

Associations: Raynaud's phenomenon, sicca syndrome, anxiety/depression, irritable bowel syndrome.

Modulating factors: Temperature/humidity change, stress, fatigue.

Diagnosis: This is based on finding a number of separate characteristic tender points—when palpated with the thumb to give a pressure of about 4kg. There are 11 pairs to look for (right and left), and it is usual to have ≥15 sites affected.[3] The sites are:

1 Occiput at the suboccipital muscle insertion.
2 Low cervical at anterior aspect of intertransverse spaces at C5–7.
3 Trapezius at the mid point of the upper border.
4 Supraspinatus origins above the scapula spine near medial border.
5 2nd rib surface just lateral to 2nd costochondral junction.
6 Lateral humerus epicondyle 2cm distal to the epicondyles.
7 Gluteal at the upper outer quadrants.
8 Greater trochanter just posterior to the trochanteric prominence.
9 Knee at the medial fat pad proximal to the joint line.

The cause is unknown.

Treatment is supportive. A randomized trial has shown the benefits of electroacupuncture,[4] but its use long term has not been formally assessed. Other treatments tried: physiotherapy, NSAIDs.

1 B Svenungsson 1994 *BMJ* i 671 2 P Croft 1994 *BMJ* ii 696 3 Amercan College of Rheumatology 1990 *Arthrit Rheum* 1990 33 160 4 C Deluze 1992 *BMJ* ii 1249

Metabolic bone disease—I: Osteoporosis

Osteoporosis implies reduced bone density. If trabecular bone is mostly affected, crush fractures of vertebrae are common; if cortical bone is mostly affected, fracture of a long bone is more likely, eg femoral neck: *the* big cause of death and orthopaedic expense, especially in older women.

Prevalence: 5%. ♀/♂≈4

Risk of future osteoporotic fracture is increased if:

- Slender or anorectic
- Smoker or alcoholic
- Prolonged rest; old age
- Hyperparathyroidism
- >5mg/day prednisolone
- Vertebral deformity
- Early menopause
- Cushing's disease
- Malabsorption
- Thyrotoxicosis
- Myeloma
- Amenorrhoea
- Osteoporosis in family
- Primary biliary cirrhosis
- Rheumatoid arthritis
- Hypogonadism
- Past low-trauma fracture
- Mastocytosis (p 602)

Diagnosis: Once fractured, it is easy to look at a bone's x-ray and say that osteoporosis is present. Without the 'retrospectoscope' this is harder. Serum Ca^{2+}, PO_4^{3-} and alkaline phosphatase are normal. Measurement of bone mass (densitometry/dual-photon x-ray absorptiometry—DPXA) may be used, but its rôle is unclear: screening is probably not effective, and it is less effective than the taking into account of risk factors in the prediction of hip fracture. It provides little information about microstructure and elasticity—which are indirectly measured by utrasound attenuation. So it is suggested, as the result of a large trial (*N*=5662 women with a mean age of 80 years) that if we combine DPXA with os calcis ultrasound we can identify groups with very high or very low risk of hip fracture. NB: biopsy specimens may be unrepresentative.

Prevention and management: In those who have had fractures recommend:

- Gentle exercise (stressing bone delays mineral loss).
- If dietary Ca^{2+}↓, give effervescent calcium lactate gluconate, eg as Sandocal-1000® 1 tablet/day PO (gives 1g calcium). CI: renal failure.
- Hormone replacement therapy (HRT) reduces perimenopausal acceleration of bone loss. ►Avoid unopposed oestrogens (risks endometrial cancer). Raloxifene, a new SERM HRT, protects bones and *reduces* breast and endometrial cancer risk. See p 18. Trials of crystalline hydroxyapatite, fluoride, calcitonin, anabolic steroids and vitamin D either show no additional benefit compared with HRT, or are seriously flawed.
- In vertebral osteoporosis, consider long-term osteoclast inhibition with etidronate, eg Didronel PMO®, each pack lasts 90 days, with 14 days of etidronate (400mg/day, 2h ac; SE angio-oedema constipation, headache, paraesthesia, Ca^{2+}↓, PO_4^{3-}↑ WCC↓) + 76 tablets of 1250mg effervescent calcium carbonate. This increases bone density.[1] Alendronate ~10mg/24h ½h ac is an alternative here, and is known to reduce risk of hip and wrist fracture too (SE: rashes, constipation; oesophagitis—so patients must wash down the tablet with plenty of water, and remain sitting up for 30mins).[2]

Note: if on long-term steroids, pamidronate ↑spinal density,[3] and calcitriol 6μg/day PO prevents bone loss,[4,5] but it is not known if fractures are reduced.

Osteomalacia and **hyperparathyroidism** See *OHCM* p 648 & 546.

II: Paget's disease of bone

There is ↑bone turnover associated with abnormal hypernucleated osteoclasts[7] causing remodelling, bone enlargement, deformity and weakness. Rare if <40yrs; incidence ↑with age. It is common in temperate climes, and in Anglo-Saxons. It may be asymptomatic or cause pain ± enlargement, eg of skull, femur, clavicle, tibia ('sabre' tibia). Pathological fractures, nerve deafness (bone overgrowth) and high-output CCF occur. *X-rays:* Patchy changes in bone density (eg sclerotic 'white' vertebrae) ± remodelling. *Tests:* Plasma Ca^{2+} and PO_4^{3-} are normal; alk phos markedly raised.

Complications: Bone sarcoma occurs in ~10% of those affected for >10yr.

Treatment: In ⅓ of those in whom analgesia is inadequate, calcitonin 0.5–2u/kg/24h SC; or disodium etidronate 5mg/kg/24h PO ac for 6 mths (it ↓bone turnover; SE: , defective mineralization, fractures) may help pain and ↓alk phos (by ~50%[6]). Calcitonin SE: nausea, faintness, flushes.

*Densitometry MAY be indicated in those with:**

- Oestrogen lack which poses a substantial risk of osteoporosis:
  - –Early menopause
  - –Premenopausal amenorrhoea.
  - –Perimenopausal ladies if the result would change HRT plans.
- Vertebral osteopenia on plain x-ray.
- Some patients with vertebral deformity.
- Previous osteoporosis-related or 'low trauma' fracture(s).
- Monitoring response to osteoporosis therapy is some patients.
- Monitoring diseases associated with osteoporosis (opposite).
- Those taking long-term steroids.

Understanding Dexa bone scans: WHO osteoporosis criteria

Typical sites examined are the lumbar spine (preferably 3 vertebra) and hip. Bone mineral density (BMD, in grams/cm^2) is compared with that of young healthy women (if it is a woman being tested). The 'T-score' relates to the number of standard deviations the BMD is from the average. If the T-score is:

>0	BMD is better than the reference
0 to -1	BMD is in the top 84%: no evidence of osteoporosis
-1 to -2.5	Osteopenia, with risk of later osteoporotic complication —so consider preventive measures (see opposite).
-2.5 or worse	BMD is in the bottom 2.5% of the population: osteoporosis is present—severe if there is one or more fragility fracture.

Osteoporosis in men* Consider densitometry in those with low-trauma fractures, or osteopenia on x-ray (or if on long-term steroids): If Z=0 to –1 (or T ≥–2.5) offer lifestyle advice. If T or Z scores are more negative, do bone profile, FBC, TSH, protein electrophoresis and serum testosterone—and consider bisphosponates (eg alendronate) ± anabolic steroids.* Recheck densitometry every 1–2 years.

*1998 Consensus Guidelines (*Ger Med* **28** 50) & Arthritis & Rheumatism Council 1996

1 D Hans 1996 *Lancet* **348** 511 2 D Black 1996 *Lancet* **348** 1535 3 T Spector 1993 BMJ **ii** 519
4 P Sambrook 1993 NEJM **328** 1747 5 *An Rheumatic Diseases* 1995 **54** 783 6 J Compston 1994 i BMJ **ii** 711

Reducing pain in A&E[1]

A calm, reassuring manner and good pain relief make the procedure more pleasant for everyone. Techniques may be local or systemic:

Local

1 Injected local anaesthetic. See p 687.

2 Lidocaine (=lignocaine) cream 2.5% (Emla®) ↓pain of minor procedures. It needs to be applied 1 hour in advance (eg for elective IV cannulation).

3 Ethyl chloride sprayed onto intact skin until it looks white produces brief numbness, suitable for very minor procedures and painful injections, eg ring blocks. Do not use with cautery.

Examples of systemic techniques for the control of pain

Oral: NSAIDs (eg ibuprofen 400mg/8h PO)

Inhalational: Nitrous oxide (Entonox®), under the patient's control, can be a useful adjunct to local anaesthesia.

IV/IM: Morphine, eg 5–15mg in adults. For children, see below.

Psychological: Hypnosis may also be useful, when available.

Children in A&E

Remember, white coats can be very frightening. Toys, friendliness and a simple explanation of what is going to happen go a long way to avoid creating a lifelong fear of doctors.

- Do you need to suture a wound? Consider the alternatives (p 686).
- Do you need to inject local anaesthetic? Consider needle-free alternatives. It is rarely worth an injection for a single suture.
- If suturing is unavoidable, consider sedation: Chloral hydrate if <2yrs: 30–50mg/kg PO (max 1g). An alternative is papaveretum 7.7mg/mL: 1mL diluted with 9mL water. Dose: child up to 1 month: 0.15mL/kg IM; if 1–12 months, 0.15–0.2mL/kg IM of the above dilution. For older children (1–12yrs) use 0.02–0.03mL/kg IM of *undiluted* papaveretum 7.7mg/mL solution. Papaveretum is given with atropine 15–20µg/kg IM.

Explain gently to the child and the parents what you are going to do. Wrap the child in a blanket. Enlist enough nurses to hold the child and immobilize the part you are suturing. Warn the parents of possible distress. If they prefer not to be present, try to sit them out of earshot! Showing the child the result in a mirror, offering a big bandage and giving an 'I was brave' badge can help.

A general anaesthetic is rarely justified; if it is, the wound should probably be sutured by a plastic surgeon.

1 King's College Hospital A&E Department *Paediatric Manual*

►►Gunshot and other penetrating injuries

Murders by handguns: (Typical annual figures) Australia 13; UK 33; Sweden 36; USA 13,220.

Four cardinal rules

- ►All but superficial wounds need exploration under GA to repair or exclude damage to deep structures (and for debridement). Get expert help as it is all too easy to do further damage.
- ►Even minimal surface injury may hide much deep injury, depending on the weapon used, the mechanism of injury, and bullet speed.
- ►Most victims are young and fit with good reserves. Therefore cardiorespiratory decompensation indicates severe injury.
- ►If the weapon (eg knife) is still *in situ*, do not remove it until the patient is on the operating table—the danger is exsanguination.

Define and record each injury. Note that low velocity bullets leave dirty tracks, requiring exploration, excision, and *delayed* closure. High velocity weapons (eg military rifles) are extraordinarily destructive due to the temporary cavity caused by the missile. Ruthless and massive debridement is essential. Tetanus prophylaxis: p 686.

Chest injuries Penetration of the chest may damage pleura, lung, great vessels, heart, mediastinum, diaphragm and abdominal contents. The commonest injury is a haemopneumothorax from damage to lung and chest wall. This requires a large (adult: 32 gauge) chest drain. Any deterioration or cardiac arrest demands prompt thoracotomy. Wounds of intercostal vessels or heart can cause massive haemorrhage: if drainage is initially >1500mL, or >300mL/h, thoracotomy is needed.

Sucking chest wounds must be closed at once, eg by Vaseline® gauze pads sealed on 3 sides only (acts as flutter valve)—complete the seal when chest drain inserted. ►►Relieve tension pneumothorax by needling the chest on the side of the suspected lesion *before* inserting a 32G chest drain (*OHCM* p 356 & p 754) or doing x-rays (delay may be fatal).

Respiratory embarrassment due to pain, flail chest, or diaphragmatic injury requires intubation and ventilation. Insert a chest drain if there is any chance of a tear to lung, bronchus, or chest wall.

Cardiac tamponade 15% of deep chest injuries involve the heart.

Diagnosis: Beck's triad: rising venous pressure, falling BP, and a small, quiet heart (± pulsus paradoxus). NB: JVP may not be visible if there is hypovolaemia. ►►Pericardial aspiration is life-saving and diagnostic (and buys time before definitive anterolateral thoracotomy).

Procedure: Insert an 18G needle to the left of the xiphoid. Aim at the left shoulder, but with the needle angled downwards at 45° to the horizontal.

All these patients need: Crossmatching of ≥6 units of blood, THEN:

- At least one large-bore IV cannula for vigorous fluid replacement.
- Monitoring: vital signs; blood gases; CXR; ECG monitoring.
- ITU care with a chest drain immediately to hand, and facilities for immediate thoracotomy (eg if any deterioration, or a cardiac arrest).

Abdominal injuries All but the most superficial will need admission, and exploration, never just observation. See p 718.

Limb injury Nerves, tendons and vessels are endangered, so examine limbs in good light, testing *pulses* (their presence doesn't exclude arterial injury), *sensation* and *sweating*. Any damage found will need formal surgical repair. Direct pressure will staunch bleeding. Do not use a tourniquet: it may augment ischaemic damage, and you may forget to take it off.

The Glasgow Coma Scale (GCS)[1]

This gives a reliable, objective way of recording the conscious state of a person. It can be used by medical and nursing staff for initial and continuing assessment. It has value in predicting ultimate outcome. 3 types of response are assessed:

- **Best motor response** This has 6 grades:
  6 *Carrying out request ('obeying command'):* The patient does simple things you ask (beware of accepting a grasp reflex in this category).

  5 *Localizing response to pain:* Put pressure on the patient's finger nail bed with a pencil then try supraorbital and sternal pressure: purposeful movements towards changing painful stimuli is a 'localizing' response.

  4 *Withdraws to pain:* Pulls limb away from painful stimulus.

  3 *Flexor response to pain:* Pressure on the nail bed causes abnormal flexion of limbs: decorticate posture.

  2 *Extensor posturing to pain:* The stimulus causes limb extension (adduction, internal rotation of shoulder, pronation of forearm): decerebrate posture.

  1 *No response to pain.*

NB: record the best response of any limb.

- **Best verbal response** This has 5 grades.
  5 *Oriented:* The patient knows who he is, where he is and why, the year, season, and month.

  4 *Confused conversation:* The patient responds to questions in a conversational manner but there is some disorientation and confusion.

  3 *Inappropriate speech:* Random or exclamatory articulated speech, but no conversational exchange.

  2 *Incomprehensible speech:* Moaning but no words.

  1 *None*

NB: record level of best speech.

- **Eye opening** This has 4 grades.
  4 *Spontaneous eye opening*

  3 *Eye opening in response to speech:* Any speech, or shout, not necessarily request to open eyes.

  2 *Eye opening to response to pain:* Pain to limbs as above.

  1 *No eye opening*

An overall score is made by summing the score in the 3 areas assessed, eg: no response to pain+no verbalization+no eye opening = 3. Severe injury, GCS ≤8; moderate injury, GCS 9–12; minor injury GCS 13–15.

Note: an abbreviated coma scale, AVPU, is sometimes used in the initial assessment ('primary survey') of the critically ill

- A = **a**lert
- V = responds to **v**ocal stimuli
- P = responds to **p**ain
- U = **u**nresponsive

1 G Teasdale 1974 *Lancet* ii 81

►►Drowning

Drowning is common: the worldwide incidence is 140,000/year, second only to traffic accidents as the cause of death in those aged 1–40yrs. 40% of drownings occur in those <4yrs—little boys being particularly at risk.

Most drownings occur in drunk adults, or in children who are poorly supervised near water. It is quite common for a toddler to bath with a slightly older sibling 'in charge'—the mother thinking that as the child can sit up, he can also save himself from drowning should he topple over.

In communities wealthy enough to have many private swimming pools there are summertime spates of drownings. An adult is temporarily distracted and leaves the garden, and, on return, finds a corpse in the pool. When such a child is brought to A&E the chief concerns are:
1 Cardiac arrest **2** Hypothermia **3** Acidaemia **4** Pulmonary oedema.

Management focuses on **a**irway, **b**reathing and **c**irculation:
- Immobilize the cervical spine as you open the airway—there may have been trauma here.
- Clear vomit from mouth. Vomiting is common (much water is ingested).
- If pulseless, start cardiopulmonary resuscitation.
- Expect BP to drop after leaving the water, and be sure to transport in the horizontal position, and keep cardiovascular instability to a minimum.[1]
- In coma, intubate trachea (pre-oxygenate with 100% O_2; if hypothermic, this can induce VF). Do Glasgow Coma Scale, p 680; if <6 prognosis poor.
- Continue to ventilate with 100% O_2.
- Monitor ECG. Defibrillate if in VF (p 311). For the first shock, give ~2 joules/kg body weight (~20J at 9 months, 40J at 4yrs, 60J at 8yrs, and 80J at 12yrs). NB: defibrillation often fails until core T° >30°C. Various heroic measures have been tried without neccessarily affecting outcome[2] —eg rapid core rewarming, eg by warm-water immersion, warm IV fluids at 40°C, breathing of heated humidified gas,[3] peritoneal dialysis, thoracotomy for heart irrigation, or cardiac bypass.
- Monitor core T° & CNS signs. Cerebral oedema may occur suddenly in first 24h: no evidence supports use of dexamethasone or barbiturate coma.
- If T° <35°C, monitor rectal T° often and rewarm using high ambient T°. Circulatory support may be needed to counter rewarming vasodilatation. Measuring left atrial pressure helps guide IV fluid: too much will ↑ICP.
- Pass a nasogastric tube to relieve gastric dilatation.
- As soon as recovery is under way do U&E, blood gases and Hb.

The effects of asphyxia and fresh water overload The child usually swallows large amounts of water before final aspiration. This leads to gastric dilatation, vomiting and further aspiration—as well as to ICP↑, cerebral oedema, acute respiratory distress syndrome, haemodilution, haemolysis and hypokalaemia. To combat these, steroids and antibiotics are sometimes given, although there is no evidence of their efficacy. As the raised intracranial pressure (ICP) is due to cell death, steroids do not lower ICP (unlike the raised ICP seen with space-occupying lesions).

The diving reflex Children retain this useful adaptation to our earlier aquatic way of life. As cold water hits the face, the pulse slows and blood is diverted from limbs and muscles to vital areas (brain, kidney). Cold further reduces the metabolic rate. This is the physiological explanation for remarkable stories of recovery from prolonged (eg 20min) total immersion. It is also the reason why resuscitation of a seemingly dead child must continue for 40min before death is declared.

1 M Stoneham 1995 *Lancet* **345** 1048 2 L Spack 1997 *Pediatric Emerg Care* **13** 98 3 P Mair 1995 *Lancet* **345** 1048

►►Major injury, including blunt chest injury

This page assumes that the resuscitator has an experienced person to help him and a well-equipped resuscitation room. On hearing that a major injury is coming in, summon experienced help (eg senior traumatologist). Remember **ABC** (*a*irway, *b*reathing, *c*irculation): see opposite. If breathing spontaneously, give *all* patients O_2 at 15L/min through tight-fitting mask with reservoir. Note quality of breathing: stridor (± voice change) indicates a sternoclavicular fracture/posterior dislocation—get expert help at once as intubation may be difficult owing to tracheal compression, until the dislocation is reduced—by extending the shoulders, and grasping the clavicle with a clamp (eg towel clip) and manually reducing the fracture. Cover and seal open chest wounds on 3 sides only. ►►*Is there a tension pneumothorax?* Making this diagnosis is urgent: *don't wait for x-rays*. Its 6 signs are:

–Air hunger + respiratory distress	–Pulse↑ (+ BP↓)	–Tracheal deviation
–Breath sounds↓ on one side	–Cyanosis	–Neck vein distension

Relieve by inserting a needle (2nd intercostal space, mid-clavicular line), then:

- Set up 0.9% saline IVI; crossmatch; glucose stix.
- Use 2 big cannulae—via a cut down (*OHCM* p 698), if IV access fails.
- Take systolic BP. If <90mmHg and blood loss is the probable cause, give colloid (Haemaccel®) fast IV until BP↑, pulse↓, urine flows (>30 mL/h; catheterize at leisure—exclude urethral injury first) and crossmatched blood arrives (►ask for group-compatible blood—only takes 5–10min).
- Remove clothes (large scissors). *What are the injuries?* Do *circumferential burns* need escharotomy to relieve laryngeal pressure? Any *surgical emphysema* (chest drain may be needed). Is there a *flail chest* (a segment has no bony continuity with thorax, with paradoxical respiration)? The main problem is the injured lung, which is sensitive to *over* and *under* resuscitation; intubate and ventilate.
- *Assume spinal instability*. Before radiology, keep immobile (sandbags, collar, tape).
- Apply pressure and elevation to any actively bleeding part.
- Do level-of-consciousness (AVPU, p 680) + ECG (ST & conduction problems ≈ myocardial damage: extent is revealed via direct inspection by a thoracic surgeon).
- Falling BP + rising JVP and a quiet heart = cardiac tamponade: ►see p 679.
- Examine all peripheral pulses. 30% of fractures are missed in the resus room; x-ray cervical spine (p 726) + pelvis. *Skull x-rays may waste time*. If intraperitoneal haemorrhage is suspected, see p 718. Do blood gases and CXR; implications:
  - -If free air, needle the chest (or formal chest drain) for pneumothorax.
  - -If persistent large pneumothrax after chest drain suspect bronchial tear.

-# of ribs 1-3 ≈ ?airway/big vessel injury*	-Ribs 9–12 ≈ ?abdominal trauma
-# of >2 ribs in 2 places ≈ ?flail chest	-CXR fluid level ≈ haemothorax
-Bowel gas in chest ≈ ?diaphragm injury	-Diaphragm contour↓ ≈ ?rupture
-Coils of NGT in chest ≈ ?diaphragm injury	-Liver raised ≈ ?diaphragm injury
-# of sternum ≈ ?myocardial contusion	-Mediastinal air ≈ oesophagus tear
-Respiratory distress + CXR OK ≈ ?aspiration	-# of scapula ≈ ?airway injury
-Wide mediastinum ≈ ?aortic rupture*	-Tracheal deviation ≈ aortic injury*
-Deviation of oesophagus ≈ ?aortic rupture*	-No aortic knob ≈ ?ruptured aorta*

- Chart pulse, BP + pupil size every few mins. If pupils unequal, summon neurological help. Give mannitol 1g/kg IVI to relieve cerebral oedema, p 714.
- Head-to-toe exam ('secondary survey'). Glasgow Coma Scale (p 680).
- If fits occur give 10mg diazepam IV followed by 100mg in 500mL 5% dextrose infused at 40mL/h if they continue (children: 0.3mg/kg IV, then 50μg/kg/h IVI)—beware apnoea. If fits continue, give 40–100mL of ready prepared 0.8% chlormethiazole IVI over 10mins (kept in the fridge)—adults only. The subsequent infusion rate is determined by the response.
- In lung contusion, near-drowning or smoke inhalation, consider early high-dose steroids (methylprednisolone 30mg/kg IV).
- Give *tetanus toxoid* booster ± *human anti-tetanus immunoglobulin* (p 686).
- Get experienced help in prioritizing treatment for each specific injury.

*Have a low threshold for aortograms, especially if deceleration injury: ATLS 1997 *Manual* 6e, 135

►►1997 UK adult basic life-support algorithm[1,2]

This algorithm assumes that only one rescuer is present, with no equipment. (If a defibrillator is to hand, get a rhythm readout, and defibrillate, as opposite, as soon as possible.)

Remove yourself and the casualty from obvious dangers

↓

Check responsiveness — *(shake & shout)*

↓

Open the airway — *(head tilt/chin lift)*

↓

Check breathing — *(look, listen, feel; if breathing, place in recovery position)*

↓

Give 2 breaths — *(have up to 5 goes at giving 2 rescue breaths sufficient to raise the chest)*

↓

Assess for signs of life for 10sec only — *(look for signs of circulation; now phone for help at once)*

↙ ↘

Circulation present: Continue rescue breathing

No circulation: Compress chest & give breaths — *(100 compressions/min at ratio of 15:2 with ventilations if single rescuer; 1:5 if two. Spend <10sec to check circulation, eg carotid pulse, every minute)*

Managing the airway

- You open the airway by tilting the head and lifting the chin—but only do this if there is no question of spinal trauma.
- Use a close-fitting mask if available, held in place by thumbs pressing downwards either side of the mouthpiece; palms against cheeks.

Chest compressions

- Cardiopulmonary resuscitation (CPR) involves compressive force over the lower sternum with the heel of the hands placed one on top of the other, directing the weight of your body through your vertical, straight, arms.
- Depth of compression: ~4cm.
- Rate of compressions: 100/min.

1 A Handley 1997 *British J Anaesthesia* 79 151 2 A Handley 1993 *Resuscitation* 26 93

The stitching of wounds

1 Remove foreign bodies and all necrotic material. Clean with 1% cetrimide.
2 Control bleeding by pressure and elevation of the part. Deep absorbable stitches (eg Dexon®, Vicryl®, catgut) will aid apposition of skin edges (avoid in the hand, as may disrupt nerves).
3 Infiltrate skin to be sutured with 1% lidocaine (<3mg/kg; SE: seizures). ►***Avoid epinephrine (=adrenaline) when anaesthetizing digits.***
4 If much tension is needed, consider tension sutures or skin grafts with expert help.
5 Handle the tissues gently to prevent further injury.
6 Use interrupted stitches for closure. Start from the middle, or with any jagged edges. This aids accurate apposition.
7 Avoid eversion or inversion of the stitched skin edges.
8 Examples of which stitches to use: *Adult's face:* 5-0 monofilament nylon (remove after 5 days). *Child's face:* 6-0 monofilament nylon (remove after 3–5 days). *Other parts of children:* 5-0 catgut. The deep part will be absorbed and the top part will slough off after 10–14 days. *Adult leg:* 3-0 nylon; remove after 2 weeks. *Shin skin flaps* (after a fall on a hard object) may have a poor blood supply, especially if the length of the flap is more than twice as long as its breadth, and healing will be better with thin strips of special adhesive tape (eg Steristrip®), rather than stitches. Exact approximation of the edges is likely to be impossible, but skin grafts are rarely needed. *Adult arm, trunk, abdomen:* 3-0 silk (or equivalent). Remove after ~9 days. *Scalp:* 3-0 silk. Remove after 5 days.
9 Learn the technique from an experienced professional (eg staff nurse). Practise suturing a slashed banana skin or pig's trotter in a sterile field.
10 Dress with sterile tulle to prevent further injury.

Alternatives to suturing Suturing requires anaesthesia and leaves scars.

Skin closure strips (Steristrips®) are useful for cuts on non-hairy skin. Leave space between strips for ooze. They can also temporarily appose edges of larger wounds while you suture. Infection is less of a risk than with stitches, particularly for animal bites. *Acrylic tissue adhesive (Histoacryl®)* is quick, minimizes scarring and needs no follow-up. Wear gloves to stop your flesh sticking to the patient. Dry the wound, and align edges carefully: you cannot correct the position once the sides have touched. Apply glue thinly (use a capillary tube), and press the edges together for 30sec. *Hair:* You may be able to close minor scalp wounds by tying strands of hair across the wound.

Preventing tetanus Active immunization with tetanus toxoid is given as part of the triple vaccine during early life (p 209). Give boosters on starting school and in early (and late, eg 65yrs) adulthood. Once given 5–6 injections, revaccinate only at the time of significant injury.[1] Other boosters are not needed, risk side-effects, and may dull immunity by overstimulation.[2]

Primary adult immunization: 0.5mL toxoid IM repeated ×2 at monthly intervals.

Wounds: Any cut merits an extra dose of 0.5mL toxoid IM, unless already fully immune (a full course of toxoid or a booster in last 10 years). The non-immune will need 2 further injections (0.5mL IM) at monthly intervals. If partially immune (ie has had a toxoid booster or a full course >10 years previously), a single booster is all the toxoid that is needed.

Human tetanus immunoglobulin: This is required for the partially or non-immune patient (defined above) with dirty, old (>6h), infected, devitalized, or soil-contaminated wounds. Give 250–500 units IM, using a separate syringe and site to the toxoid injection.

► If the immune status is unknown, assume he/she is non-immune.
Routine infant immunization started in 1961, so many adults are at risk.

►Hygiene education and wound debridement are of vital importance.

1 C Bowie 1996 *Lancet* **348** 1195 2 DoH 1996 *Immunization Against Infectious Disease*, HMSO

Maximum doses of lidocaine (=lignocaine): a rough guide[1]

0.25%	1.12mL/kg
0.5%	0.56mL/kg
1%	0.28mL/kg
2%	0.14mL/kg

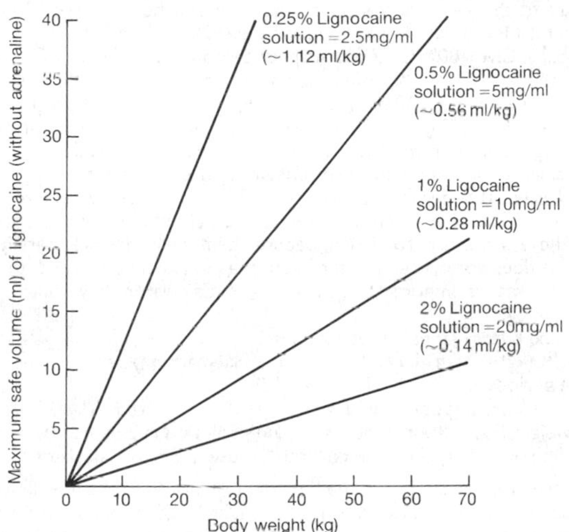

Maximum safe volume of plain lidocaine (=lignocaine) according to body weight. (Maximum safe dose of lidocaine—without epinephrine (=adrenaline) 3mg/kg, with adrenaline 7mg/kg; uses of different solutions—0.25–0.5% for infiltration and intravenous regional anaesthesia, 1% for nerve blocks, epidural anaesthesia, and intravenous regional anaesthesia, 2% for nerve blocks.)

1 D Kelly 1983 BMJ i 1784

►►Burns[ATLS]

Most hospitals do not have their own burns unit. Resuscitate and organize rapid transfer for all major burns. Always assess site, size, and depth of the burn; smaller burns in the young, the old, or at specific sites, may still require specialist help.

Assessment The size of the burn must be estimated to calculate fluid requirements. Ignore erythema. Consider transfer to a burns unit if >10% burn in children or elderly, or >20% in others. Use a Lund & Browder chart or the 'rule of nines':

Arm (all over) 9%	Front 18%	Head (all over) 9%	Palm 1%
Leg (all over) 18%	Back 18%	Genitals 1%	
	(NB: in children, head = 14%; leg = 14%)		

Estimating burn thickness: Partial thickness is painful, red, and blistered; full thickness is painless and white/grey.

Refer full thickness burns >5% of body area or full/partial thickness burns involving face, hands, eyes, genitalia to a burns unit.

Resuscitation • *Airway:* ►►Beware of upper airway obstruction developing if inhaled hot gases (only superheated steam will cause thermal damage distal to trachea)—suspect if singed nasal hairs or hoarse voice. Consider early intubation or surgical airway (*OHCM* p 799).

- *Breathing:* Give 100% O_2 if you suspect carbon monoxide poisoning (may have cherry-red skin, but often not) as $t_{1/2}$ carboxyhaemoglobin (COHb) falls from 250min to 40min (consider hyperbaric oxygen if pregnant; CNS signs; >20% COHb). ►*SpO_2 measured by pulse oximeter is unreliable* (falls, eg 3% with up to 40% COHb). Do escharotomy bilaterally in anterior axillary line if thoracic burns impair chest excursion (p 689).
- *Circulation:* >10% burns in a child and >15% burns in adults require IV fluids. Put up 2 large-bore (14G or 16G) IV lines. Do not worry if you have to put these through burned skin. Secure them well: they are literally lifelines. It does not matter whether you give crystalloid or colloid: the volume is what is important. Use a 'Burns Calculator' flow chart[1] or a formula, eg:
- *Muir and Barclay formula* (popular in UK):
  [weight (kg) × %burn]/2=mL colloid (eg Haemaccel®) per unit time
  Time periods are 4h, 4h, 4h, 6h, 6h, 12h.
- *Parkland formula* (popular in USA):
  4 × weight (kg) × %burn=mL Hartmann's solution in 24h, half given in first 8h (NB: unsatisfactory in children, so use a 'Burns Calculator').

►You must replace fluid from the time of burn, not from the time first seen in hospital. You must also give 1.5–2.0mL/kg/h 5% dextrose if Muir and Barclay formula is used. Formulae are only guides: adjust IVI rate according to clinical response and urine output (aim for >30mL/h in adults; >1mL/kg/h in children). Catheterize the bladder.

Treatment ►Do *not* apply cold water to extensive burns: this may intensify shock. Do *not* burst blisters. Covering extensive partial thickness burns with sterile linen prior to transfer to a burns unit will deflect air currents and relieve pain. Use morphine in 1–2mg aliquots IV. Suitable dressings include Vaseline® gauze, or silver sulfadiazine under absorbent gauze; change every 1–2 days. Hands may be covered in silver sulfadiazine inside a plastic bag. Ensure tetanus immunity. Give 50mL whole blood for every 1% of full-thickness burn, half in the second 4h of IV therapy and half after 24h.

1 SM Milner 1993 *Lancet* **342** 1089

Smoke inhalation

In addition to thermal injury, the problems are carbon monoxide poisoning (see opposite), and cyanide poisoning.

Cyanide poisoning is common from smouldering plastics. It binds reversibly with ferric ions in enzymes—so stopping oxidative phosphorylation and causing dizziness, headaches and seizures. Tachycardia and dyspnoea soon give way to bradycardia and apnoea. The aim is to detatch cyanide from cytochrome oxidase by making attractive ferric opportunities by producing methaemoglobin (each molecule has 3 ferric haem groups) from Hb—using amyl nitrate 0.2–0.4mL via an Ambu bag. Less safe alternatives are sodium nitrite solution (10mL of 3% IV over 3min; dimethylaminophenol (5mL of 5% IV over 1min). Also give sodium thiosulfate (25mL of 50% IV over 10min) to provide an extra source of sulfur to augment cyanide conversion to non-toxic thiocyanate. Alternatively, chelate cyanide with dicobalt edetate (20mL of 1.5% IV over 1min), followed by 50mL of glucose IV infusion 50%. (These are adult doses.)

Escharotomy

For chest escharotomy make incisions 1 and 2 first. If further expansion is needed make the others. Make incisions either side of trunk/limb or digit (one side only shown in diagrams). If it causes pain, burns are not full thickness and escharotomy is probably not needed. Substantial bleeding may necessitate covering with sterile dressings and blood transfusion.

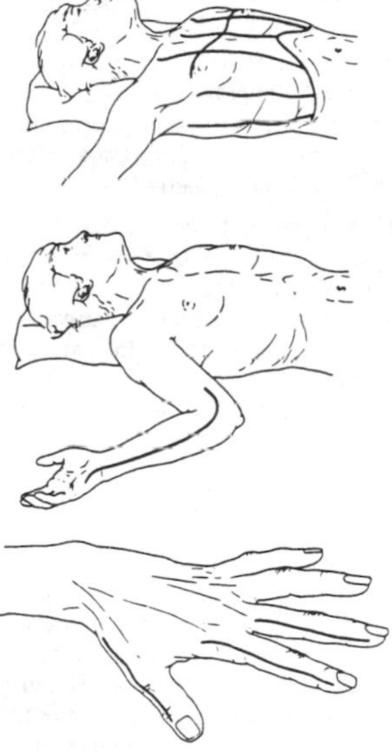

Diagrams reproduced by kind permission of the *BMJ* and C Robertson.

Fractures

Fractures may be *transverse*, *oblique*, or *spiral*. They are *comminuted* if there are >2 fragments. If broken ends protrude through the skin or into a body cavity, the fracture is *open* (an emergency). Young soft bones may bend and partially break (greenstick fractures). Compression forces yield *impacted* or *crush* fractures (in cancellous bone), and traction force causes tendons or ligaments to detach a piece of bone (*avulsion*). A *complicated* fracture causes significant damage to vessels, nerves or nearby organs. Separation of the parts is defined in terms of side-to-side *displacement*, *rotation* and *angulation* (see diagram). There may be dislocation or subluxation (partial loss of contact of joint surfaces). Ask about the degree of force which produced the injury. If it seems trivial, the bone may be diseased (*pathological* fracture, eg in secondary deposits, osteoporosis, Paget's disease—p 676).

Clinical features Pain; loss of function; tenderness; deformity; swelling; crepitus (grating of the broken ends—be gentle!).

X-rays Ask these questions: •How many fractures are there?
- Can you see the whole bone, and the joint at each end?
- How much displacement is there? In what direction?
- Are the bones normal? Look for trapped air, bone pathology and any foreign body. Are more x-rays needed (IVU, arteriogram)?

Salter and Harris classification of epiphyseal injury (See diagram)

I Seen in babies, or pathological conditions (eg scurvy).
II The commonest.
III There is a displaced fragment.
IV Union across the growth plate may interfere with bone growth.
V Compression of the epiphysis causes deformity and stunting.

Treatment •Correct shock (eg colloid IVI, 500mL/30min, until systolic BP >100mmHg); give blood if >1–1.5 litres lost, or continued bleeding. Monitor BP/15min, urine output (± CVP). Stop bleeding (may need open surgery).
- Relieve pain (eg morphine 10mg/4h IM or 1–2mg aliquots IV if shock).
- Sterile cover (eg Betadine®-soaked) over protruding bones and torn skin.
- Prevent infection: eg cloxacillin 500mg IM/IV + benzylpenicillin 600mg IV/IM; tetanus toxoid (0.5mL IM) if needed.

Methods of fracture management: Immobilize and reduce the part (if necessary, p 692), eg using a plaster of Paris cast. The problem with this method is that 'fracture disease' follows immobilization—muscle atrophy, stiff joints and osteoporosis. If possible, fractures involving joint articulations should be treated by open reduction, accurate reconstruction of the joint surfaces and fixation, such that immediate movement can occur. Otherwise, secondary osteoarthritis is inevitable. *Internal fixation:* eg with plates (eg with 10 screw-holes), nails (Küntscher) or wires (Kirschner)—of all fractures in those with polytrauma leads to large reductions in serious complications (fat embolism, acute respiratory distress syndrome, as well as lessening the time during which mechanical ventilation is needed).
External fixation uses screws into bone, a bar, and a means (cement or clamps) of attaching the bar to the screws to engage the fractured cortices. The screws may be driven through the bone and out of the far side of the limb, so that a second bar can add stability. Further rigidity is afforded by another set of screws at 90° to the first set. Because the intervention is away from the field of injury, this method is very useful when there are burns, and loss of skin and bone, or an open fracture.

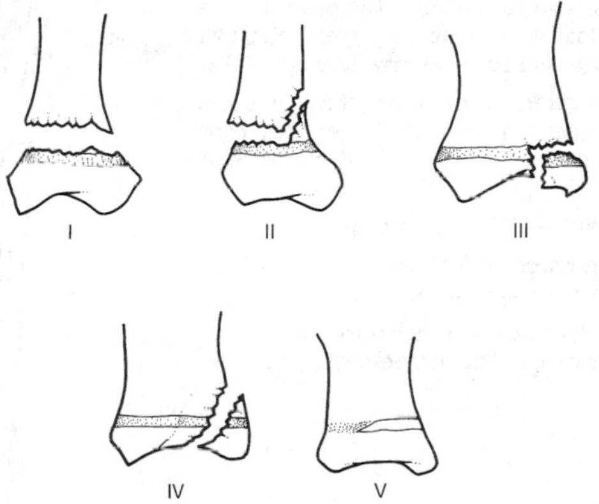
I
II
III
IV
V

Fracture reduction and traction

A displaced fracture needs realignment (reduction) unless the function and appearance of the limb are satisfactory. For example, a small displacement acceptable in a fracture of the femoral shaft might not be acceptable in the radius, where it could cause difficulty in supination. Reduction also allows freeing of any structures trapped between bone ends. Accurate reduction helps revascularization (vital in subcapital fractures of the femur) and prevents later degenerative change if fractures involve joints. Internal and external fixation has removed the need for much traction in adults, but it is still used for children.

Methods of reduction *Manipulation* under anaesthesia (most cases).
Traction This may be for subcapital femur fractures or spinal injury.
Open reduction aids accuracy, eg before internal fixation (p 690).

The next problem is to hold the reduction in place (using traction or fixation) during healing—which may take from 2 weeks (babies) to 12 weeks (a long bone in an adult).

Skin traction uses adhesive strapping to attach the load to the limb. The problems are that the load cannot be very great, and that sensitivity to the adhesive may develop.

Bone traction Using a pin through bone, greater forces can be employed (eg Steinmann pin, Gardner–Wells or Crutchfield skull calipers).

Fixed traction The Thomas' splint.

Balanced traction (below) The weight of the patient balances against the load.

Gallows traction is suitable for children up to 2 years of age. The buttocks rise just above the bed.

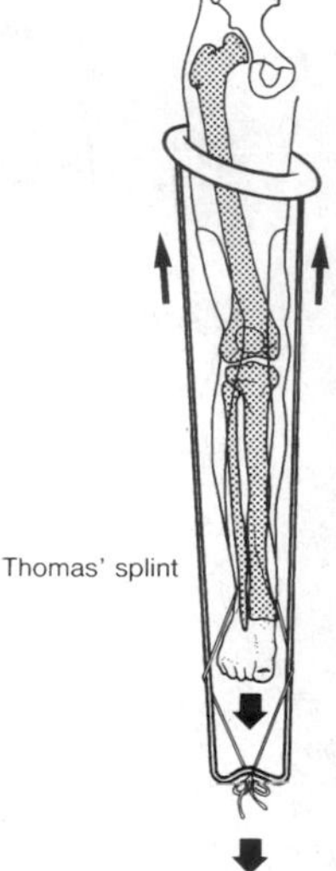

Thomas' splint

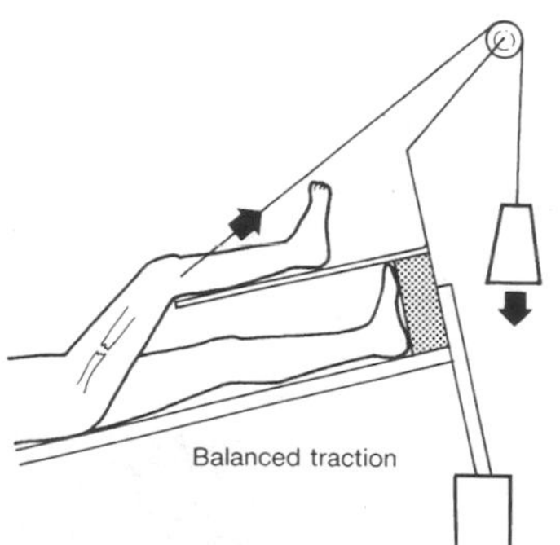

Balanced traction

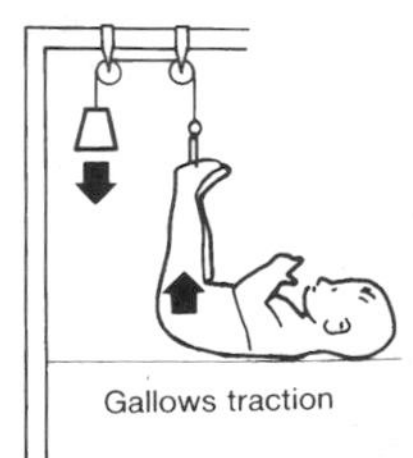

Gallows traction

Complications from fractures

Healing Haematoma → Vascular granulation tissue → Subperiosteal osteoblast stimulation → Bone matrix → Endochondral ossification → Deformable woven bone (callus) → Lamellar bone → Fracture union.

Early complications

Immediate:	*Later—local:*	*General:*
Internal or external bleeding	Skin necrosis	Venous thrombi
Organ injury, eg brain, lung	Gangrene	Pulmonary emboli
Nerve or skin injury	Pressure sores	Pneumonia
Vessel injury (limb ischaemia)	Infection [1]	Renal stones

Fat embolism: This typically occurs on day 3–10. Signs: confusion, sudden dyspnoea, hypoxia, fits, coma, fever, a petechial rash. Management: take to intensive care, summon expert help, correct shock (monitor CVP and urine output). Treat respiratory failure (*OHCM* p 352). Aim for early mobilization.

Crush syndromes and compartment syndromes: These may be a feature of any severe injury, which results in ischaemia of large amounts of soft tissue. Fluid loss, DIC and myoglobin release may lead to acute tubular necrosis. Temporary dialysis may be needed. Correct hypovolaemia vigorously. Watch urine output and plasma K^+. A patient's limbs own dead weight (eg when immobile or comatose from *any* cause) may cause a crush injury manifesting as a compartment syndrome, which is a vicious cycle of pressure → vascular occlusion → hypoxia → necrosis → increased pressure. Look for the tell-tale signs of redness, mottling, blisters, swelling, and pain on passive muscle extension. If a compartment syndrome is suspected, relieve external pressures, and measure the intracompartment pressure: if within 40mmHg of the diastolic BP, urgent fasciotomy may be needed to prevent contractures (p 616) and amputations.

Late complications • Wound sepsis (early wound cleaning is vital). Infection also complicates ~8% of closed fractures if internal fixation is used.[1]
- Failure of fixation (eg plates or nails break or dislodge).
- Joint stiffness, contractures, malalignments (malunion).
- Algodystrophy (see opposite): joint stiffness and patchy osteoporosis.
- Psychological problems in mobilizing ('compensation neurosis').
- Non-union. The signs of fracture (pain, mobility, tenderness and swelling) persist for longer than expected, eg for >3 months, in the case of a long bone in an adult (true union, with trabeculae crossing the fracture site may take much longer). If x-rays then show absence of callus (new, unremodelled bone) at the fracture site diagnose *delayed union*. If the x-ray shows that the medullary cavity has closed off, diagnose *non-union*. Non-union is commoner in cortical bone rather than in cancellous bone, where there is often impaction. Factors delaying union:

1 A fracture in a bone which has finished growing.
2 Where there is an avascular fragment (scaphoid, femoral neck).
3 Comminuted fractures, particularly if there has been infection.
4 Generalized disease (eg malignancy, infection).
5 Distraction of bone ends by muscle; open reduction ± internal fixation prevents this. NB: osteoporosis ± old age don't necessarily delay union.

Management of non-union: Rigid immobilization helps (eg internal fixation). If there is no callus, a cortical bone graft may help by providing both fixation and an osteogenic stimulus. It may be inlaid, or screwed on top of the bone ends. If realignment is not necessary a cancellous graft (using marrow-rich chips) may be used (± internal fixation). If infection is present, dead bone must be removed. Bone chips then fill in the space, which is held open by external fixation. Note: inducing an alternating electromagnetic field across the fracture appears to give encouraging results.

[1] 2g ceftriaxone IV at induction halves infection risk (to 4%)—see H Boxma 1996 *E-BM* 1 208

Algodystrophy

Synonyms[1]
Sudeck's atrophy/osteodystrophy
Reflex sympathetic dystrophy syndrome
Post-traumatic sympathetic atrophy
Shoulder–hand syndrome
Minor causalgia (causalgia means burning pain)
Post traumatic painful osteoporosis
Complex regional pain syndrome type I

Definitions 'A complex disorder of pain, sensory abnormalities, abnormal blood flow, sweating, and trophic changes in superficial or deep tissues.' The central event may be loss of vascular tone or supersensitivity to sympathetic neurotransmitters.[1,2]

Presentation This may follow weeks or months after an insult—which may be minor trauma, a fracture, zoster, or myocardial infarction.[2] Lancinating pain (which may have a trigger point) in a limb accompanies vasomotor instability. The limb may be cold and cyanosed, or hot and sweating (locally). Temperature sensitivity may be heightened. The skin of the affected part may be oedematous—and later becomes shiny and atrophic. Hyperreflexia, dystonic movements, and contractures may occur.[2]

Note that it is not the traumatized area where the symptoms occur: rather, it is some neighbouring area.

There are no systemic signs (no fever, tachycardia or lymphadenopathy). Timid, neurotic personalities are particularly affected—perhaps because of poor mobilization following the initial insult.[3]

Tests Patchy osteoporosis on x-ray, but no joint space narrowing or thinning of cartilage. Bone scintigraphy shows characteristic uniform uptake.

Treatment Refer to a pain clinic. Ordinary, standard painkillers often have little effect. Consider physiotherapy and NSAIDs. Calcitonin and postganglionic sympathetic blockade (guanethidine or bretylium[4]) have advocates. Ultimately, the condition is self-limiting.

1 D Justins 1995 BMJ ii 812 2 KP Bhatia 1995 BMJ ii 811 3 RM Atkins 1987 in OTM, 2e, OUP page 16.89 see also 3e 1996 page 3941) 4 AH Hord 1992 *Anaesthesia & Analgesia* 74 818

Trauma to the arm

Fracture of the clavicle This is common in the young, and often results from a fall on the outstretched arm (which in the elderly would be more likely to cause a Colles' fracture). A broad sling support for three weeks is usually all that is required. Fractures at the lateral end may need internal fixation.

Scapula and acromion fractures and acromioclavicular dislocation rarely require anything more than sling support. Mobilize early.

Fractures of the humeral neck Often these are impacted, and stable; if there is displacement there is risk to the brachial plexus and axillary artery. Manipulation or open reduction may be needed if there is displacement of the upper humeral epiphysis (in children) or if there is co-existing shoulder dislocation. Fractures of the head itself may result in 2–4 fragments. If three or more, internal fixation is likely to be needed.

Fractures of the humerus shaft This is often caused by a fall on an outstretched arm. Marked displacement often makes the diagnosis easy. Radial nerve injury may cause wrist-drop. Splinting with metal gutter-shaped splints and support from the wrist to the neck (collar and cuff sling) usually gives satisfactory reduction. Immobilize for 8–12 weeks.

Anterior shoulder dislocation This may follow a fall on the arm or shoulder. Signs: loss of shoulder contour (flattening of the deltoid muscle), an anterior bulge from the head of the humerus, which may also be palpated in the axilla. Damage to the axillary nerve may cause deltoid paralysis and absent sensation on a patch below the shoulder. Before reduction, x-ray (Is there a fracture too?). Relieve pain (eg parenteral opioid, and Entonox® through the procedure). Methods of reduction:
Treatment by simple reduction: Apply longitudinal traction to the arm in abduction, and replace the head of the humerus by gentle pressure.

Kocher's method: **A** Flex the elbow and put traction on the arm.
B Apply forced external rotation and **C** adduction of the point of the elbow across the chest while the arm is flexed at the shoulder.
D Now apply internal rotation, so that the volar aspect of the forearm lies on the chest. Risk: fractures of the humerus.

The Hippocratic method:[1] With the patient lying on the floor, grasp the ipsilateral wrist, and exert downward traction on the arm, with counter-traction exerted by your shoeless foot in the axilla (this method provides your only chance to lay a foot on your patient justifiably). Keep your knees and elbows straight, and lean backward. Your toes are now in a position to act as a fulcrum to relocate the head of the humerus as you slowly externally rotate the limb, and then adduct it. Offer pain relief before the manipulation. Some sources say that there is less danger to axillary vessels and the the humerus head with this method.

Surgery may be needed for recurrent dislocation (eg the Putti–Platt and Bankart reinforcement of the capsule and rotator cuff).

Posterior dislocation of the shoulder is rare, and may be caused by seizures or electroconvulsive therapy (if unparalysed). It may be hard to diagnose from an anteroposterior x-ray ('light-bulb' appearance of humeral head); lateral x-rays are essential.

1 D Fair 1993 Comments on *Pye's Surgical Handicraft* 16e, 1950, BMJ ii 808

Fractures of the elbow and forearm

The humerus *Supracondylar fractures:* The patient is usually a child who has fallen on an outstretched hand. The elbow should be kept in extension after the injury to prevent damage to the brachial artery. Median and ulnar nerve palsies are rare complications. Reduce under anaesthesia, with x-ray guidance. Avoid flexing the elbow by more than 90°. Careful post-operative observations are required. The radial pulse may not return for 24h after the reduction, although limb perfusion is usually adequate to prevent Volkmann's ischaemic contracture (p 616). Dunlop traction may be required to maintain the reduction (the elbow is held semi-extended by axial traction while a second weight is suspended over the distal end of the upper arm). Internal fixation may be required if there is much instability.

Fractures of the medial condyle: These may require surgery if manipulation fails to bring about satisfactory reduction.

Fractures of the lateral condyle: Surgical fixation will be required. Complications: cubitus valgus and ulnar nerve palsy.

T-shaped intercondylar fractures of the humerus: This is a supracondylar fracture with a further break between the condyles. The presence of a fracture may be suggested by the hoisting of the sail-shaped fat pad on the anterior aspect of the distal humerus (the 'fat pad sign'), seen on the lateral elbow x-ray—which indicates an effusion. Compare with the other elbow. If no fracture is obvious, but an effusion is present, treat initially with a broad arm sling. Re-x-ray after 10 days (when fractures are more easily seen): if clear, start mobilization. For fractures, further immobilization (± internal fixation) may be needed; physiotherapy is vital in preventing prolonged stiffness.

Fractures of the head of the radius The elbow is swollen and tender, with the movements of pronation and supination particularly painful.
X-ray often shows an effusion, but minor fractures are commonly missed. Undisplaced fractures can be treated in a collar and cuff sling—if the fracture is displaced, internal fixation or excision of the radial head may be needed. Complications: radial nerve palsy (rare).

Pulled elbow The patient is a child (1–4yrs) who has been pulled up by the arms, while being lifted in play, causing the radial head to slip out of the annular ligament. Elbow rotation (forced supination with a thumb over the radial head) may be all that is required, producing a click on reduction. X-rays are not required.

Dislocation of the elbow The patient has usually fallen on a not yet fully outstretched hand, with elbow somewhat flexed, causing the ulna to be displaced backwards on the humerus, producing a swollen elbow, fixed in flexion. Brachial artery and median nerve damage are rare. Reduction (± anaesthesia): stand behind the patient, flex the elbow, and with your fingers around the epicondyles, push forwards on the olecranon with your thumbs, and down on the forearm. Hearing a loud clunk heralds success. This may be aided by traction at the wrist from an assistant standing the other side of the trolley. Immobilize in a sling for 3 weeks.

Fractures of the olecranon are frequently part of a fracture–dislocation of the elbow. There may be wide displacement of the proximal fragment, caused by the action of triceps. Open reduction with internal fixation is often required.

Monteggia and **Galeazzi fractures** See p 754 & p 748.

Before
(radius shown alone in lateral view only)

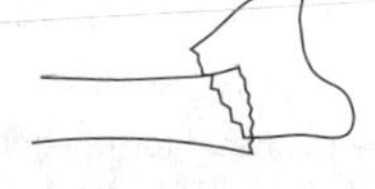

Dorsally angulated
Dorsally displaced
Loss of ulna tilt
+/− Impacted

1. Traction: distal traction should be applied to the hand either using finger traps, a pulley and weights; or directly with an assistant to provide counter-traction at the elbow. The fracture can often be felt to disimpact with a 'clunk'.
2. Exaggerate the dorsal angulation whilst maintaining distal traction. This is most easily done by keeping both thumbs on the dorsal fracture line. The intact dorsal periosteum will prevent over distraction.

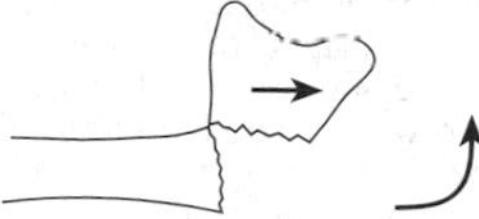

3. Correct dorsal and radial angulation, again maintaining distal traction.

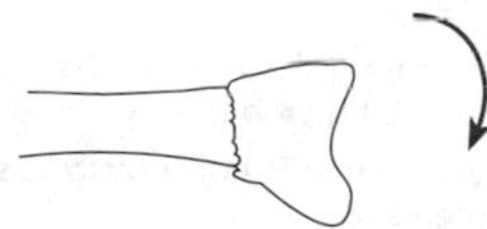

4. Apply plaster of paris (POP). Traction should be maintained whilst the POP is applied. This is most easily done by pulling on the ring and little fingers against counter-traction. This applies both palmar and ulnar forces.

→ An inability to achieve a good position may indicate soft tissue interpositioning.

→ Using adequate staff with experience saves remanipulating in theatre.

Fractures and dislocations of the wrist

Distal radial head fractures—eg Colles' fracture (common in ostoeporotic postmenopausal ladies who fall on an outstretched hand). There is backward angulation and displacement producing a 'dinner-fork' wrist deformity when viewed in pronation (the fingers are the fork's prongs). Avulsion of the styloid process of the ulna may also occur. If there is much displacement reduction will be needed, particularly if there is backward and proximal shift of the distal fragment.

Treatment: Bier's block (regional anaesthesia)—method:
►►Never use bupivacaine for a Bier's block (cardiotoxic if the cuff is inadvertently deflated). The use of a double cuff is controversial—a properly applied and checked tourniquet should suffice.

1 Place a loose tourniquet around the upper arm.
2 Empty the arm of blood either by raising above the heart for one minute or by the use of an esmarch bandage.
3 Inflate the cuff to to 100mmHg above the systolic BP.
4 Inject 30–40mL 0.5% prilocaine into a vein on the back of the hand.
5 Allow anaesthetic to develop (20–30min), then manipulate the fracture.
6 30min after the injection deflate the tourniquet. NB: Sudden early release of prilocaine into the circulation can cause fits. Other methods such as direct infiltration of the haematoma (haematoma block) are less effective.[1] The alternative is general anaesthesia.

The manipulation: Prepare a plaster back slab up to the knuckles. Ask an assistant to hold the elbow. Apply traction to disimpact the fragment and push it forwards, and towards the ulnar side. Keeping the arm under traction, apply the slab, with wrist slightly flexed and hand in ulnar deviation. Support in a sling, once an x-ray has shown a good position. Check x-ray in 5 days, when swelling has reduced. The plaster is then completed. Complications: median nerve symptoms (should resolve after good reduction); ruptured tendons; malunion; Sudeck's atrophy (p 695).

Smith's fracture distal radius (radial fragment angled *forward*). Manipulate, with the forearm held in full supination. These fractures are often unstable, and require fixation.

Bennett's fracture Carpometacarpal fracture/dislocation of the thumb. Reduce and apply a plaster cast to the extended thumb (for 4–6 weeks).

Fractures of the scaphoid This fracture, which is notoriously easy to miss on x-rays, may result from a fall on the hand.
Signs: Swelling, pain on wrist movements and tenderness on direct pressure 2cm distal to Lister's tubercle of the radius, and on proximal pressure on the extended thumb or index finger. *X-rays:* if the fracture is suspected request additional oblique 'scaphoid' views. If x-rays are –ve, and scaphoid fracture is a strong possibility, a bone scan is a good test.[2] If unavailable, put in plaster and x-ray at 2 weeks, by which time the fracture may be visible.
Treatment: Immobilize in plaster from below the elbow to beyond the knuckle (include the thumb up to the base of the nail) until union takes place (eg 8 weeks). If there is non-union, consider a bone graft or Herbert screw fixation. Complications: as the nutrient artery enters distally, there may be avascular necrosis of the proximal fragment. This may cause late degeneration in the wrist.

Dislocation of the carpus This may be anterior or posterior. Both require prompt manipulation or open reduction, and plaster immobilization for 6 weeks. Median nerve compression may occur.

1 A Cobb 1985 BMJ ii 1683   2 *Injury* 1992 23 77-9

A-P views

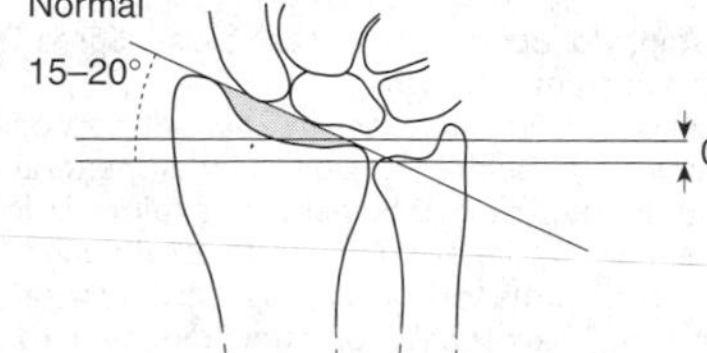

The articular surface of the radius is level with, or proud of, the ulna and is tilted towards the ulna.

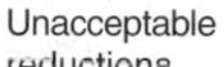

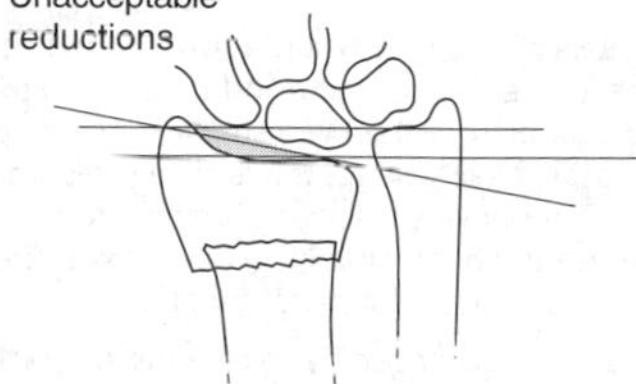

Note loss of radial length and reduction in ulnar tilt of the radius.

Lateral views

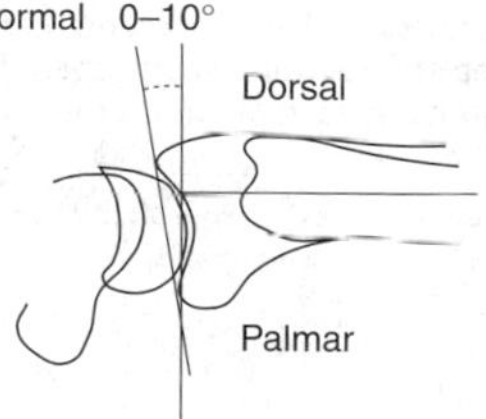

Acceptable

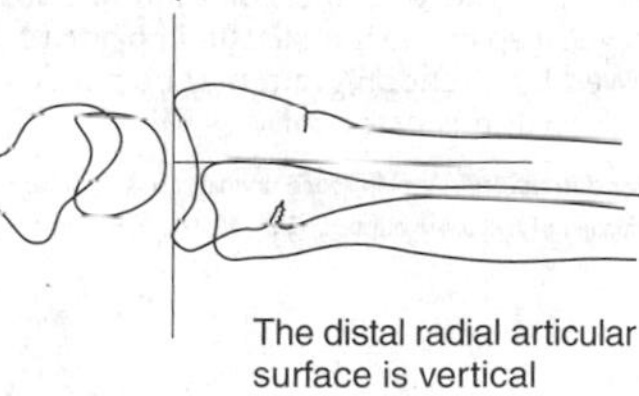

The distal radial articular surface is vertical

Unacceptable

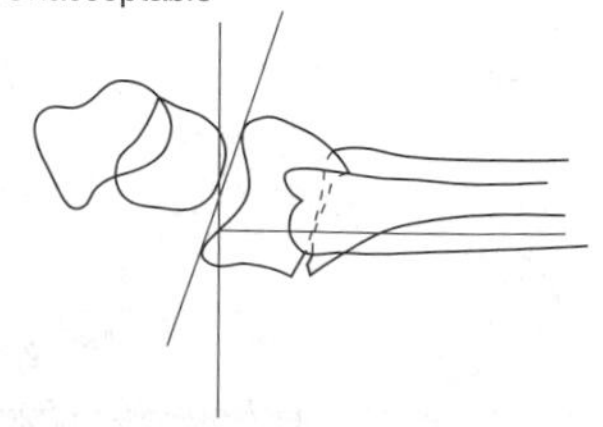

The distal radius surface is dorsally angulated. If allowed to heal in this position it will cause a marked restriction in function.

Injuries to the hand

►*There are no minor injuries to the hand.* Any breach of the integument may be the start of a chain of events which leads to loss of our most useful appendage. Contrary to beliefs of poets, our fingers are *not* protected from accidents by an invisible ring of shining:* *they are very frequently injured.*

Infections A streptococcus or staphylococcus is the usual cause. Spread may occur within a tendon sheath which may slough.
Treatment: If pus is present, take a swab. Give flucloxacillin 250mg/6h PO or erythromycin 500mg/12h PO starting 1h before surgery. Under general anaesthesia and tourniquet control, the bloodless field is explored. If necessary, the synovial sheath is excised at its proximal end. Local collections of pus can occur in tendon sheaths or palmar spaces. Surgical drainage is indicated. Any abscess (eg paronychial or subcutaneous) or infected fascial spaces must also be drained and cleaned. Sometimes primary suturing will be possible, provided that all necrotic material has been removed. A chronic 'cold' abscess of the tendon sheath suggests tuberculosis. Enlist expert help early.

Nerve injury (see p 664 and p 720) Examine sensory and motor function. Inability to lift the thumb out of the plane of the palm indicates median nerve injury (failure of abductor pollicis brevis). Nerves smaller than the digital nerve at the level of the distal interphalangeal joint are rarely reparable. Function is better if the injury is to a nerve subserving a single modality (motor or sensory), as regenerating fibres simply grow down the nearest Schwann tube (at ~1mm/day) irrespective of distal function.

Tendon injuries Failure to raise the affected finger by extending the MCP joint indicates extensor tendon division. Failure to flex the DIP joint against resistance indicates a divided flexor digitorum profundus. If this is intact, but flexion of the PIP joint is affected, there is division of superficialis. Flexor pollicis longus section leads to inability to flex the interphalangeal joint of the thumb. In general, flexor tendon injuries are best treated by primary repair. If there is loss of tendon substance, or delayed presentation, a staged repair with a silastic implant to keep the tendon sheath open, followed by a tendon graft, may be needed. Intensive hand physiotherapy with supervision is essential.

Hand incisions: A, pulp space drainage; B & B[1], lavage of flexor tendons; C, drainage of radial bursa; D, drainage of the ulnar bursa; E & E[1], for the mid-palmar space; F, drainage of the thenar space.

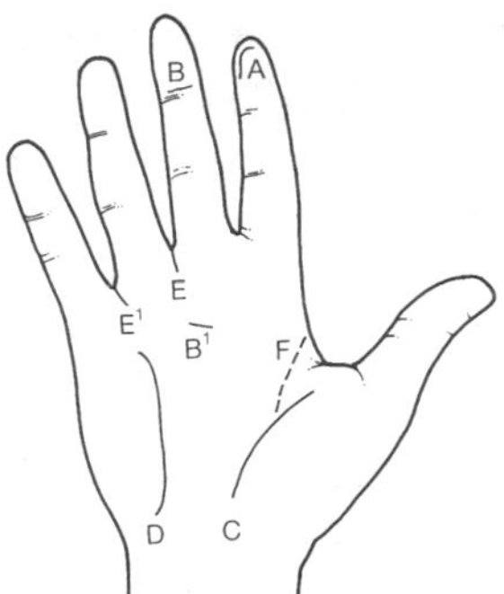

Stephen Spender 1985 *To My Daughter*
Complete Works, Faber

* *BRIGHT clasp of her whole hand around my finger*
My daughter, as we walk together now.
All my life I'll feel a ring invisibly
Circle this bone with shining . . .

Limb surgery in bloodless fields[1]

This may be achieved by using pneumatic tourniquets. The risk of inducing ischaemic changes in the limb is minimized by applying 'Bruner's rules'.

- Width of tourniquet: 10cm for the arm; 15cm for legs.
- Apply to the upper arm, or mid/upper thigh.
- Inflation—arm: 50–100mmHg above systolic BP; leg: double systolic.
- Deflation—must be within ~2 hours (3h is the absolute maximum).
- Avoid heating the limb (cooling is better, if feasible).
- Use ≥2 layers of orthopaedic wool to provide adequate padding (make sure it does not get wet with the skin preparation fluid, which should be aqueous, so that if wetting happens inadvertently, 'burns' do not occur).
- Apply only with the utmost caution to an unhealthy limb.
- Ensure the apparatus is calibrated weekly, and is well maintained.
- Document duration and pressure of tourniquet use.

1 I Braithwaite 1996 *Journal of the Medical Defence Union* **12** 14

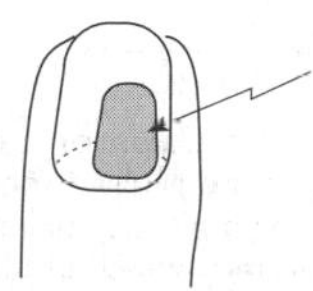

Sub-ungual haematoma

Release with needle by 'drilling' down – twiddling it between finger and thumbs; *or* by heating a paper clip to white heat and burning a hole through the nail.

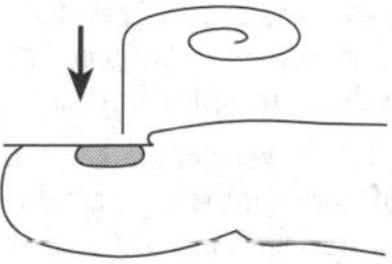

If left, the blood does not clot for up to 24hrs, therefore there is a throbbing pain due to pressure. This sometimes works (relieving the pressure) up to 2 days after the original injury.

Beware: subungual lacerations to the nail bed

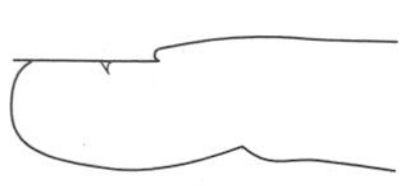

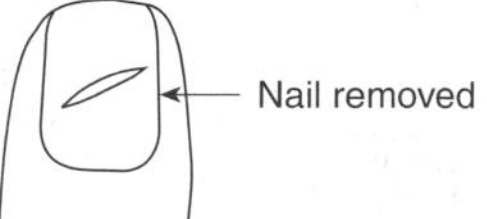

These need to be stitched, and the nail removed.
Also remove nail in case of nail bed avulsion.

Fractures in the hand

Fractures of the metacarpals These only need manipulation if there is gross displacement. The fifth metacarpal is most commonly involved, often from a punching injury. Immobilization for up to 10 days in a wool and crêpe bandage is usually all that is required, with finger movement encouraged after the first 2–3 days. Longer periods of splinting in a plaster or 'boxing glove' bandage can result in a stiff hand. Refer any fractures with obvious rotational deformity (a clinical, not a radiological decision), as this can be disabling. Rotational fractures disclose themselves by producing a rotation of the fingers (flex the fingers and look at all the nails end on); they usually require operative fixation with plate and screws, as do fractures of ≥2 metacarpals.
►Beware wounds overlying metacarpophalangeal joints—these are often from the teeth of the punched victim, are contaminated bites, and may communicate with the joint.

Fractures of the proximal phalanx Spiral or oblique fractures occurring at this site are likely to be associated with a rotation deformity—and this must be corrected. Often, the only way to do this accurately is by open reduction and fixation.

Fractures of the intermediate phalanges These should be manipulated and splinted in flexion over a malleable metal splint, and the affected finger strapped to its neighbour. The aim is to control rotation, which may interfere with subsequent finger flexion.

Fractures of the terminal phalanges may be caused by crush injuries and are often compound. If closed, symptoms may be relieved by trephining the nail to reduce swellings (a lightly-held hypodermic needle can be used as a drill, or a paper clip heated in a paraffin flame will pierce the nail). Split skin grafts from the thenar eminence may be needed for partial amputations of the finger tip.

Mallet finger The tip of the finger droops because of avulsion of the extensor tendon's attachment to the terminal phalanx. If the avulsed tendon includes a piece of bone, union is made easier—using a plastic 'mallet finger splint' or a simple wooden spatula (with adhesive felt) which holds the terminal phalanx taped in extension. Use for 6 weeks. Interphalangeal arthrodesis may be needed if active extension remains limited. A poorer outcome is associated with delay in splinting, and in those >50yrs old.

Gamekeeper's thumb This is so-called because of the rupture of the ulnar collateral ligament of the metacarpophalangeal joint of the thumb during the forced thumb abduction that occurs when wringing a pheasant's neck. The same injury is described in dry ski-slope participants who fall and catch their thumb in the matting ('Hill-end thumb'). Diagnosis can be difficult as the thumb is so painful to examine, but to miss this injury may condemn the patient to a weak pincer grip—inject 1–2mL 1% plain lidocaine (=lignocaine) around the ligament to facilitate examination. Nearly always the ligament ends are turned into the joint, and are best dealt with by open surgery and repair.

Nail avulsion

1. Warn the patient the nail may not regrow or regrow properly.
2. Ring block the finger and test it is numb.
3. Push one jaw of a small straight clamp down one side of the nail at its edge.
4. Close the clamp firmly. Warn the patient to look away.
5. Turn the clamp on its long axis as if opening a sardine can. The nail will wrap round the clamp and peel off its nail bed.
6. Having repaired the nailbed, dress the wound with some paraffin gauze, tucking some into the pocket at the base of the nailbed.

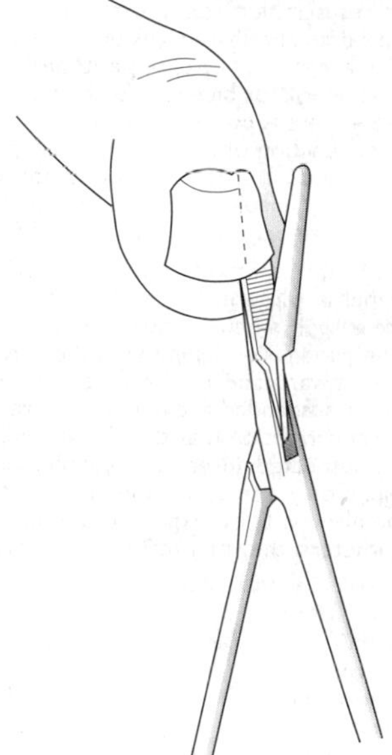

Fractures of the pelvis

► *The pelvis is like a suit of armour: after damage there is much more concern about its contents than about the structure itself.*[1] Because of the ring structure of the pelvis, single fractures are often stable and need no treatment other than a few weeks rest. In contrast, ≥2 fractures in the pelvis (with one above the level of the hip) renders the ring unstable and is a serious injury, with internal injuries in 25%. The force producing the fracture is usually compressive, eg from a traffic accident (60%) or fall. Signs to look for include bruising, perineal or scrotal haematoma, and blood at the urethral meatus.[2] *Examples:* Fractures of the ilium and pubic ramus (on one or both sides); fracture through a sacroiliac joint and a pubic ramus, as below.

Malgaigne's fracture (20% of all pelvic fractures, 60% of unstable ones): disruption of the pelvis anteriorly and posteriorly with displacement of a central fragment containing the hip joint.

Acetabular fractures Common sites: posterior lip or transverse. Two 45° oblique x-rays (± CT scans) are needed to define injuries exactly. Treatment: open reduction and reconstruction of the articular surface—to delay the onset of secondary osteoarthritis.

Complications •Haemorrhage (eg internal iliac artery). Check foot pulses, BP, CVP + urine output often. Transfusion is often needed. ►For rapid pelvis stabilizing in the resuscitation room, external fixation can be applied. This simple procedure dramatically reduces blood loss.

- Bladder rupture—may be intraperitoneal or extraperitoneal.
- Vaginal and rectal perforation—look for bleeding. Both rare.
- Trapping of the sciatic nerve—there is persistent pain.
- Urethral rupture, often at the junction of the prostatic and membranous parts in males. The appearance of a drop of blood at the end of the urethra is suggestive. He may be unable to pass urine (avoid repeated tries). On rectal exam, the prostate may be elevated out of reach.

Treatment Relieve pain and replace blood. *Ways to reduce blood loss:*[2] Avoid manipulations of the pelvis •Internally rotate both lower legs to close an 'open-book' fracture •Apply a pelvic binder •Suspend the patient in a pelvic sling promptly. The patient lies supine with the pelvis over the sling's webbing, which exerts upward and medial (thereby compressing) traction via weights and runners suspended above the bed. Traction is also applied to the legs. Surgical reconstruction may then be undertaken.

If rupture of the urethra is suspected, insert a suprapubic catheter, and ask for expert urological help. If only a small volume of urine is found, the reason may be rupture of the bladder. Enlist expert help. A cystogram may be needed. Avoid urethral catheters: they may make a false passage.

Reassuring signs on a pelvis x-ray:[2]

- Symphis pubis separation <1cm
- Integrity of superior & inferior rami
- Integrity of acetabula & femoral necks
- Symmetry of ilium & sacroiliac joints
- Symmetry of the sacral foramina, eg by evaluating the arcuate lines
- No fracture of transverse process of L5

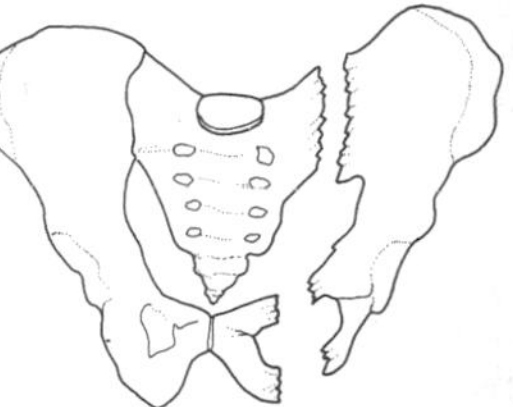

1 M Rang 1983 *Children's Fractures* p233 J Lippincott 2 ATLS 1997 *Manual* 6e, p270 ISBN 1-880696-10-X

Injury to the hip and femur

Incomplete or impacted femoral head fractures may present with coxa valgus; complete fracture with dislocation may present with coxa varus.

Intracapsular fractures occur just below the femoral head. This often causes external rotation and adduction of the leg. The injuring force may be trivial and the patient may be able to walk (but with difficulty). As the medial femoral circumflex artery supplies the head via the neck, ischaemic necrosis of the head may occur, particularly if there is much displacement. Femur fractures fill 20% of all UK orthopaedic beds. The incidence is rising (~1:100/yr in females aged 75–84). Mortality: 50%.

Treatment:

- Assess vital signs. Treat shock with Haemaccel®, but beware incipient heart failure. If present, monitor CVP.
- Relieve pain (eg morphine 0.2mg/kg IM + prochlorperazine 12.5mg IM).
- X-rays: a good quality lateral is essential to make the diagnosis if there is impaction or little displacement.
- Prepare for theatre: FBC, U&E, CXR, ECG, crossmatch 2U, consent. Tell anaesthetist about any drugs the patient is taking.
  Sort out any medical problems before embarking on surgery.
- In theatre: if displacement is minimal, either multiple screw fixation, or Garden screws. (Sliding nail plate units are not used for intracapsular fractures.) Alternatively, the head is excised and a prosthesis inserted.

Intertrochanteric–extracapsular fractures (between greater and lesser trochanters). They occur in a younger age group and, as blood supply is adequate, non-union is uncommon. *Treatment:* Traction and bed rest for 3 months—or internal fixation (eg with plate and nail or Richard's screw). The principle of the screw plate is to fix the fracture, but to allow compression by sliding.

Femoral shaft fracture ►Is the femoral artery torn? (Look for swelling and check distal pulses.) Sciatic nerve injury may also occur. The proximal bone fragment is flexed by iliopsoas, adbucted by gluteus medius, and laterally rotated by gluteus maximus. The lower fragment is pulled up by the hamstrings and adducted (with lateral rotation) by the adductors. *Treatment:* Typically, this is with a locked intramedullary nail. This is introduced proximally over a guide wire that can be manipulated across the fracture under x-ray control. This allows early mobilization. Alternative: manipulation under anaesthesia (exact reduction is not needed) with fixed traction with a Thomas knee splint, or skeletal traction, or sliding traction, with the thigh supported on a frame, or a cast brace with a hinge at the knee (this permits early weight bearing). Union takes 3–4 months. Intramedullary nail fixation allows early restoration of function.

Condylar fractures and tibial plateau fractures Being intra-articular, these demand accurate joint reconstruction to minimize secondary osteoarthitic changes.

Posterior hip dislocation These occur to front-seat passengers in car accidents, as the knee strikes the dashboard. The femoral head may be felt in the buttock. The leg is flexed, adducted and shortened. There may be damage to the popliteal division of the sciatic nerve. *Treatment:* Reduction under anaesthesia, by lifting the femoral head back into the joint. Traction (for about 3 weeks) enables the joint capsule to heal.

Fracture dislocation of the hip This is described on p 706.

Injuries of the lower leg

The patella Lateral dislocation may result from a blow to the side of the knee, causing a tear in the medial capsule and the quadriceps aponeurosis. It is an injury of young people. On examination, the knee is unable to flex. Recurrent dislocation may be related to under-development of the lateral femoral condyle. Sudden contraction of quadriceps may snap the patella transversely, whereas direct force may produce a multiple 'star-shaped' fracture (undisplaced within the quadriceps tendon).

The knee *Injury to the collateral ligaments* is common in sport, eg presenting with effusion ± tenderness over the ligament injured. Rest is needed, then firm support. If there is complete rupture, varus and valgus straining opens the joint if the knee is held in 10° flexion (and if the knee is held in extension, if a cruciate ligament is also torn).
Anterior cruciate tears: Typically, these follow posterior blows to the tibia or rotation injuries, when the foot is fixed to the ground. Signs: effusion, haemarthrosis, and a +ve 'draw' sign. (Immobilize the patient's leg by sitting on his foot, and then with the knee in 90° flexion, grip the upper tibia, and try to draw it towards you, away from the femur. Note: the reverse 'set back' suggests a posterior cruciate tear—eg after car accidents as the knee strikes the dashboard.) Do a 'pivot shift test' (p 634). Examination under anaesthesia may be needed. *Treatment:* This can be problematic. 3 weeks' rest in a plaster cylinder may help. If problems (knee instability/giving way) persist, consider reconstruction using part of the patella tendon. Physiotherapy is adequate for ~60%.

Semilunar cartilage tears: Medial cartilage tears (eg 'bucket-handle') follow forcible twists to a flexed knee (eg in football). Adduction with internal rotation causes lateral cartilage tears. Extension is limited (the knee 'locks') as the displaced segment lodges between femoral and tibial condyles. The patient has to stop what he is doing, and can only walk on tiptoe, if at all. The joint line is tender, and McMurray's test is +ve (p 634). If the 'handle' of the 'bucket' becomes free at one end ('parrot beak' tear), the knee suddenly gives way, rather than locking. *Tests:* MRI; arthroscopy. *Treatment:* Removal the damaged meniscus may be needed.

Fractures of tibia *Avulsion fractures* of the intercondylar region often occur with anterior cruciate injury. Sliding traction will be required, or surgery with open elevation of the joint surface. Fractures of the tibial shaft are unlikely to be displaced, unless the fibula is also fractured. Compound fractures are common as there is so little anterior covering tissue. Tearing of the nutrient artery may make non-union a problem in fractures of the lower third of the tibia.
Treatment: Close compound fractures as quickly as possible. Reduce under anaesthesia. The treatment of choice for closed fracture is intramedullary nailing. Open fractures are treated with external fixation or unreamed intramedullary nails. Steinmann pins are now rarely used. A supportive dressing may be sufficient for isolated fibula fractures.

Pretibial lacerations The shin (particularly if elderly) has a poor blood supply. It is vulnerable to flap wounds, eg caused by steps of buses. *Treatment:* Try hard to iron out *all* the flap, and reposition it carefully: an ideal tool is the 'wrong' end of a Vacutaine® needle, sheathed in its rubber case. The important thing is to prevent tension (tension → breakdow → plastic surgery)—so skin closure with adhesive strips (eg Steristrip®), which can be loosened if the tissues swell, is better than sutures. Dress the wound and advise a support bandage, and leg elevation. Review to check for infection, wound tension, and necrosis.

Gustilo classification of open fractures[1]

Type I Low-energy wounds <1cm long, eg caused by bone piercing skin.

Type II The wound is >1cm—typically from a higher energy wound, causing moderate soft tissue damage.

Type III Extensive soft tissue injury, which is usually >1cm long. Fractures from high speed gunshot injuries are always Type III, as are most crush injuries from fast vehicles. Fractures with significant diaphyseal bone loss are generally Type III. Type III fractures are denoted IIIB if there is extensive stripping of bone, with adequate coverage. Type IIIC implies arterial injury needing repair. (IIIA implies that there is enough soft tissue to provide adequate local coverage.)

1 Scott Kozin & Anthony Berlet 1992 *Handbook of Common Orthopaedic Fractures*, Medical Surveillance Inc

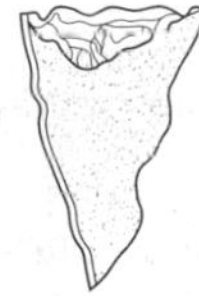

Before
Flap retracts back

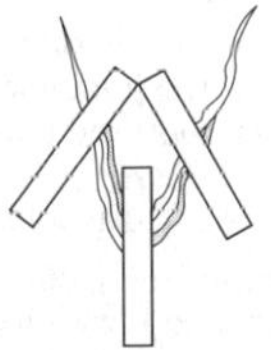

Good
No tension in flap. Held with adhesive sutures.

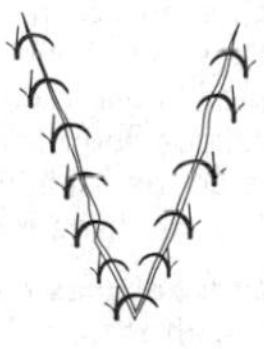

Bad
Flap stretched tight and likely to necrose.

Ankle and foot strains and fractures

Ligament strains of the ankle Twisting inversion accounts for the very common strain to the anterior talofibular part of the lateral ligament. *Signs:* Stiffness, tenderness over the lateral ligament, pain on inversion. Only if there is swelling or inability to bear weight do x-rays to rule out fracture of the lateral malleolus (p 734). *Treatment:* Simple strapping or a below-knee plaster (if there is much swelling) will be required. Complete rupture is diagnosed by stress x-rays under GA, and may need surgery. Medial deltoid ligament strains are rarer, and often need simple strapping only. Supervized walking exercises and diapulse therapy reduce symptoms. NB: minor sprains may respond to rest and simple analgesia, or a topical NSAID (eg ibuprofen, ketoprofen, or piroxicam).[1]

Malleolar and metatarsal fractures Either malleolus may be fractured by the above injuries. Rotation causes oblique lateral malleolar fracture (hard to see except on lateral x-rays), or a proximal fracture of the 5th metatarsal (avulsion by peroneus brevis). *Treatment:* Surgery to restore the length of the fibula by open reduction and fixation of the malleoli.

Eversion injuries may produce bimalleolar fractures. These are very unstable and will either require an above-knee plaster (with the knee in flexion to control rotation) or internal fixation. *Dupuytren's fracture: Distal* fibula fracture with distal rupture of the tibiofibular ligament ± fracture of the back of the lower end of the tibia (trimalleolar) with lateral displacement of the talus. *Treatment:* Open reduction + screw fixation if >⅓ of the articular surface is involved. No full weight-bearing for 7 weeks. *Maisonneuve's fracture: Proximal* fibula fracture + syndesmosis rupture, and medial malleolus fracture or deltoid ligament rupture. If 2 bones dislocate where no true joint exists, the term diastasis is used.

►Always examine the proximal fibula with 'ankle sprains'.

AO classification[2]

A Transverse fibula fracture at or below joint line.
B Spiral fibula fracture starting at the joint line with medial injury.
C1 Oblique fibula fracture above a ruptured tibiofibular ligament with associated medial injury.
C2 Maisonneuve's fracture, only the fibular fracture is more proximal.

Other fractures *Fractured neck of talus* often occurs with subtalar subluxation after forced dorsiflexion, and is a serious injury because interruption of the vessels in the sinus-tarsi may lead to avascular necrosis of the body of the talus. Treatment: Accurate reduction by manipulation and a plaster cast holding the foot in plantarflexion to maintain the reduction. If displacement of the body damages the posterior tibial artery, fixation with wires may be required, with a plaster cast for 12 weeks. *Fractures of the os calcis* are often bilateral, following a fall from a height—and may be associated with spinal fracture. *Signs:* Swelling, bruising, and inability to weight bear. ►*Does the fracture enter the subtalar joint?* This signifies a more serious injury. Treatment is often conservative, with elevation in bed until the swelling subsides. Recovery may take many months and require a subtalar arthrodesis. *Mid-tarsal dislocation* produces a painful, swollen foot. The proximal articular surface of the navicular fails to articulate with the talus. *Treatment:* Early manipulation and a plaster cast is needed. *Lisfranc dislocation of the first tarsometatarsal joint* is dangerous because it may impair the blood supply to the medial foot. *March fracture* of the second metatarsal follows stress from too much walking. Treatment: A plaster cast for 6 weeks. *Fractures of the toes:* Treatment: Simple protective dressings.

1 R Moore 1998 BMJ i 333 2 S Kozin 1992 *Handbook of Common Orthopaedic Fractures*, Medical Surveillance Inc

►►Head injury

Emergency care Do ABCs, p 685, protecting the cervical spine. Retinal vein pulsation at fundoscopy helps exclude ICP↑. ►If the pupils are unequal, diagnose rising intracranial pressure (ICP), eg from extradural haemorrhage and summon urgent neurosurgical help. Burr holes (on the side of the dilated pupil) may be needed. Other signs of ICP↑: deepening coma (or a lucid interval, then relapse), a rising BP and a slowing pulse (Cushing reflex), Cheyne–Stokes breathing, apnoea, fixed dilated pupils (ipsilateral at first) and extensor posture. Try mannitol 20% 5mL/kg IV over 15min. Enlist an anaesthetist's help with transfer to a neurosurgical centre for urgent CT ± craniotomy. Aim to offer the neurosurgeon a well-oxygenated, well-perfused brain.

Initial management Write careful notes. Record times accurately.

- High-flow inspired O_2 (F_iO_2 >0.85 + tight-fitting mask with reservoir).
- Stop blood loss. Take BP; treat shock with Haemaccel.®
- History: When? Where? How? Had a fit? Lucid interval? Alcohol?
- Search for other injuries. Do blood alcohol, gases, U&E, glucose, FBC.
- Assess level of consciousness with the Glasgow Coma Scale (p 680).
- If alert, record the most difficult thing he can do.
- Assess anterograde amnesia (loss from time of injury) and retrograde amnesia—for pre-injury events (its extent correlates with the severity of the injury, and it never occurs without anterograde amnesia).
- Examine the CNS. Chart pulse, BP, T°, respirations + pupils every 15min.
- Evaluate lacerations of face or scalp. Palpate deep wounds with sterile glove to check for step deformity. Note obvious skull/facial fractures.
- Periorbital (raccoon sign), or postauricular (Battle sign) ecchymoses.
- Check for CSF leak, from nose (rhinorrhoea) or ear (any blood behind the drum). If any present, suspect basilar skull fracture and do CT. Give tetanus and antibiotic prophylaxis, and refer at once to neurosurgeons.
- Palpate the neck posteriorly for tenderness and deformity. If detected, or if the patient has obvious head injury, or injury above the clavicle with loss of consciousness, obtain cervical spine radiographs.
- On skull x-ray (posterior/anterior, Townes', and lateral views): look for sinus fractures and intracranial air. If the pineal gland is shifted (visible if calcified) or fractures cross blood vessels (eg middle meningeal artery—the vessel of extradural haemorrhage), do a CT scan.
- Nurse semi-prone if no spinal injury. Meticulous care to bladder + airway.
- If not severely injured: sit up when headache allows (if severe, suspect a complication). Treat pain with aspirin. *Criteria for admission:* Difficult to assess (child; post-ictal; alcohol intoxication); CNS signs; severe headache or vomiting; fracture. Loss of consciousness does **not** require admission if well, and a responsible adult is in attendance.
- Complications: *early* extradural/subdural haemorrhage; fits. *Later:* subdural haemorrhage, fits, diabetes insipidus, parkinsonism, dementia.

Drowsy trauma patients (GCS <15 to >8) smelling of alcohol: Do skull x-ray (+CT if fracture or focal signs). Alcohol is an unlikely cause of coma if plasma alcohol <44mmol/L. If test unavailable, estimate alcohol from the osmolar gap (*OHCM* p 636). (If blood alcohol ≈ 40mmol/L, osmolar gap ≈ 40mmol/L.)

Improvement following impairment of brain function (concussion) Increasing pulse volume → deeper respirations → return of brainstem reflexes → eyes open → vomiting → consciousness → restlessness → complaint of headache → amnesia → post-concussional syndrome (headache, dizziness, inability to concentrate, headaches, poor memory).

Indicators of a bad prognosis Increasing age, decerebrate rigidity, extensor spasms, prolonged coma, hypertension, P_aO_2↓ (on blood gases), T° >39°C. 60% of those with loss of consciousness of >1 month will survive 3–25yrs, but may need daily nursing care.

Getting help in severe neurotrauma

Work out the Glasgow coma score (p 680) and get expert help whenever there is coma after neurotrauma; special measures may be needed, such as monitoring intracranial pressure (± ventriculostomy).

When to ventilate immediately:
Coma ≤8 on Glasgow Coma Scale (GCS)
P_aO_2 <9kPa in air (<13kPa in O_2)
P_aCO_2 >6kPa
Spontaneous hyperventilation (P_aCO_2 <3.5)
Respiratory arrhythmia, ie irregularity
Ventilate before neurosurgical transfer if:
Deteriorating level of consciousness
Bilateral fractured mandible
Bleeding into mouth, eg skull base fracture
Seizures

Inform neurosurgeon of:
Patient's age; past history
Time and mechanism of injury
Spoken or not post-injury?
GCS on admission, and now
Pupil and limb responses
BP, pulse, P_aO_2, P_aCO_2
Respiratory rate & pattern
Skull fracture/other injury
Management so far; drugs

Risk of intracranial haematoma (in adults). Fully conscious, no skull fracture = <1:1000; confused, no skull fracture = 1:100; fully conscious, skull fracture = 1:30; confused, skull fracture = 1:4.

►►Injuries to the face and neck

►*If there is airway obstruction, summon expert help promptly*. Remove blood, loose (or false) teeth, and vomit from the mouth. Lie in the semi-prone position to prevent obstruction from a swollen injured tongue, but always beware of cervical spine tauma with injuries above the clavicle. If pharynx is swelling do cricothyrotomy (*OHCM* p 799), then tracheostomy. Blood aspiration is prevented by direct pressure to the bleeding site.

Lacerations of the face Clean meticulously. Alignment of the tissues must be exact to produce a good cosmetic result.

- Complex lacerations: Is there a plastic surgeon available?
- Dog bites: give antibiotic cover (eg co-amoxiclav 1 tab/8h PO).
- Rugby player's ear: aspirate haematoma (repeat every few days) and then strap orthopaedic felt pressure pads against the head. Ruptured ear drum: advise against letting water into the meatus.
- Avulsed teeth may be replaced (p 738). If inhaled, do expiratory CXR. Bleeding socket: bite on epinephrine (=adrenaline)-soaked pads, or use sutures.
- Eye injury, nose fractures, and nose bleeds: see p 514, p 550, & p 552.

Mandible injury *Signs:* Local tenderness and swelling; jaw malocclusion; a mobile fragment; bone may protrude into the mouth in compound fractures; if comminuted, the tongue may cause airway problems.

Diagnosis: Orthopantomograph x-ray. Enlist expert dental help.

Treatment of dislocations: Place your (gloved) thumbs over the back teeth and press downwards, while at the same time levering the chin upwards with your fingers (both hands). Consider midazolam sedation: titrate up to 0.07mg/kg IV: start with 2mg over 30sec, max 1.5mg if elderly—antidote: flumazenil 0.2mg IV over 15sec, then 0.1mg every 60sec, max 1mg total.

Blows to the chin may cause fracture at the impact site, or indirect fractures near the temporomandibular joint.

Fractures: Open reduction + internal fixation with miniplates is better than wiring teeth together for 6 weeks.[1] Try to arrange this for a daytime consultant list, rather than at night.[2] Complications: infection; non-union.

'Whiplash' injury This is cervical strain caused by sudden neck flexion with rebound hyperextension. It is a common injury, often in a rear-end collision car accident. Hyperextension causes the damage—to the anterior musculoligamentous structures. Subsequent protective muscle spasm causes pain and stiffness, which may be severe. Cervical x-rays (*OHCM* p 607) may show a fragment of bone avulsed from the anterior/inferior aspect of a vertebral body. *Treatment:* Analgesia, a soft collar, and rest for 2 weeks is often advised. Gentle stretching and early mobilization may also be tried. If symptoms last for >1yr, they are likely to be permanent. ►Do not rely on plain x-rays to rule out facet joint fractures. They are more likely if the neck is rotated at the time of forced extension. Here it may be wise to ask a senior colleague if CT is indicated.[3]

Other car accident neck sprains (Seen in $^1/_3$ of car users soon after accidents.) Symptoms may be delayed—and persist for years. The best treatment may be to give NSAIDs, a cervical collar, and review in the next clinic, with referral for immediate physiotherapy if symptoms warrant this. Explain to the patient that head restraints *are* helpful—the usual mistake is that they are adjusted too low.

1 S Layton 1994 BMJ **i** 70 2 D Thomas 1995 *Health Trends* **26** 113 3 KE Jones 1993 BMJ **ii** 868

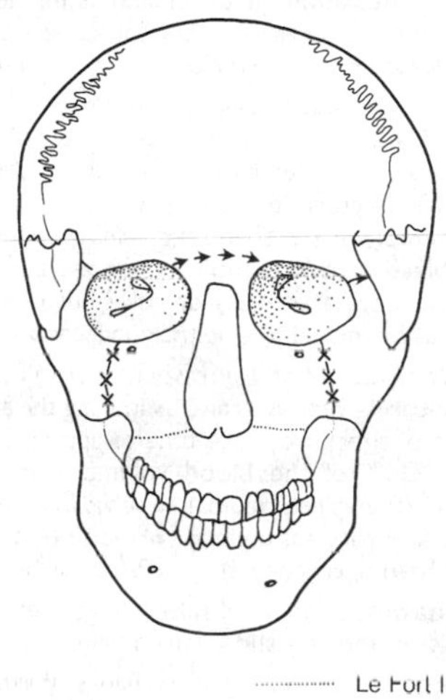

Bony injury classification of facial injuries

Le Fort I severs the maxilla's tooth-bearing part from the upper maxilla. Signs: crepitus on manipulation; epistaxis; airway compromise is rare.

Le Fort II: The middle $1/3$ of the face is driven back and down. Bite is open. The at-risk airway is cleared by lifting upper incisors forward.

Le Fort III: The fracture extends into the anterior fossa via the superior orbital margins. There may be CSF rhinorrhoea (p 550).

▸▸Abdominal injury[1,2]

Penetrating injuries mostly require prompt laparotomy/laparoscopy.[2] Assess degree of penetration (if uncertain) under local anaesthetic, by extending the wound, if necessary. Ask for expert assistance with this. Laparotomy is indicated if the posterior rectus sheath is breached.

Blunt trauma Deceleration forces may tear bowel from mesentery, liver from vena cava, or bladder from bladder neck. After blunt trauma abdomen and chest may be sites of hidden blood loss—*always* consider intra-abdominal bleeding or pelvic fracture (p 706) if BP↓ and no source of loss is found. *Key questions: Are vital signs stable?* and *Is an indication for laparotomy present?* (BP↓; GI, GU, or PR bleeding; evisceration; +ve ultrasound or peritoneal lavage). Liver, spleen, and kidneys are chiefly at risk—but remember the pancreas (amylase↑; injury may be missed by CT/ultrasound; endoscopy may be needed).

Tests CVP measurements, CT and ultrasound may all mislead. There is no substitute for monitoring vital signs and examining the abdomen *often*. In the young and fit, signs of shock may take time to appear. Systolic BP doesn't fall consistently until ≥30% of the blood volume is lost. *x-ray implications:*[1]

- Lower rib fracture (?live/spleen trauma)
- Spine fracture (?renal or pancreas trauma)
- Bowel displaced (?haemoperitoneum)
- Pelvic fracture (?rectal injury)
- Free air (?hollow viscus rupture)
- Psoas shadow↓ (retroperitoneal clot)

Signs of organ damage *Ruptured spleen:* Suggested by shock, abdominal tenderness and distension, left shoulder-tip pain, overlying rib fracture.

Any visceral injury may cause bruising in the flanks, absent bowel sounds, and muscular spasm. *GU injury* is suggested by haematuria.

Management Maintain airway; ensure adequate ventilation. Give high-flow O_2 (12–15L/min). Treat shock (p 684). Crossmatch blood. Then:

1 If the patient does not respond quickly, take straight to theatre for exploratory laparotomy (after urgent CXR to rule out pneumothorax and after passing of a nasogastric tube).

2 Baseline tests: pulse, BP, respirations, temperature, urine output.

3 Look for signs of GU injury:
- Blood at the urethral tip, signifying ruptured urethra.
- Do a rectal exam to assess bowel integrity, presence of blood, or high-riding prostate (this suggests bladder neck injury).
- Test the urine. Is there frank or microscopic haematuria?

If any suspicious signs, seek urological help to plan urethral repair. Rarely, GU trauma needs ureteroureterostomy, ureteroneocystostomy, or even kidney autotransplantation.

4 Consider peritoneal lavage (opposite, p 719) or LIF diagnostic tap.

5 Arrange a prompt exploratory laparotomy if there is:
- Shock (eg ruptured spleen)
- Peritonism (ruptured viscus)
- Penetration to unknown extent
- Air under the diaphragm on x-ray

A non-functioning kidney on IVU is a *relative* indication. *Don't* deny analgesia on finishing your assessment, simply for fear of masking signs.

6 *Blood tests:* FBC (raised WCC may occur in ruptured spleen), U&E, amylase.

7 *Radiology:* All with serious blunt trauma (eg RTA) need x-rays of cervical spine, chest and pelvis as part of their primary assessment. Abdominal films are part of the secondary assessment: consider these along with IVU, thoracolumbar spine, and other injured sites.

1 ATLS 1997 *Manual* 6e, page 270 ISBN 1-880696-10-X 2 *Br J Surg* 1993 **80** 279

Diagnostic peritoneal lavage (DPL)

Indications DPL is used to assist in the diagnosis of significant intra-abdominal injury following trauma, particularly when abdominal examination by palpation is unreliable (spinal injury; neuromuscular blocking drugs; head injury; alcohol) or difficult to interpret (pelvic, lower rib and lumbar spine fractures may produce abdominal pain and muscle guarding). It may be used to determine the cause of unexplained hypotension following trauma. It should be performed by the surgeon who is responsible for any subsequent operation.

Contraindications The need for urgent laparotomy is an *absolute* contraindication—*don't delay for* DPL. In children, abdominal CT or ultrasound, in some centres is the preferred investigation. Relative contraindications: late pregnancy, cirrhosis, known coagulation disorder.

Technique

- The bladder and stomach must be empty, so pass a urinary catheter (not if urethral trauma) and a nasogastric tube.
- Use strict asepsis and clean the abdomen in the midline below the umbilicus. Inject lidocaine (=lignocaine) *with epinephrine (=adrenaline)* ⅓ of the way between the umbilicus and the symphysis, in the midline (epinephrine limits false positives from abdominal wall bleeding).
- Incise down to peritoneum, then grasp the peritoneum with 2 artery forceps and lift clear of the bowel.
- Incise the peritoneum and pass a dialysis catheter into the pelvis.
- Aspirate for blood—if >5mL, DPL is positive. If <5mL, run in 10mL/kg of warm normal saline. Leave for 5–10min, then allow fluid to drain by hanging the bag below the level of the abdomen.

Interpretation Lavage fluid *must* be sent to the laboratory. Do not rely on naked eye appearance. *Red cells:* $>10^5/mm^3$ is positive. *White cells:* $>500/mm^3$ is positive. A positive result requires exploratory laparotomy. False negatives occur with retroperitoneal haemorrhage.

Complications Haemorrhage; organ perforation ± peritonitis; infection.

Principal source: *Advanced Trauma Life Support*, 1997, American College of Surgeons

Injury to nerves and arteries

Neurapraxia: There is temporary loss of nerve conduction often due to ischaemia following pressure (eg to the lateral popliteal nerve as it crosses the neck of the fibula, see below). In mixed nerves, the motor modality is the more vulnerable component.

Axonotmesis: There is physical damage to the nerve fibre but the endoneural tube is intact, providing guidance to the regrowing nerve. Good recovery is the rule. The growth rate is ~3 mm/day.

Neurotmesis: The whole nerve is divided and, as there is no guidance from the endoneural tube, regrowing fibrils cause a traumatic neuroma if they are unable to bridge the gap. Formal repair using 7-0 silk or nylon sutures into the perineurium may be performed at once. Problems arise in restoring independent action of the small muscles of the hand and discriminating sensation. Microsurgical funicular repair may be helpful.

Median nerve (C5–T1) This is the nerve of grasp. Injury above the cubital fossa causes inability to flex the interphalangeal joint of the index finger on clasping the hands (Ochner's test); inability to flex the terminal phalanx of the thumb (flexor pollicis longus); loss of sensation over the lateral half of the hand.

If the lesion is at the wrist, the only muscle reliably affected is abductor pollicis brevis. Test it by holding the hand palm up. Can the patient raise the thumb out of the plane of the hand? The area of sensory loss is smaller than that for higher lesions.

Ulnar nerve (C8–T1) Injury distal to the wrist produces the claw hand deformity [flexor digitorum profundus is intact, but is not countered by the small muscles of the hand—the basis of Froment's paper sign: on holding a piece of paper between thumb and finger (both hands), there is flexion of the thumb's distal phalynx on trying to pull apart. Sensory loss is over the little finger, and a variable area of the ring finger].

Radial nerve (C5–T1) This nerve opens the fist. Injury will produce wrist-drop. Test for this with the elbow flexed and the forearm pronated. Sensory loss is variable, always including the dorsal aspect of the root of the thumb.

Sciatic nerve (L4–S2) Complete lesions will affect all muscles below the knee, and sensation below the knee laterally.

Lateral popliteal (common peroneal) nerve (L4–S2) Lesions lead to equinovarus with inability to dorsiflex the foot and toes. Sensory loss is over the dorsum of the foot.

Tibial nerve (S1–3) Loss causes calcaneovalgus and inability to stand on tiptoe or invert the foot. Sensory loss over the sole.

Injuries to arteries Bleeding is usually controllable by pressure and elevation of the part. After any injury in which an artery may have been damaged, examine distal pulses carefully. If they are not felt, do not assume that this is due to spasm, but request expert help. Surgical exploration with end-to-end suture, or reversed vein grafts may be needed. The prognosis is not so bad if there are good collaterals (eg to the femoral artery, compared with the popliteal artery). *Complications:* gangrene, contractures, traumatic aneurysms, and arteriovenous fistulae.

Dermatomes

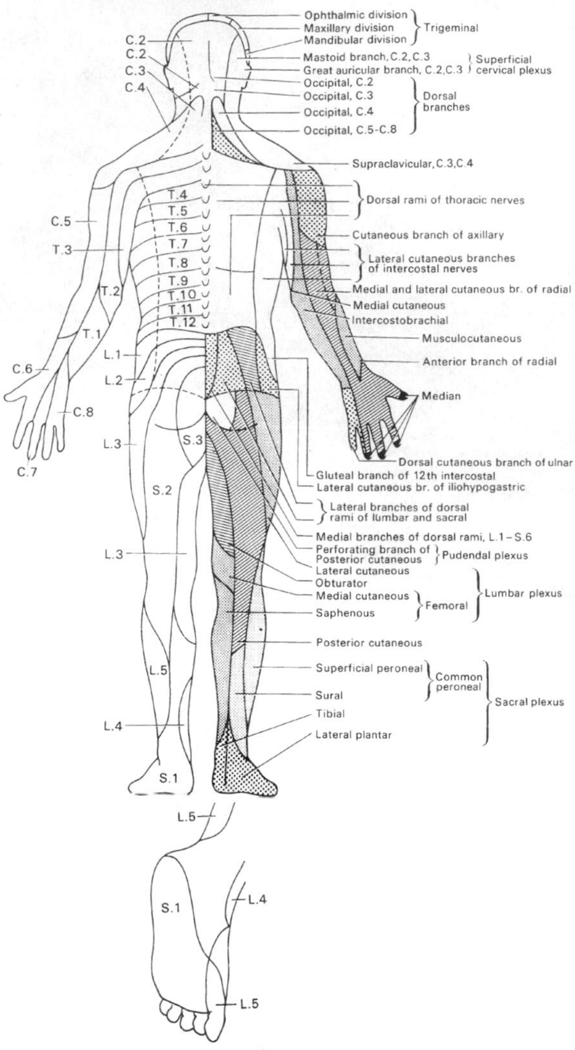

Cutaneous areas of distribution of spinal segments and peripheral nerves.

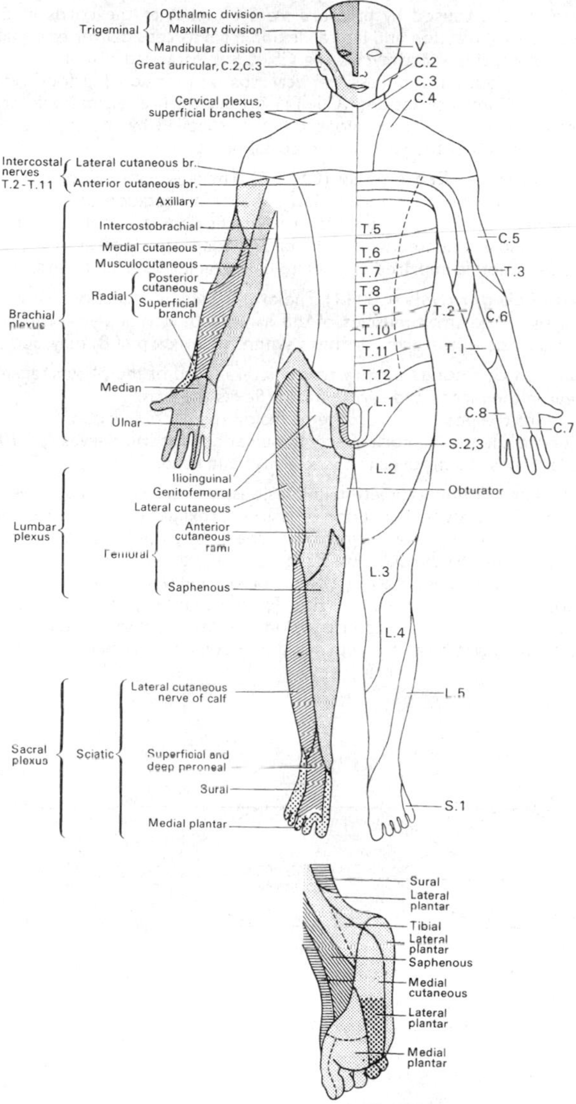

ANTERIOR ASPECT

Injuries to the brachial plexus

These may be caused by pressure from crutches to the cords in the axilla; cervical traction and lateral flexion from forceps deliveries or falls from fast-moving motorcycles (eg C5, C6 ± paralysed diaphragm); or penetrating tumours, bullets, cervical ribs or radiation (eg for breast cancer). Complete lesions (C5–T1) produce a flail, anaesthetic arm (except for a medial strip along the arm supplied by the intercostobrachial branch of the second intercostal nerve).

Root injuries—Erb's palsy (C5, C6) There is paralysis of deltoid, supraspinatus, and teres major. Because external rotation of the arm is diminished, and biceps paralysis prevents flexion, it is held internally rotated, and if adducted behind the back it adopts the 'porter's tip' position. Sensation is impaired over deltoid, lateral forearm, and hand.

Klumpke's paralysis (C8, T1) The arm is held in adduction. There is paralysis of the small muscles of the hand, with lack of sensation over the ulnar side of the arm. Horner's syndrome (*OHCM* p 488) may occur.

Injury to the cords •Injury to the lateral cord of the plexus: absent power in the biceps and carporadialis (flexes the wrist).
•Injury to the posterior cord: teres major and deltoid inaction.
•Injury to the medial cord affects the ulnar and median nerves (p 720).
•Sensation is absent over the medial arm and hand.

Recovery With incomplete trunk lesions any recovery occurs over 5 months. The prognosis is poor in lesions proximal to the dorsal root ganglion (DRG). For intradermal histamine (1%) to produce an arterial flare, the route to the DRG must be intact, so if this is present the lesion is proximal to the DRG. CSF may contain blood, and myelograms may show a leak of contrast at the injury site. Tendon transfers, shoulder arthrodesis and neurological reconstruction may be indicated. Seek expert help early. Chart recovery with serial two point discrimination tests.

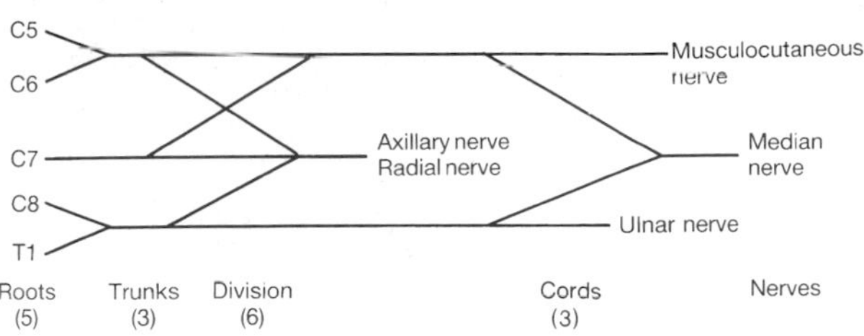

Spinal cord injury—the first day

At the site of the accident Spinal injury should be assumed to be present in any serious accident, and in all accidents when the nature of the injuring force is not known, and the patient is unconscious. This does not mean that the patient cannot be moved into the recovery position (protection of the airway is always the first priority)—but all movement should be planned. Keeping the head in neutral, the patient may be 'log-rolled' into a semi-prone position (not lateral, see p 789). For immobilization, see p 788.

Radiology Do not rely on mobile x-ray equipment; if possible, take to the radiology department, supervising all movements and the removal of sandbags and collars. The lateral view is often the most revealing (reject x-rays which do not include the C7–T1 junction). Anterior vertebral displacement of <½ the diameter of the vertebral body suggests unilateral facet dislocation. Greater displacements indicate bilateral (unstable) facet dislocations. Look for the soft-tissue shadow of a paravertebral haematoma if bony signs are minimal. Other views: anteroposterior (AP) with an open mouth view of the odontoid process, lateral tomography for the cervicothoracic junction; swimmer's view (supine, with one hand on the head and the opposite shoulder depressed to give access to the beam) to give views down to T2; '22.5°' oblique views for facet joints. Supine 45° oblique views may be more practical in severely injured patients. Thoracic, lumbar, and sacral injuries are usually shown on AP and lateral films.

Respiratory insufficiency Check vital capacity repeatedly. If <500–600mL, intubation and ventilation will be needed. Monitor blood gases. Intubation may produce vagal bradycardia, so give atropine 0.3–0.6mg IV before intubation and airway suction.

Fluid balance There is likely to be hypotension below the lesion (sympathetic interruption). This is not due to hypovolaemia, and it is dangerous to give large volumes of fluid. Use IV not oral fluids for 48h and while ileus persists. If abdominal distension causes respiratory embarrassment, pass a nasogastric tube.

The skin Turn every 2h between supine and right and left lateral positions. The Stoke Manderville bed does this electronically. Use pillows to separate the legs and maintain a lumbar lordosis.

Steroid treatment ►Methylprednisolone 30mg/kg IV stat (started within 8h of trauma) continuing with 5.4mg/kg/h IVI for 23h is known to significantly improve subsequent recovery.[1]

Anticoagulation Heparin 5000u/8h sc. Start warfarin later.

The bladder Pass a 12-gauge silicone 5mL balloon catheter before the bladder volume exceeds 500mL (overstretching of detrusor can delay the return of automatic bladder function). See p 730.

►Arrange early and expert transfer to a spinal injuries unit.
Skeletal traction will be needed for cervical injuries. Spring-loaded Gardner–Wells skull calipers are preferable to Crutchfield calipers, which need incisions.

1 M Bracken 1990 *NEJM* **322** 1405

Does this patient have a spinal cord injury?

In any unexplained trauma, suspect cord injury.

Signs to look for:[1]

- Responds to pain above clavicle
- Breathing—diaphragmatic
- Muscles—hypotonic, including reduced anal tone (do a PR)
- Reflexes—hyporeflexic
- Slow pulse and ↓BP, but in the presence of normovolaemia
- Priapism

1 http://www.trauma.org

Cord injury—functional anatomy

The 'tightest fit' between cord and canal is in the thoracic spine; this region also has the poorest blood supply. These facts explain why thoracic lesions are more likely to be complete than cervical or lumbar lesions. Ischaemic injury often spreads below the level of the mechanical injury. For the segment of the cord involved with injury at specific vertebra, see p 608.

Spinal shock (BP↓ but no tachycardia.) There is complete anaesthesia and flaccid paralysis of all segments and muscles innervated below the level affected. Tendon reflexes are absent and there is retention of urine. A 'stage of reorganization' then occurs. There is reflex emptying of the bladder and rectum, and sweat glands function. Later, flexion at the hip and knee may be brought on by stimuli (notably cold), often with emptying of the bladder and rectum (Head and Riddoch's mass reflexes). The legs may become permanently fixed in a drawn up position, with dorsiflexion of the ankles (spastic paraplegia in flexion). Over several months, the tendon reflexes return, and proprioceptive stimuli give rise to 'mass extension'.

Paraplegia/quadriplegia levels during first examination (see opposite)
►Levels vary, and can fluctuate—so frequent examinations are needed.

Raises elbow to horizontal: *deltoid* **C5**
Flexes forearm: *biceps* **C6**
Extends forearm: *triceps* **C7**
Flexes wrist and fingers **C8**
Spreads fingers **T1**

Flexes hip *iliopsoas* **L2**
Extends knee *quadriceps* **L3**
Dorsiflexes ankle *tibialis anterior* **L4**
Plantarflexes ankle *gastrocnemius* **S1**

Segment injury—A guide to possible subsequent function

C4 Can use electric chairs with chin control, operate a computer with a mouthstick, and use a 'Possum' environmental control system to turn on lights and open doors.

C5 With special devices, he can feed, wash face, comb hair, and help with dressing the upper body. He may be able to push a wheelchair along the flat, if pushing gloves are worn, and there are capstan rims on the wheels. The NHS will supply an electric wheelchair (indoor use only). Unable to transfer from wheelchair to toilet.

C6 Still needs a strap to aid feeding and washing. Dresses top half of body; helps dress lower half. Can drive with hand controls.

C7 Can transfer, dress, feed himself.

C8 Independent wheelchair life.

The occupational therapist is a key person in maximizing the levels of achievement outlined above. She is also in a position to arrange a home visit to assess the suitability of the home for wheelchair life. Grants are available from social services. She will visit with a member of the spinal injuries team, and a community liaison nurse or social worker. She can plan with local social services and the local domiciliary occupational therapist, so that the patient's (and his family's) hopes can be realized to the fullest extent. She can arrange the necessary modifications, and give invaluable professional advice about the level of independence which is realistic to strive for. As ever, the aims of the occupational therapist extend into augmenting self-esteem, and helping the patient come to terms with loss of rôle, and loss of confidence, and to mitigate the effects of disability by arranging for as much purposeful activity as possible, both in the realms of work and leisure. She will also be able to make plans for acquiring of social skills to assist the patient in his or her new way of life.

See ATLS 1997 *Manual* 6e, page 238 ISBN 1-880696-10-X

Testing sensation in dermatomes to determine the sensory level

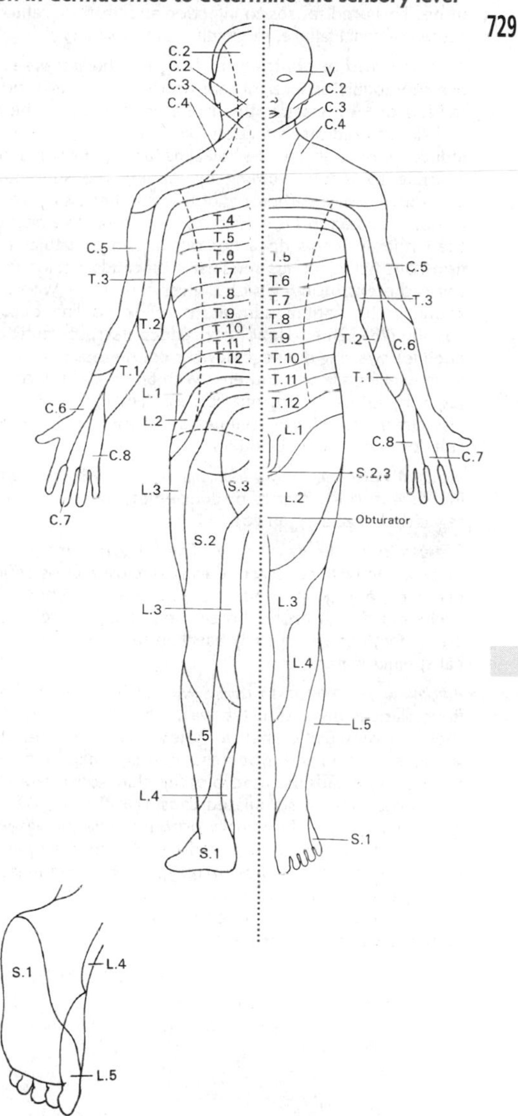

Spinal cord injury and the bladder

The problem is incontinence and reflex detrusor activity (after acontractility in the period of spinal shock) and the presence of residual urine. This predisposes to infection and ureteric reflux. These are major causes of renal failure, morbidity, and mortality.

The method of bladder drainage In the first weeks after cord injury use suprapubic or intermittent urethral catheterization with a 12 or 14 FG Nelaton® catheter, with strict asepsis. Culture the urine every week, and aim to eradicate infection (particularly important with *Proteus* which induces stones in infected alkaline urine). In some patients it may be possible to induce voiding by tapping the suprapubic area for ~20 seconds. Initially, catheterization is still necessary to drain the residual urine, but when this is <80mL (on 3 consecutive occasions), discontinue the catheter. If this does not occur, and particularly if the detrusor is non-contractile (conus medularis or cauda equina injury), intermittent self-catheterization (eg with a silver catheter in women) may be used, as soon as the patient can sit. If reflex voiding occurs, propantheline 15–30mg/8–12h PO 1h ac may reduce detrusor activity and obviate the need for wearing drainage devices continuously. The elderly may require an indwelling silicone catheter, with 6-weekly changes. Weekly washouts (eg Suby-G®) may prevent stones. Aim for an output of >3 litres/day. Use clamps to achieve volumes of 300mL. Artificial sphincters are available for acontractile bladders.

Complications *Urinary infection:* This may be prevented by a high fluid intake, ensuring effective bladder emptying and acidification of the urine (eg ascorbic acid 1g/6h PO).

Detrusor-sphincter dyssynergia: The external urethral sphincter fails to relax or actively contracts during detrusor contraction. There is poor bladder emptying and vesicoureteric reflux, predisposing to pyelonephritis, hydronephrosis, and renal failure. It is wise to do U&E, creatinine, and IVU as early baseline tests. *Treatment:* Endoscopic external sphincterotomy.

Autonomic dysreflexia: In those with lesions above the sympathetic outflow, bladder distension (eg with a blocked catheter) results in sympathetic overactivity, below the level of the lesion. There is vasoconstriction and hypertension (may cause strokes). The patient has a pounding headache, and blotchy skin above the lesion. The carotid baroreceptors are stimulated causing reflex vagal bradycardia, but the signals which would normally produce relieving vasodilatation and normotension are unable to pass down the cord. Other stimuli which may produce this effect include UTI, calculi, labour, and ejaculation. *Treatment:* Remove the cause; give nifedipine (10mg—bite the capsule) with glyceryl trinitrate 0.5mg. Phentolamine 5–10mg IV is an alternative. Sphincterotomy may prevent attacks.

9. A&E

Cord injury—physiotherapy and nursing

►*Turn every two hours to prevent pressure sores.* See p 726.

The chest Start regular physiotherapy early with coughing and breathing exercises, to prevent the sputum retention and pneumonia which are likely to follow diaphragmatic partial paralysis (eg C3–4 dislocation). If the lesion is above T10 segmental level, there is no effective coughing.

The straight lift (for transferring patients) One attendant supports the head with both hands under the neck so that the head lies on the arms. 3 lifters standing on the same side insert their arms under the patient, one at a time, starting at the top. After the lift, withdraw in the reverse order.

The log-roll 3 lifters stand on the same side of the patient. The one near the head has both arms over the patient's further arm; the middle one has one arm under the legs and the other arm holds the patient's iliac crest. The third lifter supports the calves. A fourth person controls the head and neck, and gives the command to turn. The patient is then gently rolled laterally, with pillows to support the lumbar curve and to keep the position stable.

Posture Joints need to be placed in a full range of positions. Avoid hyperextension of the knees. Aim to keep the feet flexed at 90° with a pillow between the soles and the foot of the bed. Avoid over-stretching of the soft tissues (deformity may result).

Bowels From the second day of injury gentle manual evacuation using plenty of lubricant is needed. A flatus tube may be helpful in relieving distension once the ileus of spinal shock has passed.

Wheelchairs The patient should be kept sitting erect; adjust the footplates so that the thighs are supported on the wheelchair cushion and there is no undue pressure on the sacrum. Regular relief of pressure on the sacral and ischial areas is vital. Independence in transferring to bed or toilet will be a suitable aim for some patients with paraplegia. Expert skill is needed in assigning the correct wheelchair for any particular patient.

Standing and walking Using a 'tilt table', or the Oswestry standing frame with trunk support straps, the tetraplegic patient can gain the upright posture. If the level of injury is at L2–4, below-knee calipers and crutches will enable walking to take place. If the lesion is at T1–8, 'swing to gait' may be possible. The crutches are placed a short distance in front of the feet. By leaning on them and pushing down with the shoulders, both legs may be lifted and moved forwards together.

Sport Consider archery, darts, snooker, table tennis and swimming for those with paraplegia. Many other sports may also be suitable.

Personal qualities The personal qualities of the nurse, physiotherapist, and the patient are as the important as exact anatomic lesion. There may be great mood swings from euphoria to despair as the patient accustoms himself to his loss and his new body image.

Vegetative states

'Persistent vegetative state' is a term coined to describe the behaviour of severely brain damaged people who show sleep–awake behaviour, but in whom there is absent cognition and awareness. The term is something of a misnomer, because its presence does not imply permanence (recovery of cognition may occur up to 5 years after the original insult)—and it has nothing to do with vegetables.

Persistent vegetative states are rare, and liable to misdiagnosis by non-specialist neurologists and neurosurgeons—perhaps because diagnosis depends on history and examination—requiring careful, repeated assessment and the taking into account of observations made by family and carers. ►*The harder you look, the more likely you are to find signs of active cognition, so negating the diagnosis of a vegetative state.*

One method of showing awareness and cognition is by demonstrating communication, eg by following a simple request to press a buzzer or to look at a named object.[1] These switches are particularly suited to those who can only manage a tiny amount of voluntary movement. Other ways of communicating include listener scanning: the therapist goes through A–Z slowly, and the patient buzzes when the required letter is reached. It may take weeks or months to establish that the patient can communicate. Rancho scale assessment establishes the level of cognition—from confused-and-inappropriate (level 5) to purposeful-and-appropriate (level 8).

Causes Trauma, anoxia, vascular causes, encephalitis.

Management Seek expert rehabilitative help. While waiting for any recovery, aim to provide vigorous nursing care to maintain nutrition, and to prevent pressure sores, and tracheostomy and muscle contracture complications. No drugs are known to help, although there is anecdotal evidence that bromocriptine may help.[2] Randomized trials indicate that multimodal stimulation (arousal programs) help.[3] These programmes involve stimulation of all senses every 15 minutes for up to 11 hours per day.[2]

Once it is agreed that there will be no recovery (a difficult issue), discussions about withdrawing active treatment and nutrition raise difficult ethical questions—which are only partly mitigated if the patient has an advance directive (an unlikely event). Ethicists, medical specialists, nurses, physiotherapists, judges, and the family must all be allowed to have their say. None is infallible.

1 K Andrews 1996 BMJ ii 13 2 K Andrews 1992 BMJ ii 486 3 S Mitchell 1990 *Brain Injury* 4 273

Does he need an x-ray?

In this litigious world, the conclusion that doctors should perform x-rays after even the most minor trauma may seem inescapable, even if this is recognized as 'bad medicine'—not least because one of our aims must be to reduce exposure to radiation, as well as to contain costs. However, help is at hand from bodies such as the Royal College of Radiologists, the Head Injury Working Party, and the Walton Hospital 'Guidance for x-ray referral'—which form the basis for the following advice.

Once the decision has been taken not to perform an x-ray, it is wise from a medico-legal point of view to note in the records the reason why an x-ray was not considered necessary.

Presenting conditions *Twisting injury of foot or ankle:* An x-ray is indicated if a patient cannot bear weight; one is said *not* to be indicated if he can weight-bear on the affected ankle, and if tenderness and swelling are confined to a ligament, or are absent—but all rules have exceptions, and, on occasion, we've all seen patients walk on a fractured ankle.

Crush injury to the terminal phalanx of a digit: An x-ray is not indicated in localized closed injury, provided there is pain-free movement at the distal interphalangeal joint.

Head injury: An x-ray is not indicated in the presence of only a minor scalp injury if there is:

- No loss of consciousness or amnesia.
- No abnormal neurological symptoms or signs.
- No cerebrospinal fluid rhinorrhoea or otorrhoea.
- No difficulty in assessing the patient (eg those who are not children, elderly, epileptic or intoxicated).

'Possible' neck injury in minor head injury: An x-ray is not indicated if fully conscious and no symptoms or signs related to the neck.

Nose injury: An x-ray is not indicated in the Accident and Emergency department in simple nasal injury.

Rib injury: Only a posteroanterior CXR is indicated if you suspect a pneumothorax; rib views are not needed in uncomplicated blunt injury.

Lumbar spine pain: Avoid early x-rays (in first 6 weeks) if there are no CNS signs or factors suggesting serious disease, eg trauma, fever, weight loss, anaemia, ESR raised (so do blood tests first). Each examination =2.2mSv (= 40 chest x-rays; the sievert is the SI unit of radiation absorbed by biological tissues—its abbreviation is Sv), which may be expected to cause 16 malignancies/yr in the UK at current rates of exposure. It is impossible to protect the ovaries.

Abdominal pain: Plain films are rarely needed; request an erect chest film only in suspected gastrointestinal perforation. Erect abdominal films are generally not indicated.

Foreign bodies: Always x-ray if glass possible (usually radiopaque).

Note: Lumbar spine x-rays deliver a significant dose of radiation to the gonads—similarly for skull and facial x-rays and the eyes.

These guidelines yield substantial savings in costs and in patients' waiting times, without compromizing patient care.[1]

1 S Halpin 1991 *BMJ* ii 813

Appropriate use of A&E departments

From our point of view, the ideal scenario is to have a pristine, ever-ready but empty trauma department with the doctors and nurses educating themselves (etcetera) in the coffee room, occasionally being called out by paramedics to save a few lives in a brief display of energy and technical brilliance. This is not how the public sees our rôle. If you are in shock because you have just run over a hedgehog you clearly need attention *now*. All casualty departments are abused—because it is always doctors who define what abuse is. Thus up to 70% of users have been deemed inappropriate.[1]

How to cope with inappropriate attendance

- *Triage* by a trained nurse is one way to reduce inappropriate attendance. (In the UK, triage is mandatory.) Is this condition *life-threatening*, *urgent*, *semi-urgent* or is *delay acceptable*? These are the chief categories. If the most urgent patients are seen to first, patients who do not really need to be in casualty can wait for ages, and many will begin to drift away. Note that if long waits become essential because of dealing with life-threatening conditions, this should be explained to patients (under the terms of the UK health charter—and as a matter of common courtesy).
- Another way to reduce unnecessary spending is to have primary care facilities within casualty, or, more radically, to have GPs as the casualty officers—because they use resources more sparingly and are used to dealing with mismatches between patient's expectations and reality. Is this expectation borne out in practice? In one careful randomized study of patient-contacts with casualty in Dublin ($N=4684$) GPs treating people with semi-urgent problems investigated less (by 20%) referred to other hospital services less (by 39%), admitted fewer patients (45%) and prescribed more often (43%): there were no differences in measures of outcome. It is not clear whether the more economical style of the GPs was to do with being a GP, or whether the reason was that these doctors were older and more experienced than their casualty-officer counterparts.

1 AW Murphy 1996 BMJ i 1135

Bites, stings and foreign bodies

Mammal bites All animal bites are contaminated, especially those of human animals. Clean well with soap and water, debriding if needed. See p 704. ►Avoid suturing unless cosmetically essential. Give antibiotics covering anaerobes unless very trivial if not high-risk (risk↑ if: ♀, >50yrs, asplenic, immunosuppressed/compromized, has alcoholic liver disease, or the wound is to hand or foot), eg co-amoxiclav 1tab/8h PO (clindamycin 300mg/6h PO if allergic to penicillin but beware pseudomembranous colitis). NB: bites from cats may not be as trivial as they look: they carry *Pasteurella multocida*, streps and fusibacteria. Is tetanus prophylaxis needed? Consider rabies if bitten outside UK. (Post-exposure rabies prophylaxis: phone the UK Central Public Health Lab, 0181 200 4000.)

Snake bites Britain's only poisonous snake, the adder, is very rarely lethal. Identify the species if possible and move the patient to hospital without delay. Treat shock, monitor clotting time (many venoms are anticoagulant), and watch for renal failure, respiratory paralysis and tissue necrosis. Indications for antivenom treatment include systemic envenoming, as signalled by hypotension, WCC raised—as well as local envenoming which is spreading beyond the wrist and ankle more than 4h after the bite (for bites in these locations). Give Zagreb antivenom (2 ampoules IVI at rate <1mL antivenom/min), diluted in 2–3 volumes of 0.9% saline. Use the same dose for children. It may be repeated after 1h, if there is no improvement. Have epinephrine (=adrenaline) to hand (p 303). If the bite is from a foreign snake or spider, the relevant antivenom may be found at Fazakerley Hospital Pharmacy, Liverpool (0151 525 5980). Information on identification and treatment is available (Oxford: 01865 220968 or 01865 741166; Liverpool: 0151 708 9393; London: 0171 635 9191). ►Tourniquets, incisions and sucking the wound must be avoided.

Lesser weever fish stings (*Echiicthys vipera*)—eg in barefoot UK bathers. It is not serious, and may be relieved by immersion of the leg for 5–20min in water which is as hot as can be tolerated (eg <45°C).

Scorpian bites Prazosin helps; lidocaine SC at the site relieves pain.

Bee stings Scrape out with a knife or credit card *quickly*. Pheromones released from the expiring bee will attract more bees. You may well be able to outrun them if you see them coming. NB: although always fatal to the bee, a single sting almost never kills you (risk <1 in 1,000,000)—but fatalities are likely if you receive >2000 stings. Ice ± calamine lotion help itch. Give antihistamines for severe swelling/itch. Anaphylaxis, p 303.

Airgun pellets These are common, and can be hard to remove. Deaths have occurred, eg when a pellet often enters brain through the eye; venous embolism of the pellet, which then lodges in the lungs, is reported. Get 2 x-ray views to position the foreign body. If it has just penetrated the skin, inject local anaesthetic carefully so that you can still palpate it: if you cannot remove it easily, leave it *in situ* rather than risk extensive tissue destruction trying to find it, and give antibiotics. Pellets that have tracked subcutaneously, or have penetrated deeply, must be sought.

Other foreign bodies ►Always x-ray if there may be glass in a wound. Tiny shards may be left *in situ*. Even large shards can be hard to find, needing exploration under GA to remove (also true for needles/pins stuck in the sole). ►Always x-ray the orbit if high-velocity metallic foreign body, which cannot be seen (eg grinding/chiselling injuries).

Heimlich manoeuvre and back blows See p 785.

Coin ingestion

If symptomatic, do CXR + neck x-ray (AP and lateral, to differentiate GI and respiratory tract location). Abdominal films may be needed. If below diaphragm, let it pass. If in upper 1/3 of oesophagus, remove it with an endoscope. Make sure that there are no more foreign bodies before removing the scope; if lower, repeat x-rays after 12–24h. If the coin is still in the oesophagus, remove endoscopically under GA.[1]

1 M Stringer 1991 BMJ i 1321

Common minor procedures

►When in doubt, ask the casualty sister: she will have seen it all before.

'I've hammered my finger, doctor' This usually causes a subungual haematoma—relieved by expressing the blood through a hole trephined in the nail, using a 19G needle. No force is needed: simply twiddle the needle as it rests vertically on the nail: cutting edge will make a suitable hole.

'I've swallowed a fish bone and it's stuck' Always examine the throat and tonsils carefully. Often the bone has only grazed the mucosa. Use a good light, held by sister, and grip the tongue with gauze to move it out of the way before removing any visible bones with forceps. If you fail, refer to ENT.

'My fish hook has barbed my finger' Infiltrate with plain lidocaine (=lignocaine), and push the hook on through the finger—provided no important structures are in its path. Once the barb is through, cut it off. Remove the hook by the way it entered.

'My tooth has been knocked out' After the patient sucks it clean (do not use water) transport in milk—or reinsert it, stabilizing with finger pressure (or biting). Go to a dentist for splinting.

Plaster 'back slabs' (for undisplaced forearm fractures).

- Remove anything which impairs finger circulation (eg rings).
- Protect yourself and your patient with a plastic apron.
- Measure the length for the back slab—from knuckles to just below elbow, so that the fingers and elbow will remain mobile.
- Cut a piece of plaster-impregnated bandage 5 times longer than the desired length. Fold it into 5-ply. (Fig ①, opposite)
- Cut off one corner so that it does not impinge on the thumb.
- Cut a wedge off the other end—the wedge's thick end being on the same side as the thumb. This aids elbow movement. ②
- Roll stockinette over the forearm, to well above the elbow.
- Wind a roll of wool padding over the stockingette (turns must overlap by 50%, so protecting flesh from the hard plaster. ③
- Immerse the plaster bandage in tepid water and apply it to the dorsum of the arm—without pitting it with your finger tips. ④
- Reflect the stockinette down from the elbow and up from the wrist making comfortable top and bottom ends to the plaster. ⑤
- Place a bandage right around the forearm to keep everything in place, securing its end with a strip of wet plaster. ⑥
- Setting takes place over 4min: sooner if warm water is used.
- Put the arm in a sling for 1 day—after which encourage movement of shoulder and fingers to prevent stiffness.

►*Cautions for the patient:* **1** Return immediately to A&E if the fingers go blue, swell, or you cannot move them. **2** Do not get the plaster wet. **3** Do not lift heavy weights with the hand.

How to remove a tight ring from a swollen finger Wind some cotton tape around the finger, advancing towards the ring. When it is reached, thread the tape through it. Grasp this end of the tape and unwind. This levers the ring over the PIP joint. If not, try using a ring cutter (not for brass or steel).

'I've caught my penis in my zip, doctor' Failing simple measures (copious lubrication with mineral oil), the most elegant solution to this is to cut out the bridge from the slider of the zip with strong wire-cutters as shown in the diagrams. The zip then falls apart and all that is needed is a new zip. (Beware the bridge flying off at speed: hold gauze by it.)

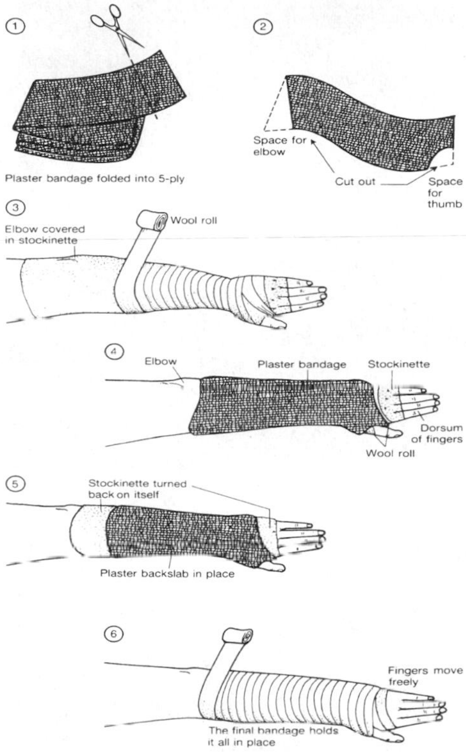

1
Plaster bandage folded into 5-ply
2
Space for elbow
Cut out
Space for thumb
3
Elbow covered in stockinette
Wool roll
4
Elbow
Plaster bandage
Stockinette
Dorsum of fingers
Wool roll
5
Stockinette turned back on itself
Plaster backslab in place
6
Fingers move freely
The final bandage holds it all in place

Strong wire cutters
Zip bridge
Zip slider
Side view
Zip slider
Zip bridge
Top view

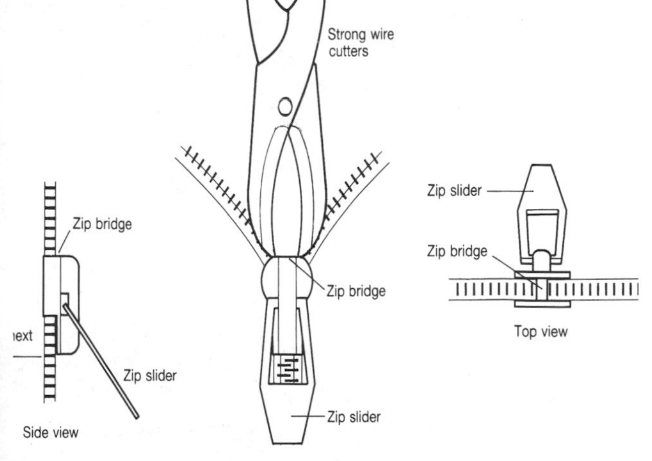

9. Orthopaedics and trauma

10. Unusual eponymous syndromes

To have any disease is a misfortune, but having a rare disease is a doubly unlucky: not only may the patient have a long wait before the diagnosis is made, but once it has been made he has to contend with his physician's lifelong morbid interest in him.

For syndromes relevant to *general medicine* and *surgery*, see OHCM p 694.

Adair–Dighton syndrome (Osteogenesis imperfecta) A metabolic bone defect (autosomal dominant) which causes fragile bones, amber or blue teeth + blue sclerae. Association: short legs and cleft palate.

Alport's syndrome Sensorineural deafness + pyelonephritis, haematuria and renal failure (glomerulonephritis + basket weaving of basement membrane). X-linked or autosomal recessive (genes *COL4A5, COL4A3* or *COL4A4*). Typical age at death (♂): 20–30yrs. *Lancet* 1997 349 1770

Asperger's syndrome This is a variety of autism in which a child (~2yrs old), shows autistic features (p 402) *without* autistic aloneness and linguistic difficulties. It carries a better prognosis than autism.

Bardet–Biedl syndrome There is retinal dystrophy, IQ↓, hypogonadism, obesity (± polydactyly) plus renal abnormalities (calyceal clubbing or blunting, calyceal cysts or diverticula, fetal lobulation). It is the absence of neurological symptoms (paraparesis) which distinguishes the syndrome from the Laurence–Moon–Biedl syndrome (which is better named the Laurence–Moon, see p 752). ♂/♀=47:41. Genetic locus: 16q13–q21 (recessive). A high incidence is found in Newfoundland (1:17,500 versus 1:160,000 elsewhere). E Hoang *Genomics* 1998 **52** 219-22.

Batten's syndrome Abnormal storage of cerebral lipofuscins causes vision↓, childhood dementia, fits, ataxia, spastic weakness, athetosis, dystonia. *Tests:* lipopigments in lymphocytes & urine. Gene on chromosome 16.

Becker's syndrome This sex-linked recessive muscular dystrophy has a slower progression than Duchenne's, but late onset + more calf enlargement in adolescence. Cause: eg lysine to glutamine dystrophin gene mutation.

Beckwith–Wiedmann syndrome Large tongue and kidneys, hemihypertrophy, microcephaly, hypoglycaemia, and omphalocoele, plus early feeding difficulties. Risk of neoplasia: 8%: half of these will be Wilms', p 220). Genes involved are at the 11p15 locus; their dysregulation may allow too much insulin-like growth factor 2 to be made. (*Lancet* 1997 349 663)

Bennett's fracture See p 700.

Bourneville's disease (Tuberous sclerosis; epiloia) There are multi-organ calcified hamartomatous tubers inherited as an autosomal dominant.
CNS: Calcified cerebral tubers (≤2cm; may transform to gliomas), ± seizures, hydrocephalus, periventricular calcification, and a low IQ.
Skin: Hypomelanic macules (Wood's lamp +ve), adenoma sebaceum (warty nasolabial angiofibromas), *café-au-lait* spots, butterfly rash, periungual fibromas, sacral plaques (Shagreen patches, like shark skin), skin tags.
Mouth: Pitted tooth enamel, gingival fibromas.
Eye: Phakomata (white or yellow retinal tumours; present in ~50%).
Bone: Sclerotic lesions, phalangeal cysts, hypertelorism.
Kidney: Polycystic enlargement,* haematuria. *Hair:* White lock.
Lungs: Honeycomb lung, pneumothorax, 'muscular hyperplasia of lung'.
Heart: BP↑, cardiomyopathy, rhabdomyomas, haemopericardium.
Lymph nodes: Castleman tumour. *Bowel:* Polyps ± Peutz–Jaegers' *OHCM* p706.
Liver and peritoneum: Carney's syndrome. *Also:* Precocious puberty.
Tests: Fundoscopy, skull views, CT/MRI, EEG, heart and renal ultrasound.
Prognosis: Usually benign; malignancy is rare.

*See D Webb 1993 *BMJ* i 1258

When entertaining the diagnosis of a rare disease. . .

- Ask whether other members of the family have been affected.
- Draw up a family pedigree (as per *OHCM* p 21).
- Have there been unexplained miscarriages or stillbirths in the family?
- Who is now pregnant (or might be or become so) in the family? In your hands you may hold vital information or vital clues which need to get to the right person at the right time: and that person may not be the person who is in front of you now. Get consent from your patient to talk to the whole family.
- Refer for genetic counselling—as per page 212.
- Is prenatal diagnosis available? If this is a critical issue, don't rely on the judgment of of a single expert. Keep on asking, as the field of prenatal tests is constantly enlarging.

Briquet syndrome (Fat file syndrome) Hypochondriasis (p 334) or 'somatization disorder' with >13 unexplained symptoms in various organs.

Bruton's sex-linked agammaglobulinaemia (♂ only) Severe infections and enlarged joints. Peyer's patches, tonsils & appendix are absent. *Cause:* One of 463 mutations in a gene coding tyrosine kinase (BTK). *Nucleic Acids Res* 1998 242

Buchanan's syndrome A single artery arises out of the base of the heart, supplying pulmonary *and* systemic vasculature. The aorta may or may not be divided. There is cyanosis from birth. Surgical correction is possible.

Capgras' syndrome The patient believes that someone well-known to him has been replaced by an exact double. It is usually, but not always, part of a psychosis. It may follow head injury or cerebral atrophy. There may be an abnormality in the right occipitotemporal area, or a pituitary tumour.

Carini's syndrome Shedding of horny layer of the dermis (alligator baby).

Castleman's disease (Angiofollicular lymph node hyperplasia) Typical presentation: an unexplained mediastinal mass on CXR (routine, or done for cough or dyspnoea). The lesion consists in a vascular tumour with satelite lymphadenopathy with pseudofollicles. There are 2 types: hyaline vascular, and plasma cell type (causes fever, anaemia, weight↓). Development of frank lymphoma is rare. POEMS syndrome may also be present (opposite).

Chediak–Higashi syndrome Immunodeficiency ± albinism, photophobia, nystagmus on exposure to light, weakness, tremor, fever, platelets↓, liver↑, ± lymphomas. Leucocytes contain gigantic peroxidase granules. *Cause:* 1q43 mutation. Fatal by ~10 years old without marrow transplantation.

Conradi–Hünermann syndrome Saddle nose, nasal hypoplasia, frontal bossing, short stature, stippled epiphyses is accompanied by optic atrophy, cataracts, mental retardation, and flexural contractures. It results from the teratogenic effects of warfarin given during the first trimester of pregnancy.

Cornelia De Lange syndrome There is short stature of unknown cause, associated with an abnormally shaped head with brows meeting in the midline. Other signs: hirsutism, low-set ears, widely spaced teeth, Simian (single) palmar crease, low IQ, fits. No chromosomal defect has been found.

Corrigan's syndrome This is congenital aortic regurgitation.

Cotard's syndrome The patient denies his existence (a nihilistic delusion) or he may believe that his bowels are rotting, or even request burial, thinking that he is a stinking corpse. According to Albert Camus 'there is in every man a deep instinct which is neither that of destruction, nor that of creation. It is simply the longing to resemble nothing'—however, our own experience suggests that making this impulse the centre of one's life is rare, even in Frenchmen. Causes of nihilism include depression, especially if over 60yrs old; alcoholism, and rarely syphilis or a parietal lobe lesion.

Crigler–Najjar syndrome Jaundice ± CNS signs appear in the first days of life due to ↓gluconyl transferase activity (?from homozygosity for genes G71R & Y486D). Liver transplantation and simpler hepatocyte transfusion are used.

Dandy–Walker syndrome Congenital obstruction of the foramina of Luschka and Magendi leads to progressive enlargement of the head, congested scalp veins, bulging fontanelle, separation of the cranial sutures, papilloedema, bradycardia. *Treatment:* Drain the CSF into a body cavity.

De Clerambault's syndrome (Erotomania) The patient is usually a single woman who is deluded that someone of a higher social status (eg a well-known politician or entertainer) is in love with her, who, for various reasons, is unable to communicate directly with her. She derives satisfaction from having been 'chosen' by him, and may make great trouble for the person by publicizing her view of his feelings towards her. In the male form, stalking may be a feature. Associations: epilepsy; a left frontal lobe lesion.

Diamond–Blackfan syndrome (Erythrogenesis imperfecta) ↓Erythroid production (Hb↓, platelets↑, MCV↑) causes pallor ± limb anomalies. Steroids and marrow transplants may be tried. *Cause:* ?deletions on 19q13. *Am J Hum Gen* 1998 1388

Helping people with Briquet's syndrome

- Give time, and don't dismiss these patients as "just the 'worried well' ".
- Explore with the patient the factors which may perpetuate the illness (disordered physiology, misinformation, unfounded fears, misinterpretation of sensations, unhelpful 'coping' behaviour, social stressors).
- Agree a management plan which focuses on each issue and makes senses to the patient's holistic view of him or herself (1997 BMJ ii 562).
- Treat any underlying depression (p 340–2); consider cognitive therapy.

Castleman's lymph node hyperplasia with POEMS syndrome

POEMS syndrome entails: **p**eripheral neuropathy, **o**rganomegaly/hyperplasia, **e**ndocrinopathy, a **m**onoclonal paraprotein, and **s**kin lesions. Interleukin-6 excess is also a feature of Castleman's disease, so also look for PUO and chronic inflammatory symptoms ± failure to thrive. Children with unexplained chronic inflammatory symptoms may need detailed soft tissue tests to reveal associated vascular tumours.

Di George's syndrome An absent thymus with hypoplasia of the parathyroid glands is associated with anaemia, lymphopenia, hypocalcaemia, and cell-mediated immune deficiency. Most are associated with a monosomy for a region of chromosome 22q11. It is thought to be related to the velocardiofacial syndrome of multiple anomalies, cleft palate, heart defects, cognitive defects, and a characteristic face. *Lancet* 1992 **i** 1138

Di Guglielmo's syndrome Red cell dysplasia with erythroid infiltration of liver, spleen and heart. Hb↓; MCV↔; WCC↓, platelets↓; LDH & B_{12}↑. Immunoperoxidase stains may show antihaemoglobin antibody. Transfusions are needed.

Duchenne's muscular dystrophy This presents in boys of 1–6yrs, with a waddling, clumsy gait. On standing, the boy uses his hands to climb up his legs (Gower's manoeuvre). Distal girdle muscles are affected late, and selective wasting causes calf pseudohypertrophy. Later wheelchairs are needed (eg at 9–12yrs). Scoliosis and many chest infections occur. Aim to keep the boy walking (eg by using knee–ankle–foot orthoses). Spinal fixation (Luque operation) or bracing reduces scoliosis. Prednisolone 0.75mg/kg/24h PO improves strength and function, but doesn't allow brace or wheelchair abandoning. There is relentlessly progressive hypoventilation: the cause of death in ~70%. A vital capacity of <700mL shows that death may be approaching. Extending life by ventilatory support is unlikely to increase its quality. Plasma creatine kinase is ↑; measure this in all boys who are not walking by 1½yrs, so that genetic advice may be given to parents (it is a sex-linked recessive). Muscle biopsy: abnormal fibres surrounded by fat and fibrous tissue. Mortality: ~75% are dead by 20yrs; 5% remain alive after 50yrs. Females only carry the disease, and ~80% will have abnormal biochemistry. Prenatal screening using gene probes is available.

Ebstein's anomaly A congenital defect with downward displacement of the tricuspid valve (± deformed leaflets) atrializing the right ventricle. There may be no symptoms, or cyanosis, clubbing, triple rhythm, systolic and diastolic murmurs. It may be associated with other cardiac malformations. *Tests:* ECG: tall *P* waves, long *P–R* interval, and right bundle branch block.

Edwards syndrome (Trisomy 18) Clinical features: a rigid baby with flexion of the limbs, mental retardation, low-set malformed ears, receding chin, protruding eyes, rocker-bottom feet, cleft lip or palate, and umbilical or inguinal hernias. A short sternum makes the nipples look widely separated. The fingers cannot be extended, and the index finger overlaps the third digit. Survival is longer in females (mean 10 months).

Ehlers–Danlos syndrome A connective tissue syndrome of soft, hyperelastic, poor-healing, easily-bruising skin ± aneurysms or GI bleeds/perforation. Joints are loose and hypermobile. Flat feet may be a feature. There are 6 types. Type II, for example, is caused by COL52A mutations, while in type IV COL381 mutations upset encoding of type III collagen. *J Med Genet* 1998 **35** 846

Eisenmenger's syndrome A congenital heart defect which is at first associated with a left to right shunt may lead to pulmonary hypertension and shunt reversal. If so, cyanosis develops (± heart failure and respiratory infections), and Eisenmenger's syndrome is present. Prognosis: poor.

Erb's muscular dystrophy (Scapulohumeral muscular dystrophy) ♂:♀≈1:1. *Onset:* 1st–6th decade. Face involvement is late. Life span is shortened, but progression is slow. *Possible cause:* Calpain gene mutation (15q). *Neurom Dis* 1996 **6** 447

Fallot's tetralogy Pulmonary stenosis, overriding aorta, interventricular defect, RVH. Presentation: cyanosis as ductus closes, dyspnoea, unconsciousness, squats at play, clubbing. CCF is rare. *Signs:* Thrill, absent pulmonary part of second sound, harsh systolic murmur at left sternal base. *Tests:* FBC: Hb↑. CXR: wooden shoe heart contour + RVH. ECG: RVH. *Prognosis:* 86% 32yr survival after corrective surgery (J Murphy 1993 *NEJM* 329 593). 'Total repair' entails closure of the VSD and removal of the pulmonary stenosis: it may result in normal life, with driving possible, provided there are no syncopal attacks.

10. Some unusual eponymous syndromes

Post-op problems: •Residual VSD + pulmonary hypertension, if big •Ventricular tachycardia •Complete heart block •Right ventricular aneurysm •IE/SBE (risk is quite low) •Dilated cardiomyopathy •Pulmonary or aortic regurgitation. NB: when pregnant (this may be unproblematic), do careful fetal echoes.

748 **Fanconi anaemia** Autosomal recessive aplastic anaemia + absence of radii, thumb hypoplasia, syndactyly, missing carpal bones, skin pigmentation, microsomy, microcephaly, strabismus, cryptorchidism, IQ↓, deafness, short stature, and ↑risk of malignancy. Survival: 70% at 5yrs post-marrow transplant (umbilical cord blood haemopoietic progenitor cells is also tried). There are 8 groups: FA-A to FA-H. FAA and FAC genes are the commonest. *Nat Genet* 1998 **20** 281

Galeazzi fracture Radius shaft fracture with distal ulna subluxation.

Ganser syndrome Disorientation plus pseudodementia with 'approximate answering', eg in answer to 'What is the colour of the chair in the corner?' was answered might be: 'What corner? I don't know what a corner is. I don't see a chair. . .' Absurd remarks only occur as answers to questions. Intellectual deficit is inconstant (hence the 'pseudo'). Hysteria, hallucinations and fluctuating consciousness are common. Often there is a preceding head injury.

Gaucher's syndrome This autosomal recessive deficiency of lysosomal acid-β-glucosidase is the most prevalent lysosomal storage disorder. Glucosylceramide accumulates in macrophage lysosomes (producing Gaucher's cells), causing face and leg pigmentation, and progressive organomegaly, with marrow and CNS infiltration. *Diagnosis:* Skin fibroblast glucocerebrosidase assay. Death is often from pneumonia or bleeding. In infantile Gaucher's, there are marked CNS signs (rigid neck, dysphagia, catatonia, hyperreflexia, IQ↓). *Treatment:* Growth, IQ, and psychomotor skills improve with human placental alglucerase (Ceredase®) which metabolizes intracellular cerebrosides in spleen and liver; dose example 60u/kg/2 weeks IVI over 4h; SE: virilization; cost to remission: ≈ £100,000 (*Lancet* 1994 ii 1679).

Hand–Schüller–Christian syndrome (Langerhans' cell histiocytosis) Synonyms: histiocytosis X, Letterer–Siwe disease, and eosinophilic granuloma of bone. Abnormal monoclonal Langerhans'-like cells are pathognomonic of this putatively neoplastic, destructive, infiltrative disease in which bone, liver, skin and spleen show necrotic (lytic) aggregates of eosinophils, plasma cells and vacuolated histiocytes. Lesions may show up on a ^{99}Technetium-labelled bone scan. It may occur in children or adults, and often starts with a polyp at the external auditory meatus. Other features:

•Fever •Dyspnoea •Bone pain •Failure to thrive
•Scalp lumps •Cord compression •Skin erosions •Pustular eczema-like rash
•Proptosis •Ear discharge •Liver/spleen↑ •Lymphadenopathy ± sinuses
•Stomatitis •Platelets↓ •Anaemia •Honeycomb lung

A lethal 'leukaemia' picture is seen in infants. *Treatment:* Bone surgery, radiotherapy, steroids or cytotoxics may induce remissions. (F Cotter 1995 *BMJ* i 74)

Hartnup's disease is a defect in tryptophan transport precipitated by light. Skin is thick, scaly, and hyperpigmented where exposed to light. *Signs:* Rashes, nystagmus, ataxia, bruxism, diplopia, insomnia, reflexes↑. *Treatment:* Give nicotinamide and vitamins from the B complex. Autosomal recessive.

Hunter's syndrome (Mucopolysaccharidosis II) Deficiency of iduronate sulfatase (sex-linked recessive, but a new mutation in 33% so usually ♂), producing deafness, IQ↓, short stature, chronic diarrhoea, an unusual face, joint stiffness, and hepatosplenomegaly—(rather like Hurler's disease, p 750 but almost always without corneal clouding, and generally pursuing a milder course). *Diagnosis* is by measuring iduronate sulfatase in the serum. *Typical age at death:* Later childhood; survival into the 30s is possible. *Pathology:* There may be translocation of a piece of the X chromosome bearing a mutant gene for iduronosulfate sulfatase (see *OTM* 3e 1996).

10. Some unusual eponymous syndromes

Huntington's disease (chorea) Prevalence: 4 to 560 per 100,000 (depends on locality). *Inheritance:* Autosomal dominant (4p16.3; CAG trinucleotide expansion/ repeats—forming the basis of a very sensitive and specific DNA test for inheritance; B Kremer 1994 *NEJM* 330 1401). The mutated gene's product is called 'huntingtin'. Unstable trinucleotide repeats also occur in myotonic dystrophy and fragile X syndrome. Unusual ethical dilemmas surround testing, as symptoms may start only after procreation has finished. Careful pre-test counselling is vital. What if a grandson wants a chance to remove the Damocles sword hanging over him, but his father does not want to do the same (if the grandson is affected, the father must be)? *Presentation:* Triad of movement abnormalities (eg hemichorea and rigidity), dementia, and a +ve family history. Personality change, self-neglect, apathy, and psychosis (rare) may preceed clumsiness, fidgets with fleeting facial grimaces (which may be mistaken for mannerisms), chorea and dementia. Memory may be relatively spared, compared with cognition. *Tests:* Mutation analysis; EEG shows reduced α-rhythms. *Treatment:* Clozapine has been found to be helpful in an open trial. Seek expert advice. *Neurology* 1994 **44** 821

Hunt's syndrome (Pyridoxine cerebral deficiency) Intractable neonatal fits cause death unless given (pyridoxine 50 mg IV under EEG control).

Hurler's syndrome (Mucopolysaccharidosis 1H) After a few months of normal growth, there is physical and mental deterioration, with hydrocephalus, thickened skin, visual disorders, hirsutism, coxa valga and nodules over the scapulae. There is deficiency of α-L-iduronidase, hence blocking degradation of dermatan sulfate and heparan sulfate, causing excess mucopolysaccharides in urine, cartilage, periosteum, tendons, heart valves, meninges and cornea. *Tests:* Skull x-ray: thickened bone, absent frontal sinuses and deformed pituitary fossa. Marrow: Reilly bodies (metachromatic inclusions) in lymphocytes and histiocytes. Death usually occurs before 10yrs of age.

Hutchinson's triad (*Congenital syphilis*) Deafness+keratitis+pointed teeth.

Ivemark's syndrome This is the association of congenital asplenia with ostium primum atrial septal defects (± pulmonary valve atresia or stenosis).

Kartagener's syndrome (Immotile cilia) is the combination of bronchiectasis, sinusitis, ♂ infertility, + situs inversus (transposed heart and abdominal organs). Otitis media and salpingitis are frequent. It results from defects in cilia function (including sperm), which also causes faulty fetal organ rotation. *Tests:* ECG: inverted P-waves in lead I, reversed R-wave progression. Genetic defects in dyneins may have a role. These large multisubunit ATPases interact with microtubules to generate cilia movement. I Milislav 1998 *Cel Motil Cytos* **39** 261

Kawasaki's disease Suspect this in anyone <9yrs old who is feverish for ≥5 days with any of: cervical lymphadenopathy (>1.5cm across), dry fissured lips, arthralgia, arthritis, palmar erythema, red eyes (uveitis), diarrhoea, a strawberry tongue, or, later, finger-tip desquamation with swelling of hands/feet ± jaundice and meningism. ►*Coronary arteritis* (similar to PAN) ± *infarction* may occur. It is commoner than rheumatic fever as a cause of acquired heart disease. It is thought of as a reaction to various infections. *Tests:* ESR/C-reactive protein↑; bilirubin↑, transaminases↑, α_2-globulin↑, platelets↑, *Differential:* Streptococcal disease, Stevens–Johnson syndrome, measles, infectious mononucleosis. *Treatment:* γ-globulin 400mg/kg/24h IVI over 3h for 3–5 days *usually* brings about a rapid (diagnostic) improvement—if not, plasma exchange may help. *Follow-up:* Echocardiogams.

Klinefelter's syndrome (XXY or XXYY polysomy + variable Leydig cell defect) This commonest cause of male hypogonadism (1:2000 births) may present at adolescence with psychopathy, learning difficulties, libido↓, gynaecomastia, sparse facial hair or complete failure of sexual maturation, infertility and small firm testes. Associations: T4↓, diabetes, asthma. Androgens and plastic surgery for gynaecomastia may help. Life span is normal, but the arm span may exceed the body length by 10cm inches.

10. Some unusual eponymous syndromes

Klippel–Feil syndrome (Autosomal dominant or recessive; candidate KFS gene on chromosome 8) Congenital fusion of cervical vertebrae, nystagmus, deafness and CNS signs. *Mirror movements* are said to occur if *voluntary* movements in a limb are *involuntarily* mimicked by another. Progressive paraplegia may occur.

Landouzy–Dejerine (Fascioscapulohumeral) muscular dystrophy Weakness of the shoulder muscles, eg on combing the hair, appears at 12–14yrs old. There is difficulty in closing the eyes, sucking, blowing and whistling. The scapulae wing and the lips pout, and the facial expression is 'ironed out'. Adult myoglobin is reduced and fetal myoglobin and sarcolemma nuclei are increased. Inheritance: often autosomal dominant.

Laurence–Moon–Biedl (Bardet–Biedl; Biedl–Bardet, p 742) syndrome The patient is usually a boy who presents with night blindness progressing to visual loss. There is obesity, polydactyly, small genitals, paraparesis and retinitis pigmentosa, squint, cataract, scanty body hair, azoospermia, IQ↓, renal anomalies (calyceal clubbing, cysts or diverticula; fetal lobulation; end-stage renal failure in 15%). Inheritance is autosomal recessive.

Leber's hereditary optic atrophy There is ↑risk of neoplasia + neuropathy mostly affecting males, with acute or subacute bilateral visual loss and central scotoma. A mutation (G→A) in mitochondrial DNA coding for a dehydrogenase enzyme has been proposed (an type of cytoplasmic inheritance).

Lesch–Nyhan syndrome ↓Hypoxanthine-guanine phosphoribosyl transferase (PP-ribose-P) leads to hyperuricaemia presenting early in boyhood (X-linked, so only fully expressed if ♂) with orange crystals in the nappy, then motor delay, IQ↓ (eg <65), torsion spasms, clonic movements, choreoathetosis, weakness, hypotonia and fits. Compulsive, agitated, self-mutilation (foot biting, head banging, face scratching—may be unilateral) then follow, as may gout, renal colic, and megaloblastic anaemia. Smiling aggression to others may occur. The chief defect might be ↓pain-consciousness *perhaps* related to dopaminergic denervation of D_1 receptors in cingulum bundle projections. Death is usually before 25yrs, from renal failure or infection. *Treatment:* Good hydration (urine flow↑). Allopurinol prevents urate stones, but not CNS signs. It has been necessary to remove teeth to stop lip mutilation. *Med Hypoth* 1998 **50** 43

Lewy-body dementia Characterized by Lewy-bodies in brainstem *and* cortex, and a fluctuating but persisting cognitive impairment, parkinsonism (p452), and hallucinations. It is a common type of dementia. Lewy bodies are eosinophilic intracytoplasmic neuronal inclusion bodies; there is overlap between Lewy-body dementia and Alzheimer's and Parkinson's diseases, making treatment hard as antiparkinsonian drugs can precipitate delusions, and antipsychotic drugs worsen parkinsonism. *J Int Neurops* 1997 **3** 179 & *Br J Psych* 1994 **165** 324

Li–Fraumeni syndrome This is a heritable condition in which families are highly susceptible to multiple malignancy at an early age. As well as being devastating for the families, it is of great interest to geneticists as families inherit a germ-line nonsense or oncogene-like mis-sense mutation in one *p*53 allele.

Lutembacher's syndrome An atrial septal defect causing mitral stenosis.

Martin–Bell syndrome (Fragile X syndrome) This semidominant condi (gene on the X chromosome; prevalence: 1:5700) is a significant caus male mental retardation. Its other features are: a low IQ (20–70), large t (>3–4mL on the Prader orchidometer), a high forehead, a big jaw asymmetry, long ears and a short temper. There is a constriction at 27 on the long arm of the X chromosome. ⅔ of carrier females h mal IQ; ⅓ are retarded. *Tests:* Prenatal cytogenetic diagnosis using f is now possible. Screening could be general or of high-risk catego lies with >1 retarded male; retarded males with large testes; autism or Prader–Willi syndrome). NB: screening for carrier statu labelling and stigmatization, and is rejected by some families. *Treat* acid may help. *BMJ* 1992 **ii** 208 & *Fragile X Syndrome*, 1992 Johns Hopl

Li Fraumeni Syndrome, p53, and the guardian of the genome

*p*53 is a vital tumour-suppressor gene (chromosome 17p13.1; encoding nuclear phosphoprotein, a transcription factor which allows passage through the cell cycle). In this syndrome, as only one allele is affected, development is normal until a spontaneous mutation affects the other allele. Somatic mutation of *p*53 occurs at both alleles in 50–80% of spontaneous human cancers. Cells with a *p*53 mutation do not pause in G1 (a phase in which DNA repair takes place, and faulty DNA purged), but procede straight to S1 (DNA replication), which is why p53 protein is known as the 'guardian of the genome').

McCune–Albright syndrome Polyosteotic fibrous dysplasia of bone, irregular areas of skin pigmentation and facial asymmetry ± precocious puberty.

Meckel's diverticulum Prevalence: ≤2%. ≤2 inches long, and >2 feet from the ileocaecal valve (antemesenteric aspect of ileum), it contains gastric and pancreatic tissue, and may be the cause of occult GI pain and bleeding (brick red stools, or dark becoming bright). This is a leading cause of rectal bleeding (± GI obstruction) in children. Diagnosis: radioisotope scan; laparotomy.

Monteggia fracture Fracture of proximal ⅓ of ulna, with angulation + radial head subluxation, caused forced pronation. Open reduction/plating is needed for good alignment (4–6 weeks in plaster), so as not to impair pronation. Wait for full union (~12 weeks) before starting normal arm use.

Morquio's syndrome (Mucopolysaccharidosis IV) Defective degradation of keratin sulfate (it is excreted in the urine) causes stature↓; deafness; weakness; a coarse, broad mouth; widely spaced teeth; pectus carinatum; aortic regurgitation—but not mental retardation. Autosomal recessive.

Moyamoya disease Intimal thickening leads to stenosis of proximal intracerebral arteries, with strokes or TIAs (alternating hemiplegia, dyspraxia, headache, or photophobia). The typical patient is a Japanese girl, with a triggering infection (eg tonsillitis). Symptoms are worsened by hyperventilation (CO_2↓ causes dangerous vasoconstriction). *Tests:* Digital subtraction angiography shows collateral vessel formation ('like a puff of smoke'). MRI or CT may show multiple infarctions in watershed areas. *Treatment:* It may resolve spontaneously. Bypass surgery may be possible.

Niemann–Pick disease (NPGD) After months or years of normal growth there is physical and mental decline, wasting ± hepatosplenomegaly from abnormal metabolism of sphingomyelin. Other signs: brown skin patches ± a cherry red spot on the macula. There are 5 types. Type D, for example, is caused by a G3097→T transversion in NPC1 gene. *Am J Hum Genet* 1998 **63** 52

Noonan syndrome Hypertrohic cardiomyopathy, VSD/ASDs, bruising (APTT↑ and ↓factors VIII, XI, XII,) associated with characteristic ptosis, downslanting eyes, low-set ears, webbed neck ± anomalies in any system. Height, IQ, and hearing are below average, but not severely so. Inheritance: autosomal dominant (gene region 12q24). Prevalence: 1:5000. *Eur J Hum Genet* 1998 **6** 32

Othello syndrome (Morbid jealousy) A lover believes against all reason that his beloved is being sexually unfaithful, and may also think that she is plotting against him, deliberately making him impotent. He may engage a detective to spy on her, and examine her underwear for signs of sexual activity. It may be primary or secondary (to alcohol, schizophrenia, neurosis, or depression). *Treatment* is difficult; get psychiatric help is needed. The condition may be deadly. '. . . Sometimes even without my having seen Albertine again . . . there would flash from my memory some vision of her with Gisèle in an attitude which had seemed innocent to me at the time; it was enough now to destroy the peace of mind I had managed to recover, I had no longer any need to go and breath dangerous germs outside, I had, as Cottard would have said, supplied my own toxin' Marcel Proust 1921, *Sodome et Gomorrhe*

Patau's syndrome (Trisomy 13) The head and eyes are small: ± defects such as absent corpus callosum and a single ventricle. Heart lesions, polycystic kidneys and cleft lip/palate are common. Hands show flexion contractures ± polydactyly with narrow fingernails. Prevalence: 1/7500 births.

Pick's dementia This often presents later than Alzheimer's disease—eg with character change associated with frontal lobe signs such as gross tactlessness. Lack of restraint may lead to stealing, practical jokes and unusual sexual adventures. Social graces are replaced by fatuous euphoria and jargon dysphasia, before intellectual and CNS deterioration occurs.

Pierre Robin syndrome Neonatal difficulty in feeding and breathing due to micrognathia (short chin) ± cleft palate or eye abnormality. Prevent the tongue slipping back by nursing on the belly (chest elevated on a pillow).

Hyperendocrinopathies, McCune-Albright, and the Taiwanese giant

In the McCune–Albright syndrome, precocious puberty is not the only endocrinopathy: hyperthyroidism and Cushing's have also been reported. In the case of the 'Taiwanese giant'[1] (an unfortunate name) excess growth hormone production has also been found. Deformities, fractures, and pain further complicate the picture (sometimes ameliorated by IV pamidronate).[2] The craniofacial fibrous dysplasia may encroach on the optic nerve, causing visual problems. GnRH analogues have been used (experimentally) to treat the precious puberty.[3]

Note that the cause is thought to be a mutation of the GNAS 1 gene coding the α subunit of the stimulatory guanine-nucleotide binding protein (G-protein). This mutation activates adenylate cyclase (∴↑intracellular cyclic AMP).[4]

1 P Szwajkun 1998 *Ann Plas Surg* 41 75
2 J Pfeilschfter 1998 *Med Klin* **15** 93
3 H Schmidt 1998 *J Ped Endo Metab* **11** 77
4 S Mandrioli 1998 *Minerva Stom* **47** 37

Pompe's glycogen storage disease (Type II) ↓Lysosomal $\alpha_{1,4}$-glucosidase activity leads to weakness and failure to thrive in early (or later) life. IQ↓ and chest infections occur. Glycogen accumulates in heart, muscle, CNS, liver, kidney and the adrenal glands. Few survive beyond infancy. Deletions/mutations in the GAA gene may be responsible. *Biochem Biophys Res Com* 1997 **235** 138

Prader–Willi syndrome Prevalence: 1 per 25,000 children. After birth there is hypotonia, epilepsy, failure to thrive, and sleepiness. The child usually has blue eyes and blond hair. Later, hyperphagia, obesity, hypogonadism, short stature and hyperglycaemia occur. *Tests:* EEG: slow spike and wave activity. 75% have a small deletion on the proximal part of the long arm of the paternally acquired chromosome 15 (15q11-q13). Most of the others have two apparently normal, but maternally acquired chromosomes 15s (maternal uniparental disomy). *Cytogenetics:* High resolution chromosome banding ± fluorescence *in-situ* hybridization with probes from the 15q11-q13 region looking for deletions and other rearrangement. NB: the gene for SNRPN RNA (small nuclear ribonucleoprotein N) is expressed thanks only to a gene on the paternally acquired chromosome 15, and its absence forms the basis of a leukocyte RT-PCR (polymerase chain reaction of reverse transcribed RNA) test.

Ramsay Hunt syndrome (Herpes zoster oticus) Severe pain in the ear, usually in elderly patients, precedes facial nerve palsy. Zoster vesicles appear around the ear, in the deep meatus, on the soft palate and in the tonsillar fossa. There may be vertigo and deafness which are both slow to resolve and may leave high tone loss. The pain usually abates after 48h.

Reye's syndrome *Presentation:* Vomiting, fever, hypotonia and stupor leading to coma and liver failure. It may have an infectious cause and/or be related to aspirin, antiemetic or antihistamine use by children. Median age of onset: 14 months (USA children are older). *Tests:* Glucose↓; transaminases↑; blood ammonium↑; INR↑. Liver biopsy: swollen, pleomorphic mitochondria (ATP↓, gluconeogenesis and ureagenesis↓).

Differential diagnosis: Inherited metabolic disorders (IMD).

Staging: The point of staging is to recognize stage 2 (or worse) which should prompt rapid referral to a tertiary centre with facilities for monitoring ICP (eg with subarachnoid bolts) and intra-arterial pressure.
Stage 2 criteria: inappropriate verbalizing, combative or stuporose, normal posture, purposeful or non-purposful response to pain, sluggish pupillary responses, intact Doll's eye reflex. *Management:* ►Correct hypoglycaemia; set up a *continuous* IVI of 10–15% glucose. Fluid restriction; do blood glucose every 2h; give vitamin K 0.25mg/kg slowly IV (monitor prothrombin time); lower ICP—see p 256. Aim for 40mmHg cerebral perfusion pressure (= systolic BP minus ICP). Control fever and seizures. *Mortality:* ~50%. *Incidence:* ~1–6 patients/10^6 children <16yrs/year. Since the widespread abandoning of aspirin for children, the incidence has fallen.

Russell Silver syndrome Asymmetrical growth/hemihypertrophy with small stature and precocious puberty. Association: Wilms'. Aberrant genomic imprinting may be to blame (http://www.asri.edu/gene-tics/brochure/agh/news/oct96/imprinting.html).

Shakhonovich 's syndrome (Hypokalaemic periodic paralysis) Attacks precipitated by: stress, menstruation, cold, large carbohydrate meals, rest after exercise or liquorice—typically starting in early morning, with flaccid paralysis, beginning in the legs, and spreading upwards. Eye movements, swallowing and speech are unaffected. Recovery takes place over 1–24h. Typical age: 7–21yrs; may have a history of migraine. During attacks muscles feel firmer than usual. Tendon reflexes are diminished. *Tests:* Serum K^+ and phosphorus usually fall during attacks. Glycosuria may be present. WCC↑ + eosinopenia. Autosomal dominant, with implication of a gene coding a1-subunits of skeletal muscle L-type calcium channel. Sporadic cases also occur. *Treatment:* Spironolactone and a very low Na^+ diet may prevent attacks. *FEBS Lett* 1996 **382** 244

Smith's fracture (reversed Colles') See p 700.

10. Some unusual eponymous syndromes

Still's disease Typically presents with systemic upset in a prepubertal girl who develops a mono- or polyarticular synovitis (may be progressive, with erosion of cartilage) ± fevers, pericarditis, iridocyclitis, pneumonitis, lymphadenopathy, splenomegaly. It accounts for 10% of all juvenile chronic arthritis. Rheumatoid factor is not present in the blood.

Other subgroups are juvenile ankylosing spondylitis, psoriatic arthritis and ulcerative colitis-associated arthritis, and juvenile-onset rheumatoid arthritis (here Rh factor +ve, and less likely to present as systemic upset).

NB: adults may get Still's disease: diagnostic criteria (*OTM*-3)—all of: daily fever >39°C; arthralgia/arthritis; Rh factor *and* antinuclear factor –ve *plus any* 2 of: WCC >15 × 10^9/L; macular/maculopapular rash; serositis (pleural or pericardial); hepatomegaly; splenomegaly; generalized lymphadenopathy—*provided* that infective endocarditis, leukaemia and sarcoid are excluded. As with all rheumatology, classification is never straightforward, and unexpected complications may occasionally occur (DIC, liver failure, renal failure, amyloid, cardiac tamponade, endocarditis, and peritonitis).

Tests: FBC: leukocytosis; ESR↑; mild anaemia; ferritin↑; LFTs↑; albumin↓. *Treatment* is supportive rather than curative. Mild exercise should be followed by one hour's rest per day. If the hips are affected, physiotherapy aims to prevent contractures by encouraging extension (eg lying prone on the floor to watch TV). Splinting, traction and non-weight-bearing exercises may be used. Hot baths relieve morning stiffness. Naproxen 5mg/kg/12h PO pc may be helpful. Give aspirin, up to 80mg/kg/day PO, to give levels <250mg/L (beware of liver and CNS toxicity). If there is severe systemic disturbance prednisolone 0.5mg/kg/day PO may be needed. For those with unremitting destructive disease, penicillamine, gold and hydroxychloroquine may help. Surgery may be needed to conserve joint function.

Sydenham's chorea (St Vitus' dance) This may start with emotional lability and a preference for being alone (± attention span↓). Next comes purposeless movement, exaggerated by tension, and disappearing on sleep, with clumsiness, grimacing, a darting lizard's tongue and unclear speech (*OHCM* p 40). It is part of rheumatic fever (in <5%, p 194), and may be the *only* feature, appearing up to 6 months after clinical and lab signs of streptococcal infection have abated. Differential diagnosis: Wilson's disease, juvenile Huntington's, thyrotoxicosis, SLE, polycythaemia, Na^+↓, hypoparathyroidism, kernicterus, encephalitis lethargica, subdural haematoma, alcohol, phenytoin, neuroleptics, benign hereditary chorea, neuroacanthosis. If needed, haloperidol, phenobarbitone, or diazepam may be tried.

Syme's amputation An amputation immediately proximal to the ankle.

Tay–Sachs disease This is an autosomal recessive gangliosidosis (Type I) which affects ~1:4000 Ashkenazic Jewish births. It is a disease of grey matter. There is reduced lysosomal hexosaminidase A. Low levels of enzyme are detectable in carriers. Children are normal until ~6 months old, when developmental delay, photophobia, myoclonic fits, hyperacusis and irritability occur. Ophthalmoscopy: cherry-red spot at macula. Death usually occurs at 3–5yrs of age. Prenatal diagnosis may be made by amniocentesis.

Tolosa–Hunt syndrome A lesion in the superior orbital fissure (or cavernous sinus) produces unilateral ophthalmoplegia with disordered sensation in the area of the first branch of the trigeminal nerve—a very convenient state of affairs for conducting cataract surgery, which may be temporarily induced by local anaesthetic agents and a longish needle.

Treacher–Collins' syndrome is the association of lower eyelid notching, oblique palpebral fissures, flattening of malar bones and absent or hypoplastic zygoma. If these are associated with mandibular defects, ear defects and deafness, it is called Franceschetti's syndrome. Mutations in the TCOF1 gene may be to blame. *Proc Nat Acad Sci USA* 1997 **94** 3110

Turner's syndrome (X0) Prevalence: 1:2500 girls. Girls lack a sex chromosome, and this is associated with short stature (<130cm)—possibly the only sign, hyperconvex nails, wide carrying angle (cubitus valgus), inverted nipples, broad chest, ptosis, nystagmus, webbed neck, coarctation of the aorta, left heart defects, leg lymphoedema. The gonads are rudimentary or absent and puberty may not occur. Mosaicism may occur (XO, XX). Typical cause of death: ischaemic heart disease. *Treatment:* Somatropin (human growth hormone) 0.14u/kg/24h sc helps prevent short stature (do not give if the epiphyses have fused). (O)estrogen therapy is controversial. Association: Crohn's disease. *Lancet* 1992 **238** 681 & *BMJ* 1994 **ii** 606

Von Gierke's syndrome (Type Ia glycogen storage disease) is the most common and severe of the glycogenoses. *Inheritance:* Autosomal recessive (gene G6Pase mutation, causing ↓glucose 6-phosphatase). *Signs:* Hypoglycaemia appearing in the first year of life, with failure to thrive, lumbar lordosis, adiposity, xanthomata over joints and buttocks, and a tendency to bleed. There is hepatomegaly but no splenomegaly. *Eur J Hum Gen* 1997 **5** 191

Werner's syndrome comprizes premature ageing, diabetes, cataracts and scleroderma-like skin changes. The responsible gene's (chromosome 8, short arm) protein unwinds DNA pairs in a disordered way. *Science* 1996 **272** 1039

Winkler's disease The typical patient is a middle-aged man with a chronic, scaly, ulcerated nodule on the helix of the right ear (or the antehelix in women)—hence its synonym: chondrodermatis nodularis helicis chronicis. Multiple lesions may occur along the ear's rim. *Cause:* Recurrent minor trauma is thought to be important. It occurs more commonly on the ear on the side of sleeping. Telephone operators are at risk, as are nuns wearing tight head dresses. It is benign. *Treatment:* Surgical excision. J Bourke 1993 *BMJ* **ii** 327

Wiskott–Aldrich syndrome is a severe X-linked primary immunodeficiency (p 201) with recurrent infections, thrombocytopenia, and eczema. Without marrow transplant, most will die before adulthood. DNA linkage helps with prenatal diagnosis. The responsible gene has been found, along with its product, known as Wiskott–Aldrich syndrome protein. Prenatal tests include direct gene analysis with single strand conformation polymorphism (SSCP) and heteroduplex formation (HD). G Wengler 1995 *Lancet* **346** 641

11. Anaesthesia

Other relevant pages: Pain relief in labour (p 114); resuscitation after delivery (p 230); neonatal ITU (p 232); ventilating neonates (p 234); major injury (p 684); choosing the correct dose of lidocaine (=lignocaine) according to body weight (p 687); pain relief in children (p 678); Bier's block (p 700).

Introduction

Anaesthesia has evolved from humble origins. It was 1842 when CW Long gave ether, but he failed to report this landmark in the relief of pain. Then, in 1844, Horace Wells used nitrous oxide for tooth extraction, and in 1846 WTG Morton gave the first surgical anaesthetic with ether. It is now a highly specialized and sophisticated specialty in its own right. While the triad of anaesthesia (hypnosis, analgesia and muscle relaxation) remains the fundamental principle behind general anaesthesia for surgery, the rôle of the anaesthetist has expanded to encompass not only the provision of ideal operating conditions for surgery, but also intensive care, resuscitation, alleviation of acute and chronic pain, and anaesthesia for diagnostic procedures. A detailed knowledge of general medicine, physiology, pharmacology and the physical properties of gases and the workings of the vast array of anaesthetic equipment are essential, in order to practise well.

►We emphasize that this short chapter is no substitute for a specialist text or for experience on the ward. The main aim is to enable understanding of the issues anaesthetists face, and to prepare one's mind for intelligent discussions on anaesthetic issues.

Pre-operative care

Aims

1 To ensure that the right patient gets the right surgery. Have the symptoms and signs changed? If so, inform the surgeon.
2 To assess and balance the risks of anaesthesia.
3 To ensure that the patient is as fit as possible.
4 To decide on the type of anaesthesia and analgesia.
5 To allay all anxiety and pain.

The pre-operative visit Assess cardiovascular and respiratory systems, exercise tolerance, existing illnesses, drug therapy and allergies. Assess past history—of myocardial infarction, diabetes mellitus, asthma, hypertension, rheumatic fever, epilepsy, jaundice. Assess any specific risks—eg is the patient pregnant? Any dental problems, or history of GI reflux?
Have there been any anaesthetic problems (nausea, DVT)? Has he had a recent GA? (Do not repeat halothane within 6 months.)

Family history Ask questions about malignant hyperpyrexia (p 772); dystrophia myotonica (*OHCM* p 470); porphyria; cholinesterase problems; sickle-cell disease (test if needed). Does the patient have any specific worries?

Drugs Ask about allergy to any drug, antiseptic, plaster.
ACE inhibitors: No special action required.
Anticoagulants: Know why he's on them. Do INR. Switch warfarin to heparin 24h pre-op. Avoid epidural/spinal blocks. Beware regional anaesthesia.
Anticonvulsants: Give the usual dose up to 1h before surgery. Give drugs IV (or by NGT) post-op, until able to take oral drugs. Sodium valproate: an IV form is available (give the patient's usual dose). Phenytoin: give IV slowly (<50mg/min). IM phenytoin absorption is unreliable.
Antibiotics: Neomycin, aminoglycosides, polymixin and tetracycline may prolong neuromuscular blockade, even *depolarizing* neuro-muscular bockers.
Beta-blockers: Continue up to and including the day of surgery as this precludes a labile cardiovascular response.
Contraceptive Pill: Don't stop except perhaps before very major surgery.
Digoxin: Continue up to and *including* morning of surgery. Check for toxicity and do plasma K^+. suxamethonium ↑serum K^+ by ~1mmol/L, and can lead to ventricular arrhythmias in the fully digitalized. Potentiation of the vagotonic effects of digitalis by halothane and neostigmine may be precipitated by an increase in calcium and low potassium.
Diuretics: Beware hypokalaemia. Do U&E (and bicarbonate).
Hormone replacement therapy: As there is no increased risk of DVT or PE, there is no need to stop these agents.
Insulin: If on long acting preparations stabilize pre-operatively on short-acting. IV 5% dextrose with KCl and insulin the morning of theatre allows accurate control. See *OHCM* p 108.
Levodopa: Possible arrhythmias when the patient is under GA.
Lithium: Stop 3 wks pre-op. It may potentiate neuromuscular blockade and cause arrhythmias. Beware post-op toxicity ± U&E imbalance; see p 354.
Monoamine oxidase inhibtors: Stop 3 weeks before surgery. Interaction with narcotics and anaesthetics may lead to hypotensive/hypertensive crisis.
Ophthalmic drugs: Anticholinesterases used to treat glaucoma (eg ecothiopate iodine) may cause sensitivity to, and prolong duration of, drugs metabolized by cholinesterases, eg suxamethonium.
Oral hypoglycaemics: No chlorpropamide 24h pre-op (long $t_{1/2}$).
Steroids: If the patient is on or has recently taken steroids give extra cover for the peri-operative period (p 763).
Tricyclics: These enhance epinephrine (=adrenaline), exerting anticholinergic effects causing tachycardia, arrhythmias and low BP.

Pre-operative examination and tests

It is the anaesthetist's duty to assess suitability for anaesthesia. Be alert to chronic lung disease, hypertension, arrhythmias, and murmurs (endocarditis prophylaxis needed?—see p 194). In rheumatoid arthritis do a lateral cervical spine x-ray to warn about difficult intubations. Post-op chest infections are *six times* more likely in smokers. Stopping smoking even 1 day pre-op is of benefit.

The *ward doctor* assists with a good history and examination—and should also reassure, inform and and obtain written consent from the patient (eg get consent for orchidectomy in orchidopexy procedures, inform thyroidectomy patients of nerve damage risk, and retrograde ejaculation with TURP). Other concerns for the house officer to address include:

- DVT prophylaxis (p 654)
- Bowel preparation
- Peri-operative x-rays
- Frozen section (liase with pathologist)
- Skin preparation
- Post-op physiotherapy

Tests Be guided by the history and examination.

- In most patients, do FBC, ward test for blood glucose, and U&E—especially important if the patient is: –On diuretics –A diabetic –A burns victim –Has hepatic or renal disease –Starved –In ileus –Parenterally fed
- If Hb < 10g/dL tell anaesthetist. Investigate/treat as appropriate.
- Crossmatching: group and save for mastectomy, cholecystectomy. Crossmatch 2 units for Caesarean section; 4 units for a gastrectomy, and >6 units for abdominal aortic aneurysm surgery.
- Specific blood tests: LFT in jaundice, malignancy or alcohol abuse. Amylase in acute abdominal pain.
  Blood glucose in diabetic patients (*OHCM* p 108).
  Drug levels as appropriate (eg digoxin).
  Clotting studies in liver disease, DIC, massive blood loss, already on warfarin or heparin. Contact lab as special bottles are needed.
  HIV, HBsAg in high-risk patients—after appropriate counselling.
  Sickle test in those from Africa, West Indies or Mediterranean area—and others whose origins are in malarial areas (including most of India).
  Thyroid function tests in those with thyroid disease.
- CXR: if known cardiorespiratory disease, pathology or symptoms.
- ECG: those with poor exercise tolerance, history of myocardial ischaemia, hypertension or rheumatic fever, and those >50yrs due to high incidence of 'silent' ischaemia.

Preparation ►Fast the patient: ie no water for 2h pre-op, no milky drinks/squash for 4h, and no solids for 6h.

Use nasogastric tube as indicated: insert *before* induction to avoid risk of aspiration *at* induction. (Technique: *OHCM* p 96.) Catheterize as indicated.

ASA classification (American Society of Anesthesiologists)

1 Normally healthy.
2 Mild systemic disease, but with no limitation of activity.
3 Severe systemic disease that limits activity; not incapacitating.
4 Incapacitating systemic disease which poses a threat to life.
5 Moribund. Not expected to survive 24h even with operation.

You will see a space for an ASA number on most standard anaesthetic charts. It is an index of health at the time of surgery. The prefix **E** is used in emergencies.

Premedication

The patient should be aware of what will happen, where he will waken and how he will feel. Premedication aims to allay anxiety and contribute to a smooth induction of anaesthesia by decreasing secretions (much less important than when ether used), promoting amnesia, analgesia and decreasing vagal reflexes. *Timing:* 2h pre-op for oral drugs; 1h pre-op if IM.

Examples for the 70kg man

- Lorazepam 2–3mg PO.
- Temazepam 10–20mg PO.
- Diazepam 5–20mg PO.

Some anaesthetists still use the traditional IM premeds. Examples:

- Morphine 10mg IM and atropine 0.6mg IM.
- Pethidine 50mg IM and promethazine 25mg IM.
- Papaveretum 15.4mg (=1mL 15.4mg/mL ampoule) with 0.4mg hyoscine hydrobromide IM; a combined ampoule is available (dose 0.5–1mL IM). Avoid the obsolete term *Om and Scop* which implies Omnopon® (now called papaveretum) given with hyoscine hydrobromide (=scopolamine hydrobromide). Noscapine (?polyploidy risk in progeny of those of child-bearing age) is not contained in papaveretum manufactured since 1993.

Examples for children

- Trimeprazine 2mg/kg as a syrup.
- Always use oral premeds in children as first choice. Children over 1yr: if IM needed, give pethidine 0.5–2mg/kg or morphine 0.15mg/kg.
- EMLA® local anaesthetic cream on at least 2 sites that may be used for IV access, and at least 1h prior to venepunture (early vasoconstriction makes venepuncture difficult before this).

Specific premedication

- Antibiotics
- Bronchodilators, eg salbutamol nebulizer
- Nitrate patches, eg Transiderm Nitro®—esp. useful in cardiac surgery.
- Steroids, eg minor operations 100mg of IM hydrocortisone 1h pre-op and 6h post-op. Major operations hydrocortisone 100mg/6h IM. Consider if adrenal insufficiency or adrenal surgery; steroid therapy for more than 2 weeks prior to surgery; or steroid therapy for more than 1 month in the year preceding surgery.

Common reasons for cancellation

- Cold or recent viral illness if still symptomatic.
- Recent myocardial infarction (significant ↑ in mortality if GA is given within 6 months—believed to be related to degree of cardiac failure).
- Patient not adequately fasted.
- U&E imbalance (particularly K^+); anaemia.
- Inadequate preparation (results not available, not crossmatched).
- Patient not in optimum condition—eg poor control of drug therapy (digoxin, thyroxine, phenytoin); exacerbation of illness.
- Undiagnosed or untreated hypertension.
- Inadequate theatre time.

Equipment

Careful checking of equipment is vital before any anaesthetic or sedative procedure. The essentials are:

- Tilting bed or trolley (in case of vomiting).
- High-volume suction with rigid Yankaeur, and long suction catheters.
- Reliable oxygen supply, capable of delivering 15L/min.
- Self-inflating bag with oxygen reservoir, non-rebreathing valve and compatible mask (a 'bag-valve-mask' system).
- Oropharyngeal and nasopharyngeal airways.
- A range of anatomical face mask sizes with harness.
- Endotracheal tubes (range) and catheter mount.
- Anaesthetic circuit.
- Laryngoscope with range of blade sizes and spare batteries.
- Intravenous infusion cannulae and fluids.
- Anaesthetic and resuscitation drugs and anaesthetic gases.
- Defibrillator.
- Monitoring equipment (may include pulse oximeter and end tidal CO_2 monitor, p 772).

Inhalational agents

These are the vapours which in clinically useful concentrations help to maintain anaesthesia and decrease awareness. In Britain they are generally added to the fresh gas flow by passing a fraction of the carrier gas (generally N_2O/O_2) through a plenum vaporizer (in which the delivery of anaesthetic vapour does not depend on the patient's respiratory effort—as it does in 'draw over' systems).

Halothane This gas has little analgesic effect. It decreases cardiac output (vagal tone ↑, leading to bradycardia, vasodilation and hypotension). It sensitizes the myocardium to catecholamines (beware in patients with arrhythmias; surgical infiltration with local anaesthetic and epinephrine). It bronchodilates so is useful in bronchospasm. It relaxes the uterus in deep anaesthesia and may lead to postpartum haemorrhage (hence 0.5% concentration used during Caesarean section). The 2 major but rare complications are malignant hyperpyrexia and hepatitis.
►Do not use halothane twice within a 6-month period.

Enflurane This is similar to the above, but less potent. Avoid in epileptics (EEG epileptiform activities seen during anaesthesia). It does not sensitize the heart to catecholamines as much as halothane.

Isoflurane This is an isomer of enflurane. Theoretically induction should be quick, but isoflurane is irritant, so coughing, laryngospasm or breath-holding may complicate the onset of anaesthesia.

Stopping inhalation reverses all the above effects—except for hepatitis resulting from drug metabolism.

The ideal IV anaesthetic agent

The ideal IV agent would be stable in solution, be water-soluble and have a long shelf-life. It would be painless when given IV; non-irritant if injected extravascularly (with a low incidence of thrombosis) with some pain (as a warning) if given intra-arterially.

- It should act rapidly within one arm–brain circulation.
- Recovery should be quick and complete with no hangover effect.
- It should provoke no excitatory phenomena.
- Analgesic properties are advantageous.
- Respiratory and cardiovascular effects should be minimal.
- It should not interact with other anaesthetic agents.
- Hypersensitivity reactions are not ideal.
- There should be no post-op phenomena, eg nausea, or hallucinations.

This perfect drug does not exist.

IV anaesthetic agents: thiopental sodium

Thiopental (=thiopentone) sodium ($t_{1/2}$=11h) When mixed with water to give a 2.5% solution this barbiturate is stable for 24–48h, so make it up daily. It has a rapid onset of action (arm–brain circulation time about 30sec). Effects last 3–8mins. Awakening is due largely to redistribution, not metabolism. Some 30% of the injected dose is still present in the body after 24h, giving rise to the hangover effect. Patients must not drive, operate machinery etc. within 24h.

Dose: eg 4–6mL of 2.5% solution (3–5mg/kg, but less in the elderly and the premedicated, and more in children who generally require 6–7mg/kg, but some children need much less, eg 2mg/kg.) Subsequent doses are cumulative. Note: thiopental (=thiopentone) sodium interacts with other drugs eg increase dose in those who consume much alcohol.

Uses: induction of GA; it is also a potent anticonvulsant.

Contraindications: •Airway obstruction •Barbiturate allergy •Fixed cardiac output states •Hypovolaemia/shock •Porphyria.

►Problems: Intra-arterial injection produces pain and blanching of the hand/limb below the level of injection due to arterial spasm, followed by ischaemic damage and gangrene—frequently following inadvertent brachial artery puncture in the antecubital fossa.

Treatment: **1** Leave the needle in the artery and inject procaine hydrochloride 10–20mL of a 0.5% solution **2** Perform, or ask an experienced colleague to perform, brachial plexus or stellate ganglion block. (These measures should dilate vessels and reduce ischaemia.) **3** Heparin IV to stop thrombus forming **4** Give pain relief **5** Postpone surgery unless desperate.

Extravascular injection produces severe pain and local tissue necrosis. Infiltrate with hyaluronidase 1500iu through the cannula.

Other IV anaesthetic agents (See p 772)

Methohexital sodium (=methohexitone) ($t_{½}$=5h) This barbiturate is like thiopental sodium (=thiopentone), but more potent, and when mixed with water it has a shelf life of 6 weeks. *Dose:* 1mg/kg at a rate of 2mg/sec. It often causes pain and involuntary movements on injection. Recovery and metabolism are swifter than for thiopental so it is more suitable for day-case patients. Contraindications are the same as for thiopentone but in addition avoid in epileptic patients as it may provoke fits in susceptible patients, although it is often used for ECT anaesthesia.

Etomidate ($t_{½}$= 3.5h) This is a carboxylated imidazole. *Dose:* 0.1–0.3mg/kg. Histamine release is not a feature; rapidity of recovery and cardiovascular stability are; therefore it is suitable for day-case surgery, the elderly and those with compromised cardiovascular systems. Be aware that this may induce involuntary muscle movements, nausea, and adrenal suppression.

Ketamine *Dose:* 0.5–2mg/kg; $t_{½}$= 22h. This is a phencyclidine derivative. There may be delay before onset of sleep. Hypertonus and salivation are problems, but there is some maintenance of laryngeal reflexes (do not rely on this). Recovery is slow. Emergence phenomena are troublesome (delirium, hallucinations, nightmares; all made worse if the patient is disturbed during recovery). Cardiac output is unchanged or increased. It is a good 'on site' or 'in the field' agent, as it can be given IM and produces profound analgesia without compounding shock. ►Avoid in the hypertensive patient, those with a history of stroke, or raised intracranial pressure (further ↑ produced), patients with a recent penetrating eye injury (risk of ↑ intraocular pressure), and psychiatric patients. Avoid epinephrine infiltrations.

Propofol This phenol derivative is the most recently introduced IV anaesthetic agent and is formulated in soya oil and egg phosphatid.

- *Dose example:* 2mg/kg; ►Rapid injection can cause cardiovascular depression (↓BP), and respiratory depression can occur when combined with IV narcotics. For sedation: 1.5–4.5mg/kg/h IVI. It acts and is metabolized quickly. Wake-up is caused by redistribution rather than metabolism. It is widely used in day-case surgery, induction and maintenance of general anaesthesia, and for sedation during regional anaesthesia, short procedures, and as a sedative in ITU. CI: the extremities of age; egg allergy.
- Its favourable recovery characteristics and antiemetic effects have made it widely popular.
- Once opened, use ampoules or discard, because of the risk of bacterial growth.
- Pain on injection occurs in up to 40% of patients. This can be minimized by either adding a small amount of lidocaine (=lignocaine) (2mL of 1%) to the propofol, or by pre-injection of a similar volume of local anaesthetic.

Neuromuscular blockers

►It is axiomatic in anaesthetic practice never to give a muscle relaxant in the presence of a compromised airway.

These drugs act on the post-synaptic receptors at the NMJ (neuromuscular junction). There are two main groups:

1 Depolarizing agents eg suxamethonium (=succinylcholine, Scoline®). These drugs depolarize the post-synaptic membrane, causing paralysis by inhibiting the normal membrane polarity. They are partial agonists for acetylcholine and cause initial fasciculation, liberation K^+, enough to raise the plasma K^+ by ~0.5–1.0mmol/L (beware in paraplegia and burns!), myoglobin and creatine kinase. Beware that K^+ liberation is increased with multiple sclerosis, Guillain–Barré, stroke, and crush injury. They also increase intra-occular pressure (eg increase risk of vitreous extrusion). 30% of patients get post-operative muscle pains. Suxamethonium is an ideal intubating agent: it has a rapid onset, a short duration of action (2–3min), and produces good relaxation. Note: a second dose, if required, should be preceded by atropine, as the vagotonic effects of suxamethonium can lead to profound bradycardia (notably in children). Beware suxamethonium (Scoline®) apnoea (p 772). Dose of suxamethonium: eg 0.6mg/kg IV. Some over-the-counter medicines and foods containing solanaceous glycoalkaloids (potatoes, tomatoes, aubergines) inhibit the beakdown of suxamethonium.[1]

2 Non-depolarizing agents These drugs compete with acetylcholine at the NMJ—but without producing initial stimulation (see suxamethonium above). Repeated doses may be given without atropine. Their action can be reversed by anticholinesterases (neostigmine). They are used during balanced anaesthesia to facilitate IPPV and surgery. Length of action and side-effects will govern anaesthetists' choices. Examples of the more common agents are:

Pancuronium Long acting (~1 hour), vagal blockade and sympathomimetic action. *Dose:* 50–100μg/kg IV then 10–20μg/kg IV as needed.

Vecuronium Lasting 20–30min, it is used if cardiovascular stability is important. No ganglion-blocking effect. *Dose:* 80–100μg/kg IV then 20–30 μg/kg IV as needed. Starting dose for infants ≤4 months: 10–20μg/kg. If over 5 months, as adult dose, but high intubation dose may not be needed. Known as the 'cleanest' of these three agents due to least histamine release.

Atracurium Lasting ~20min this causes histamine release so avoid in asthma. Metabolism is by Hoffman Elimination (spontaneous molecular breakdown), so it is the drug of choice in renal and liver failure.
Dose: 300–600μg/kg IV then 100–200μg/kg IV as needed.

1 J Hopkins 1998 *BMJ* ii 1102

Practical conduct of anaesthesia: I

The practitioner administering the anaesthetic is responsible for the suitability of the surroundings, the adequacy of the available equipment, and his own competence to deal with potential complications. Equipment *must* be checked before even the shortest anaesthetic procedure.

All anaesthetic rooms should be treated like a church—respect the contents, keep quiet unless asked to participate and follow the lead given by the (ad)minister of the anaesthetic. They differ in that hats *must* be worn, and the only person allowed to go to sleep is the patient.

Induction May be gaseous or IV (IM possible with ketamine).

Gaseous:

- Start with nitrous oxide:oxygen 60%:40% mixture. In children, it is less frightening to start with a hand cupped from the end of the circuit onto the face than to apply the mask direct to face.
- Proceed with slow, careful introduction of the volatile agent in 0.5–1% incremental doses (rapid increase in concentration is unpleasant and leads to coughing and possible laryngospasm).
- Monitor vital signs closely, as the time factor separating a struggling child from a flaccid, apnoeic, overdosed child is short.
- Establish IV access when and where appropriate, as soon as asleep.

Indications for gaseous induction:

- Any patient with airway obstruction (actual or potential, eg foreign body, tumour, or abscess).
- At the patient's request.
- Difficult IV access.

Intravenous:

- Establish IV access.
- A sleep-inducing dose of, eg thiopental (=thiopentone) sodium, is injected after a 2mL test dose to detect inadvertent arterial cannulation (p 764).
- Beware! Stimulation before anaesthesia is established can have drastic consequences (coughing, breath-holding, laryngospasm). Remember, noise is a stimulus too.

Airway control This is maintained either by holding a mask onto the face, or by intubation (p 771). To prevent airway obstruction the standard chin lift and/or jaw thrust manoeuvres are used. It may be facilitated by the use of an airway adjunct (eg oropharyngeal, or nasopharyngeal). Insertion of an airway adjunct may produce vomiting or laryngospasm. Avoid opiates with induction as they increase the risk of vomiting.

The practical conduct of anaesthesia: II

Intubation This is needed for protection of the airway in:

- Risk of vomiting/aspiration of gastric contents (eg reflux oesophagitis, abdominal disease, major trauma, non-fasted, hiatus hernia, pregnancy).

- Management of difficult airways. If difficulty is suspected, ensure senior help is available / consider fibreoptic or awake intubation
- Head and neck surgery, where masks clutter the operative field.
- Where muscle paralysis facilitates surgery, eg abdominal surgery.

► Paralysed patients cannot breathe—and so require ventilation.

Intubation requires good muscle relaxation:

- Deep anaesthesia in the spontaneously breathing patient.
- Use of short- or long-acting muscle relaxant.

Short-acting: (suxamethonium, typically ~0.6mg/kg IV) Uses: •If risk of vomiting ↑. •When difficulty with intubation is anticipated. •If the intention is to let the patient breathe spontaneously via the ET tube.

Long-acting: Numerous available, eg vecuronium 0.1mg/kg IV. They take longer to provide suitable conditions for intubation. Remember it will be at least 20min before breathing recommences, so *if there is any doubt as to the ability to maintain a patent airway, then a short-acting (or even no) muscle relaxant is more appropriate.*

Rapid sequence induction Used where the risk of vomiting is high (eg trauma, non-fasted, pregnancy >15 weeks' gestation, hiatus hernia).

- Pre-oxygenate with 100% oxygen for 3min to provide an O_2 reservoir in the lungs for use during the period of induced apnoea.
- Cricoid pressure on induction (firm backward pressure on cricoid cartilage occluding oesophagus may stop gastric reflux to larynx).
- Short-acting muscle relaxant is given immediately after induction. The trachea is intubated, and the cuff of the ET tube inflated.
- Once the ET tube is correctly positioned, cricoid pressure may be released, and a volatile agent added to maintain anaesthesia.

Maintenance of anaesthesia

1 Volatile agent added to N_2O/O_2 mixture as before. Either spontaneously breathing or ventilation, with or without opiates. If the patient is ventilated, muscle relaxants are generally used.
2 High-dose opiates with mechanical ventilation.
3 IV infusion anaesthesia, eg propofol ± opiates. The maintenance dose of propofol is 4–12mg/kg/h IVI. SE: anaphylaxis; delayed convulsions (so beware in day-case surgery).

Whatever technique is used, the dose and concentration of each agent used is adjusted according to the level of anaesthesia achieved versus the desired level. (This is determined by monitoring vital signs—eg pulse, BP, signs of sympathetic stimulation such as sweating, pupillary dilatation, lacrimation etc.)

End of anaesthesia •Change inspired gases to 100% oxygen only.

- Discontinue any infusions of anaesthetic drugs.
- Reverse muscle paralysis with neostigmine (dose 2.5mg in adults) + an anticholinergic drug to prevent its muscarinic side-effects (bradycardia, salivation), eg atropine 1.2mg IV (or glycopyrronium—preferred with neostigmine).
- Once spontaneously breathing, put the patient in the recovery position (p 789). Before the ET tube is removed the mouth and oropharynx should be cleared under direct vision.
- Administer oxygen by face mask.
- If there are no problems, transfer to the recovery room, but be prepared to reassess the patient at any time.

Intubation technique

Preparation is the key word. Always assess neck mobility, (arthritis, ankylosing spondylitis, goitre etc) pre-op. Beware the obese, short-necked, chinless patient with protruding teeth!

- ET tube sizes (mm internal diameter, ID): 9.0 in adult ♂, 8.0 in ♀. Children:
  ID = [age in years/4] + 4.5mm (*neonate = 3–3.5mm*)
  Length (oral) = [age/2] + 12.5cm
  Length (nasal) = [age/2] + 14.5cm
- Lubricate the tube, and check that its cuff and the laryngoscope work.
- Position the patient with neck flexed and head extended using a pillow ('sniffing the morning air').
- Hold the laryngoscope in the left hand, and open the mouth with the right.
- Slide the laryngoscope blade down the right side of the tongue into the vallecula (area between tongue and epiglottis), guarding the lip and teeth with the fingers of your right hand.
- Lift the laryngoscope blade upwards and away from yourself. DO NOT lever on the teeth or you may damage them.
- Lift the epiglottis from view: the cords should become visible. When they are, insert the tube with your right hand.
- Once the cuff of the endotracheal tube is beyond the cords, remove the laryngoscope; ask the assistant to inflate the cuff to prevent air leak.
- Attach to the circuit. Gently inflate lungs. Watch chest move. Do both sides move equally? Is the abdomen moving and not the chest?
- Auscultate both sides of chest. Air entry should be equal. Fix the tube with a tie, or strong tape
- Confirm correct placement with capnography. NB: the disposable end tidal carbon dioxide detector ('FEF') uses a chemical pH indicator (metacresol) to detect the presence of CO_2 in expired gases. The colour varies from mauve to yellow with inspiration and expiration (respectively). Mauve indicates a CO_2 of <0.5%; tan ≈ 0.5–2%; yellow ≈ 2–5%. The device's *cyclical* colour change may be used to distinguish oesophageal from tracheal intubation—except that gastric fluid contamination produces a *permanent* orange colour which may falsely reassure the unwary. Also, if the patient is being resuscitated with lidocaine (=lignocaine) or epinephrine (=adrenaline) given via an endotracheal tube (p 310 & OHCM p 770) a permanent yellow colour occurs. The device works for ~2h before replacement is needed.[1]

►Remember: *if in doubt, take it out.* It is safer to re-intubate than to risk leaving a tracheal tube in the oesophagus happily inflating the stomach. The tube may slip down a main bronchus (usually right). If so, withdraw the tube until both sides of the chest move equally, and air entry is equal (otherwise there is risk of collapse in the unventilated lung, or pneumothorax on the overventilated side).

If you are having problems with intubating: ►Adequate oxygenation is the first priority. •Get help •Blind nasal and fibreoptic intubation are options for the experienced •If you find you need another dose of suxamethonium, give atropine first, to prevent bradycardia •Consider a laryngeal mask. This consists of a tube with a cuff designed to sit over the larynx. The cuff takes ~30mL of air (depending on size). It is more efficient than mask ventilation (eg if arthritis prevents the neck extension needed by masks), and provides a degree, although unreliable, of airway protection. During its use, nasogastric aspiration of air may be needed, although usually only if with concomitant IPPV.

1 J Muir & M Hayes 1990 BMJ ii 4-2

Monitoring during anaesthesia

Monitoring begins prior to induction of anaesthesia and continues throughout. A warm, pink, and well-perfused patient is the aim. Sweating and lacrimation invariably indicate something is wrong.

Respirations Rate, depth (IPPV if inadequate). **BP** Intra-arterial if long procedures. **Temperature** Particularly important in infants. (Large surface area to body mass may lead to hypothermia.) A warm environment, warming blankets, warming IV fluid, are all important in long cases.

Pulse oximetry Computes pulse rate and arterial O_2 saturation, but does not obviate the need for manual pulse checks.

ECG Reveals rate, arrhythmias and ischaemia (if on correct leads).

CVP Helps differentiate hypovolaemia from ↓cardiac function. Insert when large blood loss is anticipated, or in unstable patients.

Capnography and inspired gas analysis are now widely available. A low end tidal CO_2 warns of a displaced endotracheal tube, emboli and more.

Some complications of anaesthesia

►***The commonest respiratory complication is airway obstruction due to loss of muscle tone in soft palate, or 'swallowing the tongue.'***

Atelectasis and pneumonia These are leading complications, and are partly ameliorated by good pain relief (to aid coughing) and physiotherapy, as well as antibiotics (*OHCM* p 336). Atelectasis typically occurs in the lower lobes, and prevents gas exchange, causing shunting. It is best seen on CT (not CXRs). It starts within minutes of induction, and is partly caused by using 100% O_2. In one careful study, it was prevented by using 30% O_2 at induction (just enough to cause adequate oxygenation).[1]

Laryngospasm The cords are firmly shut. Treat with 100% oxygen. Attempt to ventilate. It may be necessary to paralyse and intubate.

Bronchospasm Ensure oxygenation. If intubated check tube position (carina stimulation may be the cause: withdraw tube slightly). Check for pneumothorax. Increase concentration of volatile agent if he is 'light'). Salbutamol 250μg IV, aminophylline (p 271) + hyperventilation with 100% O_2. If persistent, give hydrocortisone 100mg IV and consider epinephrine (=adrenaline, 1–10mL of 1:10,000 IV). **Anaphylaxis** See p 303.

Shivering ± hypothermia Preventable with 'space blankets', and may be treated by radiant heat and pethidine for shivering (0.3mg/kg slowly IV). Be aware that shivering increases O_2 consumption 5-fold.

Scoline apnoea Prolonged paralysis occurs if abnormal plasma cholinesterase: ventilate until power returns: then test the patient (and family).

Malignant hyperpyrexia Uncommon, autosomal dominant condition (a candidate gene on chromosome 19 has been identified).[1] A rapid increase in body temperature (>2°C/h) is precipitated by many drugs; notably halothane and suxamethonium. Masseter spasm (after suxamethonium) may be the first indication, followed by tachycardia, mottling, hypercarbia, hyperkalaemia, arrhythmias, hypoxaemia, and acidosis.
Treatment: •Seek expert or senior advice (mortality if unrecognized ~80%; if correctly managed ~5%) which may include:
- Withdraw precipitants and stop surgery; hyperventilate with O_2.
- Actively cool the patient (ice packs, cold IV infusion etc).
- Management in ITU.
- Dantrolene 1mg/kg IV bolus and repeat as needed up to 10mg/kg.
- Mannitol for any myoglobinuria.
- Correct acidosis with sodium bicarbonate.
- Treat any hyperkalaemia (*OHCM* p 382; children p 280 this book).
- Encourage diuresis. •Insulin. •Steroids, eg hydrocortisone 100mg IV.
- Phenotype relatives (muscle biopsy response to halothane and caffeine).[2]

Awareness

Owing to neuromuscular blockade, it is notoriously difficult to diagnose awareness during anaesthesia—a most distressing state for the patient. Prevalence: ~1% in emergency/obstetric anaesthesia, as doses used are minimized, to avoid shock. It is rare otherwise (eg 0.2–0.4%).[3]

Sedation

Definition: Sedation is an induced reduction in conscious level, during which verbal contact is maintained with the patient.

Doctors in many specialities may be required to administer sedation. The doctor giving the sedation *must not* be also responsible for performing any procedure (such as manipulation of a dislocated joint). His sole responsibility is to ensure that the sedation is adequate, and to monitor the patient's airway, breathing, and circulation. Sedation is not a short cut to avoid formal anaesthesia, and it does not excuse the patient from an appropriate work-up or reasonable fasting. Monitoring is mandatory, and should include pulse oximetry.

It is easy for sedation to become general anaesthesia, with its attendant risks (see p 772). The loss of the 'eyelash reflex' (gentle stroking of the upper eyelashes to produce blinking) is a good guide to the onset of general anaesthesia.

Agents

- Diazepam (as emulsion = Diazemuls®): initial adult dose 2.5–10mg IV.
- Midazolam: 0.1mg/kg. Initial adult dose 2mg IV over 30 seconds (1mg if elderly). Further 0.5–1mg IV as needed after 2 minutes. Usual range 2.5–7mg (elderly 1–2mg). In some circumstances (eg manipulation of large joint; painful dressing changes) a narcotic analgesic may be used in addition (eg morphine in 1–2mg aliquots IV, or shorter acting opioids such as fentanyl).

Recovery from anaesthesia

- Ensure same monitoring as *during* anaesthesia.
- 40% oxygen via a face mask for >15mins to prevent 'diffusion hypoxia'—ie nitrous oxide leaves the blood faster than nitrogen from the air enters it, so greatly diluting the available oxygen in the alveoli.
- Monitor pulse and BP. • Keep the patient warm.
- Look for hypoventilation—may present as 'see-sawing respiration' (?inadequate reversal—check with nerve stimulator; narcosis — reverse opiates with naloxone—*cautiously* to minimize pain; check for airway obstruction, eg from bleeding tonsil). Ensure adequate analgesia and antiemesis.
- Return the patient to the ward when you are satisfied with his cardiovascular and respiratory status and pain relief.
- Give clear instructions on post-operative fluid regimens, blood transfusions, oxygen therapy, pain relief, and physiotherapy.

1 HU Rothen 1995 *Lancet* **345** 1387 2 F Ellis 1992 BMJ i 791 3 JG Jones 1994 BMJ ii 967

Local anaesthesia

►All regional techniques may lead to loss of consciousness or loss of airway, and so require the same facilities, expertise, and precautions as for general anaesthesia (eg full resuscitation facilities, and patient fasted).

Local anaesthesia is used either alone or to supplement general anaesthesia, the aim is to prevent or reduce nerve conduction of painful impulses to higher centres (via the thalamus), where the perception of pain occurs. (Action is by a membrane-stabilizing effect, impairing membrane permeability to sodium, so blocking impulse propagation.)

Types of local anaesthesia (LA) *Amides:*

1 Lidocaine (=lignocaine) $t_{1/2}$=2h; max dose in typical healthy adult=3mg/kg up to 200mg (500mg with epinephrine, but use with caution). Some anaesthetists use higher doses of lidocaine without epinephrine with no problems (eg 4mg/kg).
2 Prilocaine $t_{1/2}$=2h. Moderate onset. The dose is 3–5 mg/kg. (400mg is the maximum dose in adults; 600mg if used with felypressin.) Very low toxicity, so it is the drug of choice for Bier's block (IV regional anaesthesia).
3 Bupivacaine $t_{1/2}$=3h. Slow onset and prolonged duration. Maximum dose: 2mg/kg. Contraindicated in intravenous regional anaesthesia (Bier's block).

Note: 0.5% solution = 5mg/mL. 1% solution=10mg/mL. So for a 70kg man, the max dose of lidocaine is 20mL of 1% or 10mL of 2% solution. NB: lidocaine injections are less painful if they are *warm*, or at lower concentrations.

Certain commercially available preparations contain epinephrine (=adrenaline); these should be used with extreme caution, as systemic effects from the adrenaline may arise and prove hazardous, especially in CVS disease or ↑BP.

►*Epinephrine (adrenaline) is ABSOLUTELY contraindicated in digital or penile blocks, and around the nose or ears.* (Ischaemia produced may lead to gangrene.)

Esters (Infrequently used now.)

1 Cocaine. Very high toxicity. Short duration of action. Used as a paste preparation for anaesthesia and vasoconstriction prior to nasal intubation or nasal surgery.
2 Amethocaine $t_{1/2}$= 1h. Slow onset. High toxicity. *Lozenges* for buccal anaesthesia, *drops* for topical anaesthesia to eye (the eye must be covered with a patch following use), and now *topically* as an alternative to EMLA®.

Toxicity From excess dose, too rapid absorption or direct IV injection. *Features:* Perioral tingling; numb tongue; anxiety; lightheadedness; tinnitus; seizures; apnoea; collapse; direct myocardial depression; coma.

Treatment: Ensure oxygenation.
Hypotension: try IV fluids first, then consider ephedrine 5mg IV slowly, may be repeated at 3–4mins to a maximum of 30mg
Convulsions: thiopental (=thiopentone) sodium, or benzodiazepines, eg IV Diazemuls® 2.5–5mg boluses. Intubation/IPPV will probably also be needed.
CVS collapse: full resuscitation, ie intubation, epinephrine (=adrenaline), atropine, and cardiac massage as required.

Anaphylaxis (p 303) Occurs more commonly with the esters, but can occur with amides. A 2mL test dose may detect possible allergic reactions, and will also warn of inadvertent intravascular injection.

Local anaesthesia: techniques (►Bier's block: see p 700)

►Explain procedures to the patient first—their co-operation helps.

1 *Infiltration:* Use a small gauge needle. Lidocaine (=lignocaine) 0.5% most common agent. Frequent aspiration is important. Remember: after initial injection, subsequent injections through infiltrated areas hurt less. Likewise, infiltration through the cut edges of a laceration is less painful than through the skin.

2 *Topical:* Amethocaine to eye or buccal mucosa. Lidocaine 4% spray to cords prior to intubation (nil by mouth for 4h afterwards avoids aspiration).

3 *Nerve blocks:* Lidocaine (=lignocaine) 1–2%, prilocaine 0.5%, or bupivacaine 0.5%. Nerve stimulation increases success rate. It is now believed that it is the *volume* of the anaesthetic agent used, rather than the concentration *per se*, that improves anaesthesia. Hence lower concentrations can be used in larger volumes safely (eg bupivacaine 0.375%).

Femoral nerve block Direct injection, or catheter placement into the femoral sheath. Useful for fractured femur.

- Mark out the inguinal ligament (pubic tubercle to the anterior superior iliac spine). Palpate, and mark, the femoral artery.
- Insert short-bevel needle (insulated if nerve stimulator is used) 1cm lateral to the artery, just below the ligament. A 'click' is felt on traversing the skin, and again on traversing the fascia lata. Find the position either by eliciting paraesthesia, or with a nerve stimulator.
- Aspiration test, then inject eg 30–40mL 0.5% prilocaine.

Spinal anaesthesia

- Insert IV cannula and infuse 300–500mL crystalloid. Check BP.
- Sitting or left lateral position. Surgical scrub; gown & gloves. Prepare back.
- Infiltrate skin with 1–2mL 1% lidocaine (=lignocaine).
- Insert 22–25G spinal needle at L3/4 space (ie below spinal cord). Free flow of CSF confirms correct placement. Rotate the needle through 180° to ensure that all the needle aperture is in (avoids patchy blocks).
- Inject 1–3 mL 0.5% Marcain Heavy® (bupivacaine+dextrose, a hyperbaric solution that falls by gravity. This allows the height of block to be varied by posture.) Note—much less LA is required during pregnancy.
- Position patient to achieve low, high or unilateral block.
- Monitor BP—may fall; if so, give crystalloid ± vasopressors (eg ephedrine 5–30mg IV, or phenylephrine 50–100μg).

A small total drug concentration is required—producing sympathetic blockade (vasodilation, hypotension); sensory blockade (numbness); and finally motor blockade (reduction or absence of lower limb power).

Absolute contraindications to spinal anaesthesia:

- Anticoagulant states (risk pressure damage to cord from bleed).
- Local sepsis (risk of introducing infection to CSF).
- Shock or hypovolaemic states (effective reduction in circulating volume due to vasodilatation).
- Raised intracranial pressure.

Relative contraindications to spinal anaesthesia:

- Fixed output states (eg mitral stenosis, aortic stenosis).
- Neurological disease—procedure may be blamed for change in state.
- Ischaemic heart disease.
- Spinal deformity or previous surgery.
- Bowel perforation (theoretical risk of ↑parasympathetic activity, peristalsis and peritoneal soiling).

Extradural (epidural) anaesthesia

Insertion of indwelling catheter allows prolonged instillation of LA and/or opiates. Larger volumes of LA are required than with spinal anaesthesia. Lumbar most common site, but cervical/thoracic possible (needs great skill).
- Sitting or left lateral position. •Do BP. Infuse 300–500mL crystalloid.
- Aseptic technique.
- L3/4 commonest site. Infiltrate with 1–2mL 0.5% lidocaine (=lignocaine).
- Insert 18G Touhy needle until held firm in ligamentum flavum (~2–3cm).
- 'Loss of resistance' technique finds epidural space: 10mL 0.9% saline via Touhy needle is difficult to inject while in ligaments, but once in the epidural space, sudden loss of resistance enables easy injection.
- Fine-bore epidural catheter threaded, needle withdrawn, and catheter placed to needle depth plus 3–5cm.
- Aspiration test prior to 2mL test done. Wait 3min.
- Inject required dose eg 10mL 0.25% plain bupivacaine.
- Secure catheter in place.
- Monitor BP every 5min for 15min (slower onset than spinal, therefore hypotension takes longer to be revealed).

Complications of epidural anaesthesia:
- Dural puncture. CSF leak may not be obvious, hence the importance of test dose. (Ward tests for glucose will be +ve if CSF is present, but be aware that trace of blood will also be +ve). Instil one litre 0.9% NaCl/24h via the epidural filter. Push oral fluids. Nurse flat. Prescribe analgesics for headaches, laxatives to prevent constipation and straining. Blood patch may be necessary. *Inform a consultant.*
- Vessel puncture and injection. Treat with oxygen, IVI, pressor drugs, atropine if bradycardia (due to block of sympathetic outflow to heart T2–4), and remember the ABC of basic resuscitation.
- Hypoventilation. Due to motor block of intercostals. May or may not require control of ventilation.
- 'Total spinal'—ie injection of a large epidural dose into the CSF. Marked hypotension. Apnoea. Loss of consciousness. Treatment: IPPV. Treat hypotension. ►Death will occur from asphyxia if treatment is not prompt.

Caudal (sacral epidural)

- Left lateral position.
- Palpate sacral hiatus (~4–5cm above the tip of the coccyx). This is often not easy. Another method is to palpate the posterior superior iliac spines: the line joining them forms the base of an equilateral triangle with the sacral hiatus at the apex.
- Insert 21G block needle perpendicular to skin through the sacrococcygeal membrane, into the sacral canal. A 22G needle may be useful for infants.
- Aspirate, and inject up to 20mL 0.5% bupivacaine in the adult.
- If the injection is difficult (there should be no resistance), or swelling occurs, then the needle is in the wrong place—so **stop!** Withdraw the needle and start again.

Indications: •Provides anaesthesia for the sacral region.
- Useful, eg in scrotal surgery, low cavity forceps (needs experience because of risk of injecting into baby's head), hernias or haemorrhoids.

Pain

John Keats, the best known medical student to die of unrequited love, demonstrated that the life of the spirit entails the capacity to feel pain—but, as usual, Nature has been over-generous in endowing us with this capacity—so making the treatment of pain paramount: it promotes wellbeing, sleep, and the honeyed indolence preceding recovery or the easeful passage into oblivion. We tend to think simplistically about pain, assuming that when pain is submitted to us we must respond with something analgesic or anaesthetic—but there are other approaches.*

Remember also that pain relief aids physiotherapy (allowing coughing and mobility), preventing pneumonia.

Pain exacerbates hypo/hyperventilation, hypertension and tachycardia.

Methods of analgesia (See *OHCM* p 90 and *OHCM* p 688.)

1 *Oral:* Typical example: paracetamol 0.5–1g/6h. Non-steroidal anti-inflammatory drugs (NSAIDs), eg diclofenac 50mg/6h (remember danger of GI bleed, when should cover with ranitidine or misoprostol; use with caution in asthma). Opioids, eg morphine sulfate slow release (eg MST-30® or MST-100®/12h PO). NB: most opiates are poorly absorbed from the GI tract).

2 *Sublingual:* Buprenorphine (synthetic opiate; 'controlled' drug): 0.4mg/6h sublingually.

3 *Inhalational:* Nnitrous oxide/oxygen (Entonox®), useful for labour pains, changing dressings, physiotherapy.

4 *Intramuscular:* Morphine 0.2mg/kg IM. Pethidine 25–100mg IM is alternative. (Doses for typical healthy adults.)

5 *Intravenous:* Boluses or continuous infusion. Opiates (as above). Patient Controlled Analgesic System (PCAS): The patient can give himself boluses, and if this is suffcient, no background infusion of opiates is necessary. Remember to programme maximum dose limit!

6 *Regional anaesthesia:* p 776. Epidurals (opiates, or LA, boluses or continuous infusion). Numerous techniques used (intercostal nerve, brachial plexus, femoral nerve blocks). Coeliac plexus ablation with alcohol may provide 6-months' pain relief in upper GI carcinoma.

7 Transcutaneous nerve stimulation (TNS) see p 114.

Chronic pain

- Epidural steroids for chronic backache.
- Nerve blocks: either temporary (LA) or permanent (neurolytic drugs eg alcohol, phenol). Trigeminal nerve, spinal nerve, autonomic blocks (eg stellate ganglion, coeliac plexus).
- Radiofrequency lesions produce localized damage within the nervous system to block conduction.
- Hypnosis.
- Acupuncture.

**That some stream of lightning*
From the old man in the skies
Can burn out that suffering
No right-taught man denies.

But a coarse old man am I,
I choose the second-best,
I forget it all awhile
Upon a woman's breast.

Daybreak and a candle-end, WB Yeats

12. Pre-hospital immediate care

Relevant pages in other chapters:
Glasgow Coma Scale (p 680); Child Coma Scale (p 257); cardiorespiratory arrest (p 310–11 & *OHCM* p 770–1); drowning (p 683); burns (p 688); pneumothorax (*OHCM* p 798); asthma (p 270).

Definition Pre-hospital *Immediate Care* is the provision of skilled medical help at the scene of an accident or medical emergency, or while in transit to hospital.

History Baron Dominique Larrey, Napoleon's Surgeon Marshall, may have provided the first skilled help at the scene with his *ambulances volantes* ('flying ambulances'), and was the first to apply the principle of triage—to sort the injured into priorities for treatment (p 786–7).

Note The aim of this chapter is not to provide a full account of the care of *any* patient prior to hospitalization—this is by-and-large the province of the general practitioner. Rather, our aim here is to highlight those circumstances when doctor and paramedic can work together effectively to save life.

Accidents and their prevention

Road accidents affect 1 in 4 people in their lifetime. They are the most common cause of death in those <45yrs. 50% of deaths in the 15–19 age group are from road accidents. In the UK, road deaths have fallen since 1966 despite a >50% increase in numbers of licensed vehicles. There are 3621 deaths/yr (1995) and ~45,500 serious injuries/yr in the UK. Since seat belt wearing was made compulsory (1983), deaths and serious injury to car users have fallen substantially. Casualty rates per 100 million vehicle km are similar for pedal cyclists (~200 deaths/yr) and motorcyclists (596–469 deaths/yr).[1] Age is important: babies are rarely killed on roads compared with children, because their risk exposure is less. Deaths fall in middle age, rising again before falling in old age.

Alcohol is a major factor in at least 10% of all road accidents. 20% of drivers and 36% of pedestrians killed may be expected to have blood alcohol levels above the legal limit of 80mg/100mL (17.4 mmol/L). This rises to 50% of drivers and 73% of pedestrians killed between 10pm and 4am. There is some evidence that older drivers compensate to some extent for alcohol-impaired performance—by driving more carefully. Young drivers can compensate in this way, but may choose not to do so (peer group pressure or a delight in risk-taking).

Benzodiazepines, antidepressants and antihistamines have also been implicated as contributing factors to road accidents, and it is important that patients are advised not to drive while taking these. If a patient has epilepsy or diabetes with hypoglycaemic attacks (or is otherwise unfit to drive, p 468) it is his duty to inform the licensing authorities, and the doctor's duty to request him to do so.

The prevention of accidents A vital cognitive shift occurs if the word 'accident' is replaced by 'preventable occurrence', which suggests that accidents are predictable and preventable. They happen because of laziness, haste, ignorance, bad design, false economies, and failure to apply existing knowledge—more often than because of truly random events. For example, over the years, thousands of aircraft passengers have been killed because of poor design of flight decks, which could have been prevented by using simple ergonomic principles.

Various schemes have been tried to help young drivers who abuse alcohol—eg the Driver Improvement System for Traffic Violators, and rehabilitation by re-education with driving instructors. Psychotherapy is more helpful than lectures. Health education posters which picture tragic consequences to a girl- or boyfriend are successful.

Legislation is an effective means of saving lives (eg seat belt and speed laws). Alcohol laws and those governing the roadworthiness of vehicles presumably prevent accidents, but their effectiveness has not been quantified. Another effective way of reducing alcohol-related road accidents is to provide adequate lighting, eg at difficult bends or junctions. Accidents in the home may be prevented by such simple measures as child-proof containers, putting holes in polythene bags, using toughened glass throughout the home, and using cooking pans with handles turned in away from grasping toddlers.

1 Dept of Transport 1993 *Road Accidents in Great Britain 1992*, HMSO

Accident statistics (UK)

Every year about 13,000 people are killed in accidents in Great Britain. This includes 1000 children.

Deaths and other injuries (UK figures for 1995)[1,2]

On the roads	
Deaths	3621
Serious injuries	45,500
Less serious injuries	261,400
Children's deaths	270
Children seriously injured	~7000
Deaths in those >65yrs old	1004
Home-based accidents	
Deaths	4066
Other injuries	224,000
Injuries in gardens, drives and pathways	388,000
Deaths at work	376
Injuries at work (~45,000 are serious)	1,500,000

Accidents in the home Old people are particularly at risk. Over half the males and three-quarters of females who die from accidents in their homes were 65yrs old or older. About half of those old ladies falling and fracturing their femur will be dead in 6 months (p 708). The commonest cause of accidental death in children is suffocation; in the 15–44 age group it is poisoning, and in the over-45s the chief cause is falls.

Hospital attendances for accidents 7.5 million people/year in the UK attend an accident and emergency department following an 'accident'. 350,000 (4.7%) of these are admitted. One-third of accidents occur in the home, and one-quarter are in those under 5yrs old.

Many more receive treatment from their general practitioner.

Accidents in children[3]
- ~10,000 children are permanently disabled by accidents each year.
- Accidents cause 1 child in 5 to attend the A&E department each year.
- Accidents are the commonest cause of death among children aged 1–14yrs, and they cause half of all deaths in those aged 10–14yrs.

Useful addresses: •Scottish Chamber of Safety, Heriot-Watt University, Riccarton, Currie, Edinburgh EH14 4AS (UK).
- British Safety Council, 62 Chancellors Road, London W6 9RS (UK).
- Construction Health and Safety Group, St Ann's Road, Chertsey, Surrey KT16 9AT (UK); tel. 0181 741 1231.

1 Royal Society for the Prevention of Accidents (RoSPA), 1997 Edgbaston Park, 353 Bristol Rd, Birmingham B5 7ST (tel. UK 0121 248 2000) 2 Department of Transport 1992 *Road Accidents in Great Britain: 1991*, HMSO 3 APLS group 1993 *Advanced Paediatric Life Support*, BMA

12. Pre-hospital immediate care

►►Basic life support (BLS)[ALS]

Synonyms Artificial Respiration; cardiopulmonary resuscitation (CPR).

Definition BLS is the provision of life support—expired air (your own) ventilation + external chest compression, without any equipment other than a simple airway adjunct, eg a mouth shield (to protect you from vomit) or Laerdal Pocket Mask® (to facilitate contact with the patient) which should be used if available.

SAFE approach •As you approach the patient shout for help (pointing to an individual if possible, to activate him or her).
•Approach him with care—are there any hazards to yourself (p 790)?
•Free the patient from immediate danger.
•Evaluate the patient's 'ABC' (see below).

The SAFE approach

Shout for help
Approach with care
Free from danger
Evaluate ABC (Airway, Breathing, Circulation)

Establish unresponsiveness Shake gently by the shoulder while stabilising the forehead with the other hand. Ask "Are you all right?" If he responds, put in the recovery position (p 789)—if not, check for breathing.

Breathing Open and clear the airway (finger sweep; remove dental plate or *loose* false teeth—leave a well-fitting set, otherwise the mouth collapses making expired air ventilation difficult). If breathing, put in the recovery position; if not, go to get help *now*. On return, open the airway, and give 2 rescue breaths (slow inflations, just enough to make the chest rise—and achieve a tidal volume of ~400–500mL.

Circulation Feel the carotid pulse for up to 10 seconds (can be difficult, and other signs of circulation may also be used). If felt, give 10 rescue breaths, then go for help. If no pulse, give 15 chest compressions (lower ⅓ of sternum, 2 fingers' breadth above xiphisternum); depress by ⅓ of the chest's diameter, a rate of ~100/min). If there are 2 rescuers use a ratio of 1:5.

Children (1–8yrs) Same sequence, but use one hand one finger breadth above xiphisternum (rate 100/min; use ratio of 1:5 for one or two rescuers). Avoid blind finger sweep—may impact foreign body in conical upper airway; do look into the airway for easily removable foreign body. See p 310.

Infants (< 1yr) If not breathing, give 5 rescue breaths, *then* check pulse (use brachial pulse as the neck is very short). If no pulse, give 20 cycles of 1:5 ventilations-to-compressions (compression rate 100/min) *then* go for help—take the baby with you and continue BLS while phoning for help. Avoid blind finger sweeps.

►See p 310 for the algorithm of the European guidelines for basic and advanced life support.

►►Heimlich manoeuvre

Respiratory obstruction by choking on a foreign body is not an infrequent cause of death—which may be prevented by performing the Heimlich manoeuvre. If the person who is choking is conscious and standing, first ask him to bend forward and cough. If this fails, get behind him, and with your arms encircle his abdomen, mid-way between umbilicus and xiphoid process. One hand makes a fist, positioned thumb-to-abdomen. The other hand grasps this fist, and with a sharp movement presses it up and into the abdomen, to dislodge the foreign body. If the victim is already comatose, this manoeuvre can be accomplished with him lying on his back—using the heel of the hand to press with, rather than a fist. Repeated thrusts may be needed. In adults, sweep the mouth with a finger to remove the foreign body.

►Do not perform this manoeuvre on small children, instead use back blows (below) and chest thrusts (similar to cardiac compressions).

Back blows These are no better, and no worse, than the Heimlich manoeuvre in relieving foreign body obstruction. Neither should be taught or practised to the exclusion of the other. Alternate 5 back blows with 5 abdominal/chest thrusts. Use the heel of the hand to strike forcefully between the scapulae, with the patient leaning forwards.

Road accidents—1: assessment and triage

If you are the first on the scene, the following page (which assumes a highly organized response) will seem impossible on a dark night, alone. So the first priority is to get help. You may be surprised in how short a time it all becomes organized to give the picture described below. Requesting the fire service when dialing emergency services may be the quickest way to get a dozen trained first-aiders to the scene with unrivalled skill in extrication.

The distribution of trauma deaths is trimodal—*immediate* (aortic deceleration injury; severe head injury), *early* (hypoxia, and hypovolaemia), and *delayed* (sepsis; multiple organ failure). Prevention (speed restriction; road lighting; seat-belt laws; no drink-driving; air bags) is better than cure—and medical intervention is too late for the immediate deaths.

Priorities at the scene These are command, safety, communications, assessment, triage, treatment, and evacuation.

Command: Once in attendance the doctor is responsible for the provision of all medical care. He will work closely with the ambulance service, but will have supplementary skills (eg providing potent IV analgesia).

Safety: Yourself First ensure your own safety (do not approach fire or chemical hazards (p 790) until the fire service have made the area safe; wear high-visibility clothing, and carry gloves/eye protection/ear defenders).-

The scene If first to arrive, park obliquely behind the incident ('fend off') and leave hazard lights/green beacon on. The casualties Remove from any immediate danger; protect from further injury during extrication (eg cover with blanket when windows broken). ►Check for a hidden victim, eg under a car or over a wall.

Communications: Liaise with police (they are in overall command), fire service (for any hazards; they can remove the casualty quickly if he is about to die, or in a very controlled manner, eg if an isolated spinal injury, and ambulancemen (identify if they have extended skills; use appropriately). Speak to the receiving hospital by radio or cellular telephone (p 794, radio procedure), and relay the number and severity of casualties.

Assessment: Relate vehicle damage to potential injuries in the casualty ('reading the wreckage'). Is the casualty trapped—relative (cannot move a broken arm to open the door), or absolute (eg feet caught in pedals)?

Triage: From the French *trier*, to sift or sort (coffee beans), this process sorts casualties into priorities for treatment. Divide into *Immediate* (colour-code RED, will die in a few minutes if no treatment, eg obstructed airway, tension pneumothorax); *Urgent* (YELLOW, may die in 1–2h if no treatment, eg hypovolaemia); and *Delayed* (GREEN, can wait, eg minor fractures). Those who will certainly die are labelled *Expectant*—to treat them may delay you helping the salvageable, who then die unnecessarily (BLUE, but not all triage labels have this colour—use GREEN). Do not forget to label the dead (WHITE or BLACK), otherwise emergency personnel may repeatedly take a doctor to the same victim, so wasting time and resources.

Note that triage is dynamic. It starts with a brief-look assessment (see opposite), but later may involve a detailed examination. Priorities (and label colour) will change while awaiting, and after treatment.

How to triage[1]

This is a simple system: its main virtue is *speed*. All casualties should be reassessed when time and resources allow. Go through the following sequence until you arrive at a triage priority (in CAPITALS below)—assign its colour label to the casualty and move immediately to the next. Do NOT stop to treat, or you will surrender control of the incident.

1 **•Can the patient walk?**

Yes → DELAYED (Code with green label)
No → check for breathing. . .

2 **•Is the patient breathing?**

No → open the airway
Are they breathing now?
Yes → IMMEDIATE (Red)
No → DEAD (White)
Yes → count or estimate the rate (eg over 15 seconds)
<10 to >30 per minute → IMMEDIATE (Red)
10–30 per minute → check the circulation. . .

3 **•Check the circulation**

Capillary refill >2sec (or pulse >120) → IMMEDIATE (Red)
Capillary refill <2sec (or pulse <120) → URGENT (Yellow)

1 Advanced Life Support Group *Major Incident Medical Management and Support: the Practical Approach,* London 1995, BMA Publishing–also ATLS 1997 *Manual* 6e, p409 ISBN 1-880696-10-X

Equipment

In your car boot carry the following minimum equipment:

Oropharyngeal airway(s)	Laerdal pocket mask	Dressings + bandages
IV cannulae (14G+16G)	IV fluid (eg Haemaccel®)	Giving set
Sticky tape	Scissors + Torch	Fire extinguisher

You should give a high priority to making yourself safe and visible, eg: reflective jacket, hard hat, Wellington boots.

Extra equipment Cervical collars; Mini-Trach II® (cricothyrotomy kit); chest drain set; sutures; local anaesthetic; analgesia; splints; stethoscope (more a badge of office than a useful tool owing to noise).

►►First aid treatment

A: *Airway:* Remove false teeth and any vomit. Lie in the lateral position. If trapped in a car, continue to manually stabilize head and neck when a rigid collar is applied. Extricate onto a spinal board, and immobilize the head and neck with foam headblocks and securing straps.

B: *Breathing:* If spontaneous breathing give O_2 at 15L/min via tight fitting face mask with reservoir. If not breathing, ventilate mouth-to-mouth (± pocket mask); if available give 100% O_2 via bag-valve-mask and intubate the trachea. If *tension pneumothorax* suspected (cyanosis, engorged neck veins, shifted trachea), pierce chest with a large IV cannula in 2nd interspace in the midclavicular line, on the side from which the trachea is deviated. If there is an *open chest wound*, cover with an Asherman chest seal (adhesive disc with central rubber flutter valve).

C: *Circulation:* Is there a pulse? Start external cardiac massage if required. (Note that survival from traumatic cardiac arrest with no vital signs at the accident scene approaches 0%.) If there is bleeding, this will almost always be stopped by pressure and elevation of the part. Avoid tourniquets: these are often forgotten and left on too long. Insert 2 large IV cannulae (eg antecubital fossae 14G or 16G; secure these well and splint the arm, eg Armlok®) and start fluid resuscitation (eg Haemaccel®). A policeman or fireman makes a willing drip-stand. Ensure that the cannula is not pulled out when the patient is moved. Suspected internal bleeding and fractures of long bones indicate that IV fluid is needed, as blood loss may be considerable (fractured pelvis 2L, femur 1L, tibia, ankle and fractures of several ribs ~½L each). Splinting (eg one leg to the other) helps reduce blood loss as well as relieving pain.

D: *Disability:* Assess responsiveness rapidly with AVPU:

A = Alert
V = responds to Vocal stimuli
P = responds to Pain
U = Unresponsive

E: *Exposure* = head-to-toe exam (secondary survey), but is often not practiccal outside hospital. Reassess ABC; quantify coma level (adult Glasgow Coma Scale, p 680; child p 257). Remember to give analgesia (p 792).

Transport: Keep the injured warm. Procedures can be performed in moving ambulances (eg IV cannulation) if the patient can be extricated quickly.

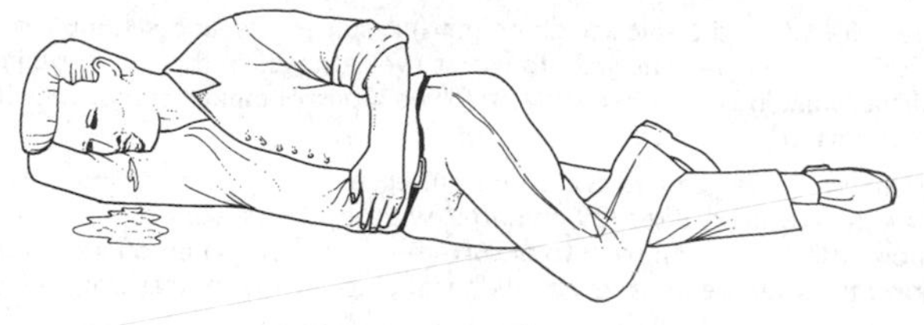

The above is one way of positioning the unconscious so vomit is not inhaled and the cervical spine is kept supported in the midline—minimizing risk of spinal cord injury. It helps if there are 2–3 people to 'log-roll' the casualty into this position, so that the neck is never out of alignment with the body. There have been reports of neurovascular risk to the arm supporting the head, so other positions are being tried, but none has been formally validated.

'Scoop and run'—or 'stay and play'?[1,2]

'Scoop and run' refers to rapid evacuation of casualties to a trauma centre (or A&E department); 'stay and play' entails detailed resuscitation at the scene of trauma. In deciding which is better, take the following into account.

- There is no single answer for all circumstances. Local geography plays a part, as does the fitness of the casualty. Only experience can tell which option is most appropriate—and luck may well play its part too.
- 'Scoop and run' and 'stay and play' are two ends of a spectrum of activity. Often a minimal amount of resuscitation can be done without causing too much delay—ie: get the best of both worlds.
- Penetrating chest injuries have been studied in a pseudo-randomized trial (*N*=289; full randomization was impossible but 'scoop and run' operated for one day, and 'stay and play' for the next). This showed that the balance of benefit probably lies in 'scoop and run' for this type of injury. Fluid resuscitation aiming for normotension without an operating theatre to hand may be dangerous, as clot may be displaced by the rising BP—with subsequent fatal haemorrhage, which could only have been prevented by major surgery. In this study, 70% in the delayed-resuscitation group survived, compared with 62% who received immediate fluid resuscitation. Duration of hospital stay was shorter for survivors in the delayed-resuscitation group. However, it is noteworthy that the results only achieved significance when pre-op and post-op deaths were pooled,[2] and that rates of complications were similar in the two groups (eg respiratory distress syndrome, coagulopathy, wound infection, and pneumonia).

1 WH Bickell 1994 *NEJM* **331** 1105–9 2 JH Siegel 1995 *NEJM* **332** 681

Road accidents—2: hazards and extrication

Hazards

790 *Fire:* <5% of road traffic accidents (RTAs) result in fire, and <1:500 result in significant burns. The world's worst ever RTA was in the Salang tunnel, Afghanistan, in November 1982, involved a petrol tanker explosion with an estimated 1100–2700 killed.

Electricity: Power shorts are common, eg from bird strike, and power may be restored after 20 minutes without investigation—you must phone the power company to ensure the source is turned off. High tension cables can be lethal even when standing several metres away.

Rail: An electrified rail may be short circuited by a bar carried by the fire service, or the operating rail authority. Remember that cutting power does not stop diesel locomotives that may also operate on the same line: trains may be stopped by signal lights, red flags, or a series of charges placed on the rail—the noise warns the driver.

Chemical: Lorries carrying hazardous loads are required to display an orange 'HAZCHEM' board (see opposite). This contains information on how to fight a fire, what protective equipment to wear, if the chemical can be safely washed down the storm drains, and whether to evacuate the area (TOP LEFT); a United Nations (UN) product identification number of four digits (MIDDLE LEFT)—eg 1270 = petrol; a pictorial hazard diamond warning (TOP RIGHT); and an emergency contact number (BOTTOM). A white plate means the load is non-toxic. The European 'Kemler' plate contains only the UN product number (BOTTOM) and a numerical hazard code (TOP—note repeated number means intensified hazard).

As a concession to freight carriers, mixed loads of <500kg need only be identified by a plain orange square at the front and rear.

To obtain information about the chemical at the scene of an accident look at the transport emergency card (TREM card) carried in the driver's cab; the fire service will be linked with CHEMDATA—a computer database at the national chemical information centre at Harwell; alternatively phone a Poison's Information Centre (eg 0171 635 9191), or the company.

►*Do not* approach a chemical incident until declared safe by the fire service.

Principles of extrication

- Stabilize the vehicle where it lies—movement may exacerbate injury.
- Make the vehicle safe—switch off ignition; immobilize the battery; swill away any petrol.
- Identify the time-critical patient—some will die unless rapidly removed from the vehicle, at whatever cost.
- Read the wreckage—relate the damage of the vehicle to potential injuries: steering wheel deformed = chest injury; dashboard intrusion = patella/femur fracture ± posterior dislocation of the hip. Bodies are softer than metal: major bodywork distortion = major injury.
- The easiest way to enter a car is through the door—try this before removing the windscreen or the roof!
- Remove the wreckage from the casualty, not the casualty from the wreckage; don't try to manouevre the casualty through too small a hole.
- Don't move from one entrapment situation straight into another—if necessary spend a short time stabilizing the patient before moving into the back of the ambulance.

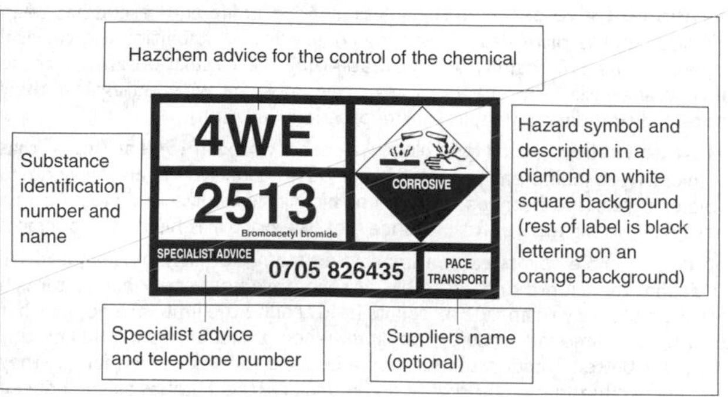

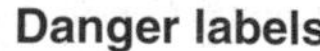

Danger labels

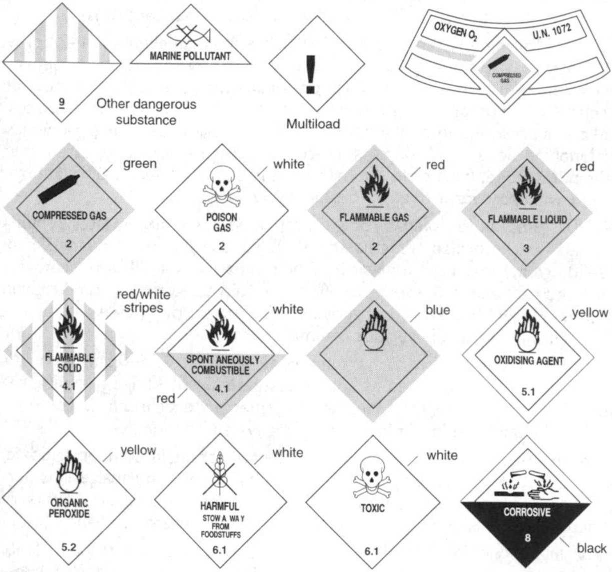

Pre-hospital analgesia

Why should I give pain relief? There are more than humanitarian reasons for giving analgesia. Catecholamines released with pain may further reduce peripheral perfusion and oxygen delivery in hypovolaemic shock, or increase myocardial oxygen demand following myocardial infarction.

When do I give pain relief? Unless all hope of life and rescue has been abandoned, the priorities of securing an airway and stabilizing the cervical spine, maintaining ventilation, and optimizing the circulation always come before analgesia. The effects of any drugs must be weighed against their potential side-effects (respiratory depression; sedation).

How do I relieve pain? *Psychological:* Beecher noted in 1944 at Anzio* that soldiers were indifferent to serious injury. This is unlikely in an RTA victim: a soldier is released from war horrors by his injuries, but an RTA victim is just beginning his nightmare. Reassurance that 'the doctor is here' is important.

Splintage: Simple splints can be improvised from clothing; an uninjured leg can splint the injured one. Inflatable air splints are not very robust, although are light and easy to apply. Box splints (fold around the limb) are popular but poorly accommodate a deformed limb, when a vacuum splint (full of tiny beads) is better. Traction splints should be used for a fractured femur: they also reduce blood loss, morbidity, and mortality (the Thomas splint reduced mortality of open fractured femur from 80% to 20% in World War I).

Gaseous: Nitrous oxide provides comparable analgesia to 10mg morphine. It is mixed with 50% O_2 as Entonox® or Nitronox® in blue cylinders with a white top. It separates at –6°C (O_2 on top). *Do not* use if Caisson disease suspected ('the bends', p 802), or pneumothorax (may tension).

Opioids: Morphine is the gold standard. Give in small aliquots (1–2mg) IV. Do not give IM in trauma victims or myocardial infarction—poor peripheral perfusion results in erratic absorption. Naloxone (0.4–1.2mg IV) must be available when opioids are given pre-hospital. Nalbuphine is a synthetic opioid and a prescription-only medicine: it is increasingly used by paramedics. Nalbuphine dose: small aliquots, up to 10–20mg slowly IV, repeated after 30min if needed; for a child the max dose is 0.3mg/kg. As a partial antagonist, it will compete with any morphine given later.

NSAIDs: IM NSAIDs (diclofenac 75mg IM, repeated once only, eg after 30min if needed—or ketorolac 10mg IM stat then 10–30mg/2–6h as needed, max 60–90mg/day) may have a place in simple musculoskeletal pain, removing the need to monitor the sedative effects of opioids. Ketorolac can be given IV over ≥15sec, but avoid in hypovolaemia, labour, or known asthmatics, and so has little place in serious trauma.

Ketamine: This is a potent, short-acting analgesic at 0.25–0.5mg/kg IV. At higher doses it can be used as sole anaesthetic agent (2mg/kg IV will produce 5–10min of surgical anaesthesia); 'emergence delirium' is common unless a benzodiazepine (midazolam ~2mg IV) is also given.

Sedation: An anxious or aggressive patient is often in pain or hypoxic. Reassurance, a clear airway with supplemental oxygen and analgesia is better than sedation, although this is needed rarely: give small aliquots of midazolam (p 716, up to 1.5mg in elderly—have flumazenil to hand).

Local anaesthesia: Peripheral nerve blocks aid release of a trapped limb. Femoral nerve block is most used and provides complete analgesia (anaesthesia) for femoral fractures (less effective for low shaft fracture). Locate the artery in the groin and put 10–20mL 1% plain lidocaine (=lignocaine) in a fan shape *lateral* to the artery. Aspirate frequently to avoid intravascula injection. Maximum dose <3mg/kg or 0.28mL/kg of 1%.

*Anzio, 33 miles south of Rome, was a crucial Allied beach-head in the recapturing of that 'Eternal City' (5/6

12. Pre-hospital immediate care

Communications

The radio net A radio user is identified by a 'call sign'. Messages are usually passed through a central controller (call sign 'control', or 'zero') without being able to hear other users—'two frequency simplex'; but on some nets all users can hear and talk directly to each other—'single frequency simplex'.

Radio voice procedure It takes practice to be comfortable with speaking into a radio. *Rhythm* should be steady; *speed* is slower than normal speech; *volume*—do not shout or whisper; *pitch* should be raised if the voice is gruff. Remember: 'RSVP'.

Using a radio Switch on and check battery light (switch off to change battery). Listen (single frequency) or look at the 'channel busy' light (two frequency)—you do not want to interrupt any message. Wait 1–2sec after pressing the transmit button before speaking, or the important first few words are lost. Release the transmit button after speaking, or you will prevent others from transmitting. VHF radios have a longer range than UHF.

Constructing a radio message To *initiate* a message say the receiver's call sign then your own. Say 'over' to indicate when the receiver should reply. To *continue* a message always start with your own call sign when you speak. To *end* a transmission say 'out'.

Example: 'Zero from Mike One, message over.'
'Zero, go ahead over.'
'Mike One, moving now to new location out.'

There is much local variation in this procedure. Remember that anyone can be listening: don't be a comic ('Send the rover over, over'); don't swear; address by appointment rather than name.

Key words Spell long or difficult words using the NATO phonetic alphabet (see opposite)—you do not want an 'empty box' when you asked for 'Entonox'. Long numbers (drug dose; grid reference) are given whole, then digit by digit (eg 1000 = 'one thousand, figures one-zero-zero-zero'). 'Roger' or 'OK' means you have understood; 'say again' means repeat the message ('Repeat' is the order for artillery to fire again and is avoided, at least on military networks!). ETA/ETD are common abbreviations for estimated time of arrival/departure. Avoid radio gibberish ('roger dodger/ten four/over and out'; 'negative' and 'positive' for 'yes' and 'no').

Telephone

Cellular telephones are useful for pre-hospital communication. However, in major incidents all cells are rapidly utilised (often by the press). In the UK, on application to the Cabinet Office the telephone may be registered to operate on a number of restricted cells in cases where the system is overloaded—this is ACCess OverLoad Control (ACCOLC).

Rank structure

Epaulette	*Police*	*Fire*	*Ambulance*
2 pips	Inspector	Station Officer	Officer band 1
3 pips	Chief inspector	Asst. Divisional Officer	Officer band 2
Crown	Superintendent		
Laurel 'U'		Asst. Senior Officer	
Laurel 'U' around pip		Divisional Officer	

Fire Service helmets:

Colour	*Black bands*	*Rank*
Yellow	Nil	Firefighter
Yellow	One thin	Leading fireman
Yellow	Two thin	Sub-officer
White	One thin	Station Officer
White	One thick	Assistant Divisional Officer
White	One thick, one thin	Divisional Officer

The NATO phonetic alphabet

ALPHA	BRAVO	CHARLIE	DELTA
ECHO	FOXTROT	GOLF	HOTEL
INDIA	JULIET	KILO	LIMA
MIKE	NOVEMBER	OSCAR	PAPA
QUEBEC	ROMEO	SIERRA	TANGO
UNIFORM	VICTOR	WHISKEY	XRAY
YANKEE	ZULU		

Radio procedure—number pronunciation

1 WUN
2 TOO
3 THUREE
4 FOWER
5 FIYIV
6 SIX
7 SEVEN
8 ATE
9 NINER

...ne major incident

...ning For a hospital to be prepared to cope with multiple casualties ...re must be planning. Each hospital will produce a detailed *Major ...cident Plan*, but additionally the tasks of key personnel can be distributed on individual *Action Cards*.

At the scene A medical incident officer (MIO) will be requested from Hospital or BASICS scheme (British Association for Immediate Care—usually GPs). Mobile medical teams (eg A&E senior doctor/surgeon + anaesthetist + 2 to 4 nurses) should come from hospitals not accepting the main casualties. BASICS doctors should be requested to the scene by radio via the ambulance station). Further BASICs doctors make valuable treatment officers, as they arrive.

Safety: Is paramount—your own and others. Be visible (luminous monogrammed jacket) and wear protective clothing where appropriate (safety helmet; waterproofs; boots; respirator in chemical environment).

Triage: See p 786.

Communications: Are essential. The police are in overall control of the scene. Each emergency service will dispatch a control vehicle and will have a designated incident officer for liaison. Support medical staff from hospital report to the medical incident officer: his job is to assess then communicate to the receiving hospital the number and severity of casualties, to assess need for further medical teams, to oversee triage and treatment (with the Ambulance Incident Officer). He must resist temptation to treat casualties as this compromises his rôle.

Equipment: Must be portable (in small cases/backpacks) and include: triage labels, intubation and cricothyrotomy equipment; intravenous fluids (colloid); bandages and dressings; chest drain (plus flutter valve); amputation kit (when required ideally two doctors should concur); drugs—*analgesic:* morphine; *anaesthetic:* ketamine (p 792); *specific antidote* if a chemical threat; cardiac resuscitation drugs; drugs to cover common medical emergencies: eg GTN spray, salbutamol inhaler; limb splints; defibrillator/monitor; ± pulse oximeter; 'comfort bag' for staff and others (£1 coins, sweets, toilet paper etc).

Evacuation: Remember: with immediate treatment on scene, the priority for evacuation may be reduced (eg a tension pneumothorax—RED—relieved can wait for evacuation—becomes YELLOW), but those who may suffer by delay at the scene must go first (eg unconscious closed head injury; myocardial infarct). Send any severed limbs to the same hospital as the patient, if possible keeping them on ice (not *in* ice as freezing harms tissues).

At the hospital a 'major incident' is declared. A control room is established and the medical coordinator ensures staff have been summoned, nominates a triage officer and supervises the best use of inpatient beds, intensive care and theatre resources. When the incident is declared clear of casualties, the major incident may still continue for some time at the hospital.

Principal source: T Hodjetts 1996 *Major Incidents* in *ABC of Major Trauma*, 2e, BMA Publishing

12. Pre-hospital immediate

...icopter transport[1]

...is often better to spend 30 minutes transporting a seriously injured ...rson to a well-resourced hospital/trauma centre with consultants stand-...ng by, than to spend 10 minutes transporting such a person to a small A&E department where the most skilled help is not *immediately* available.

The importance of helicopters for casualty rescue/transport is increasingly recognized—but be aware of their limitations. Helicopters may be used for transporting casualties to hospital, or for interhospital transfer. *Advantages:* Speed over long distances; access to remote areas; delivery of highly trained doctors and special equipment to the scene—eg ready to intubate, paralyse and ventilate, and give mannitol IVI if head injury.[2] *Disadvantages:*

- Mid-air crashes in air ambulances have occurred, and are hard to survive.
- Cost: helicopters are the most expensive method of casualty evacuation.
- Noise and general stress, leading to anxiety and disorientation and hampering communication—reassure and provide with a headset.
- Vibration exacerbating bleeding and pain from fracture sites.
- Cold—beware in those hypothermic rescues from sea or mountain.
- Problems related to altitude; aircraft limitations, eg weather, landing site, limited carriage space (especially if additional medical personnel).
- Police craft will not allow ECG monitor/oximeter due to magnetic radiation.
- Many published reports or the advantages of air ambulances lack rigour.[2]

NB: the gains of helicopter transfer depend on how many severe injuries occur. One UK study[3] concluded that at best only ~13 lives would be saved per year in the London area if it was reserved for the severest cases—Injury Severity Score (ISS, p 800) >15; in lesser trauma, there is evidence that outcome is *less* good.[3]

Helicopter safety •Always approach from the front of the aircraft, in full view of the pilot. Secure loose items, eg headgear.
- Do not enter/leave the rotor disc area without permission (thumbs up signal from pilot). Lower your head in the rotor disc area.
- Do not touch the winch strop/cable until the earthing lead has contacted the ground. Also, be sure to avoid the tail rotor.
- Make sure no-one is smoking within 50 metres of the aircraft.

Problems of altitude Hypoxia is unlikely unless there is cardiac or lung disease, anaemia, shock or chest trauma, as helicopters rarely fly high enough to produce a significant fall in P_aO_2.

Reduction in atmospheric pressure results in an expansion of enclosed gases on ascent. This produces pain in blocked sinuses, expansion of a pneumothorax, abdominal wound dehiscence (avoid flying for 10 days post surgery if possible) and renewed bleeding from a peptic ulcer. Remember drips may slow down.

On descent, beware of endotracheal tube cuffs and military antishock trousers (MAST) deflating significantly (particularly if applied at altitude eg on hillside). Rapid descent may induce barotrauma.

Specific problems •Decompression sickness (p 802): if air is breathed under pressure (divers), nitrogen dissolves in blood and tissues. On rapid ascent after a dive the nitrogen will come out of solution as bubbles, producing joint pains ('the bends') ± urticaria, CNS defects and shortness of breath. ►Do not fly if dived <30m within last 12h or >30m within 24h.
- Ischaemic chest pain or infarction is not a contraindication to flying.
- Psychiatric illness (eg mania) may preclude safe air transport.
- Burns over 20% require preflight insertion of a nasogastric tube as a precaution against gaseous expansion of an ileus.

1 Br Assoc Immed Care 1990 *Monogr.* 4 2 C Naylor 1996 *Lancet* 347 1348 3 J Nicholl 1995 BMJ ii 217

12. Pre-hospital immediate care

Trauma scoring

Essence Trauma scoring can be used at the roadside to predict the probability of survival (Ps), and thus the severity of injury, which may influence where to take the patient (nearby district general hospital, regional hospital, or Trauma Centre?). Retrospectively, physiological data may be combined with an anatomical injury score to compare performance (expected *vs* actual survivors) between hospitals.

Trauma Score (TS): The original score introduced in 1981 in USA to allow paramedics to make an objective decision on whether patient needed Trauma Centre facilities. Measures respiratory rate + effort; systolic BP; capillary refill; Glasgow Coma Scale (GCS). Maximum score 16. Score ≤13 means mortality ≥10%—USA take to Level I Trauma Centre; UK take to large hospital and alert trauma team en route.

Revised Trauma Score (RTS): Measures respiratory rate, systolic BP, and GCS only: other parameters were found to be poorly reproducible on analysis of a large North American database. Each parameter has values coded to give score of 0–4. These scores are multiplied by a weighting coefficient, then added together to produce the RTS—it is not a suitable roadside tool. RTS has a more reliable correlation with Ps than does TS.

Triage Revised Trauma Score (TRTS): This uses the same coded values of respiratory rate, systolic BP, and GCS from the RTS, but a fall by one point in any parameter is taken as significant (thus TRTS ≤11 is significant). This is the most useful pre-hospital trauma triage tool.

Limitations: These scoring systems are not validated for the very young or elderly; up to 20% may be underscored on their initial assessment (if attended rapidly, before physiological decompensation).

Injury Severity Score (ISS) TS, RTS, and TRTS use physiological variables to predict Ps. Anatomical injury (data from operation or postmortem notes) can also be used—injuries are scored from 1 (minor) to 6 (fatal) using tables from the Abbreviated Injury Scale (AIS). The body is divided into 6 regions and the 3 highest scores from different regions are squared and added. Maximum score is 75 (5 squared × 3) since AIS6 in any body region is fatal—and therefore awarded a score of 75. ISS correlates closely with Ps. ISS ≥16 implies mortality ≥10% and is termed 'major trauma'.

Limitations: Injuries can be difficult to code; isolated head injury with AIS of 3 has high mortality, but is excluded from 'major trauma' outcome analysis.

TRISS methodology Trauma audit programmes are established in USA and UK—Major Trauma Outcome Study (MTOS). TRISS is a complex formula incorporating RTS, ISS, patient age, and whether blunt or penetrating trauma. It is poor at predicting an individual's outcome, but will allow comparison of overall performance between hospitals, or the same hospital following an intervention (eg introduction of trauma team). ASCOT (a severity characterization of trauma) has recently been claimed to offer a more reliable formula.

Z and M statistics These are used to compare the outcome in different populations. *Z statistic* measures the difference between the actual and predicted number of deaths. *M statistic* (the 'injury severity match') compares the range of injury severity to the main database—if $M < 0.88$, Z is invalid.

Blast injury

Blast injury may be encountered in domestic (eg gas explosion) or industrial (eg mining) accidents or as the result of a terrorist bomb. Terrorism worldwide is responsible for 10,000 injured or killed in the last 20 years and 95% of casualties are from bombs. Death may occur without any obvious external injury, often due to air emboli, the correct cause first being recognized by Pierre Jars in 1758 as a 'dilatation d'air' (ie blast wave). Explosions cause injury in six ways:

1 **Blast wave** A transient (milliseconds) wave of overpressure expands rapidly away from the point of explosion, its intensity inversely proportional to the distance cubed. It produces: (a) cellular disruption at air–tissue interface ('spalling'), ie perforated ear-drum at 100kPa, 'blast lung' at 175kPa; (b) shearing forces along tissue planes: submucosal/subserosal haemorrhage; (c) re-expansion of compressed trapped gas: bowel perforation, fatal air embolism (coronary artery or cerebral).
Blast lung is often delayed (up to 48h). It is **rare** in survivors—only 0.6%. Suspect it if there is a perforated drum, but this is **not** a prerequisite (as position of drum in relation to blast wave is critical). Intra-alveolar haemorrhage causes acute respiratory distress syndrome (*OHCM* p 350).

2 **Blast wind** Air displaced by the explosion will totally disrupt a body in the immediate vicinity. Others may suffer avulsive amputations. Bodies can be carried by the wind with deceleration injuries on landing. Glass, wood, stones and other objects are also carried and act as secondary missiles.

3 **Missiles** Penetration or laceration from missiles are by far the commonest injuries. Missiles arise from the bomb (casing or preformed fragment—nails, nuts and bolts), or are secondary (as above, glass and wood particularly).

4 **Flash burns** These are usually superficial and occur on exposed skin (hands/face) in those close to explosion.

5 **Crush** Injuries result from falling masonry.

6 **Psychological** Acute fear and panic is the aim of the terrorist. Later, Chronic intrusive thoughts, anxiety and poor concentration may form the basis of a post-traumatic stress disorder (PTSD, p 347).

Treatment Approach the same as any major trauma with priority to airway and cervical spine control, breathing and circulation with haemorrhage control. Rest and observe any suspected of exposure to significant blast, but without other injury. Sudden death or renal failure may follow release of a limb after prolonged crush (hyperkalaemia and myoglobinuria): ensure continuous ECG and adequate hydration. Facial burns may compromise airway, which should be secured by intubation or surgical airway (*OHCM* p 753). Psychological support will be required.

Principal source: S Mellor, *Blast injury* in I Taylor, C Johnson (eds) 1991 *Recent Advances in Surgery 14*, Churchill Livingstone, London 53–68

Diving accidents

Thousands go diving every year for recreation. Because of speedy world travel, complications of diving may present to doctors miles from diving centres: for this reason we all need to be familiar with the contraindications and complications of diving, *whatever* our specialty. Do not underestimate the stress of diving: a depth change of 7 metres produces changes in ambient pressure equal to a trip from sea level to the top of Everest. *

Contraindications to diving •Asthma; COAD •Pneumothorax history •Migraine + vomiting attacks •Epilepsy •Angina; arrhythmias •Otitis (media or externa) •Ménière's disease •Perforated ear drum •Hypoglycaemia risk (eg DM) •Pregnancy •Bleeding disorders •Patent foramen ovale*

Complications of diving •Barotrauma •Decompression sickness •Drowning (p 682) •Air embolism •Pulmonary oedema •Marine bites or stings (p 736) •Hypothermia •Nitrogen narcosis

Decompression sickness[1] Nitrogen is more soluble in lipid than in water, so as N_2 tension increases, it accumulates in CNS, marrow and fat. Symptoms appear from 1–36h after surfacing. Risk factors: multiple dives, ignoring proper decompression stops, rapid ascent, previous decompression sickness, alcohol ingestion, subsequent ascent to high altitude (p 798).

Presentation:[2] •Vomiting •Mood changes •Deafness/nystagmus •Throbbing muscle/joint pains •Cough; chest pain •Fits; CNS signs •Migrating skin mottling/rashes •Cyanosis; shock •Cognitive changes •Pruritus; paraesthesiae •Osteonecrosis •Headache

Management: Speed of response is vital. If recompression starts ≤30mins after the onset of symptoms, 80% will respond; if 6h delay, only 50% respond. If air embolism is suspected, place on the left side and give 100% O_2 (15L/min through tight-fitting face mask with reservoir). Seek expert help. Transfer to a hyperbaric facility.[2] If airlift needed, maximally pressurize the cabin, if the route does not allow flying at sea-level. Transport the breathing apparatus and his diving partner (will give the history, but may himself also be at risk).[2] If there is hypothermia, expect BP to drop after leaving the water, and be sure to transport in the horizontal position, and keep cardiovascular instability to a minimum

Preventing diving accidents •Augment swimming fitness.
- Avoid dehydration (no alcohol or caffeine for >24h before the dive).
- Do the deepest part of the dive first. Time your ascent.
- Make a safety stop at 4.5 metres. Avoid remaining under water for longer than is recommended by decompression tables or dive computers.
- Rest before the dive. •Keep warm during the dive.
- After the dive avoid sitting still for long periods (decreases regional blood flow and nitrogen removal). Avoid boarding aircraft for 12h.

*See M Knauth 1997 BMJ i 689 & 701: ►This careful MRI study in 160 asymptomatic scuba divers found multiple brain lesions (?akin to multi-infarct dementia) associated with a patent foramen ovale (or other shunt) allowing paradoxical embolism of venous nitrogen bubbles (venous bubbles occur after ascent from as little as 3 metres (these bubbles are normally filtred by the lungs).

1 A Newman 1993 *Scientific American Medicine* ed. E Rubenstein and D Federman, New York ISBN 0 89454 031 0 and JJ Sykes 1994 BMJ i 1483 2 *Telephone numbers:* UK: Hyperbaric Medicine Unit's diving doctor 01224 681818; Royal Navy: 01705 822351 or 01705 818888. USA: Diving Accident Network (919 684 8111) or US Navy 904 234 4351 or Air Force (512 538 3281 or 512 536 3278)

12. Pre-hospital immediate care

►►Thrombolysis at home?

There is agreement that the sooner thrombolysis is used to relieve myocardial infarction the better (only 2 of the earlier thrombolysis trials have been equivocal on this point[1,2]). Once myocardial infarction is suspected, the chief goal is to relieve pain, correct arrhythmias, and to get patients to where thrombolysis can be started *urgently*. Only fire, exsanguination, or cardiorespiratory arrest should distract from ruthlessly pursuing this goal. We need to take steps to measure and reduce the time taken from contact with the patient to starting thrombolysis—the 'door to needle' time. This is not controversial: but the question now being asked is whose needle (GP or hospital?) and which door (the patient's front door, or the hospital door?). Should we assume that home use of thrombolysis would not much affect the outcome? Would such a strategy lead inevitably to the dangerous, inappropriate use of thrombolysis, and could it cause fatal delay in getting sick patients to hospital? The answer to all these questions is probably 'No' ($P <.04$)—in the light of a reasonably large (N=311) randomized trial on UK patients.[3] This shows that early thrombolysis (30u anistreplase IVI over 5min, *OHCM* p 593) can halve mortality—and significantly improve all measures of outcome—compared with giving thrombolysis as fast as possible, once the patient is in hospital.

In this trial, patients were given a twin pack of 2 injections, one was marked to be given at home and the other in hospital. One contained anistreplase and the other a placebo, and they were randomized between being the home injection or the hospital injection, so patients received two injections, one of which was active, and what was varied was its timing. The median delay between patient-contact and needle was 53min for general practitioners; patients had to wait a further 2h for the hospital injection, with most of this delay being within the hospital rather than in transit (despite the fact that the practices from which patients came were fairly remote from hospital (mean = 36 miles). Almost no patient (0.6%) had a hospital injection within 2h of symptom onset, but 61% had their home injection within this time—and the subgroup having thrombolysis within this time did best of all (in other words, instead of a dose–response curve, there is a time–response curve).

Note that the general practitioners were as adept at diagnosing myocardial infarction as their hospital counterparts—the main difference being that their assessment was much faster (door-to-needle time of 43min compared with a calculated 87min). Note that only one patient admitted with a suspected coronary could be assigned with confidence to another diagnosis during the admission procedure. NB: criticisms of this study included the following: some patients may have had unstable angina, not infarction;[4] many possible patients may not have been recruited to the trial;[5] and the number of deaths was small; making it possible that the lowering of morality was exaggerated.[6]

►►The vital point is that thrombolysis needs to be delivered with military precision and determination—with one part of our mind devoted to time-auditing our actions, and eliminating all non-essentials. Hence our uncharacteristic use of the word 'ruthless' above. Whether in general practice or in hospital, we have a duty to adapt our working practices to fast-track patients with chest pain to ensure they receive the care they need quickly. Do not think of this as a chore: it can be a luxury to free our minds and actions of the myriad distractions which ensnare an average day on call, and so save life.
Other care must also be prompt (*OHCM* p 280): reassurance, pain relief, arrhythmia correction, trinitrate spray, O_2, and the chewing of aspirin.

1 AIMS Trial 1988 *Lancet* i 545 **2** RG Wilcox 1988 *Lancet* ii 525 **3** E-BM 1997 **2** 160 & *Grampian Region Early Anistreplase Trial* (GREAT) 1992 BMJ ii 548 **4** J Sanderson 1992 BMJ ii 1014 **5** A Round 1992 BMJ ii 1014 **6** A Pell 1992 BMJ ii 1014—also SM Cobb 1994 BMJ i 216 and European MI Project Group 1993 NEJM **329** 383. To decipher cardiovascular trials acronyms, see TO Cheng *Am J Cardiol* 1992 **70** 1512

12. Pre-hospital immediate care

The last page

It is a pleasure to end this work with a chapter which is really a new beginning: the patient on his way to hospital. So far we have concentrated on what we can bring to the patient; but now let us turn to what the patient brings to us. All too often time and circumstance lead us to the view that patients are tireless devourers of our energies, and that for all practical purposes, we must go on giving until we die, or give up the unequal struggle with Nature and her diseases. This is to ignore the view that patients can be a source of nutrition: not just in the sense of providing us with our daily bread and butter, but also in the sense of nourishing our personalities. They do this by telling us about ourselves. You may think that you are kind and wise, or clumsy and inadequate, and it takes our patients to disabuse us of these illusions, and to show us that some days we are good, and some days we are bad. Thanks to our patients, we never stay the same. After practising medicine for a decade or so, our minds become populated by the ghosts of former patients, beckoning us, warning us, reminding us of the things we cannot control—and the ideals to which we aspire. We are lucky to work in a profession in which experience counts for more than knowledge, and it is to augment this thirst for experience that we urge our readers to turn away from learning by rote: let us read novels, cultivate our friends, travel far and wide—and try to keep forever curious, for then, if we are lucky, we stand to gain that priceless therapeutic asset: a rich and compassionate personality, and we will be all the more inclined to reformulate this tiresome and inconvenient patient who now confronts us into a lovable series of imperfections, joined together by bits of glory.

12. Pre-hospital immediate care

Index

Entries in **Bolder type** denotes emergency topics.

F

G

I

J

K

L

M

N

O

Q

R

S

T

U

V

W

X

Y

Z

The OUP
Medical Editor's Competition

The authors would like a new editor to join them for the next edition of this book. If you are interested in taking on this time-consuming task please submit (before December 1999) three new or adapted pages from this edition to: Drs Collier and Longmore, Science and Medical Department (AFL), Oxford University Press, Great Clarendon Street, Oxford OX2 6DP, UK.

Reference intervals—biochemistry

See p 292 for children and p 81 for obstetric reference intervals

►*All laboratory discourse is probabilistic.* ►Drugs may interfere with any chemical method; as these effects may be method-dependent, it is difficult for us to be aware of all possibilities. If in doubt, discuss with the lab.

Substance	*Specimen*	*Normal value*	*Your hospital*
Adrenocorticotrophic hormone	P	<80ng/L	
Alanine aminotransferase (ALT)	P	5–35IU/L	
Albumin	P¶	35–50g/L	
Aldosterone	P**	100–500pmoL/L	
Alkaline phosphatase	P¶	30–300IU/L (adults)	
α-fetoprotein	S	<10ku/L	
α-amylase	P	0–180 Somogyi u/dL	
Angiotensin II	P**	5–35pmol/L	
Antidiuretic hormone (ADH)	P	0.9–4.6pmol/L	
Aspartate transaminase	P	5–35IU/L	
Bicarbonate	P¶	24–30mmol/L	
Bilirubin	P	3–17µmol/L (0.25– 1.5mg/100 /mL)	
Calcitonin	P	<0.1µg/L	
Calcium (ionized)	P	1.0–1.25mmol/L	
Calcium (total)	P¶	2.12–2.65mmol/L	
Chloride	P	95–105mmol/L	
*Cholesterol	P	3.9–7.8mmol/L	
VLDL	P	0.128–0.645mmol/L	
LDL	P	1.55–4.4mmol/L	
HDL	P	0.9–1.93mmol/L	
Cortisol	P	a.m. 450–700nmol/L midnight 80–280nmol/L	
Creatine kinase (CK)	P	♂ 25–195IU/L; ♀ 25–170	
Creatinine (*related to lean body mass*)	P¶	70–≤150µmol/L	
Ferritin	P	12–200µg/L	
Folate	S	2.1µg/L	
Follicle-stimulating hormone (FSH)	P/S	2–8u/L (luteal): ovulatory peak 8–15 follicular phase, & ♂: 0.5–5 postmenopausal: >30	
Gamma-glutamyl transpeptidase	P	♂ 11–51; ♀ 7–33IU/L	
Glucose (fasting)	P	3.5–5.5mmol/L	
Glycated (glycosylated) haemoglobin	B	5–8%	
Growth hormone	P	<20mU/L	
Iron	S	♂ 14–31µmol/L; ♀ 11–30	
Lactate dehydrogenase (LDH)	P	70–250IU/L	
Lead	B	<1.8mmol/L	
Luteinizing hormone (LH)	P/S	premenopausal: 3–13u/L follicular: 3–12 ovulatory peak: 20–80 luteal: 3–16 postmenopausal: >30	
Magnesium	P	0.75–1.05mmol/L	
Osmolality	P	278–305mosmol/kg	
Parathyroid hormone (PTH)	P	<0.8–8.5pmol/L	
Phosphate (inorganic)	P	0.8–1.45mmol/L	
Potassium	P	3.5–5.0mmol/L	
Prolactin	P	♂<450 u/L; ♀<600 U/L	
Prostate specific antigen	P	0–4 nanograms/mL	
Protein (total)	P	60–80 g/L	
Red cell folate	B	0.36–1.44 µmol/L (160–640 µg/L)	
Renin (erect/recumbent)	P**	2.8–4.5/1.1–2.7 pmol/mL/h	